BRS
BOARD REVIEW SERIES

Microbiology and Immunology

SEVENTH EDITION

BRS

Microbiology and Immunology

SEVENTH EDITION

Dwayne M. Baxa, PhD
Associate Professor
Department of Foundational Medical Studies
Oakland University William Beaumont School of Medicine
Rochester, Michigan, USA

Tracey A. H. Taylor, PhD
Associate Professor
Department of Foundational Medical Studies
Oakland University William Beaumont School of Medicine
Rochester, Michigan, USA

. Wolters Kluwer

Philadelphia • Baltimore • New York • London
Buenos Aires • Hong Kong • Sydney • Tokyo

Acquisitions Editor: Crystal Taylor
Development Editor: Deborah Bordeaux
Editorial Coordinator: Priyanka Alagar
Marketing Manager: Danielle Klahr
Production Project Manager: Frances M. Gunning
Manager, Graphic Arts & Design: Stephen Druding
Art Director: Jennifer Clements
Manufacturing Coordinator: Margie Orzech
Prepress Vendor: S4Carlisle Publishing Services

Seventh Edition

9 8 7 6 5 4 3 2 1

Printed in Mexico

Library of Congress Cataloging-in-Publication Data

ISBN-13: 978-1-975220-45-7
ISBN-10: 1-975220-45-5

Cataloging in Publication data available on request from publisher.

shop.lww.com

QUADM0824

The authors dedicate this book to their many students who have been a source of engagement, pride, and enjoyment over the years, and to their many colleagues whose research and insight have resulted in the knowledge described herein.

Acknowledgments

The authors are grateful for the excellent medical illustration skills of Audrey Bell, medical illustrator, Mary Hooker for her help with organizing the authors, and Doug Gould for his support of this venture. And very importantly, the authors want to thank their families for continued support and patience. The authors are also grateful to the authors of previous editions of this resource: Louise Hawley, Richard Zeigler, and Benjamin Clarke.

How to Use This Book

This concise review of microbiology and immunology and its online resources is designed specifically for medical students to successfully prepare for Step 1 of the United States Medical Licensing Examination (USMLE), as well as other examinations for health professional students. This newest edition remains a succinct description of the most important microbiologic and immunologic concepts, as well as a review of critical details needed to understand important human infections and the immune system's function and malfunction.

ORGANIZATION

Facilitates Use by Either a Bug Approach or Systems Approach

The book is divided into 14 chapters of content, starting with basic information and leading quickly to the level of detail and comprehension needed for Step 1 and similar educational goals. Following an introductory chapter, for each major category of microbes (eg, bacteria, viruses, fungi, and parasites), there is a fundamental chapter followed by an organ-system infectious disease approach. Items covered are critical signs/symptoms, epidemiology, etiology, pathogenesis of infections, mechanisms for preventing infection, and means of identifying and diagnosing the causative agent. Similarly, the topic of immunology has been reorganized into Chapters 10 and 11 that provide a fundamental chapter for immunology followed by a new chapter describing immunologic disorders. A new chapter has been added to this edition (Chapter 12), which focuses on vaccination, immunization, and viral therapeutics. Chapter 13 (*Clues for Distinguishing Causative Infectious Agents*) presents the diseases a second time, this time utilizing an organ system–based approach presented by text and graphic flow-charts starting with symptoms frequently mentioned in case-based questions. An updated Chapter 14 is also new in this edition and it describes clinical laboratory diagnoses for infections and immunologic disorders. Tables listing agents associated with different types of rashes are available. Also included are detailed summary tables of the characteristics and details of the different agents causing meningitis, encephalitis, upper and lower respiratory infections, and pneumonias.

Including both an outline format and applicable detailed text facilitates rapid review of important information. Each chapter is followed by review questions and answers, with explanations that reflect the style and content of the USMLE. These questions are available online as well. We have added four separate comprehensive examinations at the end of the book. Each contains 40 USMLE-style multiple-choice questions, with some questions containing relevant images. We recommend that students perform each block under examination conditions. By allocating the standard of 90 seconds per question, each block should take 60 minutes. Each of the numbered practice assessment items is followed by answers with explanations in the end section. We feel that this self-assessment tool will help students diagnose their weaknesses prior to, during, and after reviewing microbiology and immunology. The *Comprehensive Exam* questions (accessible online as well) are not mixed with the chapter questions so they can be saved for use after initial study.

Suggestion for increasing your retention: use two cover sheets (one to move down a page and a top one to move left to right) on tables and diagrams to see if you can predict the content in each section before reading the section. We also strongly suggest that students physically write down and commit to an answer when using practice questions to get a realistic view of their comprehension.

KEY FEATURES

- Dual approach (bug and system) in one small book along with new online resources allows flexibility in study and self-testing to improve retention.

- Updated four-color tables and figures in every chapter summarize essential information for quick recall.
- End-of-chapter review tests feature updated USMLE-style questions.
- Four USMLE comprehensive exams (each should take 60 minutes to complete the 40 questions) with explanations are included in blocks of similar size to USMLE Step 1.
- Updated and current information is provided in all chapters.

We wish you well in your study, exams, and future practice!

Dwayne M. Baxa, PhD
Tracey A. H. Taylor, PhD

Contents

4.   VIRUSES   103

5.   SYSTEM-BASED AND SITUATIONAL VIRAL INFECTIONS   130

6.   MYCOLOGY   157

1

General Properties of Microorganisms

I. THE MICROBIAL WORLD

A. Microorganisms

1. Those that infect humans include eukaryotes, prokaryotes, viruses, viroids, and prions (Figure 1.1).
2. Are classified according to their structure, chemical composition, and biosynthetic and genetic organization.

> **• • • Clinical Pearl**
>
> Of the nearly 1,500 known human pathogens, approximately 40% are bacteria, 15% are viruses/viroids/prions, 20% are fungi, and the remainder are parasites.

B. Eukaryotic cells (Table 1.1)

1. Contain organelles and a nucleus bounded by a nuclear membrane.
2. Contain complex phospholipids, sphingolipids, histones, and sterols.
3. May lack a cell wall (plant and some fungal cells have a cell wall).
4. Have multiple diploid chromosomes and nucleosomes.
5. Have relatively long-lived messenger RNA (mRNA) formed from the processing of precursor mRNA, which contains exons and introns.
6. Have 80S ribosomes. Transcription and translation are uncoupled with transcription generally in the nucleus and translation in the cytoplasm.
7. Include **animalia**, **protozoa**, and **fungi**.
   a. Organisms in the **kingdom Animalia** contain multicellular, medically important species that are human parasites.
   b. Organisms in the **kingdom Protozoa** contain unicellular, medically important species that are human parasites.
   c. Organisms in **kingdom Fungi.**
      (1) Have ergosterol as the dominant membrane sterol.
      (2) May be **monomorphic,** existing only as single-celled **yeasts** or multicellular, filamentous **molds**.
      (3) May be **dimorphic,** existing as **yeast or mold forms depending on temperature and nutrition**.
      (4) May have both asexual and sexual reproduction capabilities. Deuteromycetes, or fungi imperfecti, have no known sexual stages.

C. Prokaryotic cells (see Table 1.1)

1. Have no organelles, no membrane-enclosed nucleus, and no histones; in rare cases, contain complex phospholipids, sphingolipids, and sterols.
2. Have 70S ribosomes composed of 30S and 50S subunits.
3. Have a cell wall composed of peptidoglycan-containing muramic acid.
4. Are haploid with a single chromosome.

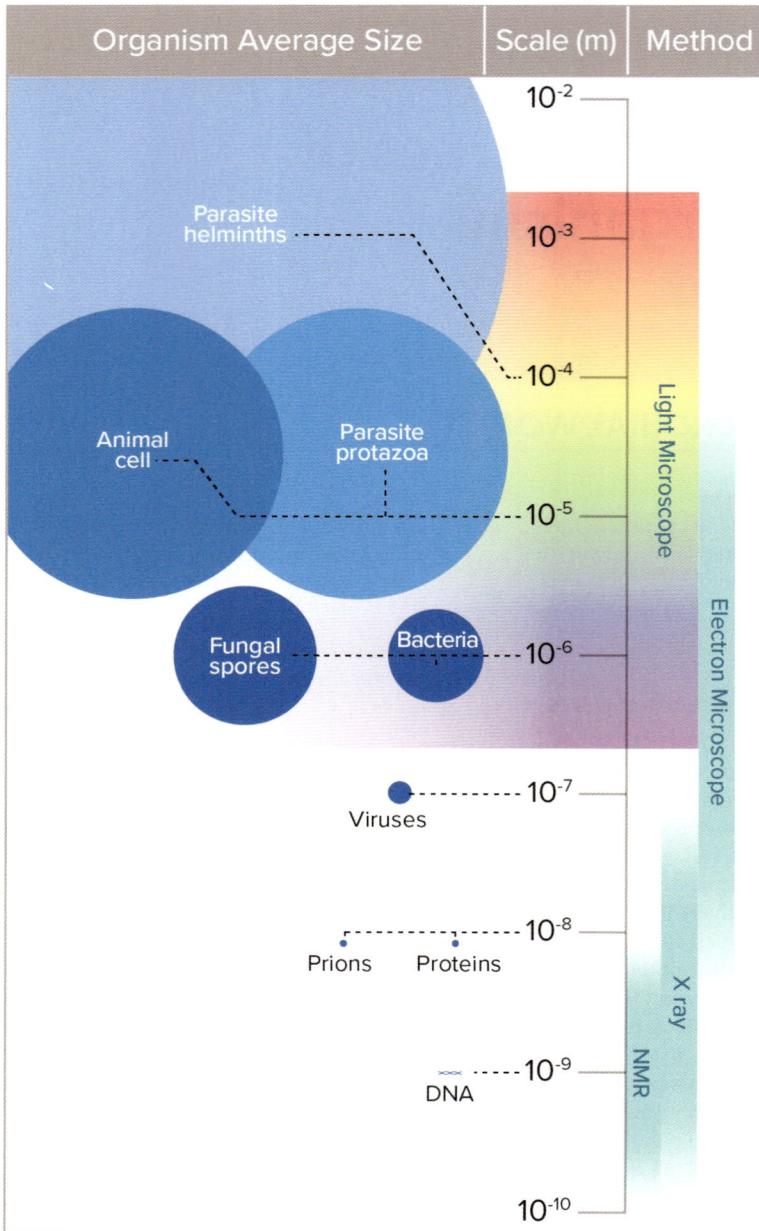

FIGURE 1.1. General Sizes of Microorganisms. Note that most microorganisms of human importance can be visualized by light microscopy. DNA and protein are also shown for comparison.

   5. Transcription and translation may be coupled, occurring simultaneously in the cytoplasm at times of rapid growth.
   6. Include **typical bacteria, mycoplasmas,** and **obligate intracellular bacteria**.
      a. Typical bacteria
         (1) Have a cell wall.
         (2) May be normal flora or pathogenic in humans.
         (3) Are classified as gram positive or gram negative.
         (4) Do not have a sexual growth cycle; however, some can produce asexual spores.
      b. Mycoplasmas

Table 1.1 Components of Microbial Cells

Structure	Composition	Virus	Gram-Positive Bacteria	Gram-Negative Bacteria	Mycoplasmas	Chlamydia[a]	Rickettsia[a]	Fungi	Parasites[b]
Envelope capsule	Polysaccharide or polypeptide	–	+ or –	+ or –	–	–	–	– or +[c]	–
Wall									
Chitin	Poly-N-acetylglucosamine	–	–	–	–	–	–	+	+ or –
Peptidoglycan	Poly-N-acetylglucosamine-N-acetylmuramic acid tetrapeptide	–	+	+	–	–	+	–	–
Periplasm	Proteins and oligosaccharides	–	–	+	–	+	+	–	–
Lipoprotein	Lipoprotein	+ or –	–	+	–	+	+	–	+
Outer membrane	Proteins, phospholipids, and lipopolysaccharides	+ or –	–	+	–	+	+	–	+
Matrix	Proteins	+ or –	–	–	–	–	–	–	–
Appendages									
Pili	Protein	–	+ or –	+ or –	–	–	–	–	–
Flagella	Protein	–	+ or –	+ or –	+	–	–	–	+ or –
Cell membrane	Proteins and phospholipids	–	+	+	+	+	+	+ (plus ergosterol)	+

[a]Obligate intracellular pathogens.
[b]Protozoan and/or metazoan.
[c]*Cryptococcus neoformans* is the only medically important fungus with a capsule.

(continued)

Table 1.1 Components of Microbial Cells (Continued)

Structure	Composition	Virus	Gram-Positive Bacteria	Gram-Negative Bacteria	Mycoplasmas	Chlamydia[a]	Rickettsia[a]	Fungi	Parasites[b]
Cytosol									
Organelles	Proteins, phospholipids, and nucleic acids	–	–	–	–	–	–	+	+
80S ribosomes	Protein and RNA	–	–	–	–	–	–	+	+
70S ribosomes	Protein and RNA	–	+	+	+	+	+	–	–
Genetic material									
Nucleus	Proteins, phospholipids, and nucleic acids	–	–	–	–	–	–	+	+
Nucleoid	Protein and nucleic acids	–	+	+	+	+	+	–	–
Nucleocapsid	Protein and nucleic acids	+	–	–	–	–	–	–	–
Plasmids	DNA	–	+ or –	+ or –	+ or –	+ or –	+ or –	+ or –	–
Transposons	RNA	– or +	+	+	–	+	+	+	+ or –
Dormant structures									
Reproductive spores	All cellular components	–	–	–	–	–	–	+	– or +
Endospores	All cellular components	–	+ or –	–	–	–	–	–	–
Cysts	All cellular components	–	–	–	–	–	–	–	– or +

[a]Obligate intracellular pathogens.
[b]Protozoan and/or metazoan.
[c]*Cryptococcus neoformans* is the only medically important fungus with a capsule.

        (1) Are the smallest and simplest of the bacteria that are self-replicating.
        (2) Lack a cell wall.
        (3) Are the only prokaryotes that contain **sterols**.
   c. Obligate intracellular bacteria include *Rickettsia* and *Chlamydia*.
        (1) *Rickettsia* are incapable of self-replication and depend on the host cell for adenosine triphosphate (ATP) production.
        (2) *Chlamydia* are bacteria-like pathogens with a complex growth cycle involving intracellular and extracellular forms. They depend on the host cell for ATP production.

D. Viruses

  1. Are not cells and are generally not visible with the light microscope with some exceptions (eg, giant viruses).
  2. Are **obligate intracellular parasites**.
  3. Contain no organelles or biosynthetic machinery, except for a few enzymes.
  4. Contain either RNA or DNA as genetic material.
  5. Are called **bacteriophages** (or **phages**) if they have a bacterial host.

E. Viroids

  1. Are not cells and are not visible with the light microscope.
  2. Are **obligate intracellular parasites.**
  3. Are single-stranded, covalently closed, circular RNA molecules that exist as base-paired, rod-like structures.
  4. The only currently known human disease is caused by hepatitis D virus (HDV), which is a viroid enclosed in a hepatitis B virus capsid.

F. Prions

  1. Are infectious particles associated with subacute progressive, degenerative diseases of the central nervous system (eg, Creutzfeldt-Jakob disease).
  2. Co-purify with a specific glycoprotein (Prion Protein or PrP) that has a molecular weight of 27 to 30 kDa. They are resistant to nucleases and may be resistant to proteases (isoform dependent). However, their infectivity may be reduced with proteases and other agents that inactivate proteins.
  3. Are altered conformations of a normal cellular protein that can autocatalytically form more copies of itself.

II. HOST-PARASITE RELATIONSHIP

A. Normal flora consist mainly of bacteria, but fungi and protozoa may be present in some individuals. They can provide useful nutrients (eg, vitamin K) and release compounds (eg, colicins) with antibacterial activity against pathogenic bacteria.

> **• • • Clinical Pearl**
>
> Most normal flora reside on the outer and inner surfaces of the body. Gastrointestinal (GI) normal flora bacterial numbers are highest, as the GI tract is the closest to the anal opening.

  1. They reside on the skin, mouth, nose, oropharynx, GI tract, urethra, and vagina.
  2. Normal flora may cause disease if they invade normally sterile areas of the body or are not properly controlled by the host immune system.

B. Microbial pathogenicity refers to a microbe's ability to cause disease, which depends on genetically determined virulence factors. A microbe's pathogenicity is related to its:
  1. Entry.
  2. Colonization.

3. Escape from host defense mechanisms.
4. Multiplication.
5. Damage to host tissues.

C. Virulence factors are chromosomal and extrachromosomal (plasmid) gene products that affect aspects related to an organism's:
   1. Invasion properties.
   2. Adherence and colonization.
   3. Host tissue damage induced by toxins, immune system reactions, and intracellular growth.
   4. Ability to elude host defense mechanisms.
   5. Antibiotic resistance.

III. STERILIZATION AND DISINFECTION

A. Terminology
   1. Sterility—total absence of viable microorganisms as assessed by no growth on any medium.
   2. Bactericidal—kills bacteria.
   3. Bacteriostatic—inhibits growth of bacteria.
   4. Sterilization—removal or killing of all microorganisms.
   5. Disinfection—removal or killing of disease-causing microorganisms.
   6. Sepsis—infection.
   7. Aseptic—without infection.
   8. Antisepsis—any procedure that inhibits the growth and multiplication of microorganisms.

B. Kinetics of killing
   1. Killing is affected by the medium, the concentration of organisms and antimicrobial agents, temperature, pH, and the presence of endospores.
   2. Killing can be exponential (logarithmic); it can result in a killing curve that becomes asymptotic, requiring extra considerations in killing final numbers, especially if the population is heterogeneous relative to sensitivity.

C. Methods of control
   1. Moist heat (autoclaving at 121 °C/250 °F for 15 minutes at a steam pressure of 15 pounds per square inch) kills microorganisms, including endospores.
   2. Dry heat and **incineration** are both methods that oxidize proteins, killing bacteria.
   3. Ultraviolet radiation blocks DNA replication.
   4. Chemicals.
      a. Phenol is used as a disinfectant standard that is expressed as a phenol coefficient, which compares the rate of the minimal sterilizing concentration of phenol to that of the test compound for a particular organism.
      b. Chlorhexidine is a diphenyl cationic analog that is a useful topical disinfectant.
      c. Iodine is bactericidal in a 2% solution of aqueous alcohol containing potassium iodide. It acts as an oxidizing agent and combines irreversibly with proteins. It can cause hypersensitivity reactions.
      d. Chlorine inactivates bacteria and most viruses by oxidizing free sulfhydryl groups.
      e. Quaternary ammonium compounds (eg, **benzalkonium chloride**) inactivate bacteria by their hydrophobic and lipophilic groups, interacting with the cell membrane to alter metabolic properties and permeability.
      f. Ethylene oxide is an alkylating agent that is especially useful for sterilizing heat-sensitive hospital instruments. It requires exposure times of 4 to 6 hours, followed by aeration to remove absorbed gas.
      g. Alcohol requires concentrations of 70% to 95% to kill bacteria given sufficient time. Isopropyl alcohol (90%-95%) is the major form in use in hospitals.

Directions: Each of the numbered items in this section is followed by answer choices. Select the *one best* lettered answer in each case.

1. A pharmaceutical company has developed a new compound that is well tolerated by the body and inhibits synthesis of the sterol ergosterol. To which type of microorganism should screening of anti-infectious agent activity be directed?

(A) Bacteria
(B) *Chlamydia* species
(C) Fungi
(D) *Rickettsia* species
(E) Viruses

2. In which type of microorganism are 50S ribosomal subunits found?

(A) Bacteria
(B) Fungi
(C) Prions
(D) Protozoa
(E) Viruses

3. Which type of microorganism does the normal flora of the large intestine consist mainly of?

(A) Bacteria
(B) Fungi
(C) Protozoa
(D) Viruses
(E) No microbial agents

4. What is the minimal concentration of alcohol necessary to kill bacteria and enveloped viruses?

(A) 30%
(B) 40%
(C) 50%
(D) 60%
(E) 70%

5. Which type of microorganism are human obligate intracellular pathogens that depend on the host cell for ATP production?

(A) Bacteriophages
(B) *Mycoplasma* species
(C) Prions
(D) *Rickettsia* species
(E) Viroids

6. Dimorphism is a characteristic of which type of microorganism?

(A) Bacteria
(B) Fungi
(C) Prions
(D) *Rickettsia* species
(E) Viruses

7. A new infectious agent has been isolated from deer ticks. It lacks a cell wall but has 70S ribosomes. What type of agent is this most likely?

(A) Bacterium
(B) *Chlamydia* species
(C) *Mycoplasma* species
(D) *Rickettsia* species
(E) Virus

8. The infectious agent associated with Creutzfeldt-Jakob disease is extremely hardy, but it can be inactivated by which of the following?

(A) Catalases
(B) Hyaluronidases
(C) Nucleases
(D) Phospholipases
(E) Proteases

9. By which method does quaternary ammonium compounds inactivate bacteria?

(A) Altering metabolic properties of membranes
(B) Binding irreversibly to DNA
(C) Denaturing proteins
(D) Inactivating 50S ribosomes
(E) Oxidizing free sulfhydryl groups

Answers and Explanations

1. **The answer is C.** [Table 1.1; I B 7 c (1)] Fungi have ergosterol as their dominant membrane sterol. Mycoplasmas are the only prokaryotes with sterols in their cytoplasmic membrane, but they do not synthesize their own sterols.

2. **The answer is A.** [Table 1.1; I C 2] Bacteria have 70S ribosomes composed of 30S and 50S subunits. Fungi and protozoa have 80S ribosomes, and prions and viruses do not have ribosomes.

3. **The answer is A.** [I C 6 a (2); II A] Bacteria form the majority of the normal flora of the large intestine. Other types of human infectious agents are not usually present except in times of disease.

4. **The answer is E.** [III C 4 g] An alcohol concentration of 70% to 95% is necessary to kill bacteria.

5. **The answer is D.** [Table 1.1; I C 6 c] Chlamydia and Rickettsia are obligate intracellular pathogens because they depend on the host cell to provide them with ATP.

6. **The answer is B.** [I B 7 c (3)] Certain species of pathogenic fungi are dimorphic (ie, existing as yeast or mold forms depending on their environment).

7. **The answer is C.** [Table 1.1; I C 6 b] Mycoplasmas are the only microbes that lack a cell wall, but they do have 70S ribosomes.

8. **The answer is E.** [I F 2] The infectious agent of Creutzfeldt-Jakob disease is a prion that is inactivated by proteases.

9. **The answer is A.** [III C 4 e] The hydrophobic and lipophilic portions of quaternary ammonium compounds react with the lipid components of the bacterial membrane so that it can no longer perform its normal metabolic and permeability functions, thus killing the cell.

2

Bacteria

I. BACTERIAL STRUCTURE

A. Shape. Along with other properties, shape is used to identify bacteria. It is determined by the mechanism of cell wall assembly.
1. Bacterial shape can often be determined with appropriate staining and a light microscope.
2. **Types**
   a. **Round** (singular coccus, plural cocci).
   b. **Rod-like** (singular bacillus, plural bacilli).
   c. **Spiral** (spirochete or spirillum).
3. Cocci and bacilli often grow in doublets (diplococci) or chains (streptococci or streptobacilli). Cocci that grow in clusters are called staphylococci.
4. Some bacterial species are **pleomorphic** (single bacterial species with more than one shape), such as *Bacteroides* spp.
5. Antibiotics that affect cell wall biosynthesis (eg, penicillin) may alter a bacterium's shape.

B. Components of a typical bacterial cell
1. **Genetic material:** In bacteria, the genetic material is generally called a **nucleoid** or **nuclear body**. As bacteria do not contain organelles, the genetic material is not surrounded by a nuclear membrane nor does it contain a mitotic apparatus. The nucleoid consists of polyamine and magnesium ions bound to negatively charged, circular, supercoiled, double-stranded DNA; small amounts of RNA; RNA polymerase; and other proteins.
2. **Cytoplasm**
   a. Bacterial cytoplasm contains ribosomes and various types of nutritional storage granules.
   b. It contains **no organelles**.
3. **Ribosomes:** Bacterial ribosomes contain proteins and RNAs that differ from those of their eukaryotic counterparts.
   a. Bacterial ribosomes have a sedimentation coefficient of 70S and are composed of 30S and 50S subunits containing 16S, and 23S and 5S RNA, respectively.
   b. Many antibiotics target ribosomes, inhibiting protein biosynthesis. Most antibiotics selectively target 70S ribosomes (e.g., erythromycin) but not 80S ribosomes.

> **••• Clinical Pearl**
>
> Even though the difference between bacterial ribosomes and eukaryotic ribosomes seems small, it is enough of a difference that antibiotics that target ribosomes can inhibit protein synthesis in bacteria but have no/little effect on human cells (ie, side effects).

4. **Cell (cytoplasmic) membrane**
   a. **Structure:** The cell membrane is a typical phospholipid bilayer that contains the following components:
      (1) Cytochromes and enzymes involved in electron transport and oxidative phosphorylation.

(2) Carrier lipids, enzymes, and **penicillin-binding proteins** (**PBPs**) involved in cell wall biosynthesis.

(3) Enzymes involved in phospholipid synthesis and DNA replication.

(4) Chemoreceptors.

b. Functions

(1) Selective permeability and active transport facilitated by membrane-bound permeases, binding proteins, and various transport systems.

(2) Site of action of certain antibiotics such as polymyxin.

5. Mesosomes are controversial structures that are **convoluted invaginations** of the plasma membrane.

a. Septal mesosomes occur at the septum (cross-wall); **lateral mesosomes** are nonseptal.

b. Function in DNA replication, cell division, and secretion.

6. Plasmids

a. Plasmids are small, circular, nonchromosomal, double-stranded DNA molecules that are:

(1) Capable of self-replication.

(2) Most frequently extrachromosomal but may become integrated into bacterial genome.

b. Function: contain genes that confer protective properties such as antibiotic resistance, virulence factors, or transmissibility to other bacteria.

7. Transposons

a. Transposons are small pieces of DNA that move between and within the genome of bacteria and plasmids; they do not self-replicate.

b. Functions

(1) Code for antibiotic resistance enzymes, metabolic enzymes, or toxins.

(2) May alter expression of neighboring genes or cause mutations to genes into which they are inserted.

8. Cell envelope (Figures 2.1 and 2.2)

a. General structure: The cell envelope is composed of the macromolecular layers that surround the bacterium. It includes:

(1) A cell membrane and a peptidoglycan layer (except *Mycoplasma* spp.).

(2) An outer membrane layer in gram-negative bacteria.

(3) A capsule, a glycocalyx layer, or both (in some bacteria).

(4) Antigens that frequently induce a specific antibody response.

b. Cell wall

(1) The *cell wall* refers to that portion of the cell envelope that is **external to the cytoplasmic membrane** and **internal to the capsule or glycocalyx**.

(2) It confers osmotic protection and Gram-staining characteristics.

(3) In **gram-positive bacteria**, it is composed of:

(a) Peptidoglycan.

(b) Teichoic and teichuronic acids.

(c) Polysaccharides.

(4) In **gram-negative bacteria**, it is composed of:

(a) Peptidoglycan.

(b) Lipoprotein.

(c) An outer phospholipid membrane that contains lipopolysaccharide (LPS).

c. Peptidoglycan (also called **mucopeptide** or **murein**) is unique to prokaryotes. It is found in all bacterial cell walls except *Mycoplasma* spp.

(1) Structure

(a) This complex polymer consists of a backbone of alternating *N*-acetylglucosamine and *N*-acetylmuramic acid and a set of identical tetrapeptide side chains.

(b) The tetrapeptide side chains are attached to the *N*-acetylmuramic acid and are frequently linked to adjacent tetrapeptides by identical peptide cross-bridges or by direct peptide bonds.

(c) The β-1,4 glycosidic bond between *N*-acetylmuramic acid and *N*-acetylglucosamine is cleaved by the bacteriolytic enzyme **lysozyme** (found in mucus, saliva, and tears).

(d) It may contain **diaminopimelic acid**, an amino acid unique to prokaryotic cell walls.

Gram-Positive Cell Envelope

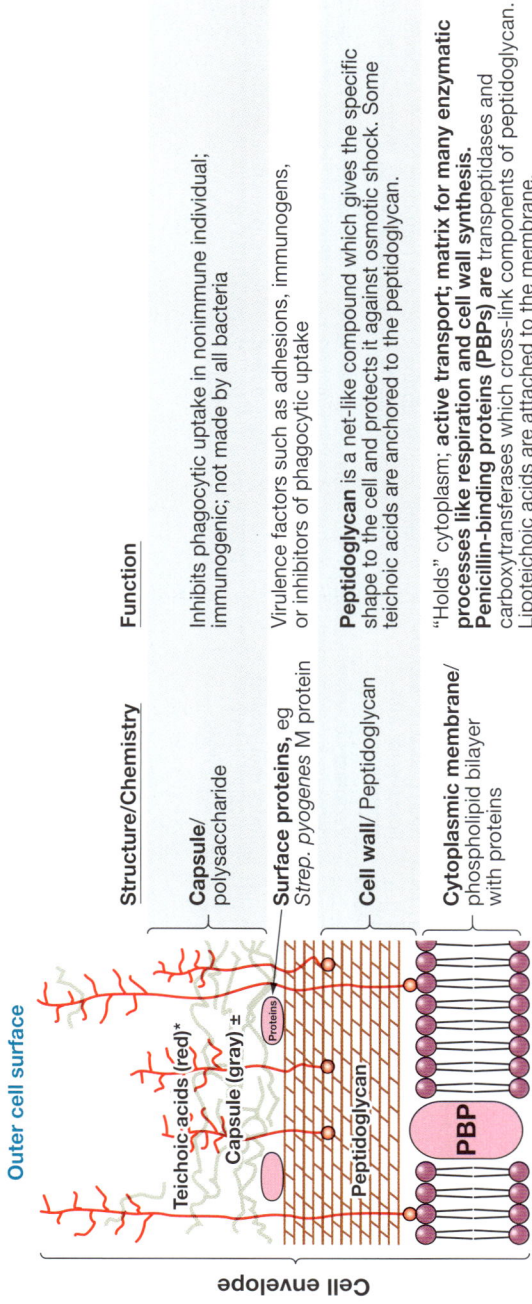

Structure/Chemistry	Function
Capsule/ polysaccharide	Inhibits phagocytic uptake in nonimmune individual; immunogenic; not made by all bacteria
Surface proteins, eg *Strep. pyogenes* M protein	Virulence factors such as adhesions, immunogens, or inhibitors of phagocytic uptake
Cell wall/ Peptidoglycan	**Peptidoglycan** is a net-like compound which gives the specific shape to the cell and protects it against osmotic shock. Some teichoic acids are anchored to the peptidoglycan.
Cytoplasmic membrane/ phospholipid bilayer with proteins	"Holds" cytoplasm; **active transport; matrix for many enzymatic processes like respiration and cell wall synthesis. Penicillin-binding proteins (PBPs) are** transpeptidases and carboxytransferases which cross-link components of peptidoglycan. Lipoteichoic acids are attached to the membrane.

* Teichoic acids (shown in red) are found only in gram-positive cells.

FIGURE 2.1. Gram-positive cell envelope showing structures and describing their chemistry and function. (Updated from Hawley LB. *High-Yield Microbiology and Infectious Diseases.* 2nd ed. Lippincott Williams & Wilkins; 2007.)

Gram-Negative Cell Envelope

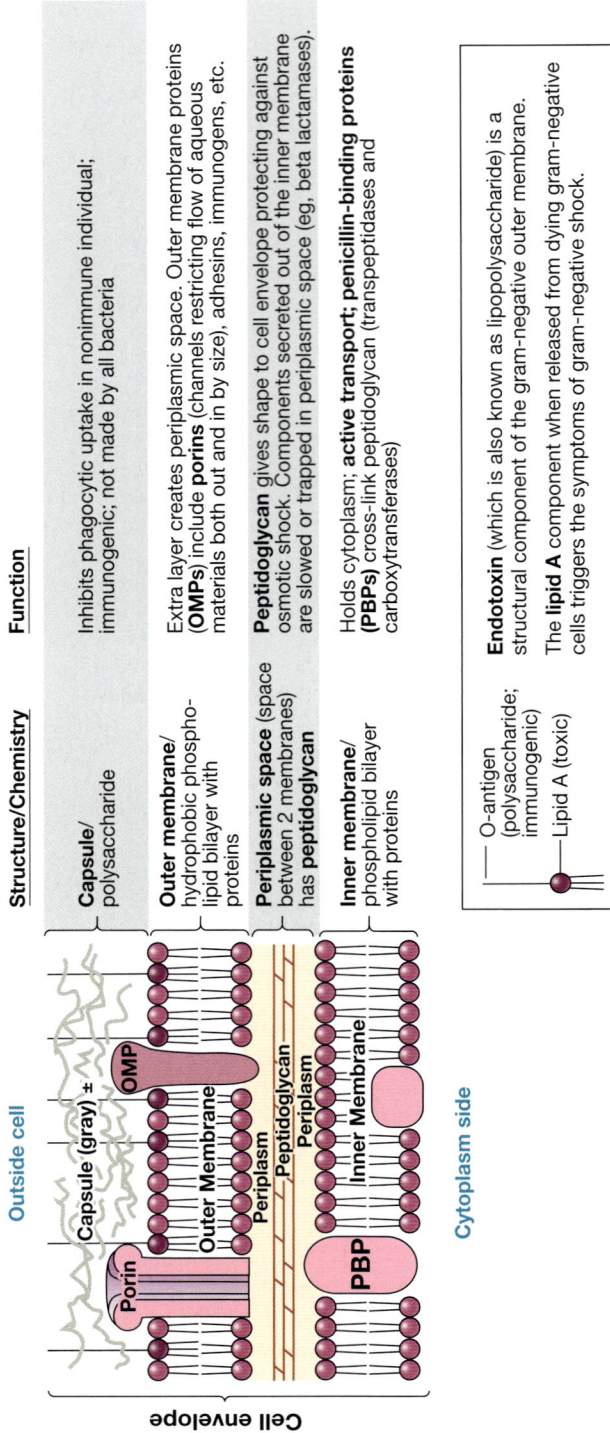

Structure/Chemistry	Function
Capsule/polysaccharide	Inhibits phagocytic uptake in nonimmune individual; immunogenic; not made by all bacteria
Outer membrane/hydrophobic phospholipid bilayer with proteins	Extra layer creates periplasmic space. Outer membrane proteins (**OMPs**) include **porins** (channels restricting flow of aqueous materials both out and in by size), adhesins, immunogens, etc.
Periplasmic space (space between 2 membranes) has **peptidoglycan**	**Peptidoglycan** gives shape to cell envelope protecting against osmotic shock. Components secreted out of the inner membrane are slowed or trapped in periplasmic space (eg, beta lactamases).
Inner membrane/phospholipid bilayer with proteins	Holds cytoplasm; **active transport; penicillin-binding proteins (PBPs)** cross-link peptidoglycan (transpeptidases and carboxytransferases)

O-antigen (polysaccharide; immunogenic)

Lipid A (toxic)

Endotoxin (which is also known as lipopolysaccharide) is a structural component of the gram-negative outer membrane.

The **lipid A** component when released from dying gram-negative cells triggers the symptoms of gram-negative shock.

FIGURE 2.2. Gram-negative cell envelope showing structures and describing their chemistry and function. (Updated from Hawley LB. *High-Yield Microbiology and Infectious Diseases.* 2nd ed. Lippincott Williams & Wilkins; 2007.)

ER.

(2) Peptidoglycan is the site of action of certain antibiotics, such as **penicillin** and the **cephalosporins**.

(3) In gram-positive bacteria, it comprises up to 50% of the cell wall. In gram-negative bacteria, it comprises 2% to 10% of the cell wall.

d. **Teichoic** and **teichuronic acids** are water-soluble polymers, containing a ribitol or glycerol residue linked by phosphodiester bonds.

  (1) They are found in **gram-positive** cell walls or membranes.

    (a) Teichoic acid is found in cell walls and is chemically bonded to peptidoglycan.

    (b) **Lipoteichoic acid** is found in cell membranes and is chemically bonded to membrane glycolipid, particularly in mesosomes.

  (2) Functions

    (a) Contain important bacterial surface antigenic determinants; lipoteichoic acid helps anchor the wall to the membrane.

    (b) May account for 50% of the dry weight of a gram-positive cell wall.

e. **Lipoprotein** is found in **gram-negative** bacteria.

  (1) Lipoprotein cross-links the peptidoglycan and outer membrane.

  (2) A peptide bond links the lipoprotein to diaminopimelic acid residues of peptidoglycan tetrapeptide side chains; the lipid portion is noncovalently inserted into the outer membrane.

f. The **periplasmic space** is found in **gram-negative** cells.

  (1) It is the area between the cell membrane and the outer membrane.

  (2) Hydrated peptidoglycan, as well as hydrolytic **enzymes** including β-**lactamases**, **specific carrier molecules**, and oligosaccharides are found in the periplasmic space.

g. An **outer membrane** is found in **gram-negative** cells.

  (1) **Structure:** The outer membrane is a phospholipid bilayer in which the phospholipids of the outer leaflet are replaced by LPSs.

    (a) It contains embedded proteins, including matrix **porins** (nonspecific pores) and some non-pore proteins (phospholipases and proteases).

    (b) It may contain transport proteins for small molecules.

  (2) Functions

    (a) Protects cells from harmful enzymes and some antibiotics.

    (b) Prevents leakage of periplasmic proteins.

h. **Lipopolysaccharide** is found in the outer leaflet of the outer membrane of **gram-negative** cells.

  (1) Structure

    (a) LPS consists of three main components: **lipid A** (several long-chain fatty acids attached to phosphorylated glucosamine disaccharide units), a **core**, and an immunogenic polysaccharide repeating unit called the **O antigen**.

    (b) It is negatively charged and noncovalently cross-bridged by divalent cations.

  (2) Functions

    (a) LPS is also called **endotoxin**; the toxicity is associated with the lipid A.

    (b) Contains major surface antigenic determinants, including **O antigen**.

i. **Protein secretion systems** play a major role in bacteria interacting with their environment and helping to determine pathogenicity, particularly in gram-negative bacteria.

  (1) Distribution

    (a) Gram-negative bacteria have at least six classes of systems; gram-positive bacteria have an additional unique class and some of the other six classes. The types are numbered (eg, type III secretion system or T3SS).

    (b) Some gram-negatives contain more than one type of secretion system in a class (*Salmonella typhimurium* has two types of T3SS coded on different pathogenicity islands).

  (2) **Structure:** There are some simple systems like T1SS that consist of transporters, outer membrane factors, and membrane fusion proteins, while others (T3SS, T4SS, and T6SS) involve a transmembrane structure (**injectosome**) that consists of more than 25 proteins.

  (3) Functions

    (a) Transport proteins or nucleic acids (T4SS) to outside of cell, periplasm, or inside host cells.

    (b) Transported proteins can be surface proteins like adhesins or toxins and effector proteins that modify the host-cell physiology, causing pathologic consequences.

9. External layers
  a. Surface proteins
    (1) Antiphagocytic proteins are external to the cell wall of some gram-positive bacteria, such as the **M protein** of *Streptococcus pyogenes.*
    (2) Function as **adhesins** facilitating tissue colonization with several species (eg, *Staphylococcus aureus* [fibronectin-binding proteins] and *S. pyogenes* [F proteins]).
  b. Capsule
    (1) The capsule (see Figures 2.1 and 2.2) is a well-defined structure of polysaccharides surrounding a bacterial cell and is external to the cell wall. One exception to the polysaccharide structure is the poly-D-glutamic acid capsule of *Bacillus anthracis.*
    (2) Functions to **protect** bacteria from **phagocytosis** and plays a role in bacterial **adherence**.

• • • Clinical Pearl

Here is a mnemonic that may be helpful to remember some medically important bacteria (and one fungus) that produce capsules: **E**ven **S**ome **S**uper **K**illers **H**ave **P**retty **N**ice **B**ig **C**apsules:

- *Escherichia coli.*
- *Streptococcus pneumoniae.*
- *Salmonella* spp.
- *Klebsiella pneumoniae.*
- *Haemophilus influenzae.*
- *Pseudomonas aeruginosa.*
- *Neisseria meningitidis.*
- *Bacteroides fragilis.*
- *Cryptococcus neoformans.*

---

  c. Glycocalyx
    (1) The *glycocalyx* (also known as *slime layer*) refers to a loose network of polysaccharide fibrils that surrounds some bacterial cell walls. It is synthesized by surface enzymes.
    (2) Functions as an adhesin and contains prominent antigenic sites.
10. Appendages
  a. Flagella are protein appendages for locomotion and contain prominent antigenic determinants.
    (1) They consist of a basal body, hook, and a long filament composed of a polymerized protein called **flagellin**.
    (2) Flagella may be located in only one area of a cell (**polar**) or over the entire bacterial cell surface (**peritrichous**).
  b. Pili (fimbriae) are rigid surface appendages composed mainly of the protein **pilin**.
    (1) Types
      (a) Common pili (adhesins) are involved in bacterial adherence and gram-positive cell conjugation. These pili are the colonization antigens or **virulence factors** associated with some bacterial species, such as *S. pyogenes* and *Neisseria gonorrhoeae.*
      (b) Sex pili are involved in attachment of donor and recipient bacteria in gram-negative cell conjugation.
11. Endospores
  a. General characteristics: Endospores are formed as a survival response to certain adverse nutritional conditions, such as depletion of a certain resource. These **metabolically inactive bacterial cells** are highly resistant to desiccation, heat, and various chemicals. They are helpful in identifying some species of bacteria (eg, gram-positive *Bacillus* spp. and *Clostridium* spp.).
  b. Structure
    (1) Endospores possess a core that contains many cell components, a spore wall, a cortex, a coat, and an exosporium.
    (2) The core contains **calcium dipicolinate**, which aids in heat resistance.
  c. Function: Endospores germinate into vegetative cells under favorable nutritional conditions after an activation process that involves damage to the spore coat. Spores are not reproductive structures.

12. **Biofilms** are aggregates of bacterial cells that form in soil and marine environments and the surface of **medical implant devices** (eg, prostheses). They enhance nutrient uptake and often exclude antimicrobials. Bacteria within these organized structures often communicate using **quorum sensing**.

C. Bacterial nomenclature

1. Streptococcaceae is a formal family name. ("-aceae" indicates it is a bacterial family.)
2. Streptococci is a common name, which could refer to the family, species, or any chain of cocci, depending on the context. These are not italicized.
3. *Streptococcus* is a formal genus name. *Note*: It is optional to italicize a genus name alone but the formal genus and species binomial should always be italicized. Colloquial (common) names are not italicized. If all of the answer choices to a question on an examination are italicized, they are formal Latin bacterial, fungal, or parasitic names. The abbreviation "spp." used after a genus name indicates the species of that genus.
   Streptococcus pneumoniae is a formal genus and species name. (The genus name is capitalized, and species name is not capitalized.)
4. *S. pneumoniae* is a formal abbreviation. *Strep. pneumo.* is colloquial usage; however, it is more precise since "*S.*" could also refer to *Staphylococcus*.
5. Pneumococcus is an informal nickname for *Strep. pneumoniae*.
6. The term *complex* is used for a series of species so closely related that they do not need to be distinguished in the lab (ie, *Mycobacterium avium-intracellulare* complex or MAC).

II. BACTERIAL GROWTH AND REPLICATION

A. Growth

1. **General characteristics of bacterial growth**
   a. Bacterial growth refers to an increase in bacterial cell numbers (multiplication), which results from a programmed increase in bacterial biomass.
   b. Bacterial reproduction is by **binary fission**, characterized by the parameter **generation time** (the average time required for cell numbers to double).
   c. Growth may be determined by measuring **cell concentration** (see next) or **biomass density** (dry weight or protein determinations).
   d. It usually occurs asynchronously (ie, all cells do not divide at precisely the same moment).
2. **Cell concentration** may be measured by:
   a. **Viable** cell counts involving serial dilutions of the sample, followed by a determination of colony-forming units (CFUs) on an agar surface.
   b. **Particle cell counting** or **turbidimetric density** measurements (include both viable and nonviable cells).
3. **Bacterial growth curve** (Figure 2.3)
   a. The bacterial growth curve involves the inoculation of bacteria from a saturated culture into fresh liquid media. It is unique for each particular nutritional environment.
   b. It is frequently illustrated in a plot of logarithmic number of bacteria versus time; the **generation time** is determined by the time necessary for cells to double in number during the log phase of growth.
   c. The bacterial growth curve consists of **four phases:**
      (1) **Lag**—metabolite-depleted cells adapt to the new environment; cells detoxify medium and/or synthesize new enzymes, and increase in size for division.
      (2) **Exponential or log**—cell biomass is synthesized by cell division at a constant rate; cells in this stage are generally more susceptible to antibiotics.
      (3) **Stationary**—cells exhaust essential nutrients or accumulate toxic products; in general, the rate of cell growth equals the rate of cell death.
      (4) **Death or decline**—cells may die due to buildup of toxic products in this closed system.

Bacterial Growth and Division

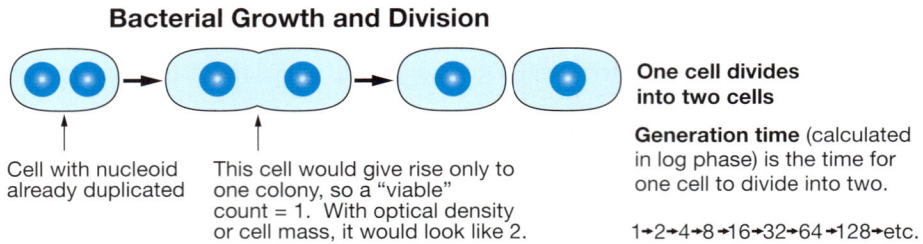

One cell divides into two cells

Cell with nucleoid already duplicated

This cell would give rise only to one colony, so a "viable" count = 1. With optical density or cell mass, it would look like 2.

Generation time (calculated in log phase) is the time for one cell to divide into two.

$1 \rightarrow 2 \rightarrow 4 \rightarrow 8 \rightarrow 16 \rightarrow 32 \rightarrow 64 \rightarrow 128 \rightarrow$ etc.

Growth Curve

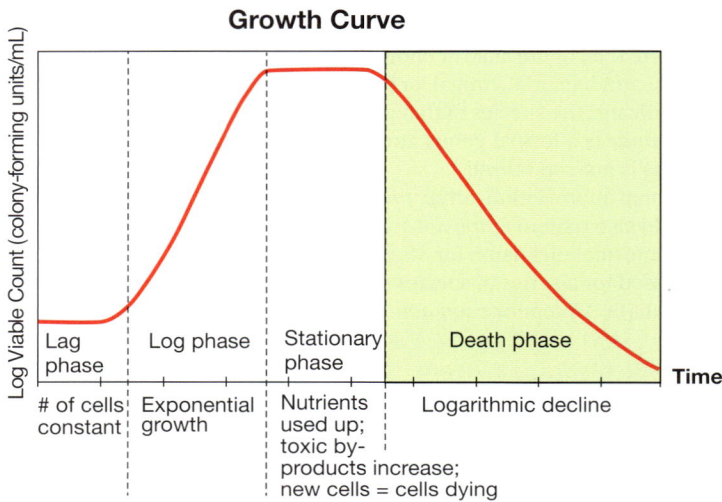

Log Viable Count (colony-forming units/mL)

Time

Lag phase | Log phase | Stationary phase | Death phase

# of cells constant | Exponential growth | Nutrients used up; toxic by-products increase; new cells = cells dying | Logarithmic decline

FIGURE 2.3. Bacterial growth and division. Binary fission (which is asexual) and typical growth curve. (Updated from Hawley LB. *High-Yield Microbiology and Infectious Diseases.* 2nd ed. Lippincott Williams & Wilkins; 2007.)

4. Synchronous growth

  a. This type of growth refers to an artificial situation in which all the bacteria in a culture divide at the same moment. It may be achieved by several methods, including thymidine starvation (thymidine-requiring bacteria), alternate cycles of low and optimal incubation temperatures, spore germination, selective filtration of old (large) and young (small) cells, and "trapped cell" filtration.

B. Cultivation

1. General characteristics of bacterial cultivation

  a. Bacterial cultivation refers to the propagation of bacteria based on their specific nutrition, pH, gas, and temperature preferences.

  b. It is performed in either liquid (broth) or solid (agar) growth medium and requires an environment that contains:

  (1) Carbon source.
  (2) Nitrogen source.
  (3) Energy source.
  (4) Inorganic salts.
  (5) Growth factors.
  (6) Electron donors and acceptors.

C. Oxygen metabolism

1. General characteristics of oxygen metabolism

  a. Oxygen is not required by all bacteria and is toxic to many bacteria; therefore, some bacteria require one or more enzymes to grow in the presence of toxic by-products such as superoxide ion (O_2) and hydrogen peroxide (H_2O_2).

     b. Superoxide dismutase is an enzyme in aerobes, and facultative and aerotolerant anaerobes that allow them to grow in the presence of the superoxide free radical, carrying out partial detoxification: $2O_2^- + 2H^+ \rightarrow H_2O_2 + O_2$.

     c. Catalase or **peroxidase** enzymes degrade hydrogen peroxide in the reaction: $H_2O_2 + H_2A^* \rightarrow 2H_2O + A$, where if H_2A^* is hydrogen peroxide, A is O_2.

  2. Obligate aerobes: require oxygen for growth (cannot survive in the absence of O_2); produce superoxide dismutase and catalase, which protects them from toxic O_2^-.

  3. Obligate anaerobes: are killed by the O_2; grow maximally at a pO_2 concentration of less than 0.5% to 3%; and lack superoxide dismutase, catalase, and cytochrome c oxidase (enzymes that destroy toxic products of oxygen metabolism).

  4. Facultative anaerobes: grow in the presence or absence of oxygen; also called facultative aerobes or facultative; produce superoxide dismutase and catalase; can use both aerobic and anaerobic metabolism depending on the presence or absence of oxygen.

  5. Aerotolerant anaerobes: resemble facultative bacteria but use anaerobic metabolism (ie, are not able to use O_2); produce superoxide dismutase and catalase.

  6. Microaerophilic organisms: grow maximally at a pO_2 concentration of less than 20% and produce small amounts of superoxide dismutase and catalase; use aerobic metabolism.

D. Nutritional requirements

  1. Heterotrophs require preformed organic compounds (eg, sugar, amino acids) for growth. All known bacterial pathogens exhibit heterotrophic metabolism.

  2. Autotrophs do not require preformed organic compounds for growth because they can synthesize them from inorganic compounds and carbon dioxide.

E. Growth media (Table 2.1)

  1. Minimal essential growth medium

     a. This medium type contains only the primary precursor compounds essential for growth.

     b. Bacteria grown in this medium must synthesize most of the organic compounds required for growth.

     c. Generation time is relatively slow.

  2. Complex growth medium

     a. This medium type contains most of the organic compound building blocks (eg, sugars, amino acids, nucleotides) necessary for growth.

     b. Generation time for a bacterium is faster relative to its generation time in minimal essential medium.

     c. Fastidious bacteria may be grown in this medium type.

  3. Differential growth medium

     a. This medium type contains a combination of nutrients and pH indicators to allow the visual distinction/differentiation of bacteria that grow on or in it.

     b. Colonies of particular bacterial species may have a distinctive color.

  4. Selective growth medium

     a. This media type contains compounds that prevent the growth of some bacteria while allowing the growth of other bacteria (in other words, selecting for the growth of some bacteria).

     b. High salt concentration, dyes or sugars, antibiotics, or pH is used to achieve selectivity.

  5. Enrichment growth medium

     a. This media type contains additional compounds that enhance the growth of certain bacteria.

F. Metabolism

  1. General characteristics

     a. Bacterial metabolism is the sum of **anabolic processes** (synthesis of cellular constituents requiring energy) and **catabolic processes** (breakdown of cellular constituents with concomitant release of waste products and energy-rich compounds), and can vary depending on the nutritional environment.

Table 2.1   Common Growth Medias

Media	Common Bacteria Identified	Identification Mechanism
Blood agar	Hemolytic bacteria (staphylococcal and streptococcal species) Complex growth media for many bacteria	Red blood cells (RBCs) in nutrient agar base provide identification of α-hemolytic (green zone around colonies; partial hemolysis) and β-hemolytic (clear zone around colonies; complete hemolysis). Differential
Hektoen enteric agar	Enteric gram-negative rods (*Escherichia coli*, *Klebsiella*, *Salmonella*, and *Shigella*)	Contains bile salts, thiosulfate, ferric ammonium citrate, lactose, and sucrose. Gram-positives are inhibited. Lactose/sucrose fermenters and H_2S producers are observed with a color change. Selective and differential
MacConkey agar	Enteric gram-negative rods (*E. coli*, *Klebsiella*, *Salmonella*, *Shigella*, and *Proteus*)	Contains bile salts, crystal violet, lactose, and neutral red pH indicator. Bile salts and crystal violet inhibit gram-positives; only gram-negatives that ferment lactose give the colonies a color. Selective and differential
Löwenstein-Jensen media	*Mycobacterium* spp.	Glycerol, egg-potato media (provides fatty acids and proteins) containing malachite green dye, penicillin, and nalidixic acid to inhibit gram-positive and some gram-negative organisms. Selective
Chocolate agar	*Haemophilus* spp. *Neisseria* spp.	Blood agar containing gently heat-lysed RBCs to provide nutrients. Enrichment
Thayer-Martin medium	*Neisseria* spp.	Variant of chocolate agar with antibiotics to inhibit most normal respiratory and genital flora. Selective
Charcoal-yeast extract agar	*Legionella* spp.	Media that contains activated charcoal and antibiotics for the selective enhancement of growth of *Legionella* bacteria. Enrichment
Regan-Lowe media	*Bordetella* spp.	Contains lysed horse blood, charcoal, starch, and nicotinic acid to support the growth of *Bordetella pertussis*. Enrichment
Thiosulfate-citrate-bile salts-sucrose (TCBS), alkaline medium	*Vibrio* spp.	Selective media for growth of *Vibrio* species. Differential due to fermentation of sucrose: *V. cholerae* are yellow, other *Vibrio* spp. are green. Selective and differential

    b. Bacterial transport systems are generally required for metabolism and involve membrane-associated binding or transport proteins for sugars and amino acids.
        (1) Energy is frequently required to concentrate substrates inside the cell.
        (2) Transport is usually inducible for nutrients that are catabolized; glucose, which is constitutive, is an exception.
        (3) Phosphotransferase systems are frequently used for sugar transport.
  2. Carbohydrate metabolism
    a. Fermentation is a method of obtaining metabolic energy that is characterized by **substrate phosphorylation** and is generally carried out in the absence of oxygen (by anaerobes, facultative organisms in the absence of oxygen, and aerotolerant organisms).
        (1) Adenosine triphosphate (ATP) formation is not coupled to electron transfer.
        (2) An organic electron acceptor (eg, pyruvate) is required.
        (3) Specific metabolic end products are synthesized, which may aid in the identification of bacterial species.

    b. Respiration refers to the method of obtaining metabolic energy that involves **oxidative phosphorylation** and is generally carried out by organisms in the presence of oxygen (aerobes, facultative organisms in the presence of oxygen, and microaerophiles).

      (1) ATP is formed during electron transfer and the reduction of gaseous oxygen in aerobic respiration.

      (2) A cell membrane electron transport chain composed of cytochrome enzymes, lipid cofactors, and coupling factors is used during this process.

  3. Regulation

    a. Regulation of enzyme activity

      (1) Enzymes are **allosteric proteins**, susceptible to binding of effector molecules that influence their activity.

      (2) Feedback inhibition involves the end product.

      (3) Substrate-binding enhancement regulates catalytic activity.

    b. Regulation of enzyme synthesis may involve the following mechanisms:

      (1) Allosteric regulatory proteins that activate (**activators**) or inhibit (**repressors**) gene transcription.

      (2) End-product feedback repression of biosynthetic pathway enzymes.

      (3) Substrate induction of catabolic enzymes.

      (4) Attenuation control sequences in enzyme messenger RNA (mRNA).

      (5) Catabolite repression, which is under positive control of the **catabolite activator protein** (**CAP**).

    c. Pasteur effect is caused by oxygen blocking the fermentative capacity of **facultative bacteria**. The energy needs of the bacteria are met by using less glucose during aerobic growth.

G. Cell wall synthesis (Figure 2.4)

  1. Cell wall synthesis involves the cytoplasmic synthesis of peptidoglycan subunits, which are translocated by a membrane lipid carrier and cross-linked to the existing cell wall by enzymes associated with the plasma membrane of gram-positive bacteria or found in the periplasm of gram-negative bacteria.

  2. In gram-positive cells, it involves the covalent linkage of teichoic acid to *N*-acetylmuramic acid residues.

  3. In gram-negative cells, three components (lipoprotein, outer membrane, LPS) are added, whose constituents or subunits are synthesized on or in the cytoplasmic membrane and assembled outside of the cell.

  4. Some steps of peptidoglycan synthesis are the targets of antibiotics.

III. GRAM-POSITIVE BACTERIA

> **• • • Clinical Pearl**
>
> Most cocci of medical importance are gram positive. If "-*coccus*" is in the genus name, it is gram positive. Exceptions to this rule are the gram-negative cocci: *Neisseria* and *Moraxella*.

A. General characteristics

  1. Gram-positive bacteria have highly cross-linked, **multilayered (usually thick) peptidoglycan cell walls** that trap the large Gram crystal violet-iodine complex staining them deep **purple**.

  2. Teichoic acids are linked to either the cytoplasmic membrane (**lipoteichoic acids**) or the cell wall peptidoglycan. **Teichoic acids are unique to gram-positive bacteria** and play roles in **adherence** and **triggering gram-positive shock** as the cell wall is broken down.

  3. A variety of cell surface proteins are present and are often species specific.

  4. Gram-positive bacteria have **no outer membrane** and therefore no hydrophobic barrier to limit access of larger antibiotics to the peptidoglycan.

B. Major genera of gram-positive bacteria

  1. Genus: ***Staphylococcus***. Common name: Staphylococci

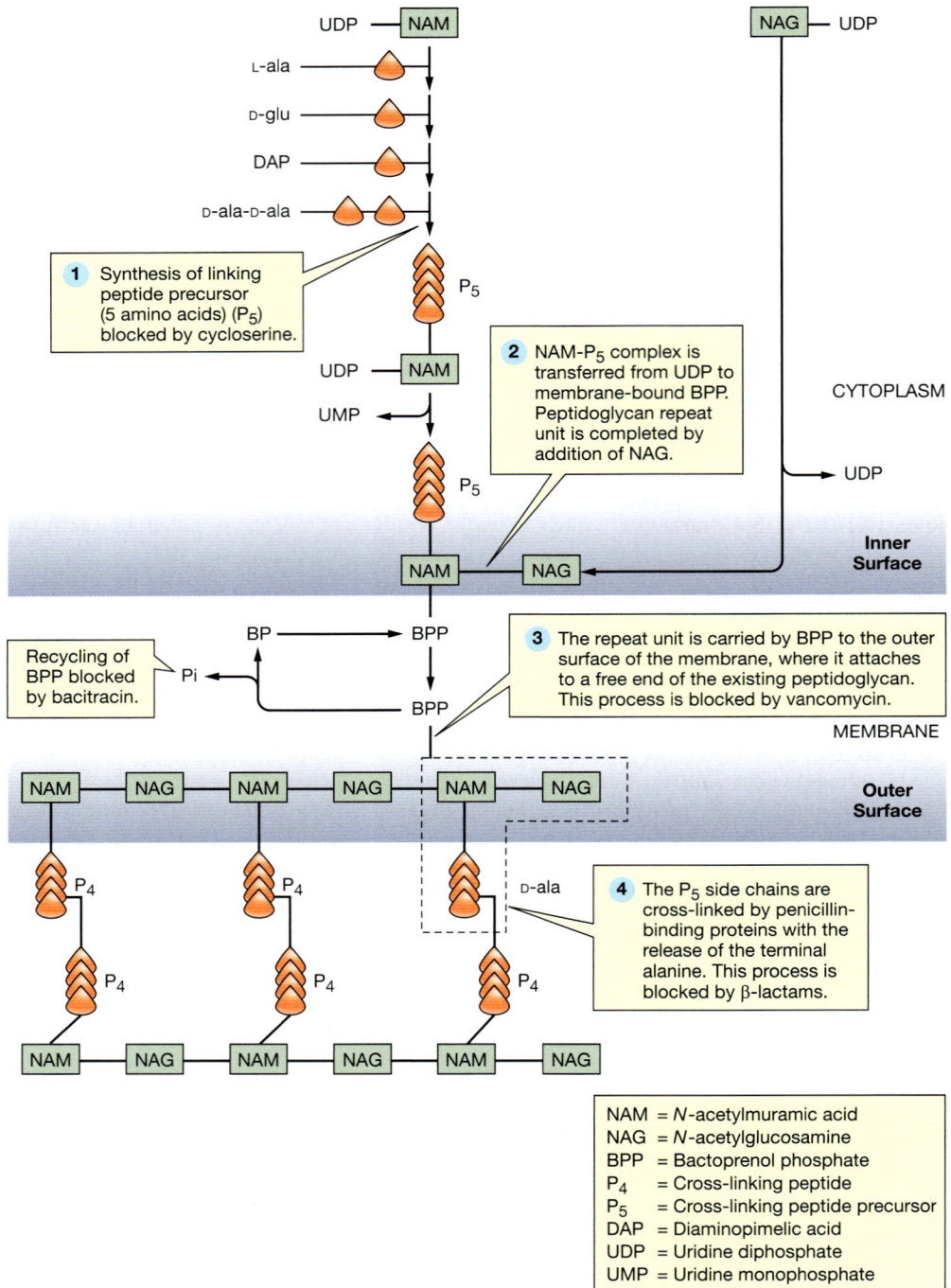

FIGURE 2.4. Synthesis of peptidoglycan.

Within the figure:

UDP — NAM

L-ala
D-glu
DAP
D-ala-D-ala

P5

1 Synthesis of linking peptide precursor (5 amino acids) (P5) blocked by cycloserine.

UDP — NAM
UMP

P5

NAG — UDP

2 NAM-P5 complex is transferred from UDP to membrane-bound BPP. Peptidoglycan repeat unit is completed by addition of NAG.

CYTOPLASM

UDP

NAM — NAG

Inner Surface

BP → BPP

Recycling of BPP blocked by bacitracin.

Pi

BPP

3 The repeat unit is carried by BPP to the outer surface of the membrane, where it attaches to a free end of the existing peptidoglycan. This process is blocked by vancomycin.

MEMBRANE

NAM — NAG — NAM — NAG — NAM — NAG

Outer Surface

P4   P4   P4   D-ala

4 The P5 side chains are cross-linked by penicillin-binding proteins with the release of the terminal alanine. This process is blocked by β-lactams.

P4   P4   P4

NAM — NAG — NAM — NAG — NAM — NAG

NAM = N-acetylmuramic acid
NAG = N-acetylglucosamine
BPP = Bactoprenol phosphate
P4 = Cross-linking peptide
P5 = Cross-linking peptide precursor
DAP = Diaminopimelic acid
UDP = Uridine diphosphate
UMP = Uridine monophosphate

Features
- **a. Gram-positive cocci** generally in tight grape-like clusters, singlets, pairs, or short chains.
- **b. Catalase positive**, breaking down hydrogen peroxide into water and oxygen.
- **c. Facultative anaerobes**, producing energy more efficiently aerobically.
- **d. Haloduric** (salt tolerant).
- **e.** Speciated medically based on **coagulase and hemolysis**.

Table 2.2 Medically Important *Staphylococcus* Species

Major Species	Location of Human Colonization	Identifying Characteristics[a]	Disease Associations
Staphylococcus aureus	Most common in the mucosa of the anterior nares; ↑s on cutaneous surfaces of health care workers, injection drug users, people with diabetes, etc	Coagulase positive β-Hemolytic	Cutaneous infections (impetigo, abscesses, cellulitis) Endocarditis, bacteremia Pneumonia Toxic shock syndrome Food poisoning
Staphylococcus epidermidis	Normal cutaneous flora	Coagulase negative Nonhemolytic (γ)	Opportunist requiring entry (surgical, catheter, shunt, prosthetic devices) causing septicemias, endocarditis, wound infections
Staphylococcus saprophyticus	Urinary mucosa colonization	Coagulase negative Nonhemolytic (γ)	Urinary tract infection, most commonly in young sexually active females

[a]All staphylococci are catalase positive.

Table 2.2 lists important medical species.
2. Genus: ***Streptococcus***. Common name: Streptococci
   Features
   a. **Gram-positive cocci in chains or pairs**.
   b. Distinguished from staphylococci based on the catalase test. **Streptococci are catalase-negative, aerotolerant anaerobes** that grow in full oxygen but ferment both in the presence and absence of oxygen.
   c. Subdivided or speciated by three different systems: serology, hemolysin production, and biochemical properties.
      (1) **Serology using Lancefield antibodies to cell wall carbohydrates.**
         (a) Streptococci that are positive for these carbohydrates are classified into Lancefield serogroups (eg, group A strep). There are more than 20 groups.
         (b) Bacteria that have these cell wall carbohydrates produce a pyogenic reaction.
         (c) Some α-hemolytic streptococci including *S. pneumoniae* and the viridans streptococci lack these cell wall carbohydrates. They are not grouped using Lancefield antibodies and are not pyogenic.
      (2) **Hemolysin testing:** There are three major types of hemolysis on blood agar plates: γ-Hemolysis is no hemolysis (the bacteria do not lyse the red blood cells in the media), α-hemolysis is partial hemolysis (the bacteria lyse some of the red blood cells, giving a greenish hue), and β-hemolysis is complete hemolysis (the bacteria lyse all of the red blood cells, so there is a clearing around the bacterial growth). See Figure 2.5.
      (3) **Biochemical tests:** Additional tests used in speciation include the CAMP (Christie–Atkins–Munch-Peterson) test, growth sensitivity to optochin, bile lysis, or growth inhibition by bacitracin.
   d. Streptococci are mainly opportunists but can cause disease if they gain entry into the body. Table 2.3 lists important medical species.
3. Genus: ***Enterococcus***. Common name: Enterococci
   Features
   a. **Catalase-negative, facultative anaerobes** fermenting even in the presence of oxygen.
   b. **α-Hemolytic** or **nonhemolytic (γ), gram-positive cocci** in chains that have the **Group D streptococcal cell wall carbohydrate**. Formerly classified as *Streptococcus* spp.

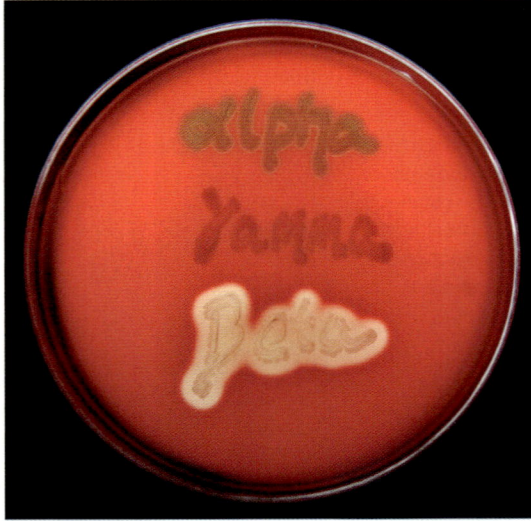

FIGURE 2.5. Hemolysis. Examples of the different types of hemolysis. (Top) α-**hemolysis** is partial hemolysis of the red blood cells with a change in the color of hemoglobin resulting in a translucent area with a greenish coloration. (Middle) γ-**hemolysis** is no hemolysis. (Bottom) β-**hemolysis** is complete lysis of the red blood cells, which results in a transparent area around the colony. (From Engleberg NC, Dirita V, Dermody TS. *Schaechter's Mechanism of Microbial Disease*. 5th ed. Wolters Kluwer Health; 2013.)

   c. Part of the normal human gastrointestinal (GI) flora.
   d. Tolerant of high concentrations of bile salts and NaCl.
   e. Have a high level of **drug resistance** that continues to increase due to efficient acquisition of plasmid transposon genes for drug resistance.
   Table 2.3 lists important medical species.

4. Genus: *Peptostreptococcus*
   Features
   a. Peptostreptococci are obligate **anaerobic streptococci**.
   b. They are part of the normal flora of the oral, intestinal, and genitourinary (GU) tracts.
   Table 2.3 lists important species distinctions and major diseases of the streptococci and its relatives.

5. Genus: *Bacillus*
   Features
   a. Gram-positive, spore-forming rods that may form chains. Although spores survive for decades in dry environments, they quickly germinate in rich moist conditions (eg, a macrophage) into metabolically active vegetative cells.
   b. They are **aerobes** (or facultative anaerobes) and grow well in ambient air.
   c. Cause anthrax (*Bacillus anthracis*) and food poisoning (*Bacillus cereus*).

6. Genus: *Clostridium*. Common name: Clostridia
   Features
   a. Gram-positive, spore-forming rods that can form chains, **anaerobic**.
   b. Cause botulism (*Clostridium botulinum*) characterized by a flaccid paralysis; gas gangrene and food poisoning (*Clostridium perfringens*); and tetanus (*Clostridium tetani*), characterized by rigid spasms.

7. Genus: *Listeria*. *Listeria monocytogenes* is the only human pathogen.
   Features
   a. Short gram-positive, nonspore-forming rods with weak β-hemolysis on blood agar.
   b. Motile in broth by characteristic **tumbling motility**.
   c. Facultative intracellular pathogens; they move from cell to cell by actin polymerization, which may propel the bacterium directly into an adjoining cell without exposure to extracellular milieu.

Table 2.3	Medically Important Streptococci and Other Gram-Positive, Catalase-Positive Cocci	
Major Species (Lancefield Group, if Applicable)	**Identifying Characteristics**	**Disease Associations**
Streptococcus pyogenes (Group A)	β-Hemolytic Bacitracin sensitive	Pharyngitis, scarlet fever Impetigo/cellulitis/fasciitis/erysipelas Postinfectious sequelae: acute glomer-ulonephritis, rheumatic heart disease
Streptococcus agalactiae (Group B)	β-Hemolytic Bacitracin resistant Colonizes 15%-20% of pregnant women	Neonatal septicemia, pneumonia, and meningitis Urinary tract infections in pregnant females
Streptococcus pneumoniae	α-Hemolytic Sensitive to optochin Lysed by bile No cell wall carbohydrates (no serogroup)	Otitis, sinusitis Lobar pneumonia Meningitis
Viridans streptococci	Normal oral flora α-Hemolytic (or nonhemolytic) Not inhibited by optochin Not lysed by bile No cell wall carbohydrates (no serogroup)	Major role in dental caries (*Streptococcus mutans*) Role in periodontal disease Endocarditis
Enterococcus faecalis or *Enterococcus faecium* (Group D)	Gastrointestinal tract flora; drug resistance	Endocarditis Urinary tract infections Septicemia
Peptostreptococcus spp.	Anaerobic streptococci	Opportunists

  d. Grows in the cold, unlike most nonspore-forming pathogens. *L. monocytogenes* is found in animal feces, rotting vegetation, and occasionally in soft cheeses, deli meats, and cabbage.
  e. Causes mild gastroenteritis, as well as septicemia in pregnant females, leading to potential fetal septicemia or meningitis, and may cause meningitis in immunocompromised patients.
8. Genus: ***Corynebacterium***
  Features
  a. Club-shaped, **gram-positive, nonspore-forming rods**.
  b. Found in characteristic arrangement of cells that may resemble broken sticks, historically called *Chinese character-like*.
  c. Aerobic and nonmotile.
  d. Part of **normal flora**; the nontoxin-producing corynebacteria found in the normal microbiota are typically called **diphtheroids**.
  e. **Toxin-producing *Corynebacterium diphtheriae*** causes diphtheria, and other *Corynebacterium* spp. cause infections via catheters and foreign bodies in immunocompromised hosts.
9. Genus: ***Actinomyces***
  Features
  a. **Anaerobic, gram-positive rods** with some branching; nonmotile.
  b. Found in crevices between teeth and gums and in the female genital tract.
  c. **Not acid-fast**

(1) Related to mycobacteria: have a similar cell wall but lack the extremely long-chain fatty acids found in the mycobacterial cell wall. They have shorter fatty acid chains.

d. Cause cervicofacial or pelvic infections following trauma that has resulted in necrotic tissue; colonies formed in tissue are sometimes described as "sulfur" granules.

10. Genus: *Nocardia*

Features

a. Gram-positive filamentous bacteria breaking up into **rods**.

b. Aerobic soil organisms.

c. Weakly or **partially acid-fast**.

d. Related to mycobacteria: cell wall with shorter chain mycolic acids.

e. Cause tuberculosis (TB)-like (but not contagious) bronchopulmonary disease in immuno-compromised patients.

11. Genus: *Mycobacterium*

Mycobacteria are considered gram positive even though they do not reliably Gram stain well. They are presented later with poorly Gram-staining bacteria. (See section V on Poorly Gram-Staining Bacteria.)

IV. GRAM-NEGATIVE BACTERIA

● ● ● **Clinical Pearl**

Most bacilli of medical importance are gram negative; however, there are more exceptions than for the gram-positive cocci. Exceptions to this rule are the gram-positive bacilli: *Actinomyces, Bacillus, Clostridium, Corynebacterium, Lactobacillus, Listeria, Nocardia,* and *Propionibacterium.*

A. General characteristics

1. Cell envelope has a **thin peptidoglycan layer** linked to an **outer membrane**; the peptidoglycan is not highly cross-linked, so on decolorization with alcohol the outer membrane is damaged and gram-negative cell walls easily lose the large Gram crystal violet/iodine dye complex, thereby becoming colorless until counterstained **red** with safranin.

2. Outer membrane has LPS, which is released on the death of the cell and has a toxic lipid A component. Entrance of aqueous materials across this outer membrane is through porin channels.

B. Major genera of gram-negative bacteria

1. Genus: *Neisseria*

Features

a. Aerobic, gram-negative, oxidase-positive diplococci occurring as pairs with flattened adjoining sides.

b. All species metabolize glucose.

c. The two pathogens in this genera are distinguished by maltose fermentation: **meningococcus** ferments **maltose**; **gonococcus** does not.

d. Sensitive to cold and drying.

e. Colonize mucosal surfaces (both nonpathogenic and pathogenic *Neisseria*).

f. Cause pneumonia, septicemia, and meningitis (*N. meningitidis*) and cervicitis, urethritis, proctitis, and conjunctivitis (*N. gonorrhoeae*).

2. Genus: *Moraxella* (*Moraxella catarrhalis*)

Features

a. Strictly aerobic, oxidase-positive, gram-negative diplococci.

b. Part of **normal oral flora**.

c. May cause otitis or sinusitis in healthy individuals; bronchitis and bronchopneumonia primarily in patients with chronic obstructive pulmonary disease (COPD).

3. Genus: *Brucella*

Features

a. Strictly **aerobic, gram-negative coccobacilli** (**or short rods**).

b. **Fastidious**; require special enriched media and 7 to 10 days to grow.

c. **Facultative intracellular pathogens** that infect **animals**; humans are infected by direct contact with infected animals; ingestion, inhalation, or implantation of contaminated materials; or in laboratory accidents. Incidence in the United States is lower than in developing countries as animal disease has been largely eradicated through vaccination and destruction of infected animals.

d. Cause brucellosis (undulant fever).

4. Genus: *Francisella*
   Features
   a. Strictly **aerobic, gram-negative coccobacilli**.
   b. **Fastidious**; require cysteine and several days for culture.
   c. Cause tularemia, a **zoonotic** disease seen mainly in rabbits, rodents, and hunters.

5. Genus: *Bordetella*
   Features
   a. Strictly **aerobic, gram-negative coccobacilli**.
   b. *Bordetella pertussis* is transmitted from person to person; humans can acquire kennel cough (*Bordetella bronchiseptica*) from animals.
   c. Very sensitive to drying and inhibitors in normal media; require special media (Bordet-Gengou, charcoal blood agar, Regan-Lowe) to grow.
   d. Causes **whooping cough** (*B. pertussis*) and a milder version (*Bordetella parapertussis*).

6. **Gram-negative, nonfermenting (aerobic) rods:** *Pseudomonas*, *Burkholderia*, and *Acinetobacter*
   a. Genus: *Pseudomonas*
   Features
   (1) Small, **polar-flagellated, gram-negative rods ubiquitous** in soil and water.
   (2) **Oxidase positive**.
   (3) Cause pneumonia and septicemia in individuals with cystic fibrosis and immunocompromised patients (especially those with neutropenia); cellulitis, and septicemia in burn patients; cellulitis in feet with foreign body trauma; otitis and eye infections.
   b. Genus: *Burkholderia*
   Features
   (1) **Gram-negative opportunists** found in moist environments, similar to *Pseudomonas*.
   (2) Cause infections in individuals with cystic fibrosis and immunocompromised patients (*Burkholderia cepacia* complex).
   (3) *Burkholderia pseudomallei* cause melioidosis, an infectious disease endemic in Southeast Asia.

7. **Gram-negative, nonmotile, fastidious rods:** *Haemophilus*, *Pasteurella*, *Coxiella*, *Bartonella*, and *Legionella*
   a. Genus: *Haemophilus*
   Features
   (1) **Gram-negative, pleomorphic** rods (elongated forms in culture but very short rods/coccobacilli in cerebrospinal fluid [CSF]).
   (2) **Fastidious:** *H. influenzae* requires **X** (**hemin**) and **V** (**nicotinamide adenine dinucleotide [NAD]**) factors on nutrient agar and grows well on chocolate agar. Do not grow on blood agar.
   (3) Strains without capsules (non-typeable) are part of the normal flora.
   (4) *H. influenzae* **type b** strains are encapsulated and cause meningitis or esophagitis in infants and toddlers who have not been vaccinated; some strains cause conjunctivitis and otitis; may cause bronchitis in patients with COPD.
   b. Genus: *Pasteurella*
   Features
   (1) **Gram-negative coccobacilli**, colonize the mouths of healthy animals (normal oral flora).
   (2) *Pasteurella multocida* may cause cellulitis in humans following untreated animal bites.

    c. Genus: *Coxiella*

Features

      (1) Gram-negative rod, obligate intracellular microorganism, but cannot visualize by Gram stain.

      (2) *Coxiella burnetii* is the causative agent of **Q-fever** (pneumonitis, atypical pneumonia, hepatitis), a **zoonotic** infection (usually from domestic mammals) with a small infectious dose.

    d. Genus: *Bartonella*

Features

      (1) Gram-negative, slightly curved rod, aerobic but slow-growing and difficult to visualize on Gram stain.

      (2) *Bartonella henselae* is the causative agent of **cat scratch fever** (skin and eye rash), spread by cat scratches.

    e. Genus: *Legionella*

Features

      (1) Gram-negative, short **rod**, but often cannot visualize by Gram stain because rods are too thin so other methods are used (eg, direct fluorescence antibody [FA] staining).

      (2) Obligate aerobes and **facultative intracellular** organisms.

      (3) Grow in amoeba in streams, survive in water to contaminate water lines (eg, grocery store vegetable sprayers, dental water lines, etc) and air-conditioning cooling tanks.

      (4) Fastidious: utilize **proteins** rather than carbohydrates as an energy source; **charcoal-yeast extract** (**CYE**) **agar** contains cysteine and is the selective isolation medium.

8. Family: **Enterobacteriaceae,** including *Escherichia, Klebsiella, Shigella, Yersinia, Proteus, Salmonella,* and *Serratia.*

    a. General characteristics

      (1) Gram-negative rods that **ferment glucose.**

      (2) Facultative anaerobes; oxidase negative.

    b. Genus: *Escherichia*

Features

      (1) Ferment lactose as well as glucose.

      (2) Major component of **normal colon flora.**

      (3) Motile. Have antigens that may be used in identification: **O antigen** (cell envelope), **H antigen** (flagella), and **P antigen** (pili).

      (4) May or may not have a capsule (K antigen), depending on the strain.

      (5) Cause urinary tract infections, septicemia, neonatal septicemia and meningitis, several GI tract diseases and peritonitis following bowel perforation.

    c. Genus: *Klebsiella*

Features

      (1) Ferment lactose as well as **glucose.**

      (2) Highly **motile**; found in the human colon and in water.

      (3) Produce **copious** amounts of **polysaccharide capsule** (K antigen) for a **mucoid** colony phenotype.

      (4) Are opportunists; cause hospital-acquired and ventilator-associated pneumonias.

    d. Genus: *Shigella*

Features

      (1) Do not ferment lactose.

      (2) Nonmotile because they lack flagella (no H antigens).

      (3) Do not produce H_2S.

      (4) Have **no animal reservoirs**, only human hosts.

      (5) Invade M cells of the intestine and then move into adjoining cells via **actin polymerization** (similar to *Listeria*).

    e. Genus: *Yersinia*

Features

      (1) Coccobacilli; show enhanced **bipolar** staining (looks like a safety pin).

      (2) Do not ferment lactose.

      (3) Nonmotile (no flagella or H antigens).

      (4) Do not produce H_2S.

(5) Are endemic in rodents in the southwestern United States (desert); vector is the rodent flea; cause plague (***Yersinia pestis***).

   f. Genus: ***Proteus***
   Features
   (1) Motile with **swarming motility** (peritrichous flagella, H antigen).
   (2) Do not ferment lactose.
   (3) Produce **urease** and H_2S.
   (4) Cause urinary tract infections and infections in immunocompromised patients.

   g. Genus: ***Salmonella***
   Features
   (1) **Highly motile** (capsule antigen of *Salmonella typhi* is called Vi antigen rather than H), **do not ferment lactose**.
   (2) **Produce H_2S.**
   (3) Have more than 2,000 serotypes; most classified as *Salmonella enterica* serovar x where the "x" is the former species name.
   (4) Have animal reservoirs except for *S. enterica* serovar typhi (eg, *S. typhi*), which is strictly a human pathogen.

   h. Genus: ***Serratia***
   Features
   (1) Slow lactose fermenting.
   (2) Some lab strains produce a **red pigment** (rarely during infection).

9. Family: **Vibrionaceae**, including ***Vibrio*** and ***Aeromonas***.
   a. General characteristics
   (1) **Comma-shaped or curved gram-negative rods with polar flagella**.
   (2) Facultative anaerobes, oxidase positive.
   (3) Found in aquatic environments and cause GI and wound infections.
   b. Genus: ***Vibrio***
   Features
   (1) Curved rods, some requiring salt (halophilic) to grow, live in aquatic habitats.
   (2) Cause cholera (mainly O1 and O139 and strains of ***Vibrio cholerae***), gastroenteritis (***Vibrio parahaemolyticus***), and cellulitis or hepatitis/septicemia (***Vibrio vulnificus***).
   c. Genus: ***Aeromonas.*** Ubiquitous; grow in fresh and salt water (opportunists).

10. **Gram-negative spiral-shaped rods:** ***Campylobacter*** and ***Helicobacter***
   a. General characteristics
   (1) **Capnophilic** (require elevated CO_2) and **microaerophilic** (grow only in the presence of low oxygen).
   (2) **Fastidious** (require special media) partially because they **do not metabolize carbohydrates** either oxidatively or by fermentation.
   b. Genus: ***Helicobacter***
   Features
   (1) Grow at 37 °C.
   (2) ***Helicobacter pylori*** colonizes the human gastric tract with potential to cause ulcers and stomach cancer.
   c. Genus: ***Campylobacter***
   Features
   (1) Grow at 42 °C.
   (2) Cause inflammatory diarrhea (***Campylobacter jejuni***).

11. **Gram-negative anaerobes:** ***Bacteroides***, ***Prevotella***, ***Porphyromonas***, and ***Fusobacterium***
   a. General characteristics
   (1) Anaerobes are prominent colonizers of mucosal surfaces of the oropharynx, female genital tract, and intestines, and thus cause endogenous infections, which are generally **polymicrobial** (involving more than one genus or species). Infections often result following growth in tissues by GI obstruction or surgery, diverticulitis, bronchial obstruction, tumor growth, or ulceration of the GI tract.
   (2) Anaerobes outnumber aerobes 1,000:1 in the gut and 100:1 in the mouth. They comprise 99% of the total fecal flora (estimated 10^{11}/g of stool in the large bowel).

    b. Genus: *Bacteroides*

    Features

        (1) Slender, gram-negative rods that stain pale red and have endotoxin with reduced toxicity compared with other gram-negative bacteria.

        (2) Part of normal GI tract flora.

        (3) Have a **capsule** as the major virulence factor.

        (4) Resistant to bile, so they are prominent colonizers of the intestine.

        (5) Although other species of *Bacteroides* are more prevalent in the GI tract, *B. fragilis* are prominent in infections.

    c. Genera: *Prevotella* and *Porphyromonas* are pigmented, **gram-negative anaerobes** found in oropharyngeal mucosa.

    d. Genus: *Fusobacterium:* **fine needle-like gram-negative anaerobes** that are part of the normal oral flora.

V. POORLY GRAM-STAINING BACTERIA

Many bacteria cannot be reliably visualized on Gram stain. These include many of the following groups of bacteria: **spirochetes**, **rickettsias**, **chlamydiae**, **mycoplasmas**, and **mycobacteria**. Most are too thin in diameter for the light microscope to resolve the color inside of the cell. The mycobacterial wall inhibits uptake of the dyes. Stains such as silver, Giemsa, or FA stains, which deposit on the surface of the cell, are generally used for these organisms.

A. Spirochetes: *Treponema, Leptospira,* and *Borrelia*

  1. General characteristics

    a. Spiral-shaped (or corkscrew-shaped) bacteria, technically **gram negative**.

    b. Endoflagella (also called axial filament) run from one end of each bacterium to the other, beneath the outer membrane, creating a springing motility.

    c. Not reliably seen by Gram stain (due to their small diameter), but because they have a thin, flexible peptidoglycan layer covered with an outer membrane, they are considered gram negative. FA and dark-field microscopy are used to visualize material from lesions.

    d. Classified by their tightness of coiling, cell diameter, and presence of terminal hooks into three major genera of medical importance.

  2. Genus: *Treponema*

    Features

    a. Very thin with **tight coiling** and no terminal hooks.

    b. Difficult to culture in the clinical lab; often listed as obligate pathogens (but are generally extracellular).

    c. Cause **syphilis** (*Treponema pallidum*) and related diseases.

  3. Genus: *Leptospira*

    Features

    a. Very thin with **tight coiling** and **hooks on the ends**.

    b. Cause leptospirosis, a **zoonotic** disease transmitted by animal urine in water.

  4. Genus: *Borrelia*

    Features

    a. Larger in diameter and more **loosely coiled** than the treponemes or leptospires.

    b. Cause **Lyme disease** (*Borrelia burgdorferi*) and relapsing fever (other *Borrelia* species).

B. Order: Rickettsiales

  1. General characteristics

    a. Obligate intracellular parasites.

    b. Survive only a short time outside of the host cell.

    c. Transmitted by **arthropod vectors** and most are maintained in nonhuman reservoirs.

2. Genera: *Rickettsia* and *Orientia*
   Features
   a. Obligate intracellular organisms that **escape the phagosome** into the cytosol of the host cell for replication.
   b. Have animal hosts and **tick** vectors.
   c. **Infect and kill endothelial cells**, causing capillary leakage and vasculitis; cause serious systemic diseases like **Rocky Mountain spotted fever** (*Rickettsia rickettsii*) and scrub typhus (*Orientia tsutsugamushi*).
3. Genera: *Ehrlichia* and *Anaplasma*
   Features
   a. Obligate intracellular organisms that **replicate in vacuoles** of **white blood cells**.
   b. Have animal hosts and **tick** vectors.
   c. Cause human monocytic ehrlichiosis (*Ehrlichia chaffeensis*) and human granulocytic anaplasmosis (*Anaplasma phagocytophilum*; *Ehrlichia phagocytophila*).

Important *Rickettsiales* are listed with their reservoirs, vectors, and diseases in Table 2.4.

Table 2.4	Important Rickettsial Species			
Group	**Disease Associations**	**Organism**	**Vector**	**Clinical Presentation**
Anaplasmosis	Primarily northeast and north central United States	*Anaplasma phagocytophilum*	*Ixodes* and perhaps other ticks	Human granulocytic anaplasmosis (HGA) = systemic disease from destruction of granulocytes; fever, malaise, myalgias, with thrombocytopenia
Ehrlichiosis	Primarily in southeast and south central United States	*Ehrlichia chaffeensis*	Ticks (*Amblyomma*)	Human monocytic ehrlichiosis (HME) = disease similar to HGA, but thrombocytopenia is not as common and monocytes infected.
Typhus	Epidemic (worldwide) or sylvatic typhus (eastern United States)	*Rickettsia prowazekii*	Human body lice or flying squirrels (possible role of fleas)	Trunk rash, progressing to extremities; gangrene, shock, hemorrhages in kidney, heart, brain, and lungs; milder disease in the United States
	Endemic	*Rickettsia typhi*	Rat fleas	Trunk rash, progressing to extremities (less severe than epidemic typhus)
Spotted fevers	Rocky Mountain spotted fever	*Rickettsia rickettsii*	Dog and wood ticks (*Dermacentor*)	Rash on extremities, progressing to trunk, fulminant vasculitis
	Rickettsialpox	*Rickettsia akari*	Mites	Rash similar to chickenpox (benign course), adenopathy, eschar at bite site

C. Order: Chlamydiales
  1. General characteristics
   a. Obligate intracellular organisms, unable to generate ATP.
   b. Have an inner and outer membrane but **no peptidoglycan**. Proteins in the outer membrane of the elementary bodies are extensively cross-linked, providing some rigidity.
   c. Transmitted directly from **person to person** by respiratory droplets or direct mucosal contact, or during the birth process.
   d. Two morphologic forms:
    (1) The **infectious form** is the **metabolically inert elementary body**. It has surface ligands that bind to human host cells, triggering uptake.
    (2) In human cell phagosomes, the elementary bodies develop into **reticulate bodies**, which replicate by binary fission.
   e. Molecular studies indicate two genera of medical importance (***Chlamydophila*** and ***Chlamydia***), but medically they are often all called genus *Chlamydia*. The species is identified by nucleic acid techniques.
   f. Most commonly diagnosed using **FAs** on specimens or gene probes. Can be identified by growth in tissue cells, direct FA staining, or polymerase chain reaction (PCR).
  2. Cause pneumonia (***Chlamydophila pneumoniae***, ***Chlamydophila psittaci***, and ***Chlamydia trachomatis***) and sexually transmitted diseases and eye infections (***C. trachomatis***).

D. Family: Mycoplasmataceae. Genera: *Mycoplasma* and *Ureaplasma*
  1. General characteristics
   a. Smallest extracellular bacteria.
   b. Lack a cell wall; are very flexible and able to pass through filters that are 0.4 μm (traps most other bacteria).
   c. Contain sterols in their cell membrane; however, they cannot synthesize sterols so mycoplasmas acquire them from hosts or specialized media.
   d. Facultative anaerobes except for ***Mycoplasma pneumoniae***, which is an obligate aerobe.
   e. Spread by **direct contact** or **respiratory droplets**.
   f. Bind to the exterior of cells and **damage epithelium**.
   g. Fastidious and slow to grow even on cholesterol-containing medium, so diagnosis is usually clinical or serologic with PCR.
   h. Cold agglutinins (autoantibodies agglutinating red blood cells at 4 °C) may be present after 1 to 2 weeks of clinical disease. Titers greater than 1:32 are generally considered positive. Complement fixation is more sensitive.
  2. *M. pneumoniae* causes respiratory tract infections; ***Mycoplasma hominis*** and ***Ureaplasma urealyticum*** may be involved in GU tract infections.

E. Genus: *Mycobacteria*
  1. General characteristics
   a. Poorly Gram-staining, thin bacilli.
   b. Have a **waxy cell surface** containing a thin triple layer of peptidoglycan linked to and covered with long-chain fatty acids (**mycolic acids**). The waxy cell envelope has the following features:
    (1) Porin proteins allow transport of aqueous materials across the hydrophobic envelope.
    (2) Confer resistance to drying, allowing respiratory droplet nuclei (the dried remains of respiratory droplets) to spread in air handling systems.
   c. Aerobic bacteria; when in granulomas, the metabolism slows but they release antigens that stimulate the continued remodeling of the granuloma. If the immune system begins to fail, the granuloma wall thins and may erode, exposing the organism to oxygen and triggering new growth and spread.
  2. *Mycobacterium tuberculosis* and ***Mycobacterium bovis*** (both cause **TB**).

3. *Mycobacterium kansasii* or *Mycobacterium avium-intracellulare* (also known as *Mycobacterium avian* complex [**MAC**]): grouped as **nontuberculous mycobacteria** or atypical mycobacteria or mycobacteria other than tuberculosis (MOTTS). These opportunists cause respiratory diseases in patients with low CD4$^+$ counts. They are **not contagious from person to person** and are acquired from showers or dust.
4. *Mycobacterium leprae* causes leprosy.

VI. BACTERIAL VIRUSES

A. General characteristics: Bacteriophages are bacterial viruses that are frequently called **phages**.
1. These obligate intracellular parasites are host-specific infectious agents for bacteria.
2. **Bacteriophage virions** are complete (genetic material and capsid) infectious particles.
3. Major components are protein and RNA or DNA.

B. Genetic classes of bacteriophages
1. *RNA phages* refer to all phages with RNA as their genetic material. The RNA is usually single-stranded and can act as polycistronic mRNA.
2. *DNA phages* refer to all phages with DNA as their genetic material. Some of the nucleic acid bases may be unusual (eg, 5-hydroxymethylcytosine or 5-hydroxymethyluracil).
   a. Two classes are recognized: **virulent** and **temperate**, depending on whether their pattern of replication is strictly **lytic** (virulent) or alternates between lytic and **lysogenic** (temperate).

C. Bacteriophage replication
1. **General characteristics:** Phages replicate using the biosynthetic machinery of the host cell. During replication, the phage genome is injected into the host cell. (Filamentous phages are the exception.)
   a. The basic sequence of events is adsorption; penetration; phage-specific transcription, translation, or both; assembly; and release.
   b. It is initiated by the interaction of phage receptors and specific bacterial surface receptor sites.
   c. For lytic phages, replication is usually complete in 30 to 60 minutes.
2. **Lytic replication** (also known as *productive replication*) occurs when a virulent virus replicates in a permissive host (Figure 2.6A) and may also occur with temperate phages.
   a. Strains of bacteria can be identified based on their lysis by a selected set of phages, a process called **phage typing**.
   b. **Generalized transducing phages** may be generated (see VII B 3).
3. **Lysogenic replication** occurs in **temperate phages** (eg, *E. coli* phage λ) (see Figure 2.6B).
   a. The synthesis of a phage-specific **repressor protein** inhibits phage-specific transcription, thus limiting phage-specific protein synthesis. If the phage repressor protein is destroyed, the phage can revert to lytic replication.
   b. **Prophage** (phage DNA) is incorporated into specific sites in the host-cell DNA. The prophage is passed to succeeding generations of the bacteria.
   c. **Specialized transducing phages** may be generated.
   d. Lysogenic replication may result in **lysogenic phage conversion**, a change in the phenotype of the bacteria as a result of limited expression of genes within a prophage. This mechanism occurs in the following situations:
      (1) In *Salmonella*, O polysaccharides are changed when lysogenized by the temperate bacteriophage ε.
      (2) Conversion of nontoxigenic strains of *Corynebacterium diphtheriae* to toxin-producing strains.
      (3) Conversion of nontoxigenic *C. botulinum* types C and D to toxin-producing strains.

Lytic Replication of Phage

Bacterial virus
= bacteriophage
= phage

1 Bacteriophage infects by binding to specific receptor on bacterial envelope and injecting DNA. DNA circularizes.

Bacterial DNA
(heavier line)

Phage DNA circularizes
(thin line)

2 Early functions: synthesis of mRNAs and proteins to shut off bacterial cell function and to make enzymes and factors to replicate phage DNA

Early proteins

Early mRNA

3 Phage DNA is synthesized.

4 Late mRNA and proteins (primarily structural proteins) are synthesized.

Phage DNA

5 Assembly

6 Normal infective (non-transducing) phage is released by lysis.

7 This phage packaged **bacterial DNA** in its head by mistake. It is called a **transducing phage.** Because any gene can be incorporated (depending on what bacterial DNA is incorporated), it is called a **generalized transducing phage.**

A

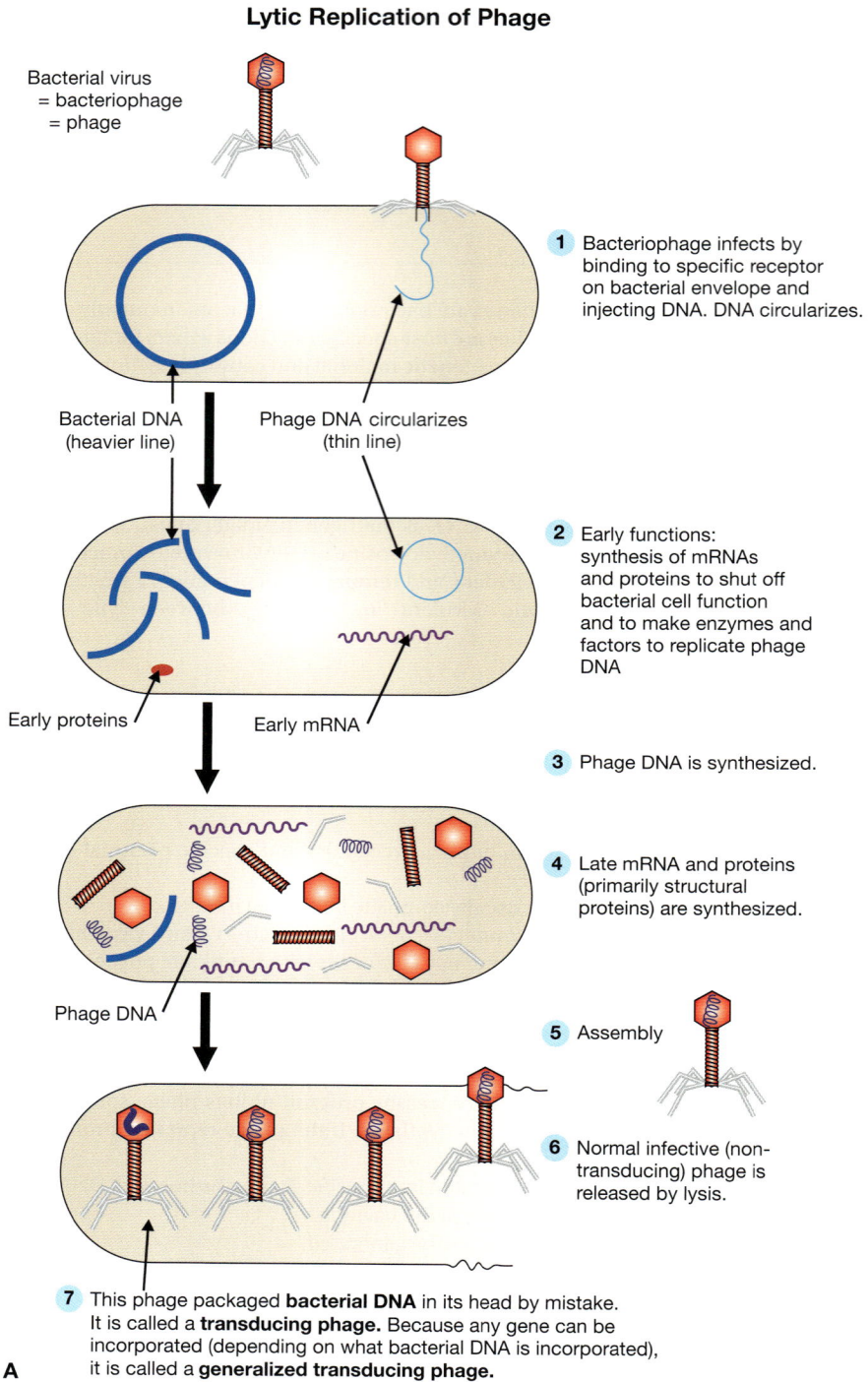

FIGURE 2.6. **Bacteriophage Replication.** A. Lytic replication. Note that this productive cycle always occurs in the virulent phage and may also occur in the temperate phage. B. Temperate phage infection: lysogeny. Transduction: induction/excision of prophage. If the repressor in a lysogenized cell is damaged by ultraviolet light, cold, or alkylating agents, the cell is "induced" into active virus production, which begins with the excision of the prophage DNA. Excision is the reverse of site-specific integration. The normal process of induction/excision of a prophage leading to active temperate phage replication is shown in (A). Aberrant excision leading to production of a specialized transducing phage is shown in (B). (Updated from Hawley LB. *High-Yield Microbiology and Infectious Diseases.* 2nd ed. Lippincott, Williams & Wilkins; 2007.)

Lysogenic Replication of Phage

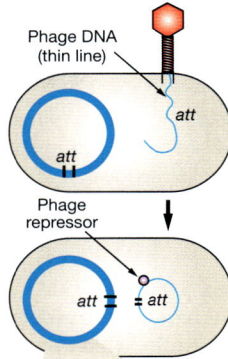

Phage DNA
(thin line)

att

att

1 The temperate phage lambda (λ) is shown. Lambda phage binds to specific receptors on the bacterial cell surface and injects phage DNA, which circularizes. The λ DNA contains the *att* gene.

Phage
repressor

att ⇌ *att*

2 If functional repressor protein is made quickly enough, it inhibits transcription of structural proteins and active production of virus, allowing the virus DNA to integrate.

Phage could have gone into lytic life cycle if repressor protein synthesis was slower.

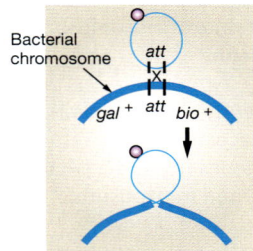

Bacterial
chromosome

att

gal + *att* *bio* +

3 Enlarged view of **integration of lambda DNA:** Note that both molecules of DNA have a small area of homology (*att* sites) where the pairing and crossing over occur. This is an example of site-specific recombination where the whole molecule is integrated rather than an exchange taking place. Note that *att* site is between the bacterial genes *gal* and *bio*.

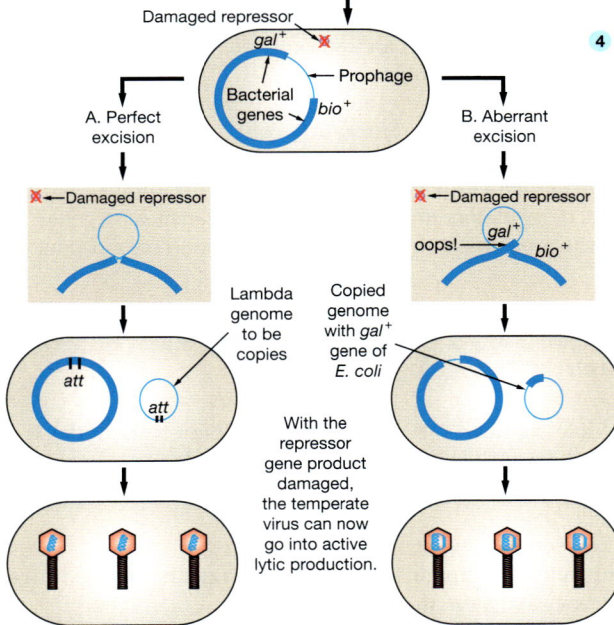

Damaged repressor

gal+

Prophage

Bacterial
genes *bio*+

A. Perfect
excision

B. Aberrant
excision

4 This is a **lysogenized cell** (state is called **lysogeny**). When host bacteria undergo replication, both the bacterial DNA and the phage DNA will be duplicated. As long as the repressor protein continues to be synthesized and is functioning, lysogeny will continue. The phage is called a prophage.

Damaged repressor

Damaged repressor

oops! *gal*+

bio+

Lambda
genome
to be
copies

Copied
genome
with *gal*+
gene of
E. coli

att

att

With the
repressor
gene product
damaged,
the temperate
virus can now
go into active
lytic production.

Only lambda DNA in all phage heads

Part of lambda DNA plus
gal+ gene in all phage heads

Normal lambda phage are generally produced. These are not transducing. If after a perfect DNA excision there is a late DNA packaging error, then a generalized transducing phage could be produced along with these normal nontransducing phage.

Specialized lambda transducing phage are produced, each of which is carrying the *gal*+ gene. (Only the *gal* **or** *bio* genes could have been picked up.)

B

FIGURE 2.6. (*continued*)

VII. GENETICS

A. **Comparison of bacterial and eukaryotic genomes.**
   1. **Eukaryotic genome**
      a. Structure: the eukaryotic genome of humans, fungi, and parasites.
         (1) Is **diploid** with two homologous copies of each chromosome, except in some fungi.
         (2) Is contained in two or more linear chromosomes located within a membrane-bound nucleus.
         (3) Contains **introns** (DNA sequences not translated into gene products) and redundant genetic information.
      b. Replication
         (1) Begins at several points along the linear DNA molecule.
         (2) Is regulated by specific gene inducer or repressor substances.
         (3) Involves a specialized structure, the **spindle**, which pulls newly formed chromosomes into separate nuclei during mitosis.
   2. **Prokaryotic genome**
      a. Structure: The prokaryotic genome is **haploid** (single, usually circular chromosome encoding several thousand genes). It may contain extrachromosomal DNA called **plasmids** and movable genetic elements called **transposons**.
         (1) Plasmids
            (a) Are DNA that replicate independently of chromosomal replication.
            (b) May exist in an **episomal** form that can integrate into the bacterial chromosome.
            (c) May carry **antibiotic resistance** genes (eg, EM-1 β-lactamase gene of *E. coli*), **toxin genes** (eg, enterotoxins of *E. coli*), and transposons.
         (2) Transposons
            (a) Are **movable genetic elements** (also called jumping genes) incapable of independent replication.
            (b) Contain insertion sequences and can transfer genetic information by insertion into bacterial chromosomes or plasmids.
            (c) May contain antibiotic resistance genes (eg, *N. gonorrhoeae*, β-lactamase) or virulence factors (eg, heat-stable enterotoxin of *E. coli*).
         (3) Pathogenicity islands
            (a) Are **groups of virulence-associated** genes that code for unique secretion systems, toxins, adhesins, or regulatory proteins and contain transposase genes.
            (b) Are associated with transfer RNA (tRNA) genes on bacterial chromosomes or plasmids.

> **• • • Clinical Pearl**
>
> Both gram-negative and gram-positive bacterial chromosomes may contain pathogenicity islands, but they are more common in gram-negative bacteria.

   b. Replication: Each double-stranded DNA circle (chromosomes, plasmids) is capable of self-replication bidirectionally ($5'$-PO_4 to $3'$-OH) from a fixed origin.

B. **Gene transfer in bacteria**
   1. **General characteristics**
      a. Genetic variability in microbes is maintained through **gene transfer** followed by **recombination** of allelic forms of genes and by gene mutation.
      b. Gene exchange may also occur as the crossing over of homologous chromosomes or by non-homologous means (eg, movement of plasmids or transposons, insertion of viral genes).
      c. It can result in the acquisition of new characteristics (eg, antigens, toxins, antibiotic resistance).
      d. There are three major mechanisms of gene transfer: conjugation, transduction, and transformation.
   2. **Conjugation** (Figure 2.7A,B) is a one-way transfer of genetic material (usually plasmids) from a donor bacterium to recipient by means of physical contact. In gram-positive cells, contact occurs between a plasmid-encoded adhesin on the donor cell and receptors on the recipient

Conjugation: F⁺ to F⁻

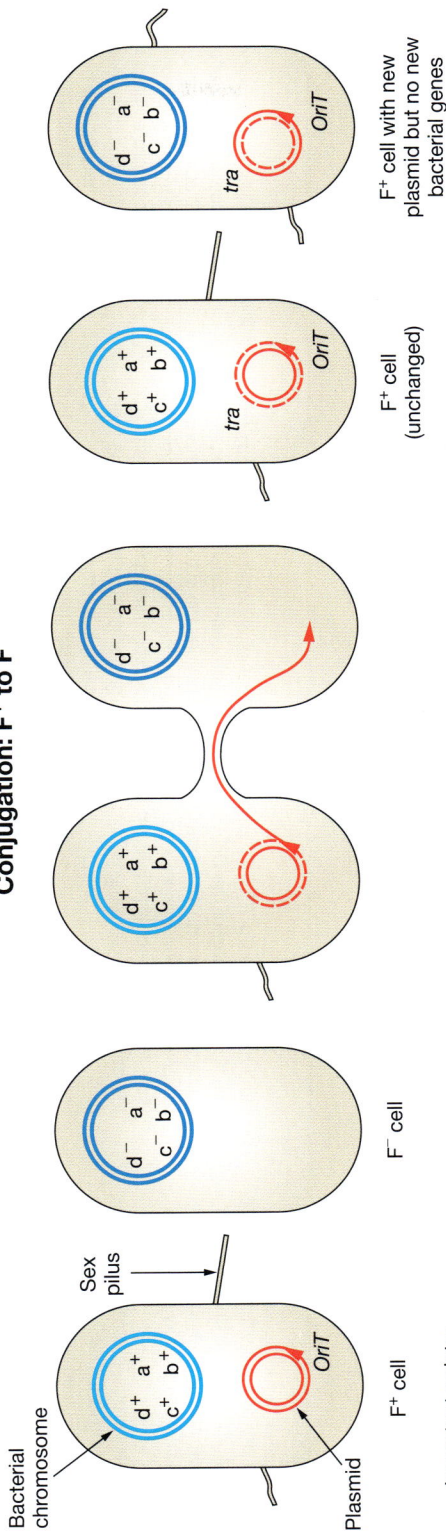

Bacterial chromosome

Sex pilus

Plasmid

OriT

F⁺ cell

F⁻ cell

Important points:

1 In the male or F⁺ parent, the fertility factor is present but free from the bacterial chromosome.

Transfer is unidirectional from F⁺ to F⁻.

OriT (origin of transfer) is transferred first, followed by the rest of the plasmid genes.

2 Note, only a single strand of the plasmid DNA duplex is transferred.

The area that is lost is reduplicated (shown as dotted lines), so that the donor always keeps the same genotype.

The last genes to be transferred are those in the *tra* region.

F⁺ cell (unchanged)

F⁺ cell with new plasmid but no new bacterial genes

3 Note that the F⁻ cell undergoes a change, from F⁻ + becoming F⁺ (male). These two F⁺ cells can no longer mate.

Note, no BACTERIAL chromosome genes are transferred.

A

FIGURE 2.7. A. Conjugation: F⁺ to F⁻ cross. B. Conjugation: Hfr to F⁻ cross. Newly synthesized DNA is shown as dashed lines. Hfr, high-frequency recombination. (Updated from Hawley LB. *High-Yield Microbiology and Infectious Diseases.* 2nd ed. Lippincott Williams & Wilkins; 2007.)

Conjugation: Hfr to F⁻

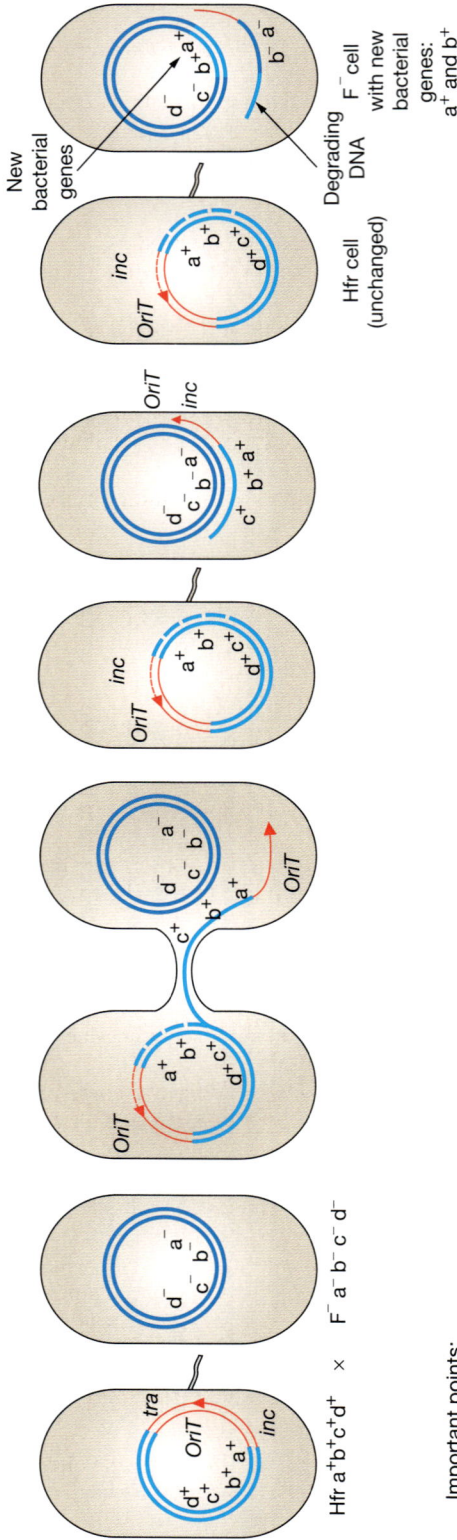

Hfr a⁺b⁺c⁺d⁺ × F⁻ a⁻ b⁻ c⁻ d⁻

Important points:

1 Hfr donor means that the fertility factor (fine red line) is already integrated into the bacterial chromosome (heavier blue line).

In this cross, plasmid genes starting at *OriT* will be transferred first, followed by the bacterial genes in linear order away from the plasmid.

2 Note that as with the F⁺ × F⁻ cross, only a single strand of the DNA duplex is transferred. The area that is transferred is reduplicated (note the rolling model at left), so that the donor genotype remains unchanged.

IF the entire chromosome were to be transferred, the last genes to be transferred would be the *tra* region.

3 It takes approximately 2 hours for a complete transfer to occur. Because the cytoplasmic bridge and DNA are so fragile, mating is normally interrupted before the transfer is complete. Assume that mating is interrupted and the recipient gets some new genes but does not become Hfr.

4 If homologous recombination occurs following conjugation, some or all of the genes transferred from the Hfr donor may be incorporated onto the F⁻ bacterial chromosome, resulting in a new genotype. The new F⁻ cell is still not able to initiate conjugation because it does not contain *oriT* or other conjugation genes.

B

FIGURE 2.7. (*continued*)

cell. In gram-negative cells, contact occurs through sex pili. Gram-negative cell conjugation typically involves one of the following types of plasmids:

    a. F (fertility) plasmids, which mediate the creation of a sex pilus necessary for conjugal transfer of the F plasmid to the recipient.

        (1) Cells that contain this plasmid are called F^+, whereas those that do not are called F^-.

        (2) The F plasmid can integrate into chromosomal DNA, creating **high-frequency recombination** (**Hfr**) donors from which chromosomal DNA is readily transferred.

    b. R factors, which contain genes for conjugal transfer and genes conferring **drug resistance**.

        (1) Resistance genes are frequently carried on transposons.

        (2) The resistance phenotype is expressed through natural selection.

3. Transduction is the **phage-mediated transfer** of host DNA sequences. It is performed by temperate and lytic phages. It occurs in two forms:

    a. In **generalized transduction**, by mistake, the phage randomly packages host bacterial DNA inside a bacteriophage coat, as was seen in Figure 2.6A. Thus the **transducing particle** can transfer any randomly packaged bacterial DNA (Figure 2.8).

    b. In **specialized transduction**, the lysogenic phage favors the transfer of host DNA segments near the site of prophage integration (Figure 2.9). Specialized transducing phages contain both viral and host genes, as was seen in Figure 2.6B.

4. Transformation (Figure 2.10) is the **direct uptake** and recombination of naked DNA fragments through the cell wall by competent bacteria.

    a. Surface **competence factors** (DNA receptor enzymes) sometimes mediate transformation. These factors are produced only at a specific point in the bacterial growth cycle.

    b. Bacteria can sometimes be induced into transformation by treatment with calcium chloride and temperature or electrical shock.

C. Gene expression

1. Transcription is the production of mRNA from DNA. A short sequence of DNA bases is unwound, and complementary ribonucleotide bases are aligned onto the DNA template.

    a. In bacteria, transcription is mediated by **RNA polymerase** and initiated by the binding of **σ factor**, a subunit of RNA polymerase, to the **promoter region** of the DNA. Transcription occurs in a $5'$-PO_4 to $3'$-OH direction.

2. Translation is the assembly of polypeptide chains from the mRNA transcript at the ribosomes.

    a. Amino acids are bound together via tRNAs in accordance with the triplet-encoded mRNA transcript.

3. Regulation of gene expression

    a. Operon model: Expression is regulated primarily **during transcription** and is determined partly by the ability of the **DNA promoter region** to bind with σ factor. Expression is facilitated or blocked by regulator proteins binding to operator sequences near the promoter. An operator controls a group of genes called an **operon**.

    b. Negative control is inhibition of transcription by the binding of a repressor protein.

    c. Positive control is the initiation of transcription in response to the binding of an activator protein.

    d. *Lac* **operon:** classic example of bacterial gene regulation.

        (1) This operon controls expression of three structural genes for lactose metabolism via a repressor protein.

        (2) Transcription is induced by the presence of lactose (allolactose), which binds to the repressor protein and frees the *lac* operator for RNA polymerase to bind.

        (3) Transcription occurs in the absence of glucose only, when cyclic adenosine monophosphate (cAMP) binds to the CAP to facilitate binding of RNA polymerase to the promoter region.

D. Mutation

1. General description: Mutation is an induced or spontaneous heritable alteration of the DNA sequence. It is the means by which variability is introduced into the gene pool and results in changes to the phenotype.

Generalized Transduction

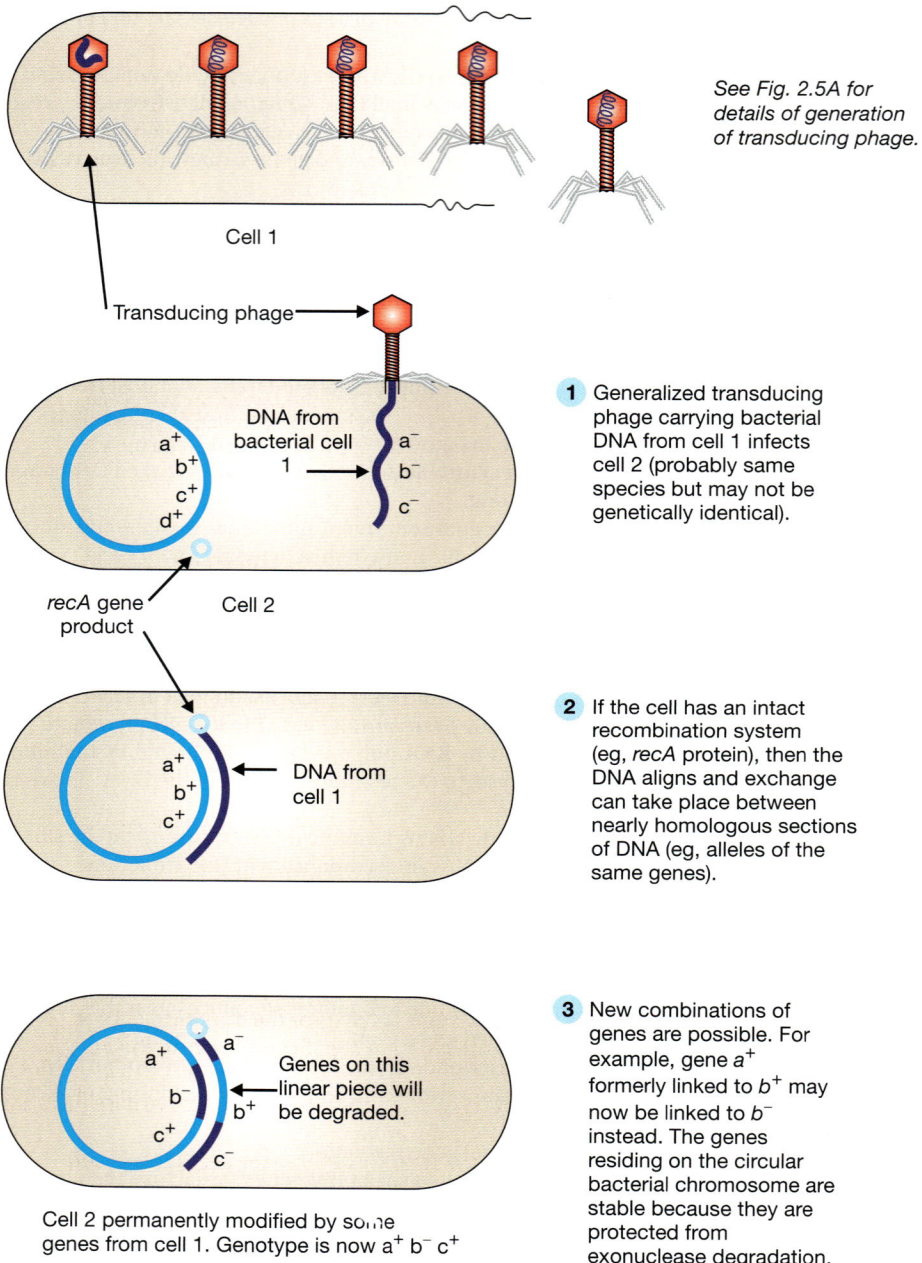

See Fig. 2.5A for details of generation of transducing phage.

Cell 1

Transducing phage ⟶

DNA from bacterial cell 1 ⟶

a⁺ b⁺ c⁺ d⁺   a⁻ b⁻ c⁻

recA gene product

Cell 2

1 Generalized transducing phage carrying bacterial DNA from cell 1 infects cell 2 (probably same species but may not be genetically identical).

a⁺ b⁺ c⁺   DNA from cell 1

2 If the cell has an intact recombination system (eg, recA protein), then the DNA aligns and exchange can take place between nearly homologous sections of DNA (eg, alleles of the same genes).

a⁺ a⁻ b⁻ b⁺ c⁺ c⁻   Genes on this linear piece will be degraded.

3 New combinations of genes are possible. For example, gene a⁺ formerly linked to b⁺ may now be linked to b⁻ instead. The genes residing on the circular bacterial chromosome are stable because they are protected from exonuclease degradation.

Cell 2 permanently modified by some genes from cell 1. Genotype is now a⁺ b⁻ c⁺

In generalized transduction, every bacterial gene has an equal chance of being incorporated into the phage head and being transferred to the next bacterial cell that is infected.

FIGURE 2.8. Generalized transduction. (Updated from Hawley LB. *High-Yield Microbiology and Infectious Diseases.* 2nd ed. Lippincott Williams & Wilkins; 2007.)

Specialized Transduction = Restricted Transduction

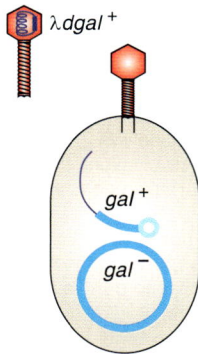

λ*dgal* $^+$

1 Specialized transducing phage created by an excisional error coming out of lysogeny to lytic replication of the phage (See Fig. 2.5B for details). This defective phage has some lambda genes and the bacterial gene *gal*$^+$.

gal$^+$

gal$^-$

2 Transducing *gal*$^+$ phage has now injected its DNA into a *gal*$^-$ cell.

Escherichia coli. gal$^-$ cell infected with a transducing phage carrying *gal*$^+$

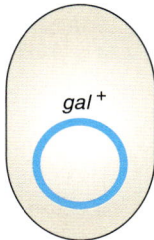

3 The phage nucleic acid recircularizes in the new cell and may either undergo reinsertion (the whole circular molecule) or homologous recombination. Either way in this cell, some *gal*$^+$ cells may result.

gal$^+$

Summary of Specialized Transduction
1. Specialized transducing phage are produced by an excisional error.

2. Only the genes that adjoin the insertion site (*att*) of a temperate phage can be integrated into the phage.

Now *gal*$^+$

3. Transduced genes may be stabilized by recombination.

FIGURE 2.9. Specialized or restricted transduction. (Updated from Hawley LB. *High-Yield Microbiology and Infectious Diseases.* 2nd ed. Lippincott Williams & Wilkins; 2007.)

a. **Frequency:** occurs approximately once for any gene in every 1 million cells.
b. **Causes:** may be caused by various mutagens, including ultraviolet light, acridine dyes, base analogs, and nitrous acid.
2. **Mutation types**
a. **Nucleotide substitutions** arise from mutagenic activity or the mispairing of complementary bases during DNA replication. These often do not significantly disrupt the function of gene products.
b. **Frameshift mutations** result from the insertion or deletion of one or two base pairs, disrupting the phase of the triplet-encoded DNA transcript.
c. **Deletions** are large excisions of DNA, dramatically altering the sequence of coded proteins. These may also result in frameshift mutations.
d. **Insertions** change genes and their products by integration of new DNA, often via transposons.
3. **Results of mutation**
a. **Missense mutations** result in the substitution of one amino acid for another. They may be without phenotypic effect (silent mutation).
b. **Nonsense mutations** terminate protein synthesis and result in truncated gene products. They usually result in inactive protein products.
4. **Reversions.** Function lost to mutation may be regained in two ways:
a. **Genotypic (true) reversion:** restoration at the site of DNA alteration.
b. **Phenotypic (suppression) reversion:** restoration of an activity lost to mutation, often by a mutation at a second site (**suppressor mutation**).

Bacterial Transformation

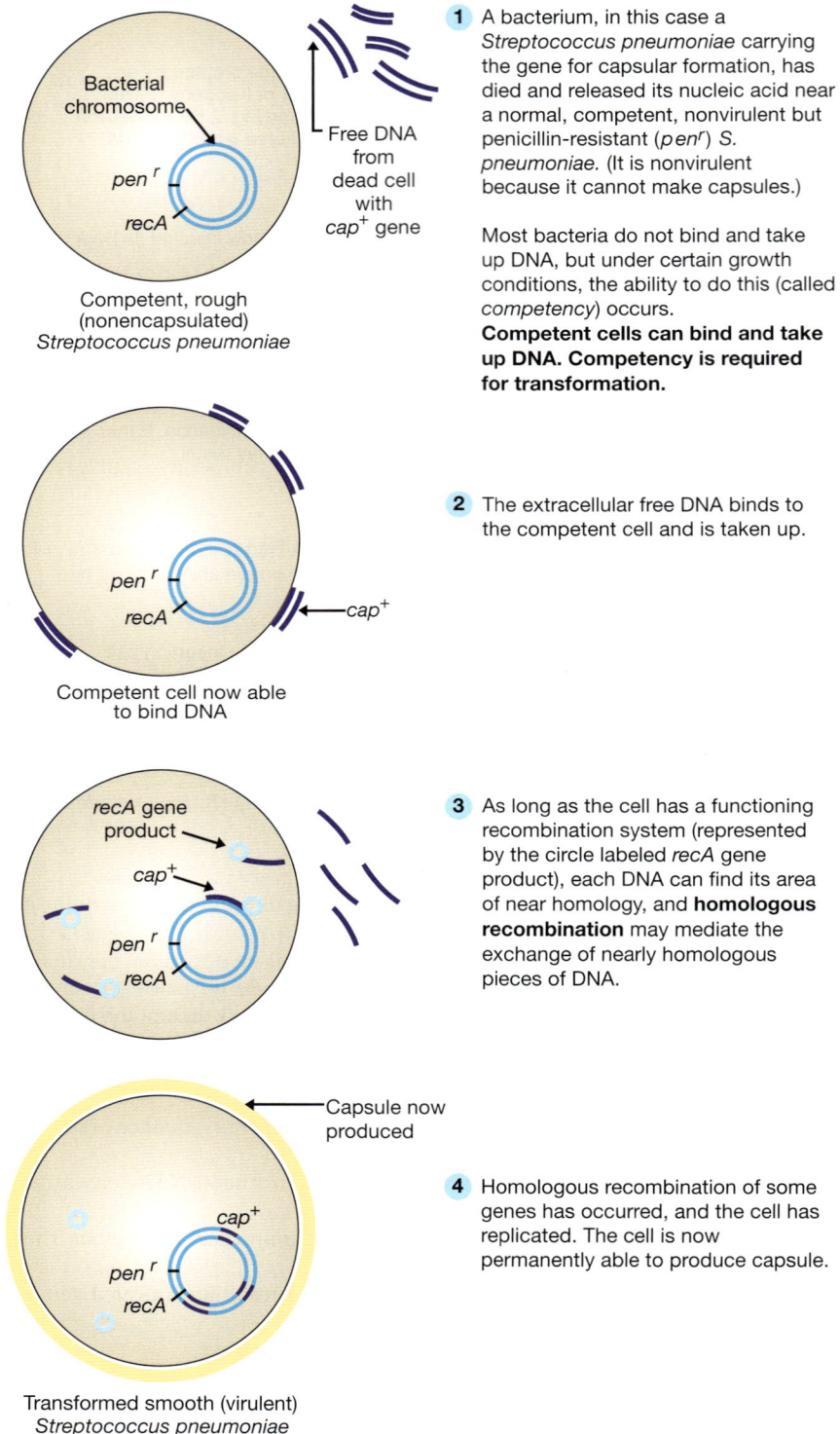

1 A bacterium, in this case a *Streptococcus pneumoniae* carrying the gene for capsular formation, has died and released its nucleic acid near a normal, competent, nonvirulent but penicillin-resistant (*pen^r*) *S. pneumoniae*. (It is nonvirulent because it cannot make capsules.)

Most bacteria do not bind and take up DNA, but under certain growth conditions, the ability to do this (called *competency*) occurs. **Competent cells can bind and take up DNA. Competency is required for transformation.**

2 The extracellular free DNA binds to the competent cell and is taken up.

3 As long as the cell has a functioning recombination system (represented by the circle labeled *recA* gene product), each DNA can find its area of near homology, and **homologous recombination** may mediate the exchange of nearly homologous pieces of DNA.

4 Homologous recombination of some genes has occurred, and the cell has replicated. The cell is now permanently able to produce capsule.

FIGURE 2.10. Gene transfer: example of bacterial transformation. (Updated from Hawley LB. *High-Yield Microbiology and Infectious Diseases.* 2nd ed. Lippincott Williams & Wilkins; 2007.)

VIII. BACTERIAL PATHOGENESIS

A. General characteristics

The pathogenesis of a bacterium depends on its virulence properties and the capabilities of the host's defense mechanism. Normal flora may become pathogenic if they gain access to normally sterile body areas or if the environmental conditions allow them to multiply to a level not controlled by the host.

B. Virulence factors

Pathogenic microbes produce virulence factors, which are gene products that enable pathogens to cause infection. These may be genetically encoded on the bacterial chromosome or located on plasmids.

1. **Structural bacterial components**, including:
   a. Antiphagocytic surface proteins and capsules.
   b. Adhesins that promote colonization.
   c. Endotoxin of gram-negative bacteria.
   d. Immunoglobulin (Ig)G antibody-binding surface proteins.
   e. Antigenic switching of surface antigens due to phase variation or antigenic variation processes.
2. **Extracellular gene products**, including:
   a. Degradative enzymes such as collagenase and hyaluronidase that facilitate tissue invasion.
   b. IgA antibody-degrading proteases.
   c. Exotoxins.
   d. Protein secretion systems.
3. **Growth properties** include the capacity for intracellular growth and the ability to form biofilms.

C. Toxins are common virulence factors produced by many pathogenic bacteria. There are two major types of bacterial toxins.

1. **Endotoxin** is the lipid A component of gram-negative bacteria. Endotoxins have the following **actions**:
   a. Induce the release of endogenous pyrogens (eg, interleukin 1 [IL-1], tumor necrosis factor [TNF], prostaglandins, etc).
   b. Increase vascular permeability.
   c. Initiate complement and blood coagulation cascades.
   d. Cause fever, hypotension, disseminated intravascular coagulation (DIC), and shock.
2. **Exotoxins** are secreted by some gram-positive and gram-negative bacteria; they may be genetically encoded on the bacterial chromosome, a plasmid, or a phage.
   a. **Actions:** Exotoxins have the following five major mechanisms of action (see Table 2.5):
      (1) Alter cellular components.
      (2) Act as **superantigens** that cause inappropriate release of cytokines.
      (3) Inhibit protein synthesis.
      (4) Increase cAMP.
      (5) Alter nerve impulse transmission.
   b. **Exotoxin structure**
      (1) Some exotoxins have an **A-B subunit structure** in which one or more B subunits are involved in binding and the A subunit possesses the enzymatic activity inside the cell.
      (2) Others are a single polypeptide with enzymatic activity or other biologic activities.
   c. **Toxoids** are chemically altered forms of toxins that may be used as immunization agents. Toxoids induce antibodies that minimize the toxin's biologic effects (eg, diphtheria and tetanus toxins).

Table 2.5   Examples of Bacterial Exotoxins

Biologic Effect	Toxin Name	Organism	Gene Location	Mechanism of Action
Alter cellular components	α-Toxin	*Staphylococcus aureus*	Bacterial chromosome	Forms pore
	Streptolysin O			Forms pore
	α-Toxin	*Streptococcus pyogenes*	Bacterial chromosome	Disrupts membranes
	Type III cytotoxin	*Clostridium perfringens*	Bacterial chromosome and plasmid	Cytoskeletal changes
	Type III cytotoxin	*Pseudomonas aeruginosa*	Phage	Alters actin cytoskeleton
		Salmonella species	Bacterial chromosomes	
Superantigens	TSST-1	*S. aureus*	Bacterial chromosome	Release of cytokines
	Enterotoxin	*S. aureus*		Release of cytokines
	Erythrogenic toxins A and C	*S. pyogenes*	Phage	Release of cytokines
			Phage	
Inhibition of protein synthesis	Diphtheria toxin	*Corynebacterium diphtheriae*	Phage	ADP ribosylation elongation factor 2
	Exotoxin A	*P. aeruginosa*	Bacterial chromosome	ADP ribosylation elongation factor 2
	Shiga toxin	*Shigella dysenteriae*	Plasmid	
	Vero toxin (also called Shiga-like toxin)	Enterohemorrhagic *Escherichia coli*	Bacterial chromosome or phage	Inactivates 60S ribosomes
				Inactivates 60S ribosomes
Increased synthesis of cAMP	Cholera toxin	*Vibrio cholerae*	Bacterial chromosome	Turns on stimulatory G protein
	LT toxin	Enterotoxigenic *E. coli*	Plasmid	Turns on stimulatory G protein
	ST toxin	*Bacillus anthracis*	Plasmid	Adenylate cyclase activity
	Anthrax toxin	*Bordetella pertussis*	Bacterial chromosome	Turns off inhibitory G protein
	Pertussis toxin			
Altered nerve impulse transmission	Tetanus toxin	*Clostridium tetani*	Plasmid	Inhibits inhibitory neurotransmitter release
	Botulinum toxin	*Clostridium botulinum*	Phage	Inhibits acetylcholine release

cAMP, cyclic adenosine monophosphate; LT, labile toxin; ST, stable toxin; TSST-1, toxic shock syndrome toxin-1.

IX. ANTIMICROBIAL CHEMOTHERAPY

A. General characteristics

1. Antimicrobial chemotherapy is based on the principle of **selective toxicity**, which implies that a compound is harmful to a microorganism but less damaging to the host.
2. The **drugs** used in antimicrobial therapy have one or more of the following properties (Figure 2.11):

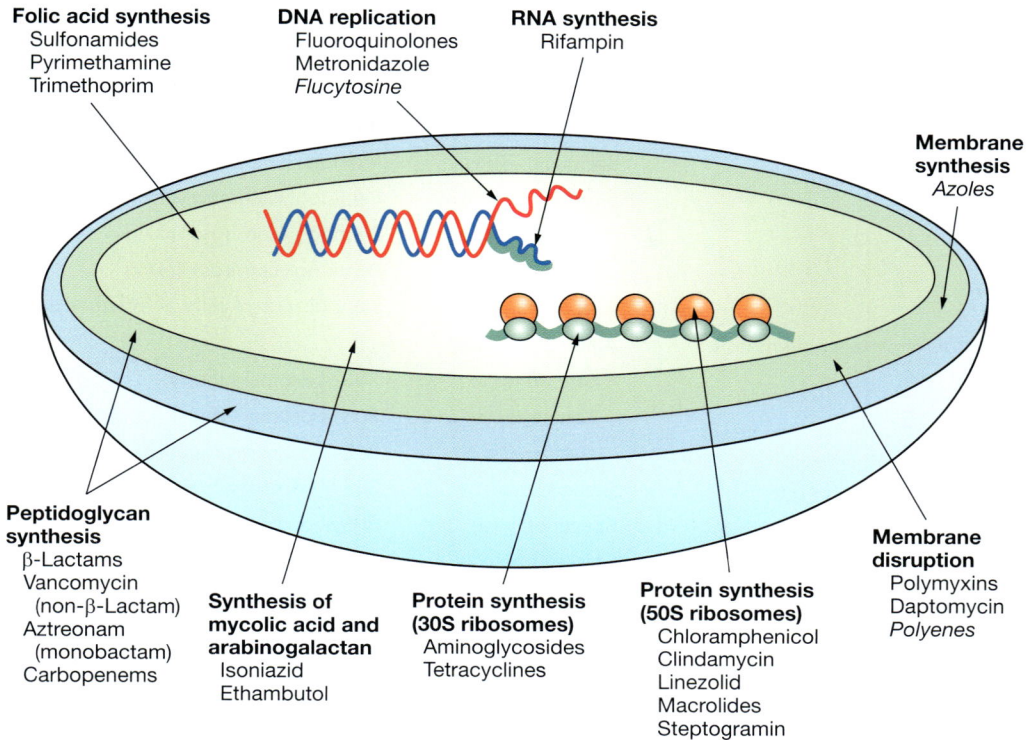

FIGURE 2.11. Sites of antibiotic activity in a typical bacterial cell with some common examples provided. Note that anti-fungal medications are listed in italics.

- **a.** Are **antimetabolites**.
- **b.** **Inhibit cell wall biosynthesis**.
- **c.** **Inhibit protein synthesis**.
- **d.** **Inhibit nucleic acid synthesis**.
- **e.** **Alter or inhibit cell membrane permeability** or **transport**.
3. Antimicrobial drugs can be either **bacteriostatic** (inhibit growth) or **bactericidal** (kill the bacterial cell).
4. Synergistic combinations of bacteriostatic drugs (eg, trimethoprim and sulfamethoxazole) are sometimes used in antimicrobial therapy.
5. **Antimicrobial activity** can be quantitated and may be modified in certain situations.
   - **a.** A **dilution** or **diffusion** test is used to determine antimicrobial activity, which is quantitated by determining the minimal inhibitory concentration (**MIC**) or minimal bactericidal concentration (**MBC**).
   - **b.** Antimicrobial activity may differ in vitro and in vivo.
   - **c.** Drug stability, pH, microbial environment, number of microorganisms present, length of incubation with drug, and metabolic activity of microorganisms can alter antimicrobial actions of certain drugs.
   - **d.** **Genetic** or **nongenetic drug resistance** may modify the antimicrobial activity of a drug for a specific bacterium.

B. Mechanisms of action (Table 2.6)
1. **Antimetabolites** are structural analogs of normal metabolites that inhibit the action of specific enzymes.
   - **a.** They include **bacteriostatic** (sulfonamide and trimethoprim) and **bactericidal** (isoniazid) drugs.
   - **b.** Some combinations of individual antimetabolites are bactericidal (eg, trimethoprim and sulfamethoxazole).

Table 2.6	Properties of Antibacterial Agents	
Mechanism of Action	**Agent**	**Site of Action**
Inhibitors of cell wall biosynthesis	Cycloserine	Peptidoglycan tetrapeptide side chain
	Bacitracin	Membrane carrier molecule
	β-Lactam penicillins	Peptidoglycan cross-linking
	Cephalosporins	Peptidoglycan cross-linking
	Carbapenems	Peptidoglycan cross-linking
	Vancomycin	Translocation of cell wall intermediates
Inhibitors of protein biosynthesis	Aminoglycosides	
	Streptomycin	30S ribosomal subunit
	Kanamycin	30S ribosomal subunit
	Gentamicin	30S ribosomal subunit
	Tetracyclines	30S ribosomal subunit
	Spectinomycin	30S ribosomal subunit
	Chloramphenicol	50S ribosomal subunit
	Erythromycin	50S ribosomal subunit
	Clindamycin	50S ribosomal subunit
	Linezolid	50S ribosomal subunit
Inhibitors of nucleic acid synthesis	Quinolones	DNA gyrase and topoisomerase IV
	Novobiocin	DNA gyrase and topoisomerase IV
	Rifampin	DNA-dependent RNA polymerase
	Metronidazole	Disrupts DNA
Inhibitors of folate metabolism	Sulfonamides	Dihydropteroate synthetase
	Dapsone	Dihydropteroate synthetase
	Trimethoprim	Dihydrofolate reductase
Inhibitor of mycolic acid synthesis	Isoniazid	Mycobacterial mycolic acid biosynthesis
Inhibitor of arabinogalactan synthesis	Ethambutol	Arabinogalactan synthesis
Alteration of cytoplasmic membrane	Polymyxins	Bacterial membrane permeability
	Colistin	Bacterial membrane permeability
	Daptomycin	Depolarization of membrane

2. **Cell wall synthesis inhibitors** are **bactericidal.**
   a. **General characteristics**
      (1) **Mechanisms of action**
         (a) β-Lactam drugs inhibit transpeptidation (cross-linking) of peptidoglycan (eg, penicillins, cephalosporins, and carbapenems).
         (b) Others inhibit the synthesis of peptidoglycan (cycloserine, bacitracin, vancomycin).
      (2) **Location of action:** These may act in the cytoplasm (cycloserine); in the membrane (bacitracin, penicillins, and cephalosporins); or in the cell wall (vancomycin).
      (3) Cell wall synthesis is required for these drugs to be effective.
   b. **Penicillins**
      (1) Are active against **gram-positive bacteria** and **gram-negative bacteria**.
      (2) React with **penicillin-binding proteins**.
      (3) Have a β-lactam ring structure that is inactivated by β-lactamases (penicillinases), which are genetically coded in some bacterial DNA or some R plasmids.

  c. Cephalosporins
    (1) Are active against both gram-positive and gram-negative bacteria.
    (2) Contain a β-lactam ring structure that is inactivated by some β-lactamases.
    (3) Are frequently used to treat patients who are allergic to penicillins.
  d. Carbapenems have a β-lactam ring fused to a five-carbon ring and are resistant to β-lactamases.
3. Protein synthesis inhibitors are frequently known as ***broad-spectrum antibiotics*** and require bacterial growth to be effective.
  a. Aminoglycosides include streptomycin, neomycin, kanamycin, and gentamicin.
    (1) These drugs are **bactericidal** for gram-negative bacteria and **bind to the 30S ribosomal subunit**, irreversibly blocking initiation of translation, or cause mRNA misreading (or both). They are not active against anaerobes or intracellular bacteria.
    (2) The effective concentration range is narrow before toxicity occurs.
    (3) Acetylation may modify their action; they also can be **rendered inactive** by **enzymes contained in R plasmids**.
  b. Tetracyclines include doxycycline, tetracycline, and minocycline.
    (1) These drugs are **bacteriostatic**, **bind to the 30S ribosomal subunit**, and prevent binding of aminoacyl tRNA to the acceptor site. They are transported out of or bound to a plasmid-derived protein in cells containing specific tetracycline R plasmids.
  c. Chloramphenicol
    (1) This drug is **bacteriostatic** for gram-positive and gram-negative bacteria, rickettsia, and chlamydia; it **binds to the 50S ribosomal subunit** and inhibits peptide bond formation.
    (2) The enzyme chloramphenicol acetyltransferase, which is carried on an R plasmid, inactivates chloramphenicol.
  d. Macrolides and **lincomycins** include erythromycin (macrolide) and lincomycin and clindamycin (lincomycins).
    (1) These drugs are **bacteriostatic** and **bind to the 23S RNA in the 50S ribosomal subunit**, blocking translocation.
    (2) In bacteria that have a mutation in a 50S ribosomal protein or that contain an R plasmid with genetic information, methylation of 23S RNA occurs, rendering these drugs ineffective by preventing the drug from binding.
4. Nucleic acid synthesis inhibitors
  a. These drugs inhibit DNA (quinolones, derivatives of nalidixic acid) or RNA (rifampin) synthesis. They are generally **bactericidal** and are quite toxic to mammalian cells.
  b. Actinomycin and mitomycin bind to strands of DNA or inhibit replication enzymes. Nalidixic acid inhibits DNA gyrase activity. Rifampin inhibits DNA-dependent RNA polymerase.
5. Mycolic acid synthesis inhibitor (**isoniazid**) is a **bactericidal** drug that inhibits mycobacterial mycolic acid biosynthesis.
6. Arabinogalactan synthesis inhibitor (**ethambutol**) is a **bacteriostatic** drug that inhibits arabinogalactan synthesis in mycobacteria.
7. Cytoplasmic membrane inhibitors
  a. These drugs are **bactericidal** and alter the permeability of the plasma membrane (polymyxin and polyenes).
  b. They are effective against gram-negative (polymyxin) and sterol-containing mycoplasma (and fungi; polyenes: nystatin and amphotericin B); used primarily as topical treatment or with severe infections.
  c. They can react with mammalian cell membranes and are therefore toxic.

C. Drug resistance (Figure 2.12)
1. Nongenetic mechanisms of drug resistance involve loss of specific target structures and may be caused by metabolic inactivity of microorganisms.
2. Genetic mechanisms of drug resistance: Common resistance mechanisms include target site mutations, drug inactivation, decreased uptake, and increased efflux. This form may result from either chromosomal or extrachromosomal resistance.
  a. Chromosomal: A chromosomal mutation may alter the structure of the receptor of the drug or the permeability of the drug.

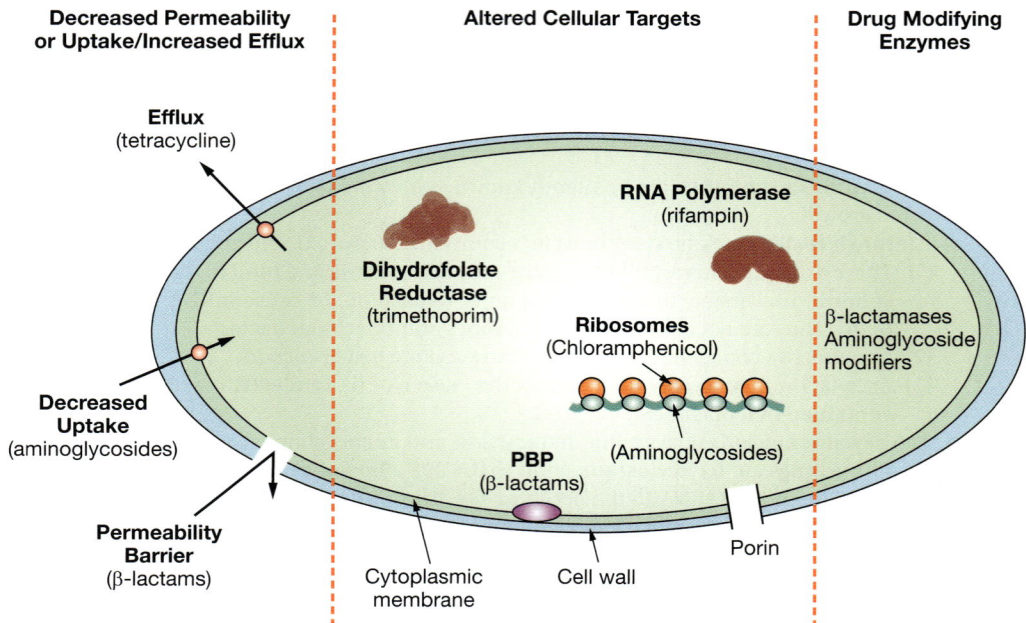

FIGURE 2.12. General mechanisms of bacterial resistance to antibacterial drugs. PBP, penicillin-binding protein.

b. Extrachromosomal

(1) A plasmid (R factor or R plasmid) that codes for enzymes may be introduced through genetic exchange; these enzymes degrade the drug (**β-lactamase**) or modify it (**acetyltransferase**). The plasmid may also code for membrane proteins that pump the drug out of the cell in an energy-dependent fashion.

(2) R factor or R plasmid

(a) Contains **insertion sequences** and **transposons**.

(b) Can acquire additional resistance genes by plasmid fusion or from transposons.

(c) Can be transmitted from species to species.

(d) Is responsible for the rapid development of multiple drug-resistant bacteria.

Directions: Each of the numbered items in this section is followed by answers. Select the *one* lettered answer that is *best* in each case.

1. Which of the following microorganisms produces a bacterial toxin with superantigen activity?

(A) *B. pertussis*
(B) *C. tetani*
(C) *E. coli*
(D) *S. aureus*
(E) *V. cholerae*

2. Thayer-Martin and Martin-Lewis media are used to isolate which of the following bacteria?

(A) *E. coli*
(B) *Mycobacteria*
(C) *Neisseria*
(D) *Salmonella*
(E) *Shigella*

3. β-Lactamases confer antibiotic resistance by which of the following methods?

(A) Altering antibiotic permeability
(B) Altering PBPs
(C) Altering 70S ribosome structure
(D) Modifying cellular RNA polymerase
(E) Modifying antibiotic structure

4. Polymers of *N*-acetylglucosamine and *N*-acetylmuramic acid are found in which of the following bacterial structures?

(A) Cell wall
(B) Glycocalyx
(C) Teichoic acid
(D) LPS

5. What is a phage that is not inactivated by proteases called?

(A) Filamentous phage
(B) Prophage
(C) Temperate phage
(D) Virulent phage

6. Which type of bacteria synthesize organic compounds from inorganic compounds?

(A) Aerobes
(B) Autotrophs
(C) Facultative anaerobes
(D) Heterotrophs
(E) Obligate anaerobes

7. Which of the following is a bacterial structure involved in adherence?

(A) Chitin
(B) Common pili
(C) LPS
(D) O-specific side chain
(E) Teichoic acid

8. Which of the following most accurately describes aminoglycoside antibiotics?

(A) Bactericidal for gram-positive bacteria
(B) Inactivated by R-factor phosphotransferases
(C) Mycolic acid synthesis inhibitors
(D) Peptidoglycan synthesis inhibitors
(E) Substances that require bacterial growth for the effect

9. *A-B subunit structure* as it relates to bacterial pathogenesis refers to the structure of which of the following?

(A) Bacterial exotoxins
(B) Gram-negative bacteria endotoxin
(C) Nucleic acid inhibitor antibiotics
(D) PBPs
(E) Resistance transfer factors

10. Which of the following display the Pasteur effect?

(A) Aerobes
(B) Autotrophs
(C) Facultative anaerobes
(D) Heterotrophs
(E) Obligate anaerobes

11. Which of the following toxins acts on synaptosomes?

(A) *C. diphtheriae* exotoxin
(B) *C. perfringens* α-toxin
(C) *C. tetani* exotoxin
(D) *E. coli* heat-labile toxin
(E) *P. aeruginosa* exotoxin

12. Which of the following most accurately describes superoxide dismutase–containing bacteria?

(A) Are frequently obligate anaerobes
(B) Grow slowly in the presence of CO_2
(C) Need superoxide to grow
(D) Produce hydrogen peroxide from hydrogen ion and the superoxide free radical (O_2^{-})

13. Which of the following processes is involved in lysogenic phage conversion?

(A) Change in bacterial phenotype due to the presence of a prophage

(B) Conversion of a prophage to a temperate phage

(C) Incorporation of a prophage into the bacterial chromosome

(D) Transformation of a virulent phage to a lysogenic phage

14. Bacteria capable of growth in a high salt concentration are best isolated in which of the following media?

(A) Complex growth media

(B) Differential growth media

(C) Minimal growth media

(D) Selective growth media

15. Which of the following best describe bacteria lacking superoxide dismutase?

(A) Aerobes

(B) Autotrophs

(C) Facultative anaerobes

(D) Heterotrophs

(E) Obligate anaerobes

16. Which of the following most accurately describes the regulation of enzyme activity in bacterial cells?

(A) Controlled by a CAP

(B) Coupled to the binding of effector molecules

(C) Involves inducer molecules

(D) Occurs via attenuation sequences

17. Which of the following best describes the bacterial plasma membrane?

(A) Contains the enzymes involved in bacterial oxidative phosphorylation

(B) Contains glycocalyx

(C) Contains matrix porins

(D) Includes endotoxin

18. Bacterial antibiotic resistance is frequently conveyed by which of the following?

(A) Intron

(B) Lytic bacteriophage

(C) R-factor plasmid

(D) Replicon

(E) Temperate bacteriophage

19. Which of the following best describes the expression of the *lac* operon?

(A) Does not involve the expression of structural genes

(B) Involves the release of allolactose from a repressor protein

(C) Must be initiated by the binding of an inducer protein

(D) Necessitates the finding of RNA polymerase followed by transcription

20. A bacteriophage containing host-cell DNA is involved in which of the following processes?

(A) Conjugation

(B) Recombination

(C) Transcription

(D) Transduction

(E) Transformation

21. The exchange of allelic forms of genes is involved in which of the following processes?

(A) Conjugation

(B) Recombination

(C) Transcription

(D) Transduction

(E) Transformation

22. Which of the following processes creates Hfr donors?

(A) Conjugation

(B) Recombination

(C) Transcription

(D) Transduction

(E) Transformation

(F) Translation

23. Toxins of enterotoxic gram-negative bacteria are transferred outside of the cell by which of the following?

(A) ATP-activated pores

(B) GTP-coupled transporters

(C) PBPs

(D) Pili

(E) Protein secretion systems

24. Which of the following best describes a mutation that rarely disrupts gene product function?

(A) Deletion

(B) Frameshift

(C) Insertion

(D) Nonsense

(E) Nucleotide substitution

25. A 21-year-old college student, who had a headache and was feeling feverish the night before, is brought this morning to the emergency department when their roommate was unable to rouse them. The student had been well until yesterday. Vital signs indicated a fever (39.8 °C/103.1 °F), tachycardia, and hypotension (BP 70/55). Remarkable on physical examination is a petechial rash (purpuric in areas) and nuchal rigidity with positive Kernig and Brudzinski signs. CSF is cloudy with high protein and low glucose. Intracellular, red diplococci are seen on Gram stain. What is the most likely causative genus?

(A) *Chlamydia*
(B) *Staphylococcus*
(C) *Streptococcus*
(D) *Mycobacterium*
(E) *Neisseria*

26. What rapid test commonly used on gram-negative rods rules out Enterobacteriaceae if positive?

(A) Catalase
(B) Chitinase
(C) Coagulase
(D) Oxidase
(E) Urease

27. A patient undergoing chemotherapy develops a cough. Acid-fast stain of the sputum shows rods and slightly longer forms, with some branching; they vary in their acid-fast reaction from one area of the slide to the next. The acid-fast stain was performed by an experienced medical technologist and, when redone, showed the same variation. A Gram stain visualized no organisms. Organism growth was aerobic. What is the most likely causative agent?

(A) *Actinomyces*
(B) *Chlamydophila*
(C) *Mycobacterium avium-intracellulare* (MAI or MAC)
(D) *Nocardia*

28. The CSF from a 2-week-old infant with meningitis shows rods with tumbling motility. These bacteria are found to be gram positive and do not form spores. What is the most likely agent?

(A) *Actinomyces*
(B) *Bacillus*
(C) *Clostridium*
(D) *Corynebacterium*
(E) *Listeria*

29. Both a 53-year-old male and his 21-year-old son present in August to their physician with fever, myalgia, and malaise, which they came down with within a few hours of each other. The son had been home in southern Minnesota for only 3 weeks to help field-train two new hunting dogs, and his father is a farmer. When asked about potential tick bites, the son had one on him, which was engorged. Platelets and granulocytes are low in each patient's blood. A Giemsa stain on a thick blood smear reveals clusters of cells resembling raspberries in granulocytes, even though nothing grows in any of the blood cultures. What genus does the causative tick-borne obligate intracellular parasite of granulocytes most likely belong to?

(A) *Anaplasma* (formerly *Ehrlichia*)
(B) *Borrelia*
(C) *Chlamydia*
(D) *Haemophilus*
(E) *Mycoplasma*

30. A full-term 6-day-old neonate is brought in with a purulent conjunctivitis that the parents noticed earlier today. On Gram stain of the purulent exudate, no bacteria are seen. Which of the following bacteria is most likely the cause of the conjunctivitis?

(A) *C. trachomatis*
(B) *E. coli*
(C) *L. monocytogenes*
(D) *N. gonorrhoeae*
(E) *S. pneumoniae*

31. An 83-year-old who lives in her own home develops pneumonia following an influenza infection. The Gram stain of her sputa is shown. What is the most likely causative agent?

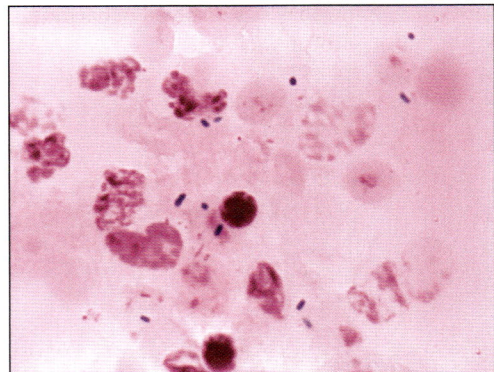

(A) *C. pneumoniae*
(B) Influenza virus
(C) *K. pneumoniae*
(D) *M. pneumoniae*
(E) *S. aureus*
(F) *S. pneumoniae*

32. What is the reagent used to distinguish staphylococci from streptococci?

(A) Hydrogen peroxide
(B) Fibronectin
(C) Fibrinogen
(D) Oxidase

33. A 14-month-old is brought to the emergency department by his parents with fever, fussiness and lethargy, and apparent headache. On examination, his neck is stiff. History reveals that the boy has not received any routine childhood vaccines. Very short gram-negative rods are seen in the CSF, so antibiotics are immediately administered. The organism grows on chocolate agar but not blood agar. No one else in the family is ill. What is the most likely causative agent?

(A) *E. coli*
(B) *H. influenzae* type b
(C) *K. pneumoniae*
(D) *N. meningitidis*
(E) *S. pneumoniae*

34. A group of organisms that are obligate intracellular pathogens transmitted by arthropod bites are most likely which of the following?

(A) Chlamydiae
(B) Enterobacteriaceae
(C) Rickettsias including *Anaplasma* and *Ehrlichia*
(D) Spirochetes including *B. burgdorferi*

Answers and Explanations

1. **The answer is D.** [Table 2.5; VIII C 2 a] *S. aureus* produces an enterotoxin and toxic shock syndrome toxin [TSST-1] with superantigen activity. *S. pyogenes* also produces toxins with this activity.

2. **The answer is C.** [Table 2.1; IV B 1] These media are variants of chocolate agar and contain antibiotics that inhibit many normal respiratory and genital bacteria but allow the growth of *Neisseria* species.

3. **The answer is E.** [IX B 2 b (3)] β-Lactamases cleave the β-lactam ring structure that is important for the antibacterial activity of penicillins, cephalosporins, monobactams, and carbapenems.

4. **The answer is A.** [I B 8 c (1) (a)] *N*-acetylglucosamine and *N*-acetylmuramic acid are polymerized to form the peptidoglycan backbone of the cell wall.

5. **The answer is B.** [VI C 3 b] A prophage is the intracellular DNA of a phage and is therefore resistant to protease degradation.

6. **The answer is B.** [II D 2] Autotrophic bacteria do not require organic compounds for growth because they synthesize them from inorganic precursors.

7. **The answer is B.** [I B 10 b (1) (a)] Common pili, adhesins, and the glycocalyx are three bacterial structures that are involved in adherence.

8. **The answer is E.** [IX B 3 a (1)] Bacteria must be actively replicating and synthesizing protein for these compounds, which bind to the 30S ribosomal subunit, to have their bactericidal effect.

9. **The answer is A.** [VIII C 2 b (1)] Many bacterial exotoxins have an A-B subunit structure in which the B subunit is involved in binding and the A subunit possesses biologic activity inside the affected cell.

10. **The answer is B.** [II F 3 c] Facultative anaerobes shift from a fermentative to a respiratory metabolism in the presence of air because the energy needs of the cell are met by consuming less glucose (Pasteur effect) under respiratory metabolism.

11. **The answer is C.** [Table 2.5] *C. tetani* exotoxin acts on synaptosomes, thereby causing hyperreflexia of skeletal muscles during tetanus infections.

12. **The answer is D.** [II C 1–6] Superoxide dismutase is found in aerobic and facultative anaerobic bacteria. It protects them from the toxic free radical ($O_2^{\cdot-}$) by combining it with a hydrogen ion to form hydrogen peroxide, which is subsequently degraded by peroxidase.

13. **The answer is A.** [VI C 3 d] *Lysogenic phage conversion* refers to a change in bacterial phenotype resulting from the presence of a lysogenic prophage of a temperate phage.

14. **The answer is D.** [II E 4] A selective growth medium that contains a high salt concentration would permit bacterial growth.

15. **The answer is E.** [II C 1–6] Superoxide dismutase, which is present in aerobes and facultative anaerobe organisms, protects them from the toxic $O_2^{\cdot-}$ radical. This enzyme is not present in obligate anaerobes.

16. **The answer is B.** [II F 3 a] The biochemical activity of an enzyme may be regulated by binding of effector molecules or by biosynthetic pathway end-product feedback inhibition. Enzyme synthesis may be controlled by inducers, attenuation sequences, or CAPs.

17. **The answer is A.** [I B 4 a (1)] The plasma membrane contains the enzymes involved in oxidative phosphorylation.

18. **The answer is C.** [VII B 2 b] R-factor (resistance) plasmids contain genes for proteins that degrade antibiotics or alter antibiotic transport, thus conferring antibiotic resistance. They also carry transfer genes, which facilitate their intercellular transfer to other genomes.

19. **The answer is C.** [VII C 3 d] The transcription of the *lac* operon is under negative control. Initiation depends on the binding of allolactose to a repressor protein. This reaction prevents the repressor from binding to the operator region, thus allowing RNA polymerase to bind and transcription to proceed.

20. **The answer is D.** [VII B 3] Bacteriophages containing portions of host-cell DNA can introduce this genetic material into new host cells via the process of transduction.

21. The answer is B. [VII B 1 a] *DNA* or *genetic recombination* is the general term used to describe the exchange of allelic forms of genes in bacteria or eukaryotic cells.

22. The answer is B. [VII B 2 a (2)] Hfr donors, which result from the integration of a fertility (F) factor into chromosomal DNA, are created by recombination.

23. The answer is E. [I B 8 i] Depending on the bacteria, one of four types of protein secretion systems of the gram-negative bacteria is responsible for transporting exotoxins to the outside of the cell.

24. The answer is E. [VII D 2 a] Nucleotide substitution and some missense mutations can be silent and not affect gene product function.

25. The answer is E. [IV B 1] Gram-negative bacteria should be described as red or pink, so the description fits a gram-negative diplococcus, which is most likely *Neisseria*. *Staph* and *Strep* would be purple, and neither *Chlamydia* nor *Mycobacterium* will show up on Gram stain.

26. The answer is D. [IV B 6 a (8) (a)] Most common gram-negative rods are oxidase positive. The major exceptions are members of Enterobacteriaceae. A catalase test (utilizing hydrogen peroxide) is most commonly used to distinguish staphylococci (+) from streptococci (−). (Most aerobes will be catalase positive and many obligate anaerobes are catalase negative.) Coagulase is used to distinguish *Staph. aureus* (+) from other medical isolates (coagulase-negative *Staph*). No medically important bacteria have chitinase. There are several medically important urease-positive bacteria, most importantly *H. pylori*, *Proteus* spp., and *U. urealyticum*.

27. The answer is D. [III B 10] Either *Nocardia* or MAI is possible from the clinical scenario, but the most likely agent from the acid-fast stain description, the focus of the question, is *Nocardia*. Also, MAI would not grow in 2 days (so some mention of time would be made) and *Actinomyces* would only grow anaerobically, which would also be stated. *Chlamydophila* would not grow except in tissue culture.

28. The answer is E. [III B 7] *Listeria* is the correct answer. Both *Bacillus* and *Clostridium* can be eliminated because they are spore-formers. *Actinomyces* and corynebacteria are both gram positive and nonmotile and are not common causative agents of neonatal meningitis. *Listeria* has a tumbling motility when grown in broth, in this case CSF.

29. The answer is A. [V B 3] Obligate intracellular bacteria transmitted through arthropods would most likely be the genera: *Rickettsia*, *Orientia*, *Anaplasma*, and *Ehrlichia*, with the latter two infecting white cells and *Anaplasma* causing the described disease (human granulocytic anaplasmosis).

30. The answer is A. [V C] Neonatal eye infections are most likely to be *C. trachomatis*, which does not show up on Gram stain. All of the remaining organisms stain well with Gram stain.

31. The answer is F. [III B 2] The most common cause of pneumonia in people over 65 years of age has generally been *S. pneumoniae*. Although the other agents also cause pneumonia, *S. pneumoniae* is the only organism that fits the descriptions of gram-positive cocci in chains. It is also quite common following influenza. If the woman had not been vaccinated for influenza, then she also may not have been vaccinated for pneumococcus.

32. The answer is A. [III B 1 and 2; Tables 3.2 and 3.3] Staphylococci are aerobic, while streptococci are aerotolerant anaerobes. Streptococci ferment even in the presence of full oxygen and lack catalase. A standard quick test is the test mixing staphylococci with hydrogen peroxide. The generation of oxygen bubbles indicates that a gram-positive coccus is *Staphylococcus* (catalase positive) rather than *Streptococcus* (catalase negative). This is called a catalase test. A coagulase test using serum to see if fibrinogen is clotted is used to distinguish the coagulase-positive staphylococci from coagulase-negative staphylococci. Oxidase is not the reagent but the reactor in the oxidase test.

33. The answer is B. [IV B 7 a] Although *H. influenzae* type b is rarely seen in vaccinated children younger than 2 years, it still occurs in unvaccinated children. The description of a chocolate agar–positive organism should suggest either *N. meningitidis* or *H. influenzae* type b. The descriptor as a short rod (from CSF) or pleomorphic rod (from culture) suggests *H. influenzae* type b. Although both *K. pneumonia* and *E. coli* (a cause of neonatal meningitis) are both gram-negative rods, neither is likely to cause meningitis in a healthy child, and, like all other Enterobacteriaceae, will grow on blood agar. *Streptococcus* is gram positive.

34. The answer is C. [V B 3] Of the choices, only the chlamydiae and rickettsias are obligate intracellular organisms. Chlamydiae are spread by direct contact or respiratory droplets, while rickettsias (the correct answer) are spread commonly by arthropod vectors. Spirochetes such as *B. burgdorferi* are not obligate intracellular pathogens and most are also not transmitted by arthropod vectors.

3

System-Based and Situational Bacterial Infections

This chapter describes major bacterial infections by organ system or situation. The majority of the information for each specific bacterium is found under the system- or situation-based disease section with which it is most closely associated, though many are mentioned in multiple systems. Four important species of bacteria are involved in so many different systems that rather than repeating the basic information for each, they are presented in the first section of this chapter under the heading "Major Recurring Species." These species are *Escherichia coli*, *Pseudomonas aeruginosa*, *Staphylococcus aureus*, and *Streptococcus pyogenes*.

Antibiotic usage has become increasingly complicated and is beyond the scope of this book. But particularly where antibiotic treatment is straightforward or there is known drug resistance or where treatment involves something in addition to antibiotics, it may be mentioned to reinforce studying of pharmacology. A summary of the major bacterial pathogens, along with distinguishing characteristics and diseases, is shown at the end of this chapter in Table 3.4.

I. MAJOR RECURRING SPECIES

Four major recurring species of bacteria are listed in this section and referred to throughout the chapter. They are *E. coli*, *P. aeruginosa*, *S. aureus*, and *S. pyogenes*.

A. *Escherichia coli*

Features

1. **Motile, lactose-fermenting** member of the **Enterobacteriaceae family** (gram-negative rod, oxidase negative, facultative anaerobe, fermenter of glucose).
2. Colonic **normal flora (NF)** (**nonpathogenic strains**) of humans and animals. May colonize the **lower urethra and vagina**. Transmitted during **birth** or via the **fecal-oral** route.

Diseases

1. *E. coli* causes **urinary tract infections (UTIs), neonatal sepsis** and **meningitis,** and **diarrheal diseases**.
2. Disease results when **NF strains enter normally sterile body sites** or **acquire virulence factors, or the host acquires a new virulent strain**.
   a. All strains have endotoxin and constitutively produce common pili that adhere to colon cells.
   b. Like other Enterobacteriaceae, *E. coli* easily receives (or donates) genetic elements from other enterobacteria.
3. **Lab ID**
   a. Grows on bile-containing differential media such as Hektoen or MacConkey.
   b. Ferments lactose and is identified by a panel of metabolic tests.
4. **Treatment:** treated (except for uncomplicated UTIs) according to drug susceptibility results.

B. *Pseudomonas aeruginosa*

Features

1. **Gram-negative rod** with polar **flagella**.
2. **Oxidase-positive** (not an Enterobacteriaceae) **aerobe** (**nonfermentative**).
3. **Pigments: fluorescein**, a fluorescent pigment, and **pyocyanin, a blue-green pigment**. Blue-green pus is a classic sign of *P. aeruginosa* cellulitis in burn patients.
4. **Ubiquitous** and widely distributed in/on **plants**, **soil**, and **water**. Rapid growth occurs even in distilled or tap water (ie, sink drains, faucet aerators, cut flowers).

Diseases

1. Pseudomonas is a frequent cause of **nosocomial infections**, with pneumonias in cystic fibrosis (CF), neutropenic, or patients on ventilation; cellulitis in burn patients; plus other infections often involving trauma (eg, nail penetrating tennis shoe to foot, eye trauma). Infections are also associated with keratitis (eye infections).
2. **Pathogenesis**
   a. The **exopolysaccharide layer (slime/capsule) inhibits phagocytic uptake** and **increases adherence** to tracheal epithelium and mucin-creating biofilms. It is **upregulated in CF biofilms**. **Pili** also aid in adherence.
   b. **Endotoxin** triggers inflammation/shock.
   c. *P. aeruginosa* exotoxin A is an **ADP-ribosyl transferase** (similar in activity to diphtheria toxin) that **inactivates EF-2** (elongation factor-2), halting protein synthesis **primarily in the liver**, resulting in liver necrosis.
   d. **Phospholipase C** damages all membranes, causing tissue necrosis; **elastase and other proteolytic enzymes** damage elastin, immunoglobulins (Igs), complement components, and collagen.
3. **Lab ID:** often iridescent sheen on colonies; fruity odor.
4. **Treatment:** drug resistance; antipseudomonal (AP) antibiotics and **susceptibility**.
   a. *Pseudomonas* has a **high inherent resistance** and also may also acquire resistance (eg, β-lactamases, decreased carbapenem entrance due to porin loss, DNA gyrase mutations (Fluoroquinolones), and aminoglycoside-inactivating enzymes). **Efflux pump** rids it of antibiotics.
   b. **AP penicillins**; **dori-, mero-, or imipenems**; **third-generation cephalosporins, tobramycin, or ciprofloxacin**; AP penicillin + tobramycin/ ciprofloxacin in serious disease.

C. *Staphylococcus aureus*

Features

1. **Catalase-positive, coagulase-positive, β-hemolytic, gram-positive coccus** found in **grapelike clusters**.
2. **Colonizes anterior nares' mucosa** (~15% of adults are carriers; shed on skin). **Increased cutaneous numbers** are found on **individuals who use needles**. Transmitted by **direct contact/ fomites** (eg, bedrails).

Diseases

1. Causes **skin/tissue/surgical infections**, **endocarditis**, infective arthritis, **osteomyelitis**, pneumonias (postinfluenza, very young patients with CF, following community-acquired methicillin-resistant *S. aureus* [MRSA] cellulitis, etc); **toxic shock syndrome (TSS)**, scalded skin syndrome, and food poisoning.
2. **Pathogenesis**
   a. **Hemolysins/cytolytic toxins** including the pore-forming exotoxin A.
   b. **Fibrinogen-binding clumping factor** allows *S. aureus* to bind to normal tissue (eg, heart), thereby facilitating damage by other toxins. This is one of many *S. aureus* MSCRAMMs (microbial surface components recognizing adhesive matrix molecules) playing roles in its ability to adhere to and cause disease in many sites.
   c. **Coagulase binds to prothrombin, triggering fibrin polymerization around** *S. aureus*, slowing clearance.
   d. Surface **protein A binds the** antibody **Fc** (fragment crystallizable) portion, **reducing opsonization** (as does the **capsule**).

  e. **Teichoic acids (lipoteichoic** and **cell wall bound)** play a role in **adherence**; when the cell wall is breaking up, lipoteichoic acids with peptidoglycan **trigger shock** via the same pathways as endotoxins.
3. **Lab ID: positive catalase and coagulase** tests; **β-hemolytic**; haloduric and ferments mannitol (**mannitol agar positive**), gold colonies.
4. **Treatment:** drug resistance is common so antibiotic susceptibility tests are often required.
  a. In the 1950s, *S. aureus* acquired a **plasmid-conferring resistance to many early antibiotics** such as tetracyclines and penicillins; these strains are known as **methicillin-sensitive S. aureus** (**MSSA**). New β-lactams (methicillin and nafcillin) were developed to treat MSSA.
  b. In the 1980s, some MSSA strains developed new cell wall synthetic enzymes (penicillin-binding proteins or PBP) made by the *mecA* **gene**, which allows these bacteria to build peptidoglycan in the presence of methicillin or nafcillin; these are the **methicillin-resistant S. aureus** (**MRSA**).
  c. Now, there are **vancomycin-intermediate S. aureus** (**VISA**) with thick cell walls that bind fairly high levels of vancomycin and **vancomycin-resistant S. aureus** (**VRSA**) with higher resistance, similar to vancomycin-resistant enterococci (VRE).

D. *Streptococcus pyogenes* (group A strep [GAS] or GABHS)

Features
1. GAS is a **β-hemolytic, gram-positive, catalase-negative, coccus in chains**.
2. Also known as *GAS* because it interacts with **Lancefield antibodies for group A cell wall carbohydrates** (the basis for the rapid antigen test).
3. **Inhibited by bacitracin** and produces L-pyrrolidone arylamidase (**PYR test positive**).
4. **Colonizes skin and upper respiratory tract mucosa.** Survives on hard surfaces; spreads by **fomites**, **respiratory droplets**, and **direct contact**.

Diseases
1. GAS causes **pharyngitis, impetigo, erysipelas, cellulitis, necrotizing fasciitis, bacteremia**, and **streptococcal toxic shock syndrome.** Some strains may cause **rheumatic heart disease** (**following untreated strep throat**) and others **poststreptococcal acute glomerulonephritis** (**post-pharyngitis or cutaneous infections**).
2. **Tissue is damaged by enzymes**, including streptolysins and streptokinase A and B, which break down clots, DNase, and hyaluronidase (the spreading factor in necrotizing fasciitis).
  a. **Streptolysin S** is a β-hemolysin.
  b. **Streptolysin O (SLO)** is an immunogenic, β-hemolysin. Antibody to SLO is a **marker** of recent mucosal infections used in the diagnosis of rheumatic heart disease (**ASO or anti-streptolysin O titer**) along with clinical symptoms.
3. **M proteins** are anchored in *S. pyogenes* cytoplasmic membranes with class I M proteins extending through the cell wall to the cell surface although class II M proteins do not.
  a. Strains causing rheumatic heart disease have exposed class I M proteins, which are responsible for cross-reactivity with human heart antigens.
  b. M-12 strains are associated with glomerulonephritis.
4. Nonimmunogenic **hyaluronic acid capsule**—inhibits phagocytic uptake until other surface components are opsonized.
5. *S. pyogenes* **erythrogenic (SPE) toxins**
  a. **SPEs** are produced only by **strains of S. pyogenes carrying a lysogenic phage**.
  b. All SPEs produce a **fine, blanching, "sandpaper" rash** on the arms and upper trunk.
  c. **SPE-A** and **SPE-C are superantigens**, nonspecifically activating large numbers of T cells, triggering proinflammatory cytokines, and ultimately producing shock and multisystem organ failure.
6. **Lab ID:** *S. pyogenes* pharyngitis: rapid antigen test and culture if negative; all other infections: culture on blood agar (BA). Isolates are β-hemolytic, catalase negative.

SYSTEM-BASED DISEASE

II. EYE INFECTIONS

While viruses are the most common cause of conjunctivitis, **bacterial conjunctivitis** tends to be more serious and is characterized by a purulent exudate, sticky eyelids, and palpebral papillae. Chlamydial (intracellular bacteria) and viral conjunctivitis are generally nonpurulent with preauricular lymphadenopathy and follicles instead of papillae. **Neonatal conjunctivitis** is acquired during birth, and onset of symptoms and microscopy suggest the etiology. The mother may be asymptomatic, but she (and her partner) also requires treatment. Etiologic diagnosis for some bacterial eye infections can be made with Gram stain, fluorescent antibody (FA) staining, antigen testing, or nucleic acid amplification testing (NAAT). **Neonatal conjunctivitis** causative agents include *Chlamydia trachomatis* **serovars D-K** and *Neisseria gonorrhoeae*. **Conjunctivitis** in adults and children can be commonly caused by *Staphylococcus* **spp.**, *Streptococcus pneumoniae*, *Haemophilus influenzae*, and less commonly by *P. aeruginosa* and *E. coli*. Symptoms are typically acute and mucopurulent with conjunctival injection and eyelid swelling (unilateral to quickly bilateral). **Adult inclusion conjunctivitis** (aka, TRIC for trachoma inclusion conjunctivitis) is caused by *C. trachomatis* serovars D-K. **Trachoma** is caused by *C. trachomatis* serovars A, B, Ba, C. **Keratitis** is most commonly caused by *P. aeruginosa* but can be caused by many other pathogens. Keratitis is characterized by eye pain and is associated with eye trauma (eg, wearing extended-wear contacts for too long, eye surgery, or contaminated eye drops) or individuals with coma who do not receive proper eye care. Finally, **styes** (hordeola) are most commonly caused by *S. aureus* or *Propionibacterium* spp. (mucocutaneous flora). External styes are inflamed swellings involving an infected eyelash follicle, usually treated with hot packs several times a day until the stye drains and resolves. Following are the primary pathogens of bacterial conjunctivitis.

A. *Chlamydia trachomatis*
   Features
   1. Small, **non–Gram-staining**, obligate intracellular pathogens.
   2. Found **only in humans; transmitted as elementary bodies** by **direct contact** (birth, sex, or genitals-to-fingers-to-own eye) or on feet of flies tracking from one eye to the next.
   Diseases
   1. Causes **disease by intracellular replication that elicits** (except in neonates) a granulomatous response; if untreated, this leads to damage that depends on body locale (eg, fallopian tube blockage may lead to infertility or ectopic pregnancy).
   2. The **three major serovar groups** each cause a different spectrum of disease; multiple serotypes of each allow reinfection.
      a. *C. trachomatis* **serovars D-K** in the United States cause **conjunctivitis** (**primarily neonatal conjunctivitis** and **adult TRIC**), genitourinary (GU) tract infection, and neonatal pneumonia. Because neonates lack a functional lymphoid system at birth, *C. trachomatis* (intracellular) conjunctivitis in neonates resembles extracellular bacterial conjunctivitis with purulence.
         (1) Neonatal conjunctivitis onset is **3 to 10 days after birth**. Clinical manifestations include **purulent exudate**, sticky eyelids, and **palpebral papillae**.
         (2) Adult inclusion conjunctivitis (**TRIC**) is usually acute and starts as mucoid. It is often unilateral and may start from a person's own genital infection or another's.
         (3) Treatment of neonatal conjunctivitis: *oral* erythromycin to prevent pneumonitis. (signs: repetitive staccato cough without wheezing; may lead to asthma) Treat mother/partner. TRIC treatment is also oral.
      b. *C. trachomatis* **serovars A, B, Ba, C** cause **trachoma**.
         (1) Trachoma initially involves all conjunctival surfaces producing an initial mucopurulent conjunctivitis. Repeated untreated infections may lead to chronic follicular

keratoconjunctivitis with pannus formation. Ultimately upper palpebral follicles enlarge, leading to distortion of the eyelid and in-turned eyelashes, causing corneal scarring and blindness.

   (2) **Trachoma** is the leading cause of infectious blindness worldwide, usually due to poverty where access to water is limited. Daily face and hand washing reduces transmission. Transmission is by hands or flies "tracking" the *Chlamydia* from eye to eye.

   c. *C. trachomatis* serovars L1, L2, and L3 cause lymphogranuloma venereum (see Sexually Transmitted Infections); not associated with eye infections.

   3. Lab ID: NAAT, which can be done on self-collected vaginal swabs or urines, has replaced cell cultures.

   4. Treatment: commonly doxycycline or a macrolide.

B. *Neisseria gonorrhoeae*
   1. Features
      a. Oxidase-positive, gram-negative diplococcus with a "paired kidney bean" morphology; **utilizes glucose** but **does not ferment maltose**.
      b. Human oculogenital **mucosal pathogen**.
   2. Diseases: hyperpurulent **conjunctivitis in neonates.**
      a. Onset **2 to 4 days after birth**. Clinical manifestations include hyperacute and **hyperpurulent** with pus reaccumulating within minutes of lavage.
      b. Eyesight is rapidly destroyed from apparent **pressure necrosis** of the corneal surfaces due to the rapid accumulation of pus under the eyelid.
      c. Prophylaxis with erythromycin or silver nitrate.
      d. Lab ID: rapidly diagnosed by Gram stain; follow-up: culture/susceptibilities.
      e. Treatment: immediate use of intravenous (IV) **ceftriaxone** *and* **lavage** to prevent loss of eyesight. Also, treat neonate for *Chlamydia* since it is more common. Treat mother/partner.

> **● ● ● Clinical Pearl**
>
> Bacterial conjunctivitis in a newborn is most commonly caused by *C. trachomatis* or *N. gonorrhoeae*; bacterial conjunctivitis in an adult is most commonly caused by *H. influenzae, S. pneumoniae*, or *S. aureus*.

C. *Staphylococcus* spp. (see I C)
Bacterial conjunctivitis in children/adults.

D. *Streptococcus pneumoniae* (aka, pneumococcus)
   1. Features
      a. Catalase-negative, gram-positive, α-hemolytic, lancet-shaped diplococcus.
      b. Oropharyngeal mucosal colonizer/opportunist.
      c. Colonizes with **protein adhesins** and **IgA protease;** reduces numbers of competing NF by production of large amounts of **hydrogen peroxide**.
      d. Thick **polysaccharide capsule** reduces the effectiveness of complement and antibodies, **decreasing phagocytic uptake; there are more than 80 different capsular polysaccharide types**.
      e. Hemolysis of red blood cells (RBCs) through **pneumolysin** and partially reduces hemoglobin seen as a green hue on blood agar plates (**α-hemolysis**).
   2. Diseases
      a. Otitis, sinusitis, **pinkeye** (aka **bacterial conjunctivitis** in children/adults); pneumonia or meningitis in unvaccinated young, old, or those with alcohol-use disorder.
      b. Lab ID
         (1) **α-Hemolytic, lysed by bile**, and **inhibited by optochin**.
         (2) (Has no cell wall carbohydrates so not typeable with Lancefield antibodies.) **Capsules are typed by the quellung reaction** (apparent capsular swelling when mixed with the matching antibody).

   c. **Treatment: penicillin resistance due to decreased binding to PBP** mandates testing.
   d. **Prevention**
      (1) A **13-valent polysaccharide-protein conjugate** vaccine (T-cell dependent) for infants.
      (2) A **23-valent polysaccharide vaccine** for patients **65 years and older** and patients who are asplenic or have diabetes, human immunodeficiency virus (HIV), chronic obstructive pulmonary disease (COPD), and so on.

E. *Haemophilus influenzae*
   1. **Features**
      a. **Gram-negative, fastidious, pleomorphic rod** (coccobacillary in cerebrospinal fluid [CSF]).
      b. Part of **NF of the upper respiratory tract**; NF strains generally do not have a capsule and are called *nontypeable*; **encapsulated virulent strains are serotyped**; all are transmitted via respiratory droplets by direct contact.
   2. **Diseases**
      a. Otitis media may be caused by any strain with or without capsule. Virulent strains with type b capsule may cause meningitis or epiglottitis in unvaccinated children, generally younger than age 5 years. *H. influenzae* type d causes exacerbations of chronic bronchitis in patients with COPD. Less common cause of **bacterial conjunctivitis** in children/adults.
      b. **Lab ID:** *H. influenzae* is **fastidious** and nonhemolytic but requires protoporphyrin and nicotinamide adenine dinucleotide (NAD) and so **does not grow on BA** but grows on (1) **chocolate agar** where RBCs are already lysed; (2) near *S. aureus* hemolysis on BA (satellite colonies); or (3) on nutrient agar with added **X** (**hematin**) and **V** (**NAD**) **factors**.
      c. **Treatment:** treated with cefotaxime or ceftriaxone (for life-threatening infections) or amoxicillin-clavulanate or oral cephalosporins for less serious infections.
      d. **Prevention**: **Hib** is a routine conjugate vaccine against type b strains of *H. influenzae*.

F. *P. aeruginosa* is more commonly associated with **trauma** (including contact lenses) or from coma (see I B) in terms of **bacterial conjunctivitis** or **keratitis** in children/adults.

G. *E. coli* is more commonly associated with **trauma** (including contact lenses) or from coma (see I A) in terms of **bacterial conjunctivitis** in children/adults.

> **• • • Clinical Pearl**
>
> Bacterial infectious conjunctivitis (pinkeye) discharge normally presents as thick and globular and yellow, white, or green; viral conjunctivitis discharge is mostly watery with a burning, sandy, or gritty feeling in one eye.

III. DENTAL DISEASE

Dental diseases include **dental plaque**, most commonly caused by **viridans group Streptococci**, and **oral abscesses and periodontal disease**, most commonly caused by **anaerobic** oral flora such as *Prevotella melaninogenica*.

A. Viridans group streptococci
   Features
   1. **α-Hemolytic streptococci** are inhibited by neither optochin nor bile soluble.
   2. Normal oral flora. The most common species are *Streptococcus salivarius*, *Streptococcus mutans*, *Streptococcus mitis*, and *Streptococcus sanguis*.
   Disease: Dental plaque
   1. *S. mutans* **(a major player)** secretes dextran and levan capsules that **adhere** the bacteria to teeth dental enamel, facilitating destruction of enamel and dissolution of underlying dentin.
   2. If not treated (removal and filling), this invasion ultimately provides access to the tooth root and bloodstream with a high risk of serious infections, including endocarditis (see section VIII on Cardiovascular Infections).

B. Anaerobes such as *Prevotella* spp.
Features
1. **Gram-negative anaerobic rod**.
2. Prominent in the gingival spaces as anaerobic oral flora. Dental abscesses are often polymicrobic.
Disease: Oral abscesses and periodontal disease
1. Also caused by **viridans group streptococci** (see III A).
2. Oxygenation of tissues is poor from poor oral hygiene. Abscesses generally require drainage to be successfully treated.

IV. EAR AND SINUS INFECTIONS

Ear infections include **otitis media** (inflammation of the **middle ear**) and **otitis externa** (inflammation of the **outer ear**). **Otitis and sinusitis** are commonly caused by **NF** or preceded by upper respiratory tract infections. Inflammation due to viral ear infection often causes blockage of sinus or eustachian tube, allowing fluid to accumulate which serves as a lush growth medium for NF whose bacterial growth creates pressure and pain. Since the bacteria do not travel through the bloodstream to reach the middle ear or sinuses, capsules are not common virulence factors. In **neonates**, bacterial otitis media is most commonly caused by *E. coli*, *S. aureus*, and *Klebsiella pneumoniae* (see VI D). In older children, bacterial otitis media is most commonly caused by *S. pneumoniae*, *H. influenzae*, and *Moraxella catarrhalis*. Pediatric pneumococcal and *Haemophilus* vaccinations have slightly reduced the incidence of acute otitis media. Otitis **externa** is most commonly caused by *S. aureus* or *P. aeruginosa*. Bacterial **sinusitis** is most commonly caused by *S. pneumoniae*, *H. influenzae*, and *M. catarrhalis*.

A. *Streptococcus pneumoniae* (see II D)
Features: Some strains are part of the NF.
Diseases: otitis media in neonates (age <6 weeks) and older children. Common cause of bacterial **sinusitis**.

B. *Haemophilus influenzae* (see II E)
Features: Nonencapsulated strains are part of normal oropharyngeal flora (vaccine is against type b strains, so NF are not affected).
Diseases: otitis media in older children. Less common cause of otitis externa. Common cause of bacterial sinusitis.

C. *Moraxella catarrhalis*
Features
1. **Gram-negative diplococcus** (microscopically indistinguishable from *Neisseria*) is found in the normal oropharyngeal flora.
2. Virulence factors include endotoxin, fimbriae, and iron-binding proteins.
Disease
1. **Otitis media** in older children. Common cause of bacterial **sinusitis**.
2. Also an opportunistic cause of pneumonia in patients with chronic lung disease.

D. *Streptococcus pyogenes* (see I D)
A less common cause of bacterial sinusitis.

E. *Staphylococcus aureus* (see I C)
NF of the oropharynx and ear canal. **Otitis media** in neonates (age <6 weeks) and common cause of **otitis externa**. Less common cause of bacterial sinusitis.

F. *Pseudomonas aeruginosa* (see I B)
NF of the ear canal. Common cause of **otitis externa**.

V. BACTERIAL PHARYNGITIS AND EPIGLOTTITIS

Pharyngitis is inflammation of the pharynx and 70% of the time, acute pharyngitis is caused by viruses. Bacterial pharyngitis is often more serious and is most commonly caused by **S. pyogenes**. Other organisms that may cause bacterial pharyngitis include *N. gonorrhoeae* (see II B), *Neisseria meningitidis* (see VII E), or *Mycoplasma pneumoniae* (see VI G). Diphtheria (also known as *membranous pharyngitis*) is caused by ***Corynebacterium diphtheriae***. Epiglottitis is a rapidly progressive cellulitis of the epiglottis and surrounding tissues that can lead to acute airway obstruction and death; it is a life-threatening emergency. **Epiglottitis** is most commonly caused by **H. influenzae type b** and less commonly by *S. aureus* (see I C) and *S. pneumoniae* (see II D).

A. *Streptococcus pyogenes*

Features: See I D: also known as *GABHS or* group A β-hemolytic streptococci.

Diseases

1. **Strep throat**
   a. **Fever, headache, and sore throat** with an **intense pharyngeal redness**/edema, creamy-yellow tonsillar exudate, cervical lymphadenopathy, and leukocytosis; with or without nausea or anorexia.
   b. May spread to sinuses or ears; in rare cases, tonsillar abscesses may occur. The extracellular agent causes disease largely through numerous virulence factors such as hemolysins.
   c. **Lab ID: Rapid strep tests** are commercially available and can be done at the bedside. If rapid tests are negative, that does not rule out GABHS because these tests are approximately 95% specific and 80% sensitive. **Throat cultures** are the gold standard.
   d. **Treatment:** condition commonly treated with penicillin. However, drug resistance testing may be required.
   e. **Serious possible complications** include acute **rheumatic fever** (see VIII F), **scarlet fever**, and **acute glomerulonephritis** (see section X on Urinary Tract Infections).

2. **Scarlet fever** (also known as scarlatina)
   a. Scarlet fever may follow a **strep throat** infection and is associated with GABHS that produces **one or more of the pyrogenic toxins** (SPE-A, -B, or -C). SPE-A and SPE-C are encoded by phages.
   b. Presents as a fine, blanching, **sandpaper rash** (largely peripheral; sometimes described as a boiled lobster appearance) that may **desquamate** and a tongue that becomes raw (**strawberry tongue**).
   c. This **systemic** infection is most commonly seen in children ages 4 to 8 years.

B. *Corynebacterium diphtheriae*

Features

1. **Gram-positive, club-shaped pleomorphic rods** often occurring in V- and L-shaped arrangements (Figure 3.1).
2. NF of the oral cavity but toxin-producing strains may cause **diphtheria**.

Disease

1. **Toxin-mediated** by **potent exotoxin** (diphtheria toxin), which damages the pharyngeal mucosa and circulates in the blood. The toxin is **only produced by strains of *C. diphtheriae*** that

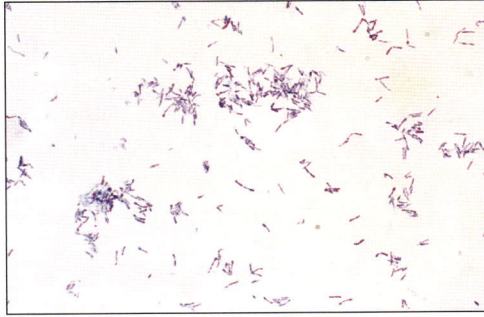

FIGURE 3.1. Photomicrograph of club-shaped, gram-positive, *Corynebacterium diphtheriae* bacilli at 1,200× magnification. (Photo courtesy of CDC Public Health Image Library [PHIL], image 1943.)

are **lysogenized by a bacteriophage carrying the *tox* gene.** Diphtheria toxin is an **ADP-ribosyl transferase** that halts eukaryotic protein synthesis by ADP-ribosylating EF-2 (host elongation factor-2).

2. **Clinical manifestations of diphtheria**
   a. Begins as **mild pharyngitis**, and the pseudomembrane may not be present initially but grows and spreads up to the **nasopharynx or down to the larynx and trachea**, resulting in a firmly adherent, **dirty gray, pseudomembrane of fibrin, dead cells, and bacteria**.
   b. **The pathogen does not disseminate** beyond the respiratory mucosa; the **toxin circulates** and causes additional signs, such as **hoarseness**, **stridor**, **myocarditis**, and, occasionally, more severe **cardiotoxicity** or **paralysis of the soft palate** and more severe **neuropathies due to the circulating diphtheria toxin's** tropism for nerves and heart. Causes **cervical adenitis** and **edema ("bull neck")**.

3. **Lab ID of *tox*-positive** strains is by culture on **Loeffler** media or **Tellurite** media (black or gray colitis) and testing for diphtheria **toxin** by the **Elek test** (agar immunodiffusion test) or **NAAT** (usually directly on the clinical isolate).

4. **Treatment:** treated with **antitoxin** and **antibiotics**.

5. **Prevention:** prevented by vaccination with an inactivated form of the diphtheria toxin (**toxoid vaccine**), **part of the DTaP (diphtheria and tetanus toxoids and pertussis) and Tdap (**tetanus, diphtheria, and pertussis**) vaccines**. All close contacts should be vaccinated.

C. *Haemophilus influenzae* **type b**

Features: See II E.

Disease: The pediatric capsular polysaccharide-protein conjugate vaccine was developed to control life-threatening acute epiglottitis and has virtually eliminated pediatric epiglottitis in vaccinated children. The vaccine is specific for type b capsule. Type a-f strains that are not type b do not often cause epiglottitis.

VI. INFECTIONS OF THE LOWER RESPIRATORY TRACT

Bacterial infections of the lower respiratory tract include **pertussis** (also known as *whooping cough*, caused by ***Bordetella pertussis***) and bacterial pneumonias.

Pneumonias may be classified by several different methods.
   a. Epidemiologic categories include **community-acquired** (defined as patient not recently in the hospital or chronic-care facility for >14 days), nosocomial (also called *health care–associated*, with ventilator pneumonias being a large concern), pneumonias in patients with compromised immunity, and aspiration pneumonias.
   b. Radiographically, categories include lobar, bronchopneumonia, interstitial pneumonia, and pneumonia with abscess or cavitation.
   c. Microbiologists and physicians may classify them as **"typical" or "atypical."** See Table 3.1.

Some pneumonias (eg, *Mycoplasma*) are caused by colonization of the upper respiratory tract, which damages the mucociliary elevator, allowing the organism to spread down the respiratory tree.

Table 3.1 General Characteristics of Bacterial Community-Acquired Pneumonia (CAP)

	Typical CAP	Atypical CAP (also known as "*Walking Pneumonia*")
Onset	**Rapid**	**Gradual** or subacute (Patients may take up to 10 d to report symptoms.)
Fever	High, with chills	Low grade
Cough	**Productive** of yellow or brown sputum	**Nonproductive, dry**, often later becomes productive
Symptom severity	Severe	Does not appear severe
Typical chest x-ray	Dense consolidation	Lack of lobar consolidation
Most common pathogens	***Streptococcus pneumoniae***	*Legionella pneumophila*
	Haemophilus influenzae	*Mycoplasma pneumoniae*
	Klebsiella pneumoniae	*Chlamydophila pneumoniae*
	Staphylococcus aureus	*Chlamydia psittaci*
Diagnosis	***Gram stain*** of sputum	Causative agents *not* visible on Gram stain of lavage fluids or induced sputum
	Growth on **blood** or **chocolate** agar	No growth on blood or chocolate agar

Others (eg, *S. pneumoniae*) depend on reduction of the cough reflex or inhalation of vomitus for the organism to make it to the alveoli. Tuberculosis (***Mycobacterium tuberculosis***), legionellosis (***Legionella pneumophila***), anthrax (***Clostridium anthracis***), some viral pneumonias, most fungal pneumonias, and **nocardial** pneumonias may be caused by organisms directly inhaled into the lungs. In addition, **C. trachomatis** (see section II on Eye Infections) is associated with **neonatal pneumonia**, acquired from an infected maternal birth canal, putting the neonate at risk for eye and pulmonary infection (atypical pneumonia characterized by a staccato cough). ***Coxiella burnetii*** (causative agent of Q fever) may also cause bacterial pneumonia. Lastly, ***P. aeruginosa*** is associated with pneumonia in individuals with compromised immunity, and also in individuals diagnosed with CF.

A. *Bordetella pertussis*

 Features

 1. **Strict aerobe**, **gram-negative coccobacillus**.
 2. **Highly infectious**, human pathogen of **ciliated respiratory epithelium**; transmitted by respiratory droplets from **infected individuals**, primarily previously vaccinated individuals whose immunity has waned. The most severe disease occurs in unvaccinated infants.

 Disease: Whooping cough (also known as **pertussis**)

 1. ***B. pertussis*** adheres to cells in the trachea and bronchi through **filamentous hemagglutinin,** cell-associated **pertussis toxin**, adherence factor protein **pertactin**, and **pili**.
 2. **Exotoxins**
    a. **Pertussis toxin**, an A-B toxin with **ADP-ribosyl transferase** activity that inhibits the negative regulator of cyclic adenosine monophosphate (cAMP), causing **an increase in cAMP** and inhibiting neutrophil functioning.
    b. **Adenylate cyclase** that enters host cells and also leads to increased cAMP levels.
    c. **Tracheal cytotoxin** (a peptidoglycan fragment) that kills ciliated respiratory cells.
 3. **Clinical symptoms of whooping cough (pertussis).**
    a. **Catarrhal stage** (lasts 1-2 weeks): mild upper respiratory tract infection with sneezing, hacking cough, low-grade fever, and runny nose.
    b. **Paroxysmal stage** (lasts 1-6 weeks): extends to the lower respiratory tract, with the characteristic **severe cough** (5-20 forced coughs per 20 seconds ending in an inspiratory whoop) producing anoxia and **vomiting**. The cough is so severe that produces eye hemorrhages and possibly the central nervous system (CNS) damage.
    c. **Convalescent stage:** less severe persistent cough.

4. **Lab ID:** Historically diagnosed by posterior nasopharyngeal cultures on **Regan-Lowe** or **Bordet-Gengou** medium. Cultures were rarely positive in vaccinated individuals or after paroxysmal cough began in unvaccinated individuals. Current diagnosis is by **NAAT** or direct fluorescent antibody (DFA) directly on nasal secretions.

5. **Prevention:** vaccination and/or antibiotic prophylaxis for exposed unvaccinated individuals.

   a. **DTaP and Tdap (D/d: diphtheria; T: tetanus; and aP/ap: acellular pertussis)** have **three pertussis components: pertussis toxoid, filamentous hemagglutinin,** and **pertactin.** These are routine pediatric immunizations with adolescent and adult boosters. It is also importantly recommended for pregnant females in the third trimester (to boost immunity transferred to their babies) or at delivery (to keep the mother from getting pertussis), as well as to grandparents, family, and caregivers having contact with infants.

B. *Streptococcus pneumoniae*

Features: See II D.

Disease: Typical community-acquired pneumonia (CAP) pneumonia

1. At highest risk are unvaccinated infants, the older adults, and persons who are immunosuppressed including those with splenic dysfunction, individuals with chronic alcohol-use disorder, and people who have had their ciliated "elevator" damaged by a viral infection, most notably influenza.

2. **Oropharyngeal colonization** is aided by **surface protein adhesins** and **IgA protease.** Large polysaccharide **capsule** (>80 serotypes) prevents or delays **phagocytosis**.

3. **Pneumococcal pneumonia** manifests with **abrupt onset, fever, chills, chest pain on inspiration, shortness of breath, and productive cough.**

4. **Lab ID:** identified by sputum Gram stain (**gram-positive, lancet-shaped diplococci**) and culture. *S. pneumoniae* is α-hemolytic on BA and is lysed by bile; its growth is inhibited by optochin. Capsular typing is by the **quellung reaction** where the binding of specific antibodies results in a refractive change.

5. **Treatment:** treated with **ampicillin, amoxicillin, or a macrolide;** however, **penicillin-resistant strains with modified PBP** are common. **Fluoroquinolones** are commonly the drug of choice for **resistant strains.**

6. **Prevention**

   a. Prevented in **infants by a polyvalent pneumococcal conjugate vaccine** producing a T-cell-dependent immunity in infants.

   b. Prevented in **adults aged over 65 years by a polyvalent capsular polysaccharide vaccine,** which is also recommended for other risk groups.

C. *Haemophilus influenzae*

Features: See II E

Disease: Typical CAP pneumonia. Capsule types a-f, but infection by type b (polyribose-ribitol phosphate; PRP) is the most common, despite the availability of a vaccine. Lab ID is by culture on chocolate agar containing hemin (X-factor) and NAD+ (V-factor).

D. *Klebsiella pneumoniae*

Features

1. **Gram-negative rod, Enterobacteriaceae** family member, **lactose fermenter** with thick **capsule** (K1 or K2).

2. Found in moist environments and in the human colon.

Disease

1. Common **ventilator-associated pneumonia** and also associated with **typical CAP,** especially for individuals with **alcohol-use disorder** (though pneumococcus is still more common) and **aspiration pneumonia**. Also causes otitis media in neonates.

2. Lobar pneumonia with a high incidence of abscesses and **thick, bloody (dark red or "currant jelly") sputum.** Because of the abscesses, fatality rates are high even if patients receive treatment.

3. **Lab ID:** gram-negative, nonmotile, lactose-fermenting, facultative, encapsulated rod.

4. Treatment: difficult because of abscesses, **drug resistance** (via extended spectrum β-lactamase [ESBL] production and carbapenem-resistant *Enterobacteriaceae* [CRE]), and because patients may be debilitated.

5. Prevention: limit respirators, keep patient upright, gloves and gowns to treat patients with CRE strains.

E. *Staphylococcus aureus*

Features: See I C.

Disease

1. Typical CAP, ventilator or **postinfluenza** pneumonias or pneumonias in individuals with **CF** (early in life) or **chronic granulomatous disease**. The older adults are at increased risk.

2. Manifests as **lobar pneumonia** with a **high rate of abscess formation, necrosis, and fatality,** especially **following influenza**.

3. Treatment: dependent on drug susceptibilities, drug resistance is common.

F. *Legionella pneumophila* and other *Legionella* species

Features

1. Gram-negative, pleomorphic rods (coccobacilli in vivo), which are **facultative intracellular pathogens of human macrophages**. They do not stain well with Gram stain in clinical specimens but stain well with silver stain.

2. Legionellae are found in **streams** as facultative intracellular parasites of amoeba; they **contaminate water systems** growing in amoeba and surviving in biofilms including hot water systems, **air-conditioning cooling towers**, grocery store produce sprayers, humidifiers, and many other standing water sources.

Disease: Legionnaires' disease (atypical CAP pneumonia)

1. Legionnaires' disease is ***not* contagious from person to person.** It causes **fibrinopurulent pneumonia** primarily in at-risk populations: individuals age 55 years or more who smoke and/or drink alcohol and/or have COPD, and patients who are immunocompromised.

2. Upon inhalation, *L. pneumophila* is endocytosed by **macrophages but survives and grows in the phagosome by inhibiting phagosome-lysosome fusion.**

3. In healthy individuals, the innate immune system (particularly tumor necrosis factor-α and **inducing iron sequestration through interferon-γ**) may limit growth of the bacteria and control infection.

4. If the immune system is unable to control intracellular replication, bacteria overgrow macrophages. Infected macrophages produce cytokines and attract blood monocytes and neutrophils into the alveolar spaces, forming microabscesses that may coalesce into **cavities**.

5. Legionnaires' disease often presents with **a triad of atypical pneumonia, major confusion,** and **diarrhea**.

6. Lab ID: Rapid immunoassay for urine antigen and NAA tests have replaced sputa stains (negative by Gram stain but positive by silver stain) or DFA stain (low sensitivity partially due to the intracellular nature). Culture on **buffered charcoal yeast extract (BCYE) agar,** which provides the required cysteine and iron, is sensitive but takes 3 to 5 days.

7. Treatment and prevention

a. Infection is commonly treated with fluoroquinolones or macrolides because *L. pneumophila* **produces β-lactamases** that inactivate cephalosporins and penicillins.

b. It can be prevented with careful maintenance of water systems, especially in hospitals.

G. *Mycoplasma pneumoniae*

Features

1. Tiny, non–Gram-staining bacterium lacking a rigid cell wall but has a triple-layered unit membrane that contains **cholesterol**; smallest free-living, self-replicating organism in nature; extracellular and pleomorphic.

2. Mucosal pathogen most frequently causes **respiratory disease in adolescents and young adults** (age <40) in outbreaks about every 4 years in crowded settings (ie, military, college dormitories).

Diseases: Bronchitis and atypical CAP ("walking pneumonia")
1. **Attaches** to upper respiratory and bronchial epithelial cells by the **P1 protein** and **releases hydrogen peroxide** and other damaging substances, triggering a largely **monocytic response** and **damaging** the respiratory epithelium (including ciliated cells)**,** producing a long-lasting, **hacking** cough. Fusion of the mycoplasma and host membrane deposits **mycoplasma antigens,** which then play a role in autoimmune-like reactions.
2. Symptoms include gradual onset of fever, throbbing headache, malaise, and severe cough (initially nonproductive). Over several weeks, interstitial or bronchopneumonic pneumonia develops; radiographic appearances vary but most commonly reveal an infiltrative pattern.
3. **Lab ID**
   a. Clinical diagnosis **confirmed by serology or NAAT.** Previously, **cold agglutinins** (IgM autoantibodies agglutinating RBCs at 4 °C) present after 1 to 2 weeks of clinical disease were used but are insensitive and not specific.
   b. **Culture** (rarely done) is **on cholesterol-containing mycoplasma medium,** taking 2 to 3 weeks and producing tiny **"fried egg" appearing colonies.**
4. **Treatment:** A macrolide, fluoroquinolone, or doxycycline over a prolonged period helps resolve manifestations. Because there is no peptidoglycan, *Mp* is *not* sensitive to β-lactams. Reinfections are common.

H. *Chlamydophila pneumoniae* (aka *Chlamydia pneumoniae*)
Features
1. **Obligate intracellular pathogen,** non–Gram-staining, pleomorphic rod with no peptidoglycan and a genus-specific lipopolysaccharide (LPS).
Disease: Atypical CAP
1. Caused by **intracellular replication** and **toxic effects of antigens.**
2. **Mild sporadic disease:** Pulmonary symptoms may include bronchitis and atypical pneumonia and possibly inflammation of vascular endothelium associated with atherosclerosis. Typical symptoms include sore throat, hoarseness, headache, and nonproductive cough.
3. **Treatment:** treated with doxycycline, erythromycin, or fluoroquinolone; resistant to all β-lactam drugs.

I. *Chlamydophila psittaci*
Features
1. **Obligate intracellular pathogen, non–Gram-staining pleomorphic rod** with **no peptidoglycan** and a genus-specific LPS.
2. **Avian pathogen** of psittacine birds (**parrots, turkeys,** and **chickens)** with outbreaks in workers in turkey production facilities (classic zoonosis).
Disease: Psittacosis (atypical pneumonia)
1. Intracellular replication and toxic effects of antigens cause psittacosis. Ranges from **subclinical to fatal pneumonia.**

J. *Coxiella burnetii*
Features
1. Small **gram-negative obligate intracellular rod** replicating in macrophage phagolysosomes; **resistant to lysosomal contents** and **drying.** Undergoes **antigenic phase variation**. Does not Gram stain.
2. Associated with domestic mammals (**sheep, cattle, goats, cats, and rabbits).** Highest numbers in products of parturition (also feces, urine, milk), which, even after drying, can be spread by **direct contact with animals** or by **contaminated soil transmitted by wind,** infecting people or animals miles away.
Disease: Q fever
1. Presents with **influenza-like symptoms with an interstitial pneumonia,** often with **hepatitis.** Chronic forms cause **cardiac problems**. Individuals who work closely with potentially infected animals are at higher risk.
2. Small infectious dose (1-10) and is a potential bioterrorism agent.

3. Lab ID: diagnosed by serology or NAAT. Is a **nationally reportable disease** in the United States. Do not culture as biosafety level 3 containment is required.

4. Treatment: acute treated with doxycycline or fluoroquinolone.

K. *Bacillus anthracis*

Features

1. **Gram-positive rod, aerobic spore former.**

2. Causes **anthrax,** a disease especially **prevalent in domestic animals** (goats, sheep, and cattle) in countries that do not vaccinate those animals. **Spores** play an important role in **transmission;** spores survive in soil or on the skin of animals for years. Humans are infected by inhalation of spores or traumatic implantation (**cutaneous anthrax**).

Disease: Pulmonary anthrax

1. **Infection starts with inhalation of spores,** which are small and light and enter alveoli, where they are engulfed by residential macrophages.

    a. In **phagocytes,** the **spores germinate** and develop into metabolically active toxin-producing vegetative cells which kill the phagocyte, **releasing the vegetative (and toxin producing) *B. anthracis* into the bloodstream.**

    b. **Vegetative cells** produce the **polypeptide capsule**, which prevents new phagocytic uptake and allows bacteria to replicate extracellularly and produce **anthrax toxin**.

        (1) The **tripartite protein exotoxin** consists of **protective antigen (PA), lethal factor (LF),** and **edema factor (EF).** PA (the B component) enhances internalization of LF and EF. **EF is a calmodulin-activated adenylate cyclase** that leads to **edema. LF is a metalloproteinase of MAPKK1 and two mitogen-activated protein kinases and interferes with signaling,** ultimately killing the cells.

2. **Clinical symptoms: abrupt onset of high fever, malaise, cough,** myalgias, **marked hemorrhagic necrosis of the lymph nodes,** massive pleural effusions, respiratory distress, and cyanosis.

3. **Lab ID:** diagnosed by microscopy of **large, "boxy" gram-positive rods** from blood; confirmed by **aerobic, nonhemolytic, nonmotile cultures on BA.** Faster methods such as **NAAT and gas chromatography to detect LF** are available from reference labs.

4. **Treatment:** Anthrax is commonly **treated with multiple drugs** including fluoroquinolones with clindamycin (to suppress toxin production) and/or rifampin but remains fatal in 50%.

5. **Prevention:** Strategies include **vaccination of domestic animals** when natural outbreaks occur; **gas sterilization of commercial wool, hair, and hides from endemic areas;** and vaccination of at-risk individuals (anthrax lab workers, farmers, animal processors, and military personnel).

L. *Mycobacterium tuberculosis*

Features

1. **Obligate aerobic bacilli** that have highly cross-linked **peptidoglycan-arabinogalactan mycolate cell walls** (~60% lipid), so are **acid-fast (AF), poorly Gram staining,** and **resistant to drying** and many chemicals. They lack endotoxin and outer membrane.

2. Human pathogens spread from person to person by dried respiratory droplet nuclei that are small enough to be directly inhaled into the lungs. Because of the resistance to drying, these nuclei persist and can also be spread by the air-handling systems of hospitals. This risk is reduced by placing all suspected patients with tuberculosis (TB) in separately exhausted, negative-pressure rooms. Bacteria are killed by ultraviolet light and can be removed from air by high-efficiency particulate air (HEPA) filters. Patients with untreated HIV infection and TB play a major role in the spread of the organism as they develop high levels of bacteria in the lungs.

Disease: Tuberculosis

1. **Primary TB infection** starts with **inhalation** of the organism into the **alveoli,** and the outcome is dependent on the individuals' immune system status.

    a. Initially, TB is **phagocytosed and moved to regional lymph nodes**, where it replicates and **kills the phagocytes.** The organisms are engulfed by lymphocytes and monocytes attracted to the site of infection. Antigen is processed and presented and a T-cell response is triggered, but generally, the organism circulates and replicates until an effective cell-mediated and tissue hypersensitivity response occurs. If the infection is not contained, miliary (disseminated) TB results.

  b. Infection stimulates a strong **cell-mediated immune response in healthy hosts,** which kills many of the organisms or successfully walls them off in **granulomas** where they may remain viable. **Granulomas** limit the oxygen to the obligate aerobic TB organisms, slowing their growth within the granuloma. Leakage of antigens from these granulomas maintains an activated immune state.

   (1) Most (90%) individuals with a primary infection will have no immediate clinical symptoms, only a positive tuberculin skin test (TST) as a marker of their primary infection.

   (2) Immediate disease occurs in individuals who cannot mount a strong cell-mediated immune response.

 2. Reactivation (secondary) TB

  a. Occurs **most commonly in the lung apices in previously sensitized individuals with a weakened immune response** (eg, malnutrition, immunotherapy). **Failure to maintain the granulomas leads to caseous necrosis, in which the center of the granuloma is liquefied, and the lesions coalesce**. Erosion exposes the organism to oxygen and it disseminates to other parts of the lung with a resulting pneumonia. Hypersensitivity leads to the **cavitation**.

  b. **TB** is characterized by chronic **cough** (often with **blood-tinged sputum**), **night sweats, fever, anorexia, and weight loss.**

 3. Lab ID

  a. Tentatively diagnosed by **microscopic demonstration of AFB (acid-fast bacilli)** in sputum, induced sputum, or gastric washings. Sputum samples may be prescreened with auramine-rhodamine fluorochrome stain; this stain is a nonspecific interaction with the waxy wall (no antibody is involved). It **requires confirmation by an acid-fast stain (AFS).**

  b. Diagnosed by **culture** in a radiolabeled broth demonstrating the metabolism of ^{14}C-**labeled palmitic acid** with release of $^{14}CO_2$. (These specimens were formerly plated on mint green **Lowenstein-Jensen agar**.) Drug susceptibilities may also be determined. Radiometric systems generally are positive in 7 to 14 days. NAAT is also available including some to identify genes involved in drug resistance.

  c. **Evaluation for TB**

   (1) **Interferon-γ release assays use TB antigen not found in nontuberculous mycobacteria including the** Bacille Calmette-Guérin **(BCG) vaccine strain**; therefore, it is better for identifying TB in BCG vaccinated persons. It does not distinguish latent from current active infection.

   (2) **Mantoux TST** with a purified protein derivative **(PPD)** of *M. tuberculosis* demonstrates that **a primary infection has occurred** and **not current disease. TST** is considered **positive if** the **zone of induration** at 48 hours measures:

    (a) **15 mm or more** if **no known exposure**.

    (b) **10 mm or more** if the patient is from a **country with high risk or with substance use disorder**.

    (c) **5 mm or more** if recent known exposure or HIV+.
       Individuals with **known tuberculous** disease **and a negative PPD** test are **anergic** to the antigen (a poor prognostic sign). TST measures delayed-type hypersensitivity.

 4. Treatment: Susceptibility tests should be done on all cultures and drug resistance is common.

  a. **Isoniazid** is the drug of choice for prophylaxis. Treatment for infection is typically with isoniazid, rifampin, pyrazinamide, and ethambutol (unless susceptibility tests indicate drug resistance).

 5. Prevention: TB is **partially prevented by the BCG vaccine**, an attenuated live strain of *Mycobacterium bovis* (the second causative agent of human TB). BCG is not recommended for countries with low TB burden (such as the United States and Canada). Alternative TB control measures include detection and treatment of latent TB.

M. *Mycobacterium avium-intracellulare* (MAI or MAC for *M. avium* complex)

  Features

 1. Non-TB (atypical) mycobacteria are indistinguishable from *M. tuberculosis* by AFS or fluorochrome stain as they are also **AFB**.

 2. MACs are **environmental organisms** found in water, soil, birds, and other animals; in humans, are **opportunists. Not contagious** from person to person.

Disease: Atypical mycobacterial pulmonary infection
1. **MAC** causes active disease only in individuals who are **immunocompromised,** generally with **CD4$^+$ cell counts below 100/mm^3 or individuals with chronic lung disease.** It is an AIDS-defining condition with a poor prognosis.
2. MAC causes a **chronic bronchopulmonary disease** characterized by **fever, night sweats, anorexia, weight loss, and diarrhea.** (The gastrointestinal [GI] tract may be the initial site of infection.)
3. **Lab ID:** diagnosed with **cultures** from **blood or tissue** using a variety of procedures, including **radiometric techniques with probes for rapid identification of growth.** Also, **AFB** by microscopy, similar to TB.
4. **Treatment:** Treat the underlying condition (ie, HIV) **plus azithromycin**.
5. **Prevention: antibiotic prophylaxis** for individuals with HIV+, started when CD4 count less than 50 to 100 cells/mm^3.

N. *Nocardia asteroids*
Features
1. **Aerobic, filamentous gram-positive,** and **partially AF** bacteria that fragment into rods. Cell wall is somewhat waxy so also withstands drying.
2. Found in the **soil**; transmitted through **inhalation** of dust or traumatic implantation.
Disease: Nocardia pulmonary disease
1. Rare cause of pneumonia with cavitation in **individuals with compromised immunity with a high rate of metastases** to the brain.
2. **Lab ID:** often not diagnosed until autopsy, but antemortem diagnosis is made using gastric washings, lung biopsy, and brain biopsy with Gram and positive modified-AFS and culture.
3. **Treatment:** treated with sulfonamides.

O. *Pseudomonas aeruginosa* (see **I B**)
May cause **pneumonia** in **burn patients and patients with CF** and **severe neutropenia.** Difficult to eradicate due to biofilm formation.

VII. NERVOUS SYSTEM INFECTIONS

Bacterial meningitis can be rapidly fatal. Presenting symptoms in **neonates** include **temperature instability and lethargy;** symptoms in **adults are generally fever, stiff neck, severe headache,** and, particularly for meningococcal meningitis, **petechiae.** Treatment must be started quickly (within 30 minutes) without waiting for lab results; if possible, CSF for culture should be obtained before starting therapy. The initial etiologic diagnosis generally can be quickly made by **Gram stain of CSF.** NAAT is also useful, especially if antibiotic treatment was started before obtaining CSF. Bacterial meningitis can be divided into three major groups:
1. **Neonatal/infant meningitis:** caused by viruses (see Chapter 5) or bacteria: *Streptococcus agalactiae* (group B; GBS [group B streptococcus]), or more rarely *Listeria monocytogenes*, *E. coli* **K1**, or even more rarely *Treponema pallidum* or *Borrelia burgdorferi*.
2. **Acute bacterial meningitis (ABM):** caused by bacteria; may be community-acquired or nosocomial ABM. Most commonly caused by *S. pneumoniae, N. meningitidis,* or *H. influenzae* (pre-vaccine in children ages 3 months to 2 years).
3. Subacute/chronic meningitis: caused by *Mycobacteria* spp. or the fungal pathogen *Cryptococcus neoformans* (see Chapter 7).

• • • Clinical Pearl

The distinction of bacterial meningitis from viral meningitis is based on CSF findings. Bacterial: elevated white cell counts, elevated protein, and lowered glucose levels. Also, often elevated serum or CSF C-reactive protein.

Bacterial CNS infections also include **abscesses**: CNS abscesses may follow trauma, surgery, sinusitis, otitis, or gingival abscesses. These are commonly mixed infections caused by oropharyngeal flora, including the gram-negative anaerobe *P. melaninogenica* (see III B) and *Fusobacterium nucleatum.*

Other neurologic manifestations of microbes include:

1. Guillain-Barré syndrome associated with previous *Campylobacter* GI infections (see section IX on Gastrointestinal Infections).
2. Bell palsy associated with Lyme disease (see XIV B).
3. Flaccid paralysis (descending) from botulinum toxin (see IX D).
4. Rigid spasm from tetanus (see XI A).

A. *Streptococcus agalactiae* (group B streptococcus or GBS)

Features

1. **β-Hemolytic, gram-positive coccus** in chains possessing the **Lancefield group B cell wall antigens** and a **polysaccharide capsule.**
2. GBS occurs frequently in vaginal and oral flora in adult females (15%-40% of females). Colonization of the maternal genital tract predisposes newborns to respiratory infections and septicemia, which may progress to **meningitis**. Prolonged labor after the rupture of the membranes increases the transmission risk.

Disease: Neonatal meningitis

1. **GBS**'s polysaccharide **capsule** inhibits phagocytic uptake.
2. **Early-onset GBS neonatal sepsis** (birth to 7 days) leading to **respiratory distress** and a high fatality rate has been reduced by intrapartum antibiotics.
3. **Much less common late-onset neonatal sepsis** (7 days to 4 months) is characterized by **meningitis,** which **commonly leads to permanent neurologic damage** and has a fatality rate of 15% to 20%.
4. **Treatment and prevention**
   a. Meningitis is commonly treated with penicillin.
   b. Early-onset GBS infections are reduced by universal **predelivery screening** of pregnant females (35-38 weeks) and **intrapartum antibiotic** treatment to prevent infection of the neonate.

B. *Listeria monocytogenes*

Features

1. **β-Hemolytic**, **gram-positive, facultative intracellular bacillus** that has **tumbling motility in broth** at room temperature and is a **psychrophile,** even growing at refrigeration temperatures (4 °C).
2. *Listeria* is found in **vertebrate feces** contaminating unpasteurized **dairy products, deli meats, and soft cheeses made from unpasteurized milk, unheated hot dogs (and the package liquid),** and **uncooked cabbage.** Pregnant females are exposed through food: Fetus is exposed to placenta infection or exposure to feces at birth.

Disease: Neonatal meningitis or meningitis in persons with compromised immunity

1. *Listeria* invades mononuclear phagocytes and epithelial cells. Inside the phagosome, *Listeria* produces **listeriolysin O,** which facilitates the rapid **egress into the cytoplasm before phagosome-lysosome fusion,** allowing protected **cytoplasmic replication.** *Listeria* is then able to "hijack" the host cell actin system to propel itself directly into adjoining cells," avoiding the extracellular environment.
2. In healthy individuals, ingestion of *Listeria* causes **transient diarrhea** with subsequent fecal carriage.
3. In **pregnant females,** *Listeria* causes **GI disease with septicemia (flu-like symptoms) and the possibility of neonatal infection** by:
   a. **Crossing the placenta,** leads to severe disease in the neonate with abscesses and granulomas throughout the body.
   b. **Fecal contamination at birth** may cause septicemia and late-onset neonatal meningitis.
4. In **patients with compromised immunity,** particularly in transplant patients, *Listeria* can cause **septicemia and meningitis.**
5. **Lab ID**
   a. **Often missed in Gram stain of CSF** because of low numbers and intracellular residence. Diagnosed by growth on BA where it is **weakly β-hemolytic** with hemolysis enhanced by growth near *S. aureus* hemolysis **(positive CAMP [Christie, Atkins, and Munch-Petersen] test).**
   b. Shows characteristic **"tumbling motility"** in 25 °C broth cultures.

   6. Prevention: prevented through limiting exposure and pasteurization. Pregnant females and patients who are immunocompromised should avoid soft cheese and raw cabbage, and heat all processed meats before eating.

C. *E. coli* (see I A). **Neonatal meningitis** is caused by birth exposure to **encapsulated (primarily K1) strains of *E. coli*.** It is treated based on susceptibility testing.

D. *Streptococcus pneumoniae* (see II D)

In addition to **pneumococcal meningitis**, pneumococcus also causes **septicemia and meningitis in the very young.** It is the **dominant cause of bacterial meningitis in adults.** It is not considered highly contagious as it must colonize the oropharyngeal mucosa, invade the bloodstream, and cross the blood-brain-barrier. Vaccination reduces the risk of infection by vaccine strains.

E. *Neisseria meningitidis*

Features

1. **Gram-negative, oxidase-positive, kidney-shaped diplococcus** with a **polysaccharide capsule** and the ability to **use both glucose and maltose. See Figure 3.2 for Gram stain.**
2. Human pathogen colonizing upper respiratory membranes. About 10% of healthy people are carriers who have sufficient immunity to block disease but still have mucosal colonization.

Disease: Meningococcal meningitis

1. Meningococcal meningitis is **most prevalent in children ages 6 months to 2 years,** with a **second peak in young adults**, especially those housed together (college students in residence halls or military recruits).
2. Organisms have more than 12 capsular serogroups; most **U.S. infections are caused by the B, C, W-135, and Y serogroups,** the B capsule being notoriously nonimmunogenic. **Serotype A** strains cause epidemics in **Africa and China.**
3. Bacteria bind to nonciliated mucosal cells via **pili** and reach the submucosa by **passing through mucosal cells**. The **capsule, IgA protease,** and **serum resistance allow this extracellular pathogen to survive in the bloodstream.** If it reaches the **blood–brain barrier, pili** and the outer membrane endotoxins (**lipooligosaccharides [LOS]**) cause **inflammation, facilitating entry of *N. meningitidis* into the CNS**. They then cause tissue necrosis, hemorrhage, circulatory collapse, intravascular coagulation, and shock.
4. *N. meningitidis* disease begins as **mild pharyngitis** with occasional slight fever but, in the immunologically naive, organisms disseminate to most tissues (especially the skin, meninges, joints, eyes, and lungs), resulting in a **fulminant meningococcemia, pneumonia,** and **meningitis** that can be fatal in 1 to 5 days.
5. Characterized by **fever, vomiting, headache, and stiff neck.** Pneumonia may be present. A **petechial eruption** develops that progresses from erythematous macules to frank purpura. **Vasculitic purpura** is the hallmark. **Waterhouse-Friderichsen syndrome** is a fulminating meningococcemia with hemorrhage, circulatory failure, and adrenal insufficiency. May result in

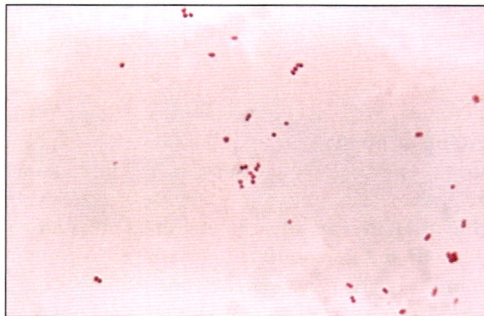

FIGURE 3.2. Photomicrograph of aerobic, gram-negative, *Neisseria meningitidis* diplococcal bacteria at 1,200× magnification. (Photo courtesy of CDC Public Health Image Library [PHIL], image 6423.)

eighth-nerve deafness, CNS damage (learning disabilities and seizures), and severe skin necrosis that may require skin grafting or amputation.

6. **Lab ID: Gram-negative diplococci** on Gram stain CSF. Culture of CSF and blood on **chocolate agar** or **Thayer-Martin agar**; antibiotic susceptibility testing is often needed.

7. **Treatment:** Meningococcal meningitis requires **rapid diagnosis, treatment,** and **prompt hospitalization.** Treated with IV ceftriaxone.

8. **Prevention: Meningococcal conjugate vaccine** includes capsules from serotypes Y, W-135, C, and A, each conjugated to protein. Recombinant protein vaccines for serogroup B are available. Approximately 50% of U.S. cases are serogroup B, whose capsule is poorly immunogenic. Routine use is recommended for high-risk children ages 2 to 10 years; all children ages 11 to 12 years; and military recruits or college students if not previously vaccinated.

F. *Haemophilus influenzae* **type** b (see II E)

Before *H. influenzae* type b vaccines, an estimated 30,000 cases per year of invasive *H. influenzae* disease occurred in infants and toddlers, including meningitis, osteomyelitis, and epiglottitis. Vaccination has almost eliminated epiglottitis. **Meningitis** occurs primarily in **unvaccinated children ages 3 months to 2 years**. Strains that cause childhood meningitis have the **type b polyribitol capsule.** (Strains without capsules are called *nontypeable*; they are part of our normal oropharyngeal flora and do not cause disease.) Meningitis is **rapidly progressive with permanent** CNS deficits (hydrocephalus, mental retardation, paresis, and speech and hearing problems) in a third of the cases.

VIII. CARDIOVASCULAR INFECTIONS

Infectious endocarditis is inflammation of the **heart endothelium** (endocardium), often involving the valves; it is a direct infection of the endocardium (classified as acute or subacute) or, in the case of rheumatic heart disease, an immune reaction to streptococcal pharyngitis. Infectious sources of endocarditis are most commonly from bacteria in the bloodsteam from brushing teeth, untreated cavities, periodontal disease, passing a hard stool, parturition, surgery, prostate exams, IV lines, IV drug use, and other related activities.

Clinical symptoms of **acute endocarditis** include high fever of unknown origin, **new** or increasing **heart murmurs**, and **fatigue.** Acute infections may occur in the healthy or predamaged heart and are most commonly caused by *S. aureus.*

Clinical symptoms of **subacute endocarditis** include slow onset **low-grade fever, with weight loss, night sweats, increasing heart sounds**, and **increasing fatigue,** commonly in someone who already has a **damaged heart.** The infectious agents are more likely to be **opportunists with less virulence,** such as **viridans streptococci,** *Streptococcus bovis* **group,** *Enterococcus* **spp., and HACEK organisms,** and require help to access the bloodstream (like a root canal).

All endocarditis agents bind to fibronectin. Fibronectin is found on prosthetic devices, on nonbacterial thrombolytic vegetations, and on the subendothelial matrix exposed by damage to the endothelium but not on the normal cardiac endothelial surface. *S. aureus* **also binds fibrinogen,** which is one of the reasons (along with invasiveness and damaging enzymes) that it can attack a healthy heart as well as a damaged heart tissue. Endocarditis may result in **vegetations,** three-dimensional bacterial growths made up of extracellular bacterial products, platelets, fibrin mesh, but few immune cells.

Endocarditis in individuals with **prosthetic** valves is often caused by *Staphylococcus epidermidis*, *S. aureus*, the fungus *Candida* spp., or gram-negative enteric bacilli. Endocarditis in individuals who utilize **IV drugs** (often from contaminated needles) is most commonly caused by *S. aureus*, and less commonly by *P. aeruginosa*, or the fungus *Candida albicans*. These infections are often **polymicrobial**.

Myocarditis is caused primarily by coxsackie viruses but can rarely be caused by disseminated *B. burgdorferi* (see XIV B), *Chlamydia* spp., or *Legionella* spp. **Pericarditis** is caused primarily by enteroviruses, but rare cases of **purulent pericarditis** (aka acute bacterial pericarditis) may be caused by *S. aureus*, *S. pneumoniae*, or other streptococci.

A. Staphylococcus aureus (see I C)

Common cause of **acute endocarditis** and endocarditis in individuals who use **IV drugs**.
Fibrinogen binding aids in binding to normal heart. However, *S. aureus* also binds to fibronectin. **Bacterial coagulase** allows **formation of fibrin clots,** which reduces access of phagocytic cells to clear *S. aureus*. *S. aureus* **cytolytic toxins** such as the pore-forming **α-toxin rapidly damage heart cells.**

B. Viridans streptococci (see III A)

1. These organisms cause **subacute** endocarditis in individuals with **damaged hearts** who either have **poor oral hygiene or have had recent dental work without prophylactic antibiotics**.
2. Viridans streptococci are not invasive, but they can bind fibronectin, a characteristic of all bacteria causing infective endocarditis.
3. Note that the **S. bovis group** are organisms formally classified as viridans group streptococci and have very similar characteristics in terms of endocarditis infections.

C. *Enterococcus faecalis, Enterococcus faecium,* and other *Enterococcus* spp.

1. Enterococci are part of the normal GI flora and are a leading cause of nosocomial infections, including **subacute endocarditis**.
2. They enter the bloodstream via microscopic bowel defects created by **cytotoxic anticancer agents or via medical manipulation of the GU or GI tract.**
3. Endocarditis is commonly seen in older males with already damaged heart tissue who have recently undergone prostate exams; mortality rates are quite high.
4. **Antibiotic resistance** is common.

D. *HACEK group*

Features

1. This is a group of **fastidious, gram-negative bacilli**:
   Haemophilus spp. (*H. parainfluenzae, H. aphrophilus, H. paraphrophilus*).
   Aggregatibacter (*Actinobacillus*) *actinomycetemcomitans*.
   Cardiobacterium hominis.
   Eikenella corrodens.
   Kingella kingae.
2. These organisms normally colonize the oral cavity (NF) and have few virulence factors. All are slow-growing in vitro so require days for isolation in the lab if needed.

Disease: Rare cause of subacute endocarditis

E. *Staphylococcus epidermidis*

Features

1. **Coagulase-negative** and **nonhemolytic staphylococci** (Gram-positive catalase positive cocci).
2. **Normal skin commensal** with little virulence but may cause infection in individuals with medical devices (eg, **artificial heart valves** or **knees, pacemakers, IV lines**). The hydrophobicity of both *S. epidermidis* and device polymers facilitates their binding; the polysaccharide slime (also known as glycocalyx or extracellular matrix) made by *S. epidermidis* serves as a "glue," **creating biofilms** that are difficult to clear without removal of the device.

Disease: Endocarditis in those with artificial heart valves

F. *Streptococcus pyogenes* (GAS) (see I D)

Disease: Rheumatic fever (acute disease)/rheumatic heart disease (chronic damaged heart)

1. **Follows untreated group A streptococcal pharyngitis** in individuals who are genetically predisposed.
2. **"Rheumatic strains" of GAS** are more likely to result in this condition. May result from anti-streptococcal antibodies (to certain epitopes of bacterial **M-protein** and **glycoprotein capsule**) **cross-reacting** with sarcolemma membrane proteins and cardiac myosin. The resulting antigen-antibody complexes initiate a damaging inflammatory process. Results in a systemic inflammatory process involving the connective tissue, heart, joints, and CNS, which may worsen with each subsequent *S. pyogenes* infection.
3. May **damage heart muscle and valves,** with **mitral stenosis** as a lesion hallmark.
4. **Lab ID**: In addition to other tests, testing for **anti-SLO** antibodies indicates a recent infection.

IX. GASTROINTESTINAL INFECTIONS

Diarrheal illness is a leading cause of death worldwide. GI infections are termed *gastroenteritis*, where common symptoms include nausea, vomiting, diarrhea, and/or abdominal pain. Diarrhea is excess fluid in the intestinal lumen that causes feces to be soft and/or runny, whereas dysentery is inflammation and/or tissue damage that results in blood and pus in feces. Lastly, enterocolitis is inflammation involving the mucosa of the small and large intestines. Bacterial GI infections can be divided into three major categories: (1) noninflammatory GI infection, usually involving a preformed toxin (called *enterotoxin*): ***S. aureus, Bacillus cereus, Clostridium perfringens, Clostridium botulinum***; (2) GI inflammatory infection which usually involves a fever: ***B. anthracis, L. monocytogenes, E. coli* ETEC (enterotoxigenic *E. coli*), EPEC (enteropathogenic *E. coli*), EAEC (enteroaggregative *E. coli*), diffusely adherent *E. coli* (DAEC), *Vibrio cholerae, Vibrio parahaemolyticus, Vibrio vulnificus***; and (3) GI invasive infection which usually involves blood and/or pus in the mucosa and systemic infection: ***Campylobacter* spp., *E. coli* EHEC (enterohemorrhagic *E. coli*), EIEC (enteroinvasive *E. coli*), *Salmonella* spp., *Shigella* spp., *Plesiomonas* spp., *Yersinia enterocolitica***. There are many other GI infections that do not fit into these categories, including antibiotic-associated colitis caused by *Clostridium difficile* (now known as ***Clostridioides difficile***), and gastritis and ulcers caused by ***Helicobacter pylori***. ***Bacteroides fragilis*** are anaerobes that are involved with GI abscesses in polymicrobial infections.

> **● ● ● Clinical Pearl**
>
> Diarrhea, which is large-volume watery stool, is usually caused by bacteria that produce enterotoxin(s) such as *E. coli* ETEC, *C. perfringens*; *Vibrio* spp., *B. cereus*; *S. aureus*; and viruses such as rotavirus, adenovirus, calicivirus, astrovirus, norovirus, and Norwalk-like virus. Diarrhea which is small volume mucoid or bloody is usually caused by invasive bacteria and is rarely viral.

A. *Staphylococcus aureus* (see I C)
1. Cause of **noninflammatory GI vomiting disease** known as ***staphylococcal food poisoning.*** Spread to food from the nares (sneezing or on hands) or from cutaneous lesions of food preparers; produces **heat-stable enterotoxins (Staph enterotoxin A or SEA) in poorly refrigerated, high-protein foods** or **cream-filled desserts** (eg, ham, custard-filled pastries, potato salad, processed meats).
2. **Staphylococcal food poisoning** results from the **ingestion of the preformed enterotoxins,** which have a CNS effect with a **rapid onset (1-6 hours)** of **nausea and GI pain.** It **resolves in less than** 24 hours without treatment.

B. *Bacillus cereus*
Features
1. **Gram-positive, spore-forming aerobe** with central spores.
2. It is found in nature, notably in rice. It germinates and produces toxins in poorly refrigerated **cooked rice (especially fried)** and also in **high-protein food** such as meat sauce and cream.
Disease: Food poisoning: watery diarrhea or vomiting (noninflammatory)
1. **Spore germination** in food process produces one of **two distinct enterotoxins:**
   a. **Type 1 disease (emetic):** emetic enterotoxin **cereulide**, which binds to the 5-HT3 receptor to induce vomiting. It is a **heat-stable** enterotoxin, associated with **high-carbohydrate** food (rice, pasta). The **emetic** illness occurs less than 6 hours after ingestion, lasts 8 to 10 hours, and is not associated with diarrhea or fever.
   b. **Type 2 disease (watery diarrhea): Heat-labile** enterotoxins HBL, NHE (non-hemolytic enterotoxin), and CytK (cytotoxin K) act to increase adenylate cyclase-cAMP in intestinal epithelial cells resulting in watery diarrhea. Associated with **high-protein** food (meat, sauces, creams). **Profuse diarrhea** occurs 10 to 14 hours after ingestion and lasts about 24 hours. There is little vomiting and no fever.

C. *Clostridium perfringens*
Features
1. **Anaerobic, gram-positive, spore-forming bacilli.**

2. Found in the **environment (soil)** and the **GI tract of humans and animals.**
3. Grows with a characteristic **double zone of hemolysis** on **anaerobic** BA.

Disease: Noninflammatory GI infection

1. Most implicated food products are **meats and gravy dishes, sometimes vegetables**. Following ingestion of the organism, alkaline conditions in the small intestine stimulate toxin formation. **Heat-labile enterotoxin (CPE or** *C. perfringens* **enterotoxin)** alters epithelial cell ion transport and membrane permeability, resulting in **watery diarrhea** when excess ions and water enter lumen. Diarrhea and abdominal cramps occur 8 to 24 hours after ingestion.
2. Food products contaminated with **large numbers of organisms** are needed to cause disease (10^8). Refrigeration prevents growth of organisms in meat, while reheating meat destroys the heat-labile enterotoxin.
3. **Pig-bel or enteritis necroticans**: **Rare** strains may also produce β-toxin, which causes a serious acute necrotizing process in jejunum. Symptoms include acute abdominal pain, vomiting, and bloody diarrhea and may cause ulceration of the small intestine and perforation of intestinal wall.

D. *Clostridium botulinum*

Features

1. **Gram-positive, spore-forming, anaerobic rod,** which **requires a low redox potential for growth** in food or tissue.
2. The spores are ubiquitous in **soil** and **dust;** they are highly resistant to heat and drying and can survive decades in dry environments.
3. Once in a moist, nutritious environment that is not too acidic, the spores germinate and develop into vegetative cells.

Disease: Foodborne botulism

1. The vegetative cells produce a potent **exotoxin** (**botulinum neurotoxin**), which is **absorbed from the GI tract into the bloodstream,** entering neurons at the myoneuronal junction. Through its endopeptidase activity, it cleaves proteins to **prevent the release of acetylcholine,** producing **flaccid muscle paralysis.**
2. **Food poisoning ("adult" botulism)**
   a. Adult botulism follows **ingestion of the preformed toxin** in contaminated food (improperly canned food, foil-wrapped potatoes, meat pies). Initial **symptoms include double vision, fixed pupils, dry mouth, dizziness, and constipation with bilateral descending paralysis**.
   b. **Treatment:** trivalent **antitoxin** to neutralize unabsorbed toxin in the bloodstream. Recovery may be slow, as nerve endings must regrow.
3. **Infant botulism** in 6-month to 2-year-old infants after **spore ingestion** (from **dust or honey**). Due to the **immature GI tract flora,** ingested spores germinate, and **vegetative cells** grow and **produce botulinum toxin in the GI tract**.
   a. **Botulinum toxin disseminates** (as described above) causing **a descending flaccid paralysis** resulting in constipation, **weak cry, and loss of eye/head/limb control,** producing a "floppy baby" and, potentially, diaphragm paralysis with death.
   b. If diagnosed and managed for respiratory arrest, infant botulism is rarely fatal. **Recovery** (prolonged but complete) **is accelerated by** one-time **use of recombinant human anti-botulinum toxin. Antibiotics are contraindicated.** Prevention is to **avoid honey**.
4. **Lab ID:** diagnosed by symptoms and the presence of the toxin in remaining food, stool, blood, or vomitus and typical electroencephalogram (EEG) results.

E. *Bacillus anthracis* (see VI K)

GI anthrax is extremely rare. Spores are ingested and germinated, and bacteria colonize lesions on the intestinal mucosa. Bacteria produce **anthrax toxins**. Symptoms include abdominal pain, nausea, vomiting and may or may not include bloody diarrhea.

F. *Listeria monocytogenes* (see VII B)

GI infections are usually a mild, watery diarrhea that is self-limiting. In some cases, it is a more systemic infection, involving fever, headache, myalgia, and abdominal cramps, but usually no vomiting. Those individuals who are immunocompromised or older adults are at risk for a more serious infection. Major risk of maternal infection during pregnancy. As with nervous system infections, pregnant females are at increased risk of infection due to the possibility of neonatal sepsis and meningitis after amniotic fluid infection. Prevention includes avoiding possibly contaminated foods, such as milk, soft cheese, undercooked meat, and raw vegetables.

G. *E. coli* **strains that cause inflammatory gastroenteritis (watery diarrhea): ETEC, EPEC, EAEC, DAEC** (see I A; all are flora of the **GI tract of humans and animals)**

    a. The final "EC" in these stands for "*Escherichia coli*," while the initial "E" stands for "entero-." These four *E. coli* strains are noninvasive and cause watery diarrhea.

    b. ETEC: colonizes the small intestine during infection (adheres via **pili**) to cause a watery diarrhea and is a common cause of **"traveler's" diarrhea.** A high infectious dose is needed for infection. These bacteria secrete two major **toxins:**

        (1) Labile toxin (LT) is an A-B toxin acting similarly to **cholera** toxin; it **catalyzes ADP-ribosylation, increasing adenylate cyclase activity. (LT is heat labile.)**

        (2) ST toxin activates guanylate cyclase, increasing cyclic guanosine monophosphate (cGMP) and resulting in hypersecretion of fluids and electrolytes. **(ST is heat stable.)**

    c. EPEC: colonizes the small intestine during infection (adheres via **bundle-forming pili**) to cause watery diarrhea and mild inflammation, and is most common in **children.** These strains do *not* produce a toxin.

        (1) These bacteria are "**attaching-and-effacing**" in the small intestine: They adhere to epithelial cells and disrupt the microvilli (effacement) and intimately adhere to host cells via a **type III secretory system** (**T3SS**) using **Tir and Intimin** that causes **actin rearrangement** and alterations in the shape of gastric epithelial cells.

    d. EaggEC or EAEC: adheres to the mucosa of the colon via **pili** and causes a prolonged **persistent** watery diarrhea (weeks in duration), and is most common in **children** and those that are **HIV positive**. These strains are also a less common cause of traveler's diarrhea from Mexico.

        (1) EAEC adheres to the mucosa and causes **enhanced mucus** production which enable **biofilm** formation on surface. These strains then produce **three toxins** that damage intestinal cells: enteroaggregative heat-stable toxin (EAST) cytotoxin, plasmid-encoded toxin (Pet), and Shigella-like enterotoxin (ShET1).

    e. DAEC: adheres to intestinal epithelial cells to cause a watery diarrhea, most commonly in **children**. These strains bind to intestinal epithelial cells and the binding elicits a host cell response of the **microvilli extending and wrapping around bacteria**. Some, but not all, strains produce a toxin (Sat) that disrupts tight junctions leading to fluid leakage from cells.

H. *Vibrio cholerae*

Features

1. Gram-negative, comma-shaped rod aquatic organisms that are **oxidase positive** and have a single **flagellum** per cell. *V. cholerae* causes cholera; most epidemics are due to biotypes cholerae El Tor, and O139. The O biotype refers to outer membrane antigens.

2. Found in and transmitted by water or under the shells of shellfish raised in contaminated water.

Disease: Cholera

1. Cholera is a **toxin-mediated** disease with the toxin produced by strains **lysogenized** by bacteriophage CTX.

    a. Cholera toxin (**choleragen**) has an A fragment (the active/toxic portion) and a B fragment (binding to cells); it specifically attaches to epithelial cells of microvilli at the brush borders of the **small intestine.**

    b. The A component is an **ADP-ribosyl transferase triggering an increase in adenylate cyclase to overproduce cAMP, which disrupts the fluid and electrolyte balance, causing hypersecretion of chloride and bicarbonate.**

2. Following ingestion of contaminated water or food, cholera has an abrupt onset of **intense vomiting and diarrhea** as the key finding. **Copious fluid loss** (15-20 L/day) leads to clear stools with flecks of mucus ("**rice-water stools**") and to rapid metabolic acidosis and hypovolemic shock. It results in remission or death after 2 or 3 days.

3. Lab ID: diagnosed by clinical presentation, combined with a history of residence in or a recent visit to an endemic area. The organism appears in the stool and can be identified by FA staining. In some cases, stool culture on **TCBS agar** (thiosulfate-citrate-bile-salt-sucrose: selective for *Vibrio* spp. and differential for *V. cholerae* vs other *Vibrio* spp.; see IX I).

4. Treatment: prompt replacement of fluids and electrolytes; the patient should appear healthier within 1 to 3 hours. Proper therapy reduces the fatality rate from 60% to 1%.

I. *Vibrio parahaemolyticus* and *Vibrio vulnificus*

1. *V. parahaemolyticus* are also marine organisms in contaminated **shellfish** (oysters) that cause relatively mild gastroenteritis (**watery diarrhea**, nausea, vomiting, fever, and chills) that is usually self-limiting. This infection is common in Japan and becoming more common worldwide due to increased consumption of raw and undercooked shellfish. Infections by this **halophilic** (salt-loving) bacteria are by the organisms adhering to the small intestine using a **T3SS** and **enterotoxin** production. TDH (thermostable direct hemolysin) targets intestinal epithelial cells, leading to **pore-forming** and cell death.

2. *V. vulnificus* contaminates some Gulf of Mexico **oyster** beds in late summer and is a leading cause of seafood-related death in the Unites States. It causes relatively **mild gastroenteritis except in people with liver disease who develop serious septicemia.** It also causes a **serious cellulitis** in cuts from shucking contaminated oysters. These bacteria adhere to intestinal epithelial cells and disrupt tight junctions via a pore-forming **toxin** (MARTX: Multifunctional autoprocessing repeats-in-toxin). Antibiotic treatment is required in serious cases.

J. *Campylobacter jejuni*

Features

1. Gram negative, curved rod with polar flagella, often occurring in "nose-to-nose" pairs with extending polar flagella described as having the appearance of "seagull's wings" (**Figure 3.3**). It is both **oxidase and catalase positive, is microaerophilic, and grows at 42 °C.**

2. Found in a wide variety of wild and domestic animals (**puppies**) and is transmitted to humans most commonly through contamination from uncooked **poultry.** Outbreaks have been caused by **unpasteurized milk.** *Campylobacter* is the most common bacteria isolated from diarrhea in the United States.

Disease: Inflammatory and invasive diarrhea

1. *C. jejuni* **invades tissue,** causing an inflammatory diarrhea with blood *and* pus. Some strains produce a **toxin** with similar activity to Shiga toxin.

2. Infections are characterized by **fever, abdominal pain,** and **bloody diarrhea. Diarrhea is a result of prostaglandin production.** It may lead to **extraintestinal** and postinfective complications, including **reactive arthritis** and **Guillain-Barré syndrome**. (About 30% of cases of Guillain-Barré syndrome are due to these bacteria.)

3. Lab ID

a. Diagnosed by the finding of numerous thin S-shaped or comma-shaped microorganisms in the stool **along with blood and excess neutrophils** (indicating invasion with inflammation).

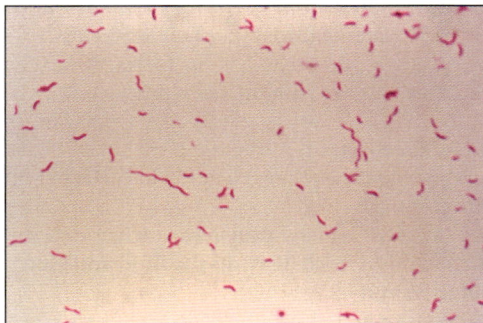

FIGURE 3.3. Photomicrograph of curved gram-negative, *Campylobacter* spp. bacilli at 1,200× magnification. (Photo courtesy of CDC Public Health Image Library [PHIL], image 6657.)

    b. Immunoassay for stool antigen.

    c. The organism is isolated on special agar (**Campy or Skirrow agar**) grown at **42 °C** (which suppresses the growth of most other GI tract flora) under **microaerophilic conditions (10% CO_2).**

4. Treatment: treated with fluid and electrolytes; the disease is generally self-limiting (lasts <1 week). In severe cases, treatment is with antibiotics.

5. Prevention: prevented by sanitation and pasteurization.

K. *E. coli* strains that cause invasive gastroenteritis (diarrhea with blood): EHEC/STEC (*Shiga-toxin producing E. coli*), and EIEC (see I A; all are flora of the **GI tract of humans and animals**).

1. EHEC (enterohemorrhagic *E. coli*) or STEC are transmitted primarily by **undercooked ground beef** and bovine fecal contamination. The dominant serotype is **O157:H7.** These strains cause **hemorrhagic colitis**: severe crampy abdominal pain, watery diarrhea followed by bloody diarrhea, with little or no fever. Children are more likely to develop the serious complication **hemolytic uremic syndrome (HUS):** The toxin also damages the kidney, and healthy children may lose kidney function within a few days.

    a. Attaches and effaces (**like EPEC** except in **the large intestine**), and secretes a **Shiga-like toxin (a cytotoxin** previously called *verotoxin*). **The toxin cleaves the intestinal cell 60S ribosome,** halting protein synthesis, **destroying the colonic mucosa,** and causing **bleeding into the intestine.** Pus is normally not present.

    b. Treatment: NO antibiotics! The Shiga-like toxin gene is a **prophage gene, but the toxin is produced only during lytic replication.** The effect of most antibiotics is to trigger lytic replication, producing more toxin (increasing risk of **HUS**) and more phage, which can infect more *E. coli* (potentially amplifying the infection).

    c. Prevention: prevented by thorough cooking of meat, pasteurizing milk and juices, and preventing bovine fecal contamination of wells.

2. EIEC (entero-invasive *E. coli*) causes **dysentery** (watery diarrhea with pus, mucus, and blood in stools; similar to *Shigella* infection) but is usually self-limiting. Often seen as sporadic outbreaks in **infants and children**. These strains invade cells of the colon, causing destruction of the intestinal mucosa and are able to spread laterally to adjacent cells. There are **no known toxins**.

L. *Salmonella* spp.

Features

1. Gram negative, motile rods; non-lactose fermenters.

2. All species from **eggs or animals as well as humans, except** *Salmonella **typhi*** and *Salmonella **paratyphi,*** which have **only human hosts.**

3. All serotypes possess **O (outer membrane) antigens used to serogroup;** may possess a **capsular (K) antigen** or the **virulence (Vi) antigen of *S. typhi*** (also a capsular antigen); they are identified further by the presence of different **flagellar (H) antigens.**

4. Important serotypes of *Salmonella enterica* include *S. typhi* and *S. paratyphi* (typhi strains)*, S. enteritidis*, *S. typhimurium*, *S. schottmuelleri*, and *S. choleraesuis* (non-typhi strains).

Disease: *Salmonella* enterocolitis (invasive gastroenteritis)

1. Mechanisms: The endotoxin causes fever, leukopenia, hemorrhage, hypotension, shock, and disseminated intravascular coagulation, and some strains may produce an exotoxin (enterotoxin). Infection is aided by antiphagocytic activity of the **capsule**, and most strains can **survive within macrophages**.

2. Enterocolitis is a **self-limiting illness** manifested by **fever, nausea, vomiting, and diarrhea** and is the most common form of salmonella infection in the United States (~2 million cases per year). Most commonly caused by non-typhi strains.

    a. Source is food contaminated by human carriers or ill individuals (particularly food handlers), exotic pets (**turtles** and snakes), or contaminated animal products (most commonly **poultry** and poultry products).

    b. Most common causes are *S. typhimurium* and *S. enteritidis,* which usually require a high infectious dose with an **8- to 48-hour incubation** period.

    c. Disease is usually characterized by **ingestion of organisms** followed by colonization of the ileum and cecum. **Penetration of epithelial cells in the mucosa and invasion, resulting in acute inflammation and ulceration with the release of prostaglandin.** Enterotoxins, resulting in activation of adenylate cyclase and increased cAMP, cause increased fluid secretion in the intestines.

3. Septicemic (extraintestinal) disease is an **acute illness,** most often of nosocomial origin, with abrupt onset and early invasion of the bloodstream.

    a. Clinical symptoms: characterized by a precipitating incident that introduces bacteria (eg, catheterization, contaminated IV fluids, abdominal or pelvic surgery), followed by a **triad of chills, fever, and hypotension.**

    b. Wide dissemination of the organisms may cause local **abscesses, osteomyelitis, and endocarditis. In patients with sickle cell disease,** *Salmonella* **osteomyelitis is a serious and recurring problem.**

    c. Septicemia is caused by *Salmonella* species as well as other Enterobacteriaceae organisms.

    d. Mortality rate is high (30%-50%) and depends on the degree of preexisting debilitation.

    e. Septicemia is **diagnosed by blood culture** because the organisms do not localize in the bowel and stool cultures are often negative.

4. Enteric fever (typhoid fever) is mainly caused by *S. typhi* with **less severe disease (paratyphoid fever)** caused by *S. paratyphi,* **both are strict human pathogens** (ie, no animal reservoirs). Most commonly caused by "typhi strains."

    a. Infection occurs through ingestion of food or water contaminated by an unknowing carrier; the organism is **highly infective even with small numbers** of bacteria (eg, 200).

    b. During the **7- to 14-day incubation** period, the organisms **multiply in the small intestine** and then **enter the intestinal lymphatics.**

    c. Dissemination into the bloodstream (and ultimately to **multiple organs**) causes malaise, headache, and gradual onset of a fever that increases during the day, reaching a plateau of 102 to 105 °F (38.8-40.6 °C) each day. **Blood cultures are positive in this first symptomatic phase** but not earlier.

    d. Multiplies in the reticuloendothelial system and lymphoid tissue of the bowel, producing **hyperplasia and necrosis of the lymphoid Peyer patches**.

    e. A characteristic **rash ("rose spots")** may appear on the trunk in the **second to third weeks**.

    f. Typically, the **disease lasts 3 to 5 weeks**; the **major complications are GI hemorrhage and bowel perforation with peritonitis**.

    g. After recovery, **3% of patients become carriers;** the organism is retained in the **gallbladder** and **biliary passages,** and cholecystectomy may be necessary.

    h. Lab ID: Salmonella are commonly first isolated in blood or bone marrow, or after 1 to 2 weeks from stool. The specimens are plated onto differential media, selective media, or both. These bacteria are non-lactose fermenters on MacConkey media and **H_2S^+**.

M. *Shigella* spp.

Features

1. Gram-negative, facultative anaerobic, nonmotile rods highly resistant to acid (including stomach acids); therefore, it takes only 100 to 200 shigellae (*Shigella flexneri, Shigella sonnei*) to successfully infect.

2. Humans are the only reservoirs (no known animals); organism is not found in soil or water unless contaminated with human fecal material.

3. Shigellae are spread by the **fecal-oral route** through poor sanitation and are readily transmitted from person to person by unrecognized clinical cases and convalescing or healthy carriers via food, fingers, feces, flies, and oral-anal sex.

4. Classification: classified into four O antigenic groups:

    a. *S. sonnei* causes mild disease; the most common cause of shigellosis in the United States.

    b. *S. flexneri* causes more severe disease; common in the United States.

    c. *Shigella boydii* causes more severe disease; rarely found in the United States.

    d. *Shigella dysenteriae* causes the most severe disease; rarely found in the United States, unless imported.

Disease: Shigellosis (inflammatory diarrhea or bacillary dysentery)

1. **All strains are invasive in the large intestine and terminal ileum.** Shigellae **traverse the M cells invading from the basal side** of the epithelial cells. In the epithelial cells, they **rearrange cellular actin to "jet propel" themselves into adjoining cells,** producing shallow ulcerations and inflammation with large numbers of (Polymorphonuclear leukocytes; "excess leukocytes"). Bloodstream invasion is rare because of shallow ulceration.
2. *S. dysenteriae* **type 1 secretes** a potent, heat-labile protein exotoxin (**Shiga toxin**), the A subunit of which **nicks the 60S eukaryotic ribosomal subunit,** causing **diarrhea** but also acting as a **neurotoxin.** Like the similar Shiga-like toxin of EHEC strains of *E. coli*, *S. dysenteriae* type 1 strains also cause HUS; however, because the Shiga-toxin gene is chromosomal, antibiotic treatment does not increase the risk of HUS.
3. **Clinical symptoms:** characterized by the sudden onset of **abdominal pain and cramps** (may be severe), **diarrhea,** and **fever** after a short incubation period (1-4 days). **Stools are liquid and scant;** after the first few bowel movements, they contain **mucus, pus, and occasionally blood.**
4. **Lab ID:** diagnosed from stool culture on differential and selective media. Rapid diagnosis can be made using NAAT. These bacteria are non-lactose fermenters on MacConkey media and **H_2S^- and nonmotile.**
5. **Treatment:** generally treated with electrolyte and fluid replacement. Only *S. dysenteriae* infections require antibiotic therapy.
6. Related to *Shigella* spp., ***Plesiomonas shigelloides*** are a rare bacterial cause of diarrhea. These bacteria are gram-negative bacilli of the Enterobacteriaceae family that are found in freshwater, freshwater fish, shellfish, and the GI tract of animals. *Plesiomonas* spp. can cause **septicemia in individuals who are immunocompromised**. These bacteria are oxidase positive, whereas *Shigella* spp. are oxidase negative.

N. *Yersinia enterocolitica*

Features

1. Aerobic **gram-negative bacilli** that are **oxidase negative** with temperature-variable motility: **motile at 25 °C and nonmotile at 37 °C.**
2. Habitat or reservoir includes domestic (especially **puppies**) and **farm animals**.
3. Transmission is via the fecal-oral route and infections are often via contaminated food (**pork**), water, and **unpasteurized milk**. Mostly infections are during **winter** months, unlike most other gastroenteritis infections.
4. These bacteria are able to survive at **cold temperatures** (including 4 °C), so refrigeration has no effect on bacterial survival.

Diseases

1. **Enterocolitis in young children:** Clinical manifestations include fever, headaches, abdominal pain, and bloody diarrhea.
2. **Appendix-like syndrome** in older children and adults. Clinical manifestations include severe right-sided abdominal pain, fever, and enlarged mesenteric lymph nodes.
3. Upon ingestion, the bacteria invade the mucosa of the terminal ileum and produce a **heat-stable enterotoxin**.
4. **Lab ID:** diagnosed from stool culture on SSDC (sodium deoxycholate and calcium chloride) or **CIN** (cefsulodin-irgasan-novobiocin) agar at 30 °C (**room temperature**). Are urease positive. Rapid diagnosis can be made using NAAT.
5. **Treatment:** Antibiotic treatment is often indicated for infants with septicemia, if disease is severe, or for appendicitis-like symptoms.

O. *Clostridioides difficile* (formerly known as *Clostridium difficile*)

Features

1. *C. difficile* **is a gram-positive, spore-forming, anaerobic rod.**
2. Colonizes 2% to 3% of healthy individuals and 5% to 15% of people who have recently had antibiotics but do not have diarrhea. Hospital environments and personnel may become contaminated with spores.
3. Many strains are **resistant to antibiotics** relative to other members of the gut flora. Antibiotic treatment kills organisms that normally restrict growth of *C. difficile*, resulting in overgrowth.

Disease: Diarrhea developing into pseudomembranous colitis (also called *antibiotic-associated diarrhea*)
1. *C. difficile* produces two toxins: An **enterotoxin (toxin A) that causes fluid accumulation and damages the mucosa of the large bowel** and a **cytotoxin (toxin B) that causes cytoskeletal changes and then kills mucosal cells.**
2. Manifests **first** as **diarrhea** and then develops into **pseudomembranous colitis**, also known as *antibiotic-associated colitis* because it follows antibiotic therapy to treat other bacterial infections.
3. **Treatment:** treated with oral rehydration and metronidazole; discontinue other antibiotics if possible; enteric isolation; avoid antimotility drugs.

P. *Helicobacter pylori*
Features
1. **Microaerophilic, gram-negative, urease-positive, spiral-shaped bacterium with multiple polar flagella** at a single pole.
2. Higher rates of infection in developing countries. Organisms persist in the **stomach**, so the rate of colonization increases with age up to middle age. Transmission is fecal or oral or by vomitus.
3. Associated with **gastritis, gastric and duodenal ulcers, mucosa-associated lymphoid tissue (MALT) lymphoma, non-Hodgkin lymphoma of the stomach, and gastric adenocarcinoma.**
Disease: Gastritis and ulcers
1. **Colonization and pathogenesis** (Note: Not all strains of *H. pylori* produce high levels of CagA [cytotoxin-associated gene A] protein or VacA [vacuolating cytotoxin A] cytotoxin):
   a. Produces **urease,** converting urea to ammonia, to facilitate survival during migration to the gastric epithelium and allowing for survival and replication in the highly acidic environment of the stomach.
   b. Penetrates the mucin with the aid of its **mucinase, spiral shape,** and polar **flagellae.**
   c. **Adhesins bind to fucose-containing receptors on gastric mucosa** (Lewis blood group antigens).
   d. Strains with the *CagA* **pathogenicity island** (a section of DNA coding for the CagA protein and a type VI injection-like secretion system) **inject CagA into epithelial cells** where it ultimately causes **cytoskeletal rearrangement.** Other proteins trigger interleukin 8 (IL-8) production, which also plays a role in the inflammatory response. High CagA producers have a higher association with inflammation and *the subsequent carcinomas.*
   e. Some produce the multifunctional **VacA, a vacuolating cytotoxin** triggering apoptosis. It has a high association with peptic ulcer disease.
2. **Clinical symptoms**
   a. **Acute infection** is characterized by epigastric pain, sometimes with nausea, vomiting, anorexia, and belching.
   b. **Chronic superficial gastritis** is caused by hypochlorhydria, which leads to persistent colonization. The immune system appears not to routinely eliminate *H. pylori.*
   c. **Peptic ulcers** are characterized by burning epigastric pain lessened by eating; they are diagnosed by invasive and noninvasive methods.
3. **Lab ID**
   a. Invasive tests on biopsy include:
      (1) **Urease test on biopsy.**
      (2) Histology (silver stain is most sensitive).
      (3) Antigen detection.
      (4) Culture at 37 °C is rarely done.
   b. Noninvasive tests include:
      (1) **Urea breath test** in which radioactive carbon-labeled urea is swallowed and urease activity is detected by the radioactive-CO_2 in the breath. A non-radioactive version is available for children and other at-risk populations.
      (2) Demonstration of **serum antibodies.**
      (3) **HpSA (helicobacter pylori stool antigen): stool antigen test.**
4. **Treatment**: treated most commonly with the combination of a proton-pump inhibitor along with amoxicillin and clarithromycin, but resistance is increasing. Success of treatment is assessed with a fecal antigen test.

Q. *Bacteroides fragilis*
Features
1. **Gram-negative, anaerobic rods** that produce some superoxide dismutase and catalase, making them somewhat resistant to short exposure to oxygen.
2. Is found in the human GI tract and female genital tract, grows rapidly under anaerobic conditions, and is stimulated by bile. It accounts for 1% of gut anaerobes along with other *Bacteroides* species.
3. It is usually involved in **polymicrobic infections** that involve more than one genus or species; consequently, therapy with several antibiotics may be necessary.

Disease: Abdominal abscesses
1. **Capsule** inhibits phagocytosis; collagenase and hyaluronidase aid its spread, but its endotoxin lacks potency, and it has no exotoxins.
2. **Abdominal abscesses** occur after damage to intestinal mucosal barriers; they are **foul smelling.**

X. URINARY TRACT INFECTIONS

Host factors that increase the risk of UTIs include obstructions, sexual intercourse, catheters, diaphragms, and voiding impairment. **Cystitis** is characterized by **painful, frequent urination; hematuria; and urgency;** it is more common in females due to the shorter urethra and proximity to the anal area. **Pyelonephritis** is infection of the kidneys commonly from an ascending UTI; it is characterized by **fever, flank pain, and tenderness and may lead to endotoxic shock.** UTIs in pregnancy, even those that are asymptomatic, can lead to pyelonephritis, often resulting in premature delivery of the fetus and so are monitored with routine prenatal care. **Prostatitis** occurs in older males.

E. coli is the most common cause of UTIs. In terms of **outpatients**, 80% of UTIs are caused by *E. coli* with minor causes including ***Staphylococcus saprophyticus, E. faecalis, Proteus mirabilis***, and other gram-negative bacilli (notably *Klebsiella* spp., *P. aeruginosa, Serratia marcescens*, and *Citrobacter* spp.). In hospital inpatients, 40% of UTIs are caused by *E. coli* with a quarter of infections caused by other gram-negative bacilli. Other causative agents include ***S. saprophyticus, E. faecalis, P. mirabilis***, and ***C. albicans.***

Acute glomerulonephritis: ***S. pyogenes* nephritogenic strains** may cause an immune complex disease **following either pharyngitis or impetigo,** even when treated.

> **• • • Clinical Pearl**
> Most (95%) of UTIs are caused by a single organism.

A. *E. coli* (see I A)
E. coli are lactose-fermenting Enterobacteriaceae (all ferment glucose, are oxidase negative, and **reduce nitrates to nitrites**). **UPEC** (uropathogenic *E. coli*) are the **most common cause of UTIs** occurring after contamination/colonization of the genital area with fecal microbiota.
Disease
1. UPEC cause cystitis through **adherence to the lower urinary tract** through mannose-sensitive **fimbriae (pili)** and inflammation from the **endotoxin.** Strains causing **pyelonephritis** have additional adhesins like **P-pili which attach to renal cell receptors.**
2. **Lab ID:** Most strains **reduce nitrate to nitrite;** therefore, urine dipstick tests for nitrites are positive as long as the urine has been in contact with the agent for a sufficient amount of time.

B. *Staphylococcus saprophyticus*
Features
1. **Coagulase-negative, catalase-positive, gram-positive staphylococcus.**
2. Causes **cystitis**, commonly in autumn in **newly sexually active adolescent females** ("honeymoon cystitis"), although *E. coli* is still more common in this population.
Disease: UTIs
1. Uncomplicated cystitis.
2. **Lab ID:** is **nitrite negative** on urine dipsticks.

C. *Proteus mirabilis*

Features

1. **Lactose-nonfermenting Enterobacteriaceae** known for characteristic **swarming motility due to peritrichous flagella.**
2. Primarily an opportunist, **transmitted via catheters**.

Disease: UTI

1. Produces a powerful **urease** that hydrolyzes urea to ammonia and CO_2, **leading to struvite kidney stones**, then to urinary tract obstruction.

D. *Enterococcus* **spp.**

Features: See VIII C. **Gram-positive coccus** of streptococcal heritage; opportunists of fecal origin.

Disease: UTI

1. Major cause of UTIs.
2. Cause endocarditis in patients with preexisting heart damage who undergo prostate surgery, cystoscopy, or urethral dilatation.
3. **Treatment:** relatively **resistant to many antibiotics**.

XI. SKIN, MUCOSAL, SOFT TISSUE, AND BONE INFECTIONS

• • • Clinical Pearl

Staphylococci and streptococci are both Gram-positive cocci and can be distinguished by the catalase test: *Staphylococcus* is catalase positive, but *Streptococcus* is catalase negative.

Many skin, mucosal, soft tissue, and bone infections involve *S. aureus* **and** *S. pyogenes* (see I C and D). **Impetigo** is an infection of the epidermis that often starts with bug bites or eczematous lesions. It is caused by *S. aureus* (characterized by **bullae**, fairly large fluid-filled vesicular lesions), *S. pyogenes* (characterized by transient vesicular lesions easily rupturing and taking on an **old**, **varnished** appearance, also described as honey crusted), and/or commonly, **mixed infections** of the two. **Folliculitis** infections are most commonly caused by *S. aureus* with the exception of "**hot-tub folliculitis**," which is caused by *P. aeruginosa* (see I B) and acquired in a contaminated swimming pool or hot tub. **Furuncles/carbuncles** (*S. aureus*) are commonly called *boils* and often start with an infected hair follicle; carbuncles are the larger, coalescing aggregates of boils. **Erysipelas** is a painful cellulitis involving blockage of the dermal lymphatics, so lesions have sharp raised borders. **Cellulitis** is infection of the deeper dermis and subcutaneous fat. Both are more commonly caused by *S. pyogenes* but may be *S. aureus*. *S. pyogenes* may cause **TSS** following invasive disease (eg, cellulitis) with encapsulated strains of M1 or M3. These strains produce SPE-A or SPE-C toxins (see I D). These toxins are **superantigens** that have direct cardiotoxicity in addition to decreasing normal liver clearance of endotoxin from the body. **Necrotizing fasciitis** involves the fascia and overlying fat. It is most commonly caused by *S. pyogenes* but may involve mixed bowel flora if the infection originates in the abdominal area. The hyaluronidase facilitates spread.

Surgical wounds: In breeching the integument, surgery raises the risk of infection even when great care is taken. The etiology varies with surgical site and hospital or clinic, but very common organisms include *S. aureus*, *S. epidermidis*, **gram-negative enteric bacteria**, *B. fragilis*, **and** *Clostridia*.

Trauma often introduces soil or plant microbes as well as normal skin, mucosal, or fecal flora into normally sterile tissues. One fairly common toxin-producing organism, *Clostridium tetani*, is often in the soil and, if not properly prevented or treated, can lead to death.

Animal bites: Because all animals, including humans, have bacteria in their mouths, all bites generally require antibiotic treatment and contain more than one organism. **Cat bites** (dominant microbe: **gram-negative** *Pasteurella multocida*) are most likely to become infected. Dog bites commonly are also infected with *Capnocytophaga canimorsus*. **Cat-scratch fever** is caused by *Bartonella henselae*.

Systemic bacterial diseases with rashes or cutaneous lesions include the following:

1. **Scarlet fever/***S. pyogenes*: Clinical symptoms are a **fine sandpaper body rash with pharyngitis** with or without nausea.
2. **TSS/***S. aureus*: Case definition requires the presence of a **diffuse macular rash that desquamates, especially on extremities.** Streptococcal TSS may also have a rash.

3. **Petechial rash with septicemia with either** *N. meningitidis* or *N. gonorrhoeae.*
4. **Secondary syphilis** (see XII C): Mucocutaneous lesions cover all surfaces **including palms and soles.**
5. **Rocky Mountain spotted fever (RMSF)** (see XIV A): Petechial rash begins on extremities and migrates to the body (**centripetal rash**); **palms and soles have a rash.** (Typhus causes a centrifugal rash.)
6. **Lyme disease: Target-shaped lesions** are found in the primary stage of the disease (see XIV B).

Osteomyelitis is infection of the bone. *S. aureus* is the most common causative agent. In **infants,** the other **agents of neonatal septicemia** (GBS and gram-negative bacilli) may also be involved. In individuals with **thalassemia or sickle cell disease,** osteomyelitis is extremely common, and it is **overwhelmingly** caused by *Salmonella* spp.

Reactive arthritis (previously Reiter's) may follow weeks *after* infections with *C. trachomatis, Campylobacter* spp., *Y. enterocolitica, Salmonella* spp., or *Shigella* spp. It is generally focused on large joints; it may be migratory and associated with cervicitis or urethritis and conjunctivitis.

Septic arthritis occurs when microbes enter the joint and the risk increases anytime there is septicemia, an artificial joint, or injection into a joint. **Gonococcal arthritis** occurs primarily as acute disease in undiagnosed/untreated young females at risk of sexually transmitted infections (STIs). It may be mono- or polyarticular. **Lyme disease** generally affects large joints and polyarticular. **Post-articular injection** infections are commonly caused by *S. aureus, S. epidermidis*, or *Pseudomonas*. **Prosthetic joints** are commonly infected by streptococci or *S. aureus* or *S. epidermidis*; these may be resistant strains.

A. *Clostridium tetani*
Features
1. **Gram-positive, spore-forming anaerobe** with **terminal spores,** resulting in a characteristic **"tennis racket"** morphologic appearance.
2. *C. tetani* vegetative cells and spores are ubiquitous in soil and are a major concern during wars and for babies born to unvaccinated mothers. Infection follows trauma where the oxygen supply to the wound is compromised.

Disease: Tetanus
1. Causes disease through **vegetative cell production of tetanus neurotoxin (TeNT; also called *tetanospasmin*). TeNT acts on synaptosomes to obliterate the inhibitory reflex response of nerve fibers, producing uncontrolled spasms**.
2. Manifests as descending muscle stiffness, **tetanospasms** of **lockjaw,** back arching (**opisthotonus**), and short, frequent spasms of voluntary muscles. Death occurs after several weeks from exhaustion and respiratory failure.
3. **Treatment:** Hospitalize and start specialized supportive care immediately. Antitoxin (**tetanus immunoglobulin [TIG]**) neutralizes unbound toxin. It is given around the wound. **Metronidazole** should be started: Dead tissue should be debrided; and vaccination should be given at a distant site from TIG.
4. **Prevention: DTaP** is a routine vaccination of infants/children, which contains the tetanus toxoid. Boosters are given every 10 years.

B. *Bacillus anthracis* (see VI K)
Disease: Cutaneous anthrax
1. Unlike *Clostridia*, *B. anthracis* can grow in very superficial wounds. However, since near eradication has occurred in animals by vaccination in the United States and gas sterilization of commercial raw wool imports, *B. anthracis* is not common in the environment. People working with imported goat and sheep products and weavers are at highest risk.
2. **Clinical symptoms**
   a. The **early papular lesion** develops into a **vesicular lesion filled with blood or clear fluid** that, due to cell death, develops **central necrosis (black eschar) with an erythematous raised margin.**
   b. Systemic disease is not present in many cases. The fatality rate is 10%.

C. *Pseudomonas aeruginosa* (see I B)

1. *Pseudomonas* is a major problem in burn patients.
2. *P. aeruginosa* is **ubiquitous** in the environment; 10% of us are transiently colonized; this colonization increases to 90% in hospitalized patients. GI colonization causes loose stools which contaminate perianal skin and spread on the skin, which is a potential source for burn colonization leading to infection. Other sources are environmental and associated with water.
3. **Blue-green pus in a burn generally indicates *Pseudomonas* infection.**
4. In **systemic infection with *P. aeruginosa*** (mainly in **patients with neutropenia or burn patients**), black skin lesions (**ecthyma gangrenosum**) that resemble anthrax develop. They start as raised and red, tumorlike lesions and then develop necrosis in the middle.
5. **Puncture wounds:** A nail that passes through the sole of a tennis shoe is most likely to cause *P. aeruginosa* cellulitis (probably from the *P. aeruginosa* inside the shoe). Some infections will progress to osteomyelitis. Tetanus risk should also be evaluated.

D. *Pasteurella multocida, Pasteurella canis*

Features

1. **Gram-negative coccobacilli, nonmotile**, facultative.
2. **Normal oral flora** of dogs, cats, other animals.

Disease: Animal bite infections

1. Cause a localized **cellulitis** and lymphadenitis following an **animal bite**.
2. Most strains are toxin producing.
3. Treatment often requires antibiotics.

E. *Capnocytophaga canimorsus*

Features

1. **Capnophilic** (requires CO_2 for growth) and slow-growing **gram-negative fusiform bacilli.**
2. **Normal oral flora** of dogs.

Disease: Animal bite infections

1. Organisms produce a substance that modifies polymorphonuclear cell chemotactic activity.
2. Infection may lead to septicemia and meningitis.

F. *Bartonella henselae*

Features

1. Aerobic, pleomorphic, short **gram-negative rods** that are **facultative intracellular** and difficult to culture and Gram stain.
2. Often visualized with **Warthin-Starry silver stain.**
3. NF in the **saliva of domestic cats**.

Disease: Cat-scratch fever

1. Symptoms include regional **lymphadenitis** after a papule at the site of a cat scratch.
2. Most common cause of unilateral regional lymphadenitis in U.S. children.
3. Also may cause **bacillary angiomatosis** and subacute bacterial **endocarditis**.

SITUATIONAL DISEASE

XII. SEXUALLY TRANSMITTED INFECTIONS

All patients with one STI should be tested for other likely STIs. Diagnostic tests may differ for different body sites; common genital sites are listed. The three major bacterial STIs are *Chlamydia*, *Gonorrhea*, and *Syphilis*.

• • • Clinical Pearl

Infections with *N. gonorrhoeae* and *C. trachomatis* present with discharge. *T. pallidum* and human papillomavirus are painless ulcers, whereas Herpes simplex virus ulcers are painful.

Bacterial vaginosis (BV) involves overgrowth of bacteria common to the NF, most notably *Gardnerella vaginalis,* a gram-variable rod, and **other anaerobes such as *Bacteroides. G. vaginalis*** is present in 20% to 40% of asymptomatic women, but almost 100% of the partners of women with BV, suggesting it is sexually transmitted. BV presents with copious amounts of an unpleasant **fishy** or musty discharge. BV is **diagnosed** by the finding of a **pH greater than 4.5, a positive amine "whiff" test** (drop of KOH on discharge will give off an amine odor), and the presence of **clue cells, which are epithelial cells coated with bacteria.**

A. *Chlamydia trachomatis*

Features: See II A. *C. trachomatis* serovars D-K are **the most common bacterial STI** in the United States.

Disease

1. High incidence of asymptomatic chronic infections, particularly in females where often infection is not obvious (so not treated) until the granulomatous response causes complications. **Reinfection is common** due to the eight serovars. Each new infection increases the risk of infertility. *Chlamydiae* are a major cause of infertility.
2. **Urethritis in males (milky discharge); urethritis, endometritis, cervicitis, salpingitis, and pelvic inflammatory disease (PID) in females; inclusion conjunctivitis in both sexes; and conjunctivitis and pneumonia in neonates. Reactive arthritis** is not uncommon several weeks after infections, particularly in males.
3. **Lab ID:** NAAT has replaced less sensitive nonamplified tests. Specimens are either first voided urine or urethral discharge for males. Results from self-collected vaginal swabs correlate well with results from physician-collected cervical swabs. DFA available.
4. **Treatment**: doxycycline or a macrolide.
5. **Prevention:** annual screening of all sexually active young people. Prevented by barrier methods.

> **• • • Clinical Pearl**
>
> *C. trachomatis* **serovars L1, L2, L3** cause the STI **lymphogranuloma venereum,** characterized by a suppurative inguinal adenitis progressing to lymphatic obstruction and rectal strictures if the disease is untreated.

B. *Neisseria gonorrhoeae*

Features: See II B. **Gram-negative, intracellular diplococci** (Figure 3.4). Infection is most common in 15- to 25-year-olds. These bacteria are sensitive to drying and cold, so transmission requires intimate contact.

Disease: Gonorrhea

1. **IgA1 protease** plays a key early role in the colonization of mucosa. **Adherence** is **through pili** (protein surface fibrils) **and other outer membrane proteins.**
   a. **Pili undergo *phase variation*** (on and off). Nonpiliation greatly reduces virulence.
   b. Pili also exhibit *antigenic variation* **by continuous genetic rearrangement.** There are 10 to 15 incomplete pilin loci (*pilS* for silent) lacking transcriptional promoter elements and one complete pilin expression locus (*pilE*). Through homologous recombination, an incomplete

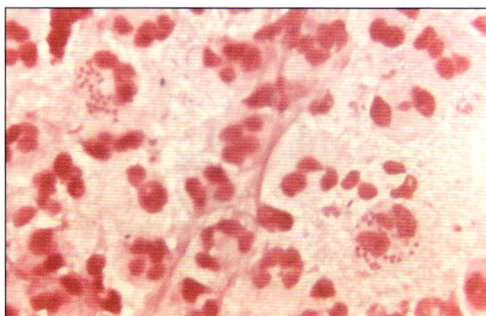

FIGURE 3.4. Photomicrograph of Gram-stained urethral discharge specimen showing gram-negative, intracellular diplococci *Neisseria gonorrhoeae* at 1,150× magnification. (Photo courtesy of CDC Public Health Image Library [PHIL], image 21362.)

gene can be recombined into *pilE*, creating millions of variants. This recombination occurs continuously and accounts for the **chronicity** of the infections, the lack of protection against subsequent infections, and why both partners need to be treated at the same time.

    c. **Outer membrane proteins** add genetic variation. They include outer membrane **porin protein (PI and PIII)** and proteins that determine **clumping (PII) or opacity.** PII-positive strains promote adherence and invasion, leading to septicemia.

  2. Attachment to the microvilli of the nonciliated cells leads to ciliary stasis and death of the ciliated cells as well as internalization of the organism. **Intracellular** gonococci replicate in vacuoles where they are protected from antibodies. Eventually they exit into the sub-epithelial connective tissue, causing inflammation and possibly gaining entrance into the bloodstream.

  3. LOS (lipooligosaccharide; a short version of LPS) stimulates TNF-α (tumor necrosis factor-α) and damage to the mucosa. Strains causing disseminated gonococcal infections have sialylation of the LOS, which provides greater serum resistance.

  4. Clinical symptoms

    a. Gonorrhea is a **mucous membrane infection,** the site dependent on patient sex, sexual practices, and strain virulence. It is **often asymptomatic in females.** Both asymptomatic and symptomatic persons may transmit the disease. Untreated/repeated infections increase the risk of infertility and predispose females to ectopic pregnancy.

    b. **Urethritis** in males is characterized by thick, yellow, purulent exudate containing bacteria and numerous neutrophils; frequent, painful urination; and possibly an erythematous meatus. Complications include **epididymitis** and **prostatitis** in males.

    c. **Endocervicitis or urethritis** in females is characterized by a purulent vaginal discharge; frequent, painful urination; dyspareunia; and abdominal pain. Approximately 50% of cases go undiagnosed. Complications include arthritis, salpingitis, pelvic inflammatory disease, sterility, and ectopic pregnancy.

    d. **Rectal infections** are characterized by painful defecation, discharge, constipation, and proctitis.

    e. **Pharyngitis** ranges from mild to severe with purulent exudate that mimics "strep" throat.

    f. **Disseminated infection** (untreated with bloodstream invasion) presents most commonly as polyarthritis or necrotic skin lesions on an erythematous base.

    g. **Ophthalmia neonatorum** rapidly leads to blindness if not properly treated immediately.

  5. Lab ID: Gonococcal infections are diagnosed with NAAT, or culture on **Thayer-Martin** (a chocolate agar with antibiotics to inhibit NF), or New York City agar. **Gram-negative intracellular diplococci** seen in urethral smears on microscopy. Culture is more common due to the need for antibiotic susceptibility testing. Patients with gonorrhea should be treated for *C. trachomatis* too.

  6. Treatment and prevention: most commonly treated with ceftriaxone; test for (and treat if positive) *C. trachomatis*. **Antibiotic resistance** is common. Prevent with condom usage.

C. *Treponema pallidum*

  Features

  1. Spirochete (**corkscrew-shaped, motile spiral bacteria** with an endoflagellum [**axial filament**] underneath the outer membrane) which is **too thin to visualize on Gram stain** but does have an outer membrane with endotoxin-like lipids. **Dark-field microscopy** is used for visualization: Figure 3.5.

  Disease: Syphilis

  1. Causes chronic, painless infections that may last 30 to 40 years if untreated. The number of organisms decreases as host defenses are stimulated, causing disappearance of symptoms; subsequently, organisms multiply and symptoms reappear.

  2. Primary syphilis: mucosal inoculation by minor trauma and replication at the site of the infection. Neutrophils, lymphocytes, and plasma cells infiltrate the site, and a **painless primary hard chancre** develops that **may heal** without treatment.

  3. Secondary syphilis: Bloodstream invasion leads to infection in almost all tissues and a papular, mucocutaneous rash over all of the body, including the palms and soles. Aggregation near vessels leads to **endarteritis and periarteritis,** resulting in inhibited blood supply and necrosis. The rash self-resolves but may reoccur.

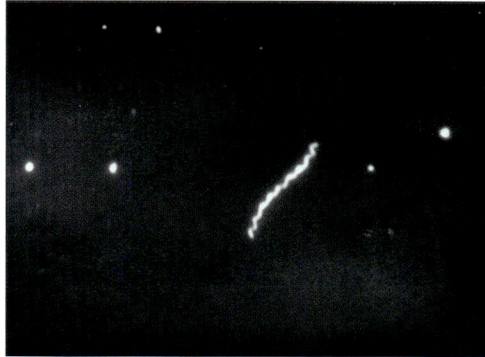

FIGURE 3.5. Photomicrograph of *Treponema pallidum* bacterium, using the dark-field microscopy technique at 400× magnification. (Photo courtesy of CDC Public Health Image Library [PHIL], image 2043.)

4. **Latent syphilis:** About two-thirds of the untreated secondary syphilis cases have persistent treponemes without symptoms.
5. **Tertiary syphilis:** About half of the individuals with latent syphilis will progress to tertiary, which is often characterized by aortitis and CNS problems, which may be fatal.
6. **In utero infection:** has severe manifestations, including abortion, stillbirth, birth defects, or latent infection (most common) with snuffles (rhinitis) followed by a rash and desquamation.
7. **Lab ID:** includes recognition of symptoms.
   a. **Microscopy (for primary)** of expressed chancre fluids is commonly done.
      (1) **Dark-field microscopy** of lesion exudate may demonstrate **corkscrew-shaped spirochetes** with "springing" motility. See Figure 3.5.
      (2) **Immunofluorescence** may be used with commercially prepared tagged antibodies: direct fluorescent Ab test for *T. pallidum* (**DFA-TP**).
   b. **Serology:** Two different antibodies are produced in response to infection. Because **(1)** each has some cross-reactivity and **(2)** only the treponemal antibodies are positive for life, it is a **positive test for each of the two types of antibodies that is diagnostic** except in tertiary, where the nontreponemal test will often be negative.
      (1) **Screening tests: nontreponemal (reaginic) antibodies.**
         (a) Triggered by *T. pallidum's* (*Tps*) *damage* to the human cells. The antigens appear to be of **mitochondrial origin and bind *Tp.*** The antibodies triggered cross-react with cow cardiolipin, which is used as an antigen in economical screening tests.
         (b) Tests are **quite sensitive but not very specific** (positive in other diseases). Confirm positive with treponemal antibody test.
         (c) **Nontreponemal antibody tests** are:
            1. **VDRL (Venereal Disease Research Laboratory)** test.
            2. **Rapid plasma reagin (RPR)** test.
         (d) **Non-treponemal antibody titers may decrease in tertiary syphilis** with or without treatment, and titers are often useful to monitor successful therapy.
      (2) **Specific tests (confirmatory): treponemal antibodies.** In screening of asymptomatic individuals, treponemal tests are used to confirm a positive nontreponemal test. For a patient with symptoms, both the screening and the more specific test would be ordered.
         (a) Treponemal antibody tests **require treponemal antigens**, so they are **more specific** and more costly.
         (b) **Treponemal antibody tests** are:
            1. **TP-PA test (treponemal particle agglutination test)** where particles have been coated with **treponemal antigens** (replacing FTA-ABS [fluorescent treponemal antibody absorption] test).
            2. ***T. pallidum* hemagglutination assay (TPHA)**.
            3. **FTA-ABS test** which is the gold standard.
         (c) Titers of treponemal antibody tests remain positive even with proper treatment.

XIII. CONGENITAL AND PERINATAL INFECTIONS

Congenital infections: A fetus is immunologically incompatible with its mother but is not rejected because of the subtle maternal immune defects and because major histocompatibility complex antigens are absent or have low density on placental cells. Placental antigens are covered with blocking antibody. Therefore, pregnant females are at increased risk of infection. If an organism is in the bloodstream, the placenta and ultimately the fetus may be infected. Some infections are transmitted during the birth process (**perinatal infections**).

> **● ● ●   Clinical Pearl**
>
> In congenital infections, the organism is able to be transmitted across the placenta to the fetus. In perinatal infections, the organism is acquired during the birthing process.

Some **bacterial congenital infections are able to cross the placenta:**
  a. *Listeria* **spp**. (see VII B).
  b. *T. pallidum* (see XII C).
Some common **bacterial perinatal infections** include:
  a. Neonatal *C. trachomatis* **D-K** eye infections or pneumonia (see II A).
  b. Neonatal *N. gonorrhoeae* ophthalmia neonatorum, which can lead to blindness (see II B).
  c. *Streptococcus algalactiae* or **GBS** septicemia and meningitis (see VII A).
  d. *E. coli* septicemia and meningitis (see I A).
  e. *L. monocytogenes* septicemia and meningitis (see VII B). (Late onset from maternal fecal colonization and exposure of the baby at birth.)

XIV. ARTHROPOD-BORNE AND ZOONOTIC DISEASES

Arthropod-borne infections are summarized in Table 3.2; **zoonoses** in Table 3.3.

A. *Rickettsia rickettsii*
  Features
  1. **Gram-negative, obligate intracellular pathogen,** with a specific predilection for **endothelial cells of capillaries.**
  2. **Tick transmitted** by bite of *Dermacentor variabilis* (**dog tick**), *Dermacentor andersoni* (**wood tick**), and *Amblyomma americanum* (**lone star tick**).
  Disease: Rocky Mountain spotted fever (RMSF)
  1. Following a tick bite, the organism **attaches to and invades vascular endothelial cells** by triggering phagocytic-like uptake and escapes the phagosome and replicates in the **nucleus and cytoplasm** where it polymerizes cellular actin to propel progeny out of the cell into the bloodstream or into neighboring endothelial cells, both facilitating spread. Peripheral vascular damage leads to symptoms. Organ damage leads to death in 20% of untreated infections.
  2. **RMSF ranges** from mild to **highly fulminant** and fatal from the damage to the vascular endothelial cells, resulting in hyperplasia, thrombus formation, inhibited blood supply, and peripheral vasculitis.
  3. **RMSF manifests** as **abrupt onset of high fever, chills, headache** (severe, frontal, unremitting), **myalgias with the macular rash, and edema starting on the extremities and spreading to the trunk; a few days later, hemorrhagic rash, stupor, delirium, and shock develop.**
  4. **Lab ID**
     a. **Diagnosis depends heavily on clinical manifestations,** especially rash and abrupt onset of fever, headache, and chills with recent exposure to ticks. Diagnosis is confirmed by immunofluorescence, enzyme immunoassay, or complement fixation tests.
  5. Treatment with antibiotics is started on suspicion. **Cell-mediated immunity and repair of the vasculature is important in recovery;** thus, older adults and those with poor cell-mediated immunity are more likely to die even with treatment.

Table 3.2   Important Arthropod-Borne Diseases

Disease	Organism	Vector	Reservoir Host	Environment/ Endemic Areas in the United States
Rocky Mountain spotted fever	*Rickettsia rickettsii*	*Dermacentor* ticks	Dogs, rodents, and ticks	Highest in Southeastern United States: Tennessee to Oklahoma but all states
Epidemic typhus	*Rickettsia prowazekii*	Flying squirrel mites/ fleas Human body lice (*Pediculus humanus*)	Flying squirrel Humans	Eastern United States War-torn countries
Human monocytic ehrlichiosis	*Ehrlichia chaffeensis*	*Amblyomma* (Lone Star) ticks and others	Various birds and mammals	South Central United States
Human granulocytic anaplasmosis	*Anaplasma phagocytophilum*	*Ixodes* ticks	White-footed mice and white-tailed deer	Northeastern and North Central United States
Lyme disease	*Borrelia burgdorferi*	*Ixodes* ticks	White-footed mice and white-tailed deer	Northeastern and North Central United States
Plague	*Yersinia pestis*	Fleas	Rodents, lagomorphs, cats	Southwestern United States: Texas to Southern California
Tularemia (also a zoonosis)	*Francisella tularensis*	Ticks, fleas, mosquitoes, trauma, ingestion, inhalation	Mainly rabbits and hares	Northern hemisphere, primarily from 30° to 71° latitude north

B. *Borrelia burgdorferi*

Features

1. **Highly motile gram-negative spirochete.**
2. Related to ***Borrelia recurrentis*** (louse borne) and the other *Borrelia* species (tick borne), all notorious for antigenic variation, which explains why these borreliae cause **relapsing fever.** *B. burgdorferi* shares the tendency for **antigenic variation.**
3. **Tick transmitted** by bite of ticks from the ***Ixodes*** genus worldwide.
   a. Life cycle of tick (eggs → larvae → nymphs → adults).
      (1) Larvae and nymphs feed on the **white-footed mouse,** the most important source of the organisms; nymphs drop on to grass and then on to humans. **Nymphs** or adults **spread disease** to humans.
      (2) Adults feed on **white-tailed deer** but also drop off on vegetation to infect humans.

Disease: Lyme disease

1. **Lyme disease** starts at the **bite site** and spreads via the **bloodstream** to other tissues, especially the **brain, heart, and joints.** It is most common during tick season (early spring through fall) in North America.
   a. The hallmark is **erythema migrans (EM), an annular lesion with a rashy border and central clearing** that spreads out from the site of the tick bite, may or may not be present. Constitutional symptoms are mild.
   b. Weeks or months later, patients experience **malaise, fatigue, headache, fever, chills, stiff neck, aches, and pains for several weeks, leading to more severe neural and cardiac problems,** including meningitis, cranial neuropathy (most commonly **Bell palsy**), radiculoneuropathy, and some cardiac dysfunction.
   c. Months or years later, **joint pain** may occur, especially in large joints, producing oligoarthritis. Intermittent bouts of arthritis may recur for 3 to 7 years. **Neural dysfunction** may lead to dementia and paralysis.

Table 3.3 Important Bacterial Zoonoses

Disease/Type	*Organism* and Features	Reservoir/Transmission
Anthrax/pulmonary Anthrax/cutaneous	*Bacillus anthracis* Gram-positive, aerobic rod	Hoofed animals and spores in animal skins or soil contaminated by sick animals/inhalation or traumatic implantation
Brucellosis/systemic	*Brucella melitensis, Brucella abortus, Brucella suis, Brucella canis*, Gram-negative rod	Goats, cattle, pigs, dogs (respectively)/contact with animals/ingestion or trauma
Campylobacter/inflammatory diarrhea	*Campylobacter jejuni* Gram-negative rod	Food contaminated with bacteria from raw chicken or other animal sources/ingestion
Cat-scratch fever/cellulitis with lymphadenopathy	*Bartonella henselae* Gram-negative rod	Cats/scratches
Erysipeloid/cellulitis (dark red) in butchers and fish mongers	*Erysipelothrix rhusiopathiae* Gram-positive rod	Raw meat or fish/trauma
EHEC/bloody diarrhea and HUS	*Escherichia coli* O157 and others with a Shiga-like toxin	Cattle/contaminated hamburger
Leptospirosis	*Leptospira interrogans* Spirochete with hooked ends	Rodent, cattle, dog urine in water/swimming or inhalation
Listeriosis/GI/septicemia	*Listeria monocytogenes* Gram-positive rod	Cabbage and deli soft cheeses and meats, unpasteurized milk and cheeses/ingestion
Listeria meningitis	Nonspore-forming rod; somewhat resistant to heat; grows in cold	Same as above
Pasteurellosis/animal bite	*Pasteurella multocida*	Oral flora of cats, dogs, and other mammals/bite
Plague/bubonic Plague/pneumonic	*Yersinia pestis*/gram-negative rod non-lactose fermenting (Enterobacteriaceae)	Rodent flea bite or inhalation from a patient with pneumonic plague
Psittacosis	*Chlamydia psittaci*/obligate intracellular pathogen	Birds, turkeys, chickens/inhalation
Q fever/pneumonia with or without hepatitis	*Coxiella burnetii* Gram-negative rod somewhat resistant to drying	Pregnant domestic animals' amniotic fluid and dried dust contaminated with *Coxiella*
Salmonellosis/diarrhea	Almost all *Salmonellae* except *S. typhi* and *S. paratyphi*	Wide variety of animals, but commonly from raw chicken/contaminates other food or eating undercooked chicken
Tularemia: ulceroglandular, pneumonic, or gastrointestinal	*Francisella tularensis* Gram-negative rod	Rabbits primarily; arthropod bite or traumatic implantation or ingestion
Vibrio cellulitis or septicemia (in people with liver disease)	*Vibrio vulnificus* Gram-negative curved flagellated rod, oxidase positive	Raw oysters from contaminated water/traumatic implantation or ingestion

2. **Lab ID: Lyme disease** is diagnosed by several methods, but clinical manifestations along with the tick bite are important.
   a. The diagnosis is confirmed most frequently by **serology**, commonly enzyme-linked immunosorbent assay (ELISA) or Western blot.
   b. The organism may be visualized by Wright- or Giemsa-stained thin blood smears for spirochetes.
   c. **Lyme urine antigen capture tests** are used primarily to follow treatment.
   d. **NAAT** is used to test joint fluid and CSF for the presence of Borrelia DNA.
3. **Prevention:** Lyme disease risk can be reduced by limiting exposure (long pants tucked in) and performing nightly tick checks in endemic areas. Antibiotic prophylaxis may be administered in some cases.

C. *Yersinia pestis*
Features
1. Pleomorphic **gram-negative rod** or coccobacilli that is a **facultative intracellular pathogen.** It is a **non-lactose-fermenting** *Enterobacteriaceae* that grow slowly on blood or MacConkey agars. It has **bipolar staining** on Giemsa or Wayson stains (looks like a closed safety pin). See Figure 3.6.
2. Endemic in the deserts of the southwestern United States in wild rodents and lagomorphs (eg, rabbits); it is **spread to humans by infected rodent flea bites.** Cats that bring infected rodents home play a role. **Pneumonic cases are highly contagious from person to person.**

Disease: Plague
1. **Pathogenesis**
   a. Produces a **coagulase** that coagulates the blood in the flea midgut, providing a fibrin clot in which *Y. pestis* (*Yp*) replicates. The starved fleas feed, regurgitating high numbers of *Yp* into the host, thereby spreading the agent.
   b. Once in the human it is **phagocytosed by PMNs and monocytes** and taken to **lymph nodes;** however, the **intracellular** organisms are able to **kill the monocytes due to V and W surface components.**
   c. The higher human temperature triggers production of the antiphagocytic **F1 capsular protein**; when the newly encapsulated organisms are released after killing the infected monocytes, the cells **replicate rapidly extracellularly in the lymph nodes,** causing inflamed swellings called *buboes* **(bubonic plague).**
   d. If the organism **invades the bloodstream (spread facilitated by the plasminogen activator),** the **envelope endotoxin** plays a major role in the peripheral vascular collapse and disseminated intravascular coagulopathy seen in plague. Thrombi formed in the pulmonary vasculature lead to the highly contagious **pneumonic plague.**
2. **Bubonic plague** is characterized by **fever** and exquisitely painful **buboes.**
3. **Septicemic plague** results from bacteria bypassing lymph nodes and multiplying in blood, **presenting as fever without a bubo.**

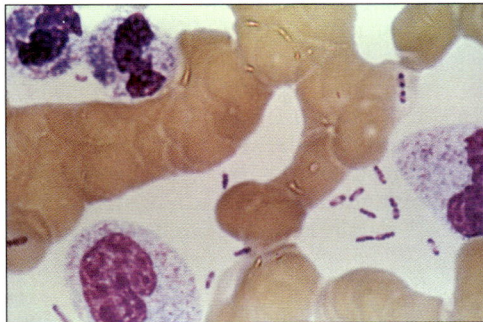

FIGURE 3.6. Photomicrograph of Wright stained blood sample, which had been extracted from a plague victim, revealed the presence of *Yersinia pestis*, whose bipolar ends were darkly stained. Note that this is not a Gram stain, so the color does not indicate the Gram reaction. Y. pestis is Gram-negative. (Photo courtesy of CDC Public Health Image Library [PHIL], image 2050.)

4. **Pneumonic plague** occurs either from bacteria seeding the lungs in bubonic plague or with respiratory exposure to *Yp*. This form is a rapidly necrotic pneumonia, with death occurring within days. It is highly contagious.

5. **Lab ID:** Diagnosis is hazardous. Bubo aspirate, sputum, and blood are stained with **Wayson stain** or **Giemsa** stain (bipolar staining) and **FAs** to confirm.

D. *Anaplasma phagocytophilum*
Features
1. **Obligate intracellular gram-negative pathogen of granulocytes**, similar to *Rickettsia* spp.
2. Endemic to the **northern United States**, and is **tick borne** by *Ixodes scapularis* and possibly other ticks. Reservoir hosts are deer, rodents, and other wild mammals.

Disease: Human granulocytic anaplasmosis (HGA)
1. **Infection starts with a tick bite.** When *Anaplasma* enters the bloodstream, it infects **granulocytes** by inducing phagocytosis and **replicates in phagosomes**.
2. **Clinical symptoms** include **fever, myalgia, headache, malaise, leukopenia,** and **thrombocytopenia,** but **rarely rash** (similar to RMSF but without the rash).
3. **Lab ID:** diagnosed by clinical symptoms and the findings of **mulberry-like clusters of cells (morulae)** in the phagosomes of granulocytes.

E. *Ehrlichia chaffeensis* or *E. ewingii*
Features
1. **Obligate intracellular gram-negative pathogen of monocytes,** similar to *Rickettsia* spp.
2. Endemic in the **southern United States;** reservoir in **white-tailed deer** and is transmitted by the *Amblyomma* **ticks (Lone Star tick).**

Disease: Human monocytic ehrlichiosis (HME) and human granulocyte ehrlichiosis (HGE)
1. As for ***Anaplasma*, it infects monocytes or granulocytes** and causes human monocytic or granulocytic ehrlichiosis.
2. HME and HGE are similar to HGA except that the thrombocytopenia may not be as severe. The organisms are also not as likely to be seen in cells.

F. *Francisella tularensis*
Features
1. **Gram-negative coccobacilli** that do not Gram stain well and cause **tularemia** (also called *deer fly fever or rabbit fever*). It is a **facultative parasite of macrophages.**
2. Found around the world in the **northern hemisphere infecting hundreds of wild animals (mainly rabbits, hares, squirrels, voles),** some domestic animals and wild birds, and over 100 arthropods. It is also found in mud and water (surviving in cold, including frozen meat). Disease acquisition is often associated with **hunting, especially rabbits.**

Disease: Tularemia
1. Infection starts at the site of entry, which may be skin (infected blood into cuts or insect bites), leading to **ulcer glandular tularemia;** inhalation of blood or respiratory secretions from a sick animal (**pneumonic tularemia**); blood in the eye (**oculoglandular tularemia**); or ingestion of undercooked meat or contaminated meat (**typhoidal tularemia**).
2. Characterized by macrophage infiltration, **granulomas,** and **necrosis of infected tissues. Regional lymph nodes become infected and suppurate.** Spread to the lungs, liver, and spleen is common.
3. Manifests as **abrupt onset of fever, headache, and regional (painful) adenopathy;** back pain, anorexia, chills, sweats, and prostration follow. The fatality rate is 1%.
4. **Lab ID:** diagnosed by **immunofluorescent stain of biopsy.** Organisms are **fastidious**, but if culture is needed, the organisms require **cysteine** for robust growth (Cysteine Heart Agar/CHA).

Table 3.4	Properties of Bacterial Pathogens	
Bacterium	**Distinguishing Characteristics**	**Diseases**
Actinomyces	Anaerobe, branching rod, Gr+ "Sulfur" granule (microcolonies) Contiguous growth through anatomic barriers Cervicofacial, thoracic, and abdominal lesions	Actinomycosis
Anaplasma phagocy-tophilum (XIV D)	*Ixodes* tick-transmitted zoonosis OIP of granulocytes; Gr− Belong to family Rickettsiaceae	Human granulocytic anaplasmosis
Bacillus anthracis (VI K)	Potent tripartite exotoxin: protective antigen, lethal factor, and edema factor Polypeptide capsule inhibits phagocytosis Spore transmission, Gr+ rod	Cutaneous or pulmonary anthrax
Bacteroides fragilis (IX Q)	Non–spore-forming pleomorphic anaerobe, Gr− Mixed infections Capsule Possesses a β-lactamase Wound debridement important	Intra-abdominal abscesses, gastrointestinal, and cellulitis
Bartonella henselae (XI F) *Bartonella quintana*	Small Gr− bacterium	Cat-scratch disease or bacillary angiomatosis (BA) Trench fever or BA
Bordetella pertussis (VI A)	Gr− rod extracellular; attaches via pili; paroxysmal cough due to toxin Toxoid part of DTaP vaccine	Whooping cough
Borrelia burgdorferi (XIV B)	*Ixodes* transmission Corkscrew-shaped motile spirochete, Gr nonstaining/−	Lyme disease
Campylobacter jejuni (IX J)	Comma-shaped rod; Gr− Animal hosts frequent cause of diarrhea Invasive Neutrophils and blood in stool	Inflammatory diarrhea
Chlamydophila pneumoniae (VI H)	OIP Elementary (infectious) and reticulate body Divides by binary fission	Atypical pneumonia
Chlamydia psittaci (VI I)	OIP, zoonotic (birds, chickens, parrots)	Atypical pneumonia nonbreaking Sudden onset
Chlamydia trachomatis (II A)	OIP Elementary (infectious) and reticulate body Divides by binary fission 15 serovars	Sexually transmitted infection (D-K): inclusion conjunctivitis PID, reactive arthritis neonatal eye, pneumonia Lymphogranuloma venereum (L1, L2, L3) Trachoma (A-C)

(continued)

Table 3.4	Properties of Bacterial Pathogens (*continued*)	
Bacterium	**Distinguishing Characteristics**	**Diseases**
Clostridium botulinum (IX D)	Spore-forming anaerobe, Gr+ Exotoxin acting at myoneural junction Suppresses acetylcholine release by peripheral nerves Produces flaccid muscle paralysis Caused by ingestion of preformed toxin or by ingestion of spores by infants	Botulism
Clostridioides difficile (IX O)	Spore-forming anaerobe, Gr+ Part of normal gastrointestinal flora Activated by antibiotic disruption of other flora Secrete an enterotoxin and cytotoxin	Gastroenteritis Pseudomembranous colitis
Clostridium perfringens (IX C)	Spore-forming anaerobe Spores introduced by severe trauma Possesses an α-toxin (lecithinase)	Gas gangrene Soft tissue cellulitis Food poisoning
Corynebacterium diphtheriae (V B)	Gr+ rod Phage-coded A/B exotoxin inhibits EF-2 Toxoid part of DTaP, Tdap, and Td vaccines	Pharyngeal diphtheria Cutaneous diphtheria
Coxiella burnetii (VI J)	Intracellular bacterium, Gr− Dust/parturition materials transmitted Absence of rash	Q fever Pneumonitis with or without hepatitis
Ehrlichia (XIV E)	*Amblyomma* tick-transmitted zoonosis OIP of monocytes Belong to family Rickettsiaceae	Human monocytic ehrlichiosis
Enterococcus (VIII C)	Formerly group D streptococci, Gr+ Most are α- or γ-hemolytic Antibiotic resistance; β-lactamase producer. Nosocomial opportunist	Urinary tract infection (UTI) Endocarditis following genitourinary (GU) manipulations
Escherichia coli (I A)	All strains possess endotoxin; Gr− rod Nonpathogenic part of normal microbiota of colon Enterotoxigenic: heat-labile toxin stimulates adenylate cyclase similar to cholera toxin; heat-stable toxin activates guanylate cyclase. Enteropathogenic: adherence to enterocytes → infantile diarrhea Enterohemorrhagic: Shiga-like verotoxin → bloody diarrhea (serotype O157) Enteroinvasive: similar to Shigella	UTIs, neonatal meningitis, sepsis Gastroenteritis Bloody diarrhea without invasion; HUS Inflammatory diarrhea
Fusobacterium nucleatum	Polymorphic, slender filaments Oral anaerobe, Gr− Synergizes with *Borrelia vincentii*	Vincent angina Brain abscess Head, neck, chest infections

Table 3.4	Properties of Bacterial Pathogens (*continued*)	
Bacterium	**Distinguishing Characteristics**	**Diseases**
Haemophilus influenzae (II E)	Gr− pleomorphic rod Antiphagocytic polysaccharide capsule Pyrogenic IgAase Grow on chocolate agar or with X and V factors. Epiglottis requires a tracheotomy. Vaccine is polysaccharide capsule linked to protein	Meningitis: type b in 3-mo- to 6-yr-old unvaccinated "kids" Chronic bronchitis: type d in COPD Epiglottitis in unvaccinated toddlers
Helicobacter pylori (IX P)	Spiral rod, polar, flagella tuft, Gr− Produces a potent urease and vacuolating cytotoxin Treat with omeprazole, amoxicillin, and clarithromycin	Gastric and peptic ulcers Increases risk for gastric adenocarcinoma
Legionella pneumophila (VI F)	Aquaphile with inhalation transmission Association with amoeba in streams Possesses a cytotoxin and endotoxin β-Lactamase producing Gr− rod Stains with Dieterle silver stain; not standard Gram stain Requires cysteine and iron for growth; intracellular parasite	Legionnaires' disease (pneumonia often with diarrhea and severe headache)
Listeria monocytogenes (VII B)	Gr+ bacillus Animal reservoirs; cold growth Infects monocytes (monocytosis) Hemolysin destroys vesicular membranes.	Gastroenteritis; septicemia Granulomas, abscesses Meningitis (newborns; transplant patients)
Moraxella catarrhalis (IV C)	Gr− diplococcus; normal oral flora	Otitis, chronic bronchitis (COPD)
Mycobacterium avium-intracellulare (VI M)	Group of acid-fast organisms; non-Gram staining Opportunist (AIDS; chemotherapy) noncontagious; drug resistance	Pulmonary disease
Mycobacterium tuberculosis (VI L)	Cell wall: peptidoglycan-arabinogalactan, mycolic acids, and so on, make all mycobacteria acid-fast and resistant to drying Cord factor (trehalose dimycolate) induces granuloma formation. Purified protein derivative (PPD) in skin test Multiple drug resistance Bacille Calmette-Guérin vaccine (attenuated)	Tuberculosis
Mycoplasma pneumoniae (VI G)	Lacks a cell wall Smallest extracellular bacterium; not an L-form Mucosal tissue tropism Requires cholesterol but cannot make it	Primary atypical pneumonia

(*continued*)

Table 3.4   Properties of Bacterial Pathogens (*continued*)

Bacterium	Distinguishing Characteristics	Diseases
Neisseria gonorrhoeae (II B)	Intracellular Gr− diplococcus Produces an IgAase and a penicillinase (plasmid) Purulent exudate Requires chocolate agar (Thayer-Martin) Oxidase positive	Urethritis, cervicitis, proctitis Pelvic inflammatory disease Conjunctivitis in newborns Septicemia, arthritis
Neisseria meningitidis (VII E)	Antiphagocytic capsule, Gr− diplococcus Endotoxin (lipooligosaccharide) IgAase Vasculitic purpura Headache and stiff neck are common.	Meningococcemia Waterhouse-Friderichsen syndrome
Nocardia (VI N)	Gr+ partially acid-fast branching rods Aerobic soil bacterium Inhalation transmission or traumatic implantation	Pulmonary infections in compromised patients; cellulitis
Prevotella melaninogenica	Anaerobic black colonies on agar Found in mouth, gastrointestinal, and GU tracts Putrid sputum Debride and drain lesion Formerly in genus Bacteroides	Oral, dental, and lung abscesses Female GU infections
Proteus mirabilis (X C)	Highly motile (swarmer) G− rods Produces urease	Pneumonia, nosocomial infections
Pseudomonas aeruginosa (I B)	Glycocalyx slime layer, Gr− Pyocyanin (blue-green pigment) Endotoxin (lipopolysaccharide) Exotoxin A (ADP-ribosyl transferase)	Burn infections/septic shock Pneumonia and septic shock in neutropenic and CF puncture wounds, ear, eye
Rickettsia rickettsii (XIV A)	*Dermacentor* tick transmission; OIP (bacterium); invades vascular endothelium	Rocky Mountain spotted fever
Salmonella (IX L)	Animal reservoirs except *Salmonella typhi*, *Salmonella paratyphi* Gr− rods; many serotypes Intracellular multiplication (facultative) Can invade bloodstream Endotoxin and Enterotoxin	Enterocolitis Septicemia Enteric fever (typhoid) Osteomyelitis in sickle cell disease
Shigella (IX M)	Gr; no known animal reservoir Pathogenic in small numbers Perpetuation by human carriers All have endotoxin and are invasive *Shigella dysenteriae* has Shiga toxin. Stools can contain mucus, pus, and blood. Bloodstream invasion is rare.	Shigellosis (inflammatory diarrhea) with shallow ulcers
Staphylococcus aureus (I C)	Grapelike cluster morphology, Gr+ cocci Antibiotic resistance Catalase and coagulase positive Enterotoxin Short incubation period for food poisoning (2-6 h)	Local abscesses, impetigo, food poisoning Endocarditis especially IV drug users Osteomyelitis Sepsis (MSSA, MRSA)

Table 3.4   Properties of Bacterial Pathogens (*continued*)

Bacterium	Distinguishing Characteristics	Diseases
Staphylococcus epidermidis (VIII E)	Gr+ cocci, normal skin flora Instrument contamination Adherence through polysaccharide slime	Endocarditis (artificial valve) infections catheter, prosthetic devices
Staphylococcus saprophyticus (X B)	Gr+, catalase-positive cocci Coagulase negative	UTIs
Streptococcus agalactiae (VII A)	Group B Streptococci, Gr+ cocci in chairs Can be part of normal vaginal and oral flora Capsule Inhibits complement	Neonatal sepsis (early and late onset) Neonatal meningitis
Streptococcus pneumoniae (II D)	α-Hemolytic Gr+ diplococcus Large antiphagocytic capsule Quellung reaction Sensitive to bile and optochin Vaccines: adult: 23 capsular serotypes; meningitis in infants and older adults Pediatric: 13-valent capsule-protein Anticapsular antibody is protective	Pneumonia Otitis media Septicemia Chronic bronchitis (COPD)
Streptococcus pyogenes (I D)	Group A M-protein (more than 80 types); anti-phagocytic β-Hemolytic Gr+ cocci Sensitive to bacitracin Erythrogenic exotoxins	Pharyngitis Scarlet fever Rheumatic fever and heart disease Acute glomerulonephritis Impetigo Cellulitis-erysipelas
Treponema pallidum (XII C)	Spirochete, not visible by Gram stain Unable to be routinely cultured Dark-field microscopy examination Serologic tests	Syphilis, 1°, 2°, 3°
Vibrio cholerae (IX H)	Comma-shaped morphology, Gr− A/B enterotoxin overproduces cAMP Vomiting and rice-water diarrhea Oral rehydration solution or IV	Cholera
Viridans *streptococci* (III A)	Noninvasive opportunist in normal oral flora, Gr+ α-Hemolytic Differentiate from *S. pneumoniae* because the viridans strep are bile insoluble and not inhibited by optochin	Endocarditis Dental caries
Yersinia pestis (XIV C)	Zoonotic disease (rats and fleas), SW United States Intracellular multiplication Fever, conjunctivitis, regional buboes, pneumonia	Bubonic plague Pneumonic plague Yersiniosis

ADP, adenosine diphosphate; AIDS, acquired immunodeficiency syndrome; cAMP, cyclic adenosine monophosphate; CF, cystic fibrosis; COPD, chronic obstructive pulmonary disease; DTaP, diphtheria and tetanus toxoids and pertussis vaccine; EF-2, elongation factor-2; Gr+, Gr−, gram positive, gram negative; GU, genitourinary; HUS, hemolytic uremic syndrome; IgA, immunoglobulin A; IV, intravenous; MRSA, methicillin-resistant *S. aureus*; MSSA, methicillin-sensitive *S. aureus*; OIP, obligate intracellular pathogen; PID, pelvic inflammatory disease; Td, Tetanus and diphtheria vaccube; Tdap, tetanus diphtheria and and acellular pertussis vaccine.

Review Test

Directions: Select the *one* lettered answer that is *best* in each case.

1. A 23-year-old man develops pneumonia and presents to the clinic. He mentions that he has recently started working on a sheep farm on the northern East Coast and started helping with lambing the day before his symptoms began. His cough produces little sputum, and a saline-induced sputum sample shows no predominant organisms either with Gram stain or with AFS. It is established that he acquired the pneumonia from parturition products from the sheep. Which agent is most likely to be the cause of his pneumonia?

(A) *A. phagocytophilum*
(B) *C. burnetii*
(C) *Rickettsia akari*
(D) *Rickettsia typhi*
(E) *R. rickettsii*

2. A 3-year-old girl is brought to the clinic by a guardian with difficulty breathing and the girl will not lie down to be examined. Acute bacterial epiglottitis is suspected, and examination of the child's epiglottis reveals it is highly inflamed. Which vaccine should this child have been given to prevent this infection?

(A) Diphtheria
(B) *H. influenzae*
(C) *N. meningitidis*
(D) Polio
(E) *S. pneumoniae* (conjugate vaccine)

3. A 22-year-old presents to the emergency department with fever and increasing dyspnea. Past medical history indicates a diagnosis of CF. A gram-negative organism is found in unusually high numbers in the pulmonary mucus. Which virulence factor is most important in colonization and maintenance of the organism in this patient's lungs?

(A) Endotoxin
(B) Exotoxin A
(C) Polysaccharide slime (alginate)
(D) Pyocyanin (blue-green pigment)

4. From the case mentioned in Question 3, exotoxin A of the causative agent most closely resembles the action of which other microbial toxin?

(A) Diphtheria toxin
(B) Heat-LT of *E. coli*
(C) Shiga toxin
(D) *V. cholerae* toxin
(E) Verotoxin

5. A 36-year-old man presents to the clinic with a cough that has been bothering him for several weeks. He says that he immigrated to the United States 15 years ago and lived in a crowded resettlement camp before arriving. He has also lost 10 pounds. A γ-interferon release blood test is positive. Which of the following factors is known to be most important in triggering the granulomatous reaction to wall off and contain the infection?

(A) Cord factor
(B) Mycolic acid
(C) PPD
(D) Sulfatides
(E) Wax D

6. A 75-year-old patient develops diarrhea 5 days after starting antibiotic treatment for a serious staphylococcal infection. What is the most likely causative agent?

(A) *C. difficile*
(B) *C. perfringens*
(C) *P. aeruginosa*
(D) *S. sonnei*

7. A 23-year-old presents to the clinic with mild gastroenteritis a few days after having a variety of sushi at a party. There is no blood or pus in the stool. Which causative agent is most likely to have caused this illness?

(A) *V. cholerae*
(B) *V. parahaemolyticus*
(C) *S. sonnei*
(D) *S. typhi*

8. A 47-year-old presents to the clinic with symptoms suggestive of the plague. Which of the following is the vector for the most likely causative agent?

(A) *Dermacentor* tick
(B) Human body louse
(C) *Ixodes* tick
(D) Rodent flea

9. A patient who had surgery to put in a pacemaker and who states he felt fine for the first 2 months now presents 3 months postoperatively with malaise and increasing fatigue. He is running a low-grade fever, tires easily, and has worsening heart murmurs. Which of the following staphylococcal organisms causes subacute bacterial endocarditis that generally occurs 2 months or more after heart surgery?

(A) *S. aureus*
(B) *S. epidermidis*
(C) *Staphylococcus haemolyticus*
(D) *S. saprophyticus*

10. A previously healthy 6-month-old boy presents with upper body weakness. He cannot hold his eyes open, his pupils do not react, and he cannot hold his head up. What is the proper treatment?

(A) Offer monitored supportive care with antibiotics
(B) Offer monitored supportive care with human anti-botulinum Ig
(C) Provide IV fluids
(D) Send him home and report back if symptoms worsen

11. A 78-year-old presents to the emergency department with a high fever, cough producing a blood-tinged sputum, and difficulty breathing. Sputum shows gram-positive cocci in pairs. What is the most important virulence factor of the causative agent?

(A) Endotoxin
(B) A phospholipase allowing escape from the phagosome
(C) Polypeptide capsule
(D) Polysaccharide capsule

12. A 45-year-old woman presents to the clinic reporting feeling febrile for several days and now presents with abdominal pain. She recently returned from a trip to Africa. Her blood cultures grow *S. typhi.* What was the most likely source of this infection?

(A) A food preparer
(B) Contact with baby goats on a farm and then eating without washing hands
(C) Raw chicken
(D) Undercooked hamburger
(E) Undercooked pork

13. A 4-day-old infant girl is brought to the emergency department by her parent, with signs of sepsis. The infant was preterm (33 weeks) and born at home to her young mother after 22 hours of labor following the rupture of the membranes. A friend had helped the mother deliver the baby. What is the best description for the agent most likely causing the sepsis if it was acquired during labor but before delivery?

(A) α-Hemolytic diplococci sensitive to both bile and optochin
(B) β-Hemolytic cocci in chains and carrying Lancefield group B antigen
(C) α-Hemolytic cocci in chains; resistant to bile and optochin
(D) Nonhemolytic organisms found as part of the normal fecal flora; resistant to bile and optochin; carries a high level of drug resistance

14. A 62-year-old man presents to the clinic with signs of a gastric ulcer. He does not regularly take nonsteroidal anti-inflammatory agents. Which characteristic plays a central role in the causative organism's ability to survive transit of the lumen to colonize the stomach?

(A) Microaerophilic lifestyle
(B) O antigens
(C) Phospholipase C production
(D) Urease production

15. A 54-year-old man develops a pyogenic infection along the suture line after knee surgery. The laboratory gives a preliminary report of β-hemolytic, catalase-positive, coagulase-positive, gram-positive cocci. Which of the following is the most likely causative agent?

(A) *M. catarrhalis*
(B) *S. aureus*
(C) *S. epidermidis*
(D) *S. agalactiae*
(E) *S. pyogenes*

16. A 24-year-old female presents with dysuria, as well as urinary urgency and frequency. A urine dipstick test is positive for both leukocyte esterase and nitrites. What genus or family is noted for the production of nitrites?

(A) *Escherichia*
(B) *Staphylococcus*
(C) *Streptococcus*
(D) *Vibrio*

17. A patient presents with rapid onset severe respiratory symptoms. Chest radiographs show a hemorrhagic lymphadenitis. The isolation of chains of fairly large, aerobic gram-positive rods that are nonmotile, some of which have started to sporulate from a patient with this presentation, should raise a major concern of which organism?

(A) *Actinomyces israelii*
(B) *B. anthracis*
(C) *C. jejuni*
(D) *C. perfringens*
(E) *H. influenzae*

18. A female patient with a new genital lesion presents to the STIs clinic. Social history reveals that she lacks health insurance and is a regular IV drug user. Syphilis is suspected. Which of the following techniques would be most appropriate to demonstrate the suspected causative agent?

(A) AFS
(B) Dark-field microscopy
(C) Electrophoresis
(D) Gram stain
(E) Immunologic test such as the VDRL

19. A healthy 7-year-old boy is brought to the emergency department by his parents in June with signs of meningitis. The family has not traveled outside the United States. No bacteria are seen on the Gram stain of the CSF, and no bacterial capsule material is present as determined by a series of latex particle agglutination tests standard to the diagnosis of meningitis. The CSF glucose level is slightly low, protein is near normal, and the white cell count is less than 500 cells/μL, mainly lymphocytes. What is the most likely causative agent?

(A) *C. pneumonia*
(B) Enterovirus
(C) *M. pneumoniae*
(D) *M. tuberculosis*
(E) *T. pallidum*

20. What is the main difference between fluorochrome staining (eg, auramine-rhodamine screening for *M. tuberculosis*) and indirect fluorescent antibody (IFA) staining?

(A) Fluorochromes are more specific and used just for *M. tuberculosis*.
(B) Fluorochrome staining is less sensitive compared to staining with light microscopy.
(C) IFAs are less specific since they use antibody to a different species' antibody (ie, rabbit antibody to human antibody).
(D) IFA's specificity is dependent on the primary antibody used; fluorochromes lack the antibody specificity.

Answers and Explanations

1. **The answer is B.** [VI J] *C. burnetii* is a rickettsia-like organism that can be spread via amniotic fluid, aerosols, or dust particles. It withstands drying and thus can be transmitted at least 10 miles by the wind.

2. **The answer is B.** [II E] Epiglottitis is a medical emergency requiring hospitalization. It can be fatal in 24 hours. Pediatric cases were almost always caused by *H. influenzae* type b and have been dramatically reduced by the conjugate vaccine.

3. **The answer is C.** [I B] *S. aureus* and *P. aeruginosa* are two primary pulmonary colonizers that cause pneumonia in patients with CF. (*Staphylococcus* is usually only in young patients with CF.) Of the two, *Pseudomonas* is gram negative. The slime material (alginate) produces the resistance to phagocytic killing and poor penetration of antibiotics to the site, which, in conjunction with the antibiotic resistance of *Pseudomonas*, makes these serious infections. All other answer choices are virulence factors of *P. aeruginosa* but are not associated with biofilm formation.

4. **The answer is A.** [I B] Both *Pseudomonas* exotoxin A and diphtheria toxin of *C. diphtheriae* inhibit protein synthesis through the inhibition of EF-2. Incorrect choices include Shiga toxin, which is a cytotoxin, enterotoxin, and neurotoxin. *V. cholerae* enterotoxin and *E. coli* LT both result in increased cAMP.

5. **The answer is A.** [VI L] *The* cord factor of Mycobacteria tuberculosis helps trigger the Th1 response, which helps contain the infection.

6. **The answer is A.** [IX O] *C. difficile* has been shown to be the major causative agent of pseudomembranous colitis, which causes diarrhea that most commonly starts after 3 to 4 days of antibiotic administration.

7. **The answer is B.** [IX I] *V. cholerae* causes classic cholera, which is not generally mild or self-limited; *V. parahaemolyticus*, in contrast, causes a relatively mild gastroenteritis and is associated with raw fish. *S. typhi* is the causative agent of typhoid. Shigellae infections are always invasive and generally will have a little pus in the stool.

8. **The answer is D.** [XIV C] Most transmission of plague in the United States is from an infected flea bite. The other route of transmission is through respiratory droplets from patients who have developed pneumonic emboli and pneumonia.

9. **The answer is B.** [VIII E] *S. epidermidis* is ubiquitous as part of the NF. Organisms are introduced into the host during invasive procedures. *S. aureus* is more likely to be acute, with high fever and damage developing more quickly.

10. **The answer is B.** [IX D] *C. botulinum* found in household dust or honey was ingested by the boy and the spores germinated in his GI tract because his NF was not sufficient to suppress the germination. It is the vegetative cells that produce the botulinum toxin. Antibiotics disrupt NF, prolonging the disease, but administration of human antitoxin can dramatically reduce the length of the hospital stay.

11. **The answer is D.** [II D] The gram-positive organism *S. pneumoniae* contains no endotoxin. It is not phagocytosed in the immunologically naive, eliminating choice B. It is the capsule that is considered the most important virulence factor.

12. **The answer is A.** [IX L] *S. typhi* has only human hosts, so this is the only possible correct answer of those listed.

13. **The answer is B.** [VII A] The mother is likely to be colonized with GBSs (*S. algalactiae*). If the labor is prolonged after rupture of the membranes, the baby is more likely to be infected. And, since she delivered before her due date and had her baby at home, she was not screened for GBSs and did not receive intrapartum antibiotics to prevent infection of the baby. The other descriptions are (A) *Enterococcus*, (B) *S. pneumoniae*, and (C) viridans strep.

14. **The answer is D.** [IX P] A major survival and virulence factor of *H. pylori* is urease, which neutralizes stomach acid to allow the organism to survive to reach the tissue.

15. **The answer is B.** [I C] Of the answer choices, only streptococci and staphylococci are gram positive. The streptococci are catalase negative and staphylococci are catalase positive. Of the two staphylococci, *S. aureus* is the β-hemolytic, coagulase-positive organism.

16. **The answer is A.** [I A] Since all *Enterobacteriaceae* generally produce nitrate reductase, they all eventually produce a positive dipstick nitrite test. *Escherichia* is the only choice belonging to this family. Other members of *Enterobacteriaceae* that cause UTIs include *Proteus* and *Klebsiella*. Staph and Strep are gram positive and *Vibrio* is a genus of gram-negative, comma-shaped bacteria. A positive nitrite test rules out *S. saprophyticus* as the cause of a UTI.

17. **The answer is B.** [VI K] *Bacillus* is the correct genus. There are two gram-positive spore-forming rods. *Bacillus* is aerobic with one species (*B. anthracis*), causing hemorrhagic lymphadenitis and pulmonary edema. The other genus with bacterial endospores, the *Clostridia*, does not grow aerobically. The other gram-positive organism listed, *Actinomyces*, often described as a branching bacterium, is also anaerobic. *Campylobacter* and *Haemophilus* are both gram negative.

18. **The answer is B.** [XII C] Notice that the question specifically asks about demonstrating the presence of treponemes and not making the diagnosis of syphilis. The lesions are still present, which suggests that it is too early for serologic methods to be reliable. *T. pallidum* is only cultured by research labs. Because treponemes are so thin in cross-section, they do not reliably show up on a Gram stain; thus, dark-field or FA (not mentioned as a choice) staining would be necessary.

19. **The answer is B.** [VII] None of the bacteria listed as choices are reliably visualized on Gram stain, and none of them are likely to cause meningitis in this scenario. It is much more likely to be a nonbacterial cause, such as an enterovirus.

20. **The answer is D.** [VI L] Fluorochrome dyes, like auramine-rhodamine screening for *M. tuberculosis*, lack the specificity of either direct or indirect FA tests because the FA tests use antibodies, making them more specific. The fluorochrome dyes are more sensitive than a comparable AFS on a bright field light microscope because they light up the microbes on a black background when viewed with the fluorescent microscope. However, the use of antibodies in the IFAs makes them highly specific.

4

Viruses

I. NATURE OF HUMAN VIRUSES

A. Virus particles are called **virions**.
   1. Virions are composed of either RNA or DNA that is encased in a protein coat called a **capsid**.
   2. They are either naked or enveloped, depending on whether the capsid is surrounded by a lipoprotein **envelope**.
   3. Virions replicate only in living cells and therefore are **obligate intracellular parasites**.
   4. Almost all cannot be observed with a light microscope. The exceptions are mimivirus, mollivirus, faustovirus, marseillevirus, and pithovirus (the giant viruses) that infect amoeba, which have been detected in human specimens.

B. Viral genome
   1. The viral genome may be single stranded or double stranded, linear or circular, and segmented or nonsegmented.
   2. Its characteristics are used as one criterion for viral classification.
   3. Viral-specific enzymes, other proteins within the virion, or both may be associated with the genome.

C. Viral capsid
   1. The capsid is composed of repeating structural units called **capsomeres,** which are protomer aggregates of **viral-specific polypeptides**.
   2. They are classified as **helical, icosahedral** (a 20-sided polygon), or **complex**; this is used as a criterion for viral classification.
   3. It serves four functions:
      a. Protects the viral genome from physical or enzymatic damage.
      b. Is the site of receptors necessary for naked viruses to initiate infection.
      c. Stimulates antibody production.
      d. Is the site of antigenic determinants important in some serologic tests.

D. The **viral nucleocapsid** refers to the capsid and enclosed viral genome and is identical to the virion in naked viruses.

E. Viral envelope
   1. The viral envelope surrounds the nucleocapsid of enveloped viruses and is composed of **viral-specific glycoproteins**, **host-cell-derived lipids** and **lipoproteins, and possibly captured host proteins.**
   2. It contains molecules necessary for enveloped viruses to initiate infection, act as a stimulus for antibody production, and serve as antigens in serologic tests; it also forms the basis of ether sensitivity of a virus due to the presence of lipids.

F. Viroporins

1. These **small, hydrophobic virus-encoded proteins** oligomerize at host-cell membranes where they are involved in enveloped virus budding and nonenveloped virus cellular lysis (see section III on Viral Replication and Genetics). They modulate host-cell permeability to ions and small molecules. They may also be involved in viral entry and genome replication.
2. They **form hydrophilic pores** that disrupt physiologic properties of the host cell, thereby contributing to viral pathogenicity such as in virus-induced apoptosis.

II. VIRAL CLASSIFICATION

Classification is based on chemical and physical properties of virions. Viruses are classified into **major families**, which are further subdivided by physiochemical and serologic characteristics into **genera**. Viruses may also be classified by their mode of replication. The Baltimore classification schema categorizes viruses by their genome (Figure 4.1).

A. DNA viruses

1. Human viruses contain double-stranded DNA (except for parvoviruses and *Anelloviridae* family members).
2. They are naked viruses (except for herpesviruses, poxviruses, and hepadnaviruses).
3. They have icosahedral capsids and replicate in the nucleus (except for poxviruses).

B. RNA viruses

1. RNA viruses contain single-stranded RNA (except for *Reoviridae* family members: reoviruses, rotaviruses, coltiviruses, orthoreoviruses, and orbiviruses).
2. They are enveloped (except for caliciviruses, picornaviruses, and reoviruses).

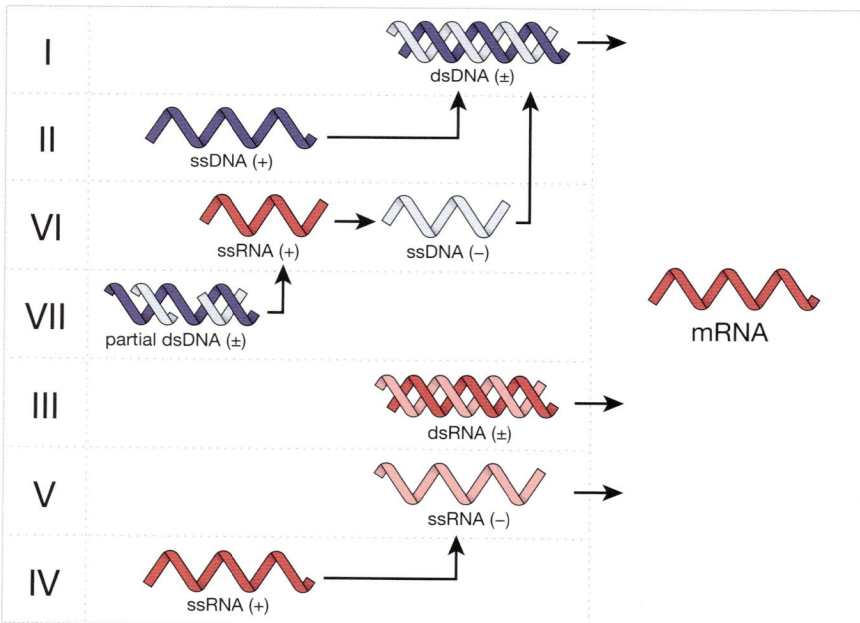

FIGURE 4.1. Baltimore classification of virus by mRNA synthesis. The Nobel laureate David Baltimore developed this model to describe both mRNA synthesis and genome replication. All virus genomes must have a path to the synthesis of mRNA for viral protein production. Group I are double-stranded DNA viruses; group II are single-stranded DNA viruses; group VI are the retroviruses that have single-stranded positive-sense RNA genome going from an RNA to DNA intermediate; group VII is a partially double-stranded DNA virus that goes from an RNA to DNA intermediate; group III are double-stranded RNA viruses; group V are single-stranded negative-sense RNA viruses; group IV are single-stranded positive-sense RNA viruses. (Created by Audrey Bell.)

3. They are known to have helical or icosahedral capsids.
4. They are classified as positive, negative, or ambisense, depending on the ability of virion RNA to act as messenger RNA (mRNA).
5. They replicate in the cytoplasm (except for orthomyxoviruses and retroviruses, which have both a cytoplasmic and a nuclear phase).

III. VIRAL REPLICATION AND GENETICS

A. **General characteristics of viral replication:** Replication occurs only in living cells. It may lead to the death of the host cell (**virulent viruses**) or may occur without apparent damage to the host cell (**moderate viruses**). Replication involves many host-cell enzymes and functions, including attachment, penetration, uncoating of the viral genome, synthesis of early proteins involved in genome replication, synthesis of late proteins (structural components of the virion), assembly, and release (Figure 4.2).

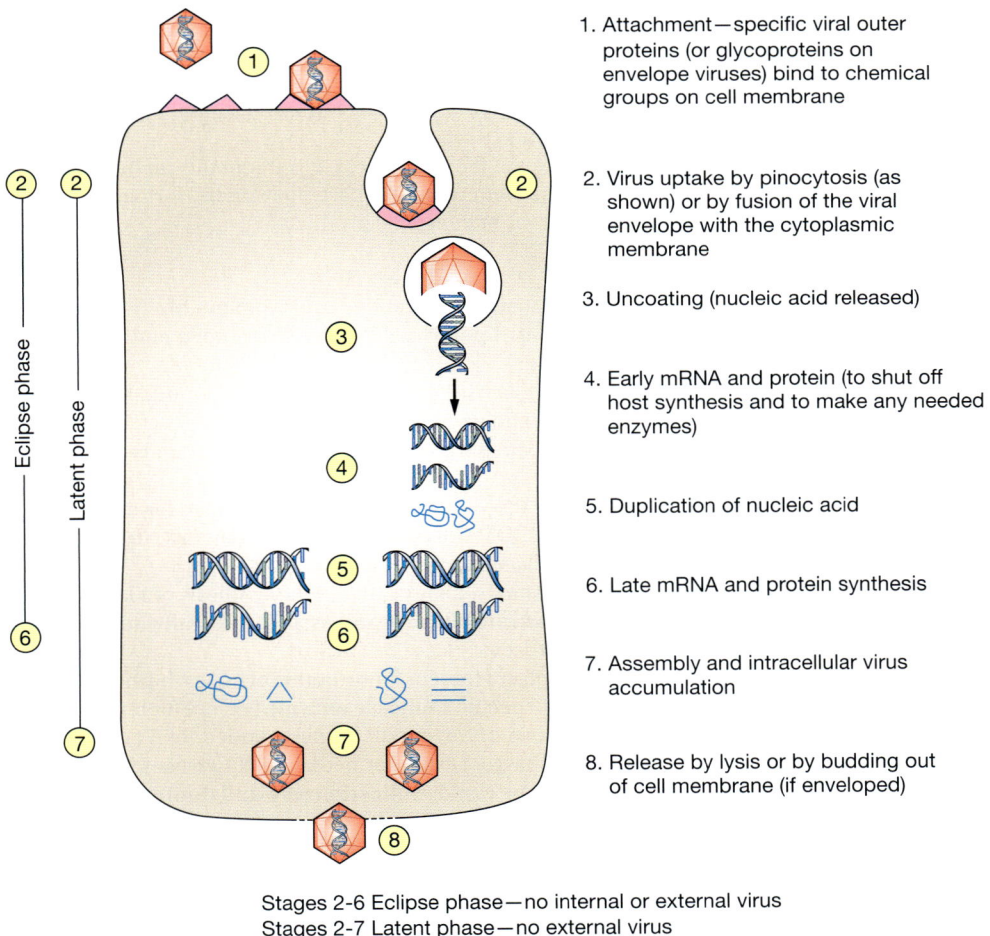

1. Attachment—specific viral outer proteins (or glycoproteins on envelope viruses) bind to chemical groups on cell membrane

2. Virus uptake by pinocytosis (as shown) or by fusion of the viral envelope with the cytoplasmic membrane

3. Uncoating (nucleic acid released)

4. Early mRNA and protein (to shut off host synthesis and to make any needed enzymes)

5. Duplication of nucleic acid

6. Late mRNA and protein synthesis

7. Assembly and intracellular virus accumulation

8. Release by lysis or by budding out of cell membrane (if enveloped)

Stages 2-6 Eclipse phase—no internal or external virus
Stages 2-7 Latent phase—no external virus

FIGURE 4.2. Viral replication: overview of a generalized infection. The eclipse phase is the time from uptake of the virus to just before the assembly of the first intracellular virus (stages 2-6). The latent phase is the time from the initial infection to just before the first release of the extracellular virus (stages 2-7). (Modified from Hawley LB. *High-Yield Microbiology and Infectious Diseases.* 2nd ed. Lippincott Williams & Wilkins; 2006:20-24.)

1. **Attachment** involves the interaction of **viral attachment proteins** (**VAPs**), **located either on the capsid or contained in the viral envelope**, and specific host-cell receptor sites. It plays an important role in viral pathogenesis, determining **viral cell tropism**; it may be inhibited by antibodies (neutralizing antibodies) against viral receptors or cellular receptor sites.
2. **Penetration** can occur by a cellular mechanism called **receptor-mediated endocytosis**, which is referred to as **viropexis** when viruses are involved. The virus envelope may fuse with the plasma membrane of the host cell.
3. **Uncoating** refers to the separation of the capsid from the viral genome. It results in the loss of virion infectivity.
4. **Budding** is the process by which enveloped viruses obtain their envelope; it confers infectivity to enveloped viruses. Budding is preceded by the insertion of virus-specific glycoproteins into the membranes of the host cell. It occurs most frequently at the plasma membrane but also occurs at other membranes.

B. Replication in DNA viruses
1. **Transcription** occurs in the host-cell nucleus (except for poxviruses) and is regulated by host-cell DNA-dependent RNA polymerases (except for virion-associated RNA polymerase as with poxviruses). It occurs in a specific temporal pattern, such as immediate early, delayed early, and late mRNA transcription. It may be followed by **posttranscriptional processing** of primary mRNA transcripts (late adenovirus transcripts).
2. **Translation** occurs on cytoplasmic polysomes and is followed by transport of newly synthesized proteins to the nucleus (except for poxviruses).
3. **Genome replication** occurs after the synthesis of the early proteins. It is semiconservative and is performed by a DNA-dependent DNA polymerase, which may be supplied by the host cell (adenoviruses) or may be virus specific (herpesviruses).
4. **Assembly** takes place in the nucleus (except for poxviruses). It is frequently an inefficient process that leads to accumulation of viral proteins that may participate in the formation of **inclusion bodies** (focal accumulations of virions or viral gene products).

C. Replication in RNA viruses
1. The **viral genome** may be single stranded or double stranded, and segmented or nonsegmented.
   a. It may have **messenger (positive-sense) polarity** if it is single stranded and able to act as mRNA (picornaviruses and retroviruses).
   b. It may have **antimessenger (negative-sense) polarity** if it is single stranded and complementary to mRNA (orthomyxoviruses and paramyxoviruses).
   c. It is **ambisense** if it is single stranded with portions of messenger polarity and antimessenger polarity (arenaviruses).
2. **Transcription** involves a viral-specified RNA-dependent RNA polymerase for all viruses, except retroviruses, which use a host-cell, DNA-dependent RNA polymerase in the nucleus. Negative-sense viruses use a virion-associated enzyme (**transcriptase**).
3. **Translation** occurs on cytoplasmic polysomes. It may result in the synthesis of a large polyprotein that is subsequently cleaved (in **posttranslational processing**) into individual viral polypeptides (eg, picornaviruses and retroviruses).
4. **Genome replication** occurs in the cytoplasm (except for orthomyxoviruses, bornaviruses, and retroviruses) and is performed by a viral-specific **replicase enzyme** (except for retroviruses). A replicative intermediate RNA structure is required for all single-stranded RNA genomes, with the exception of retroviruses which also have a DNA intermediate. **RNA viruses have a higher mutation rate than DNA viruses due to the rapid replication rate and limited proofreading capacity of viral polymerase.**

D. Genetics
1. **Phenotypic mixing** results when surface antigens from two related viruses enclose the genome of one of the viruses.
2. **Phenotypic masking (transcapsidation)** occurs when pairs or related viruses infect the same cell. It results when the genome of one virus is surrounded by the capsid or capsid and envelope of the other virus.

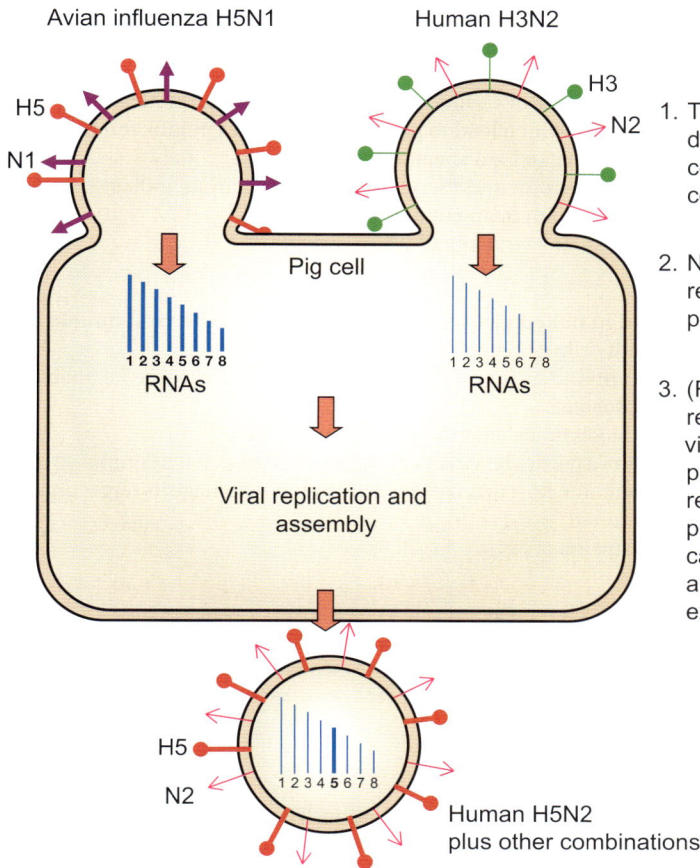

Avian influenza H5N1

Human H3N2

H5
N1
H3
N2

Pig cell

1 2 3 4 5 6 7 8
RNAs

1 2 3 4 5 6 7 8
RNAs

Viral replication and
assembly

H5
N2
1 2 3 4 5 6 7 8

Human H5N2
plus other combinations

**Genetic reassortment =
genetic shift**

1. Two influenza A viruses from
different animals co-infect one
cell. Each of the 8 RNAs carries
code for a gene product.

2. NOT SHOWN: Each virus
replicates all RNAs and all
proteins.

3. (Remember two viruses have
replicated in one cell.) In the
viral assembly, the viral RNAs
package randomly (genetic
reassortment), which may
produce a new virus that now
can infect humans (eg, H5N2)
and for which there is no preexisting immunity.

FIGURE 4.3. Major antigenic changes, called genetic shift or gene reassortment, occur when a single cell is coin-fected with two different strains of the same segmented virus. (Modified from Hawley LB. *High-Yield Microbiology and Infectious Diseases.* 2nd ed. Lippincott Williams & Wilkins; 2007.)

3. **Complementation** can occur when two mutants of the same virus or, less frequently, two mu-tants of different large DNA viruses infect the same cell. It results when one mutant virus sup-plies an enzyme or factor that the other mutant lacks.
4. **Genetic reassortment** can occur when two strains of a segmented RNA virus infect a cell. It results in a stable change in the viral genome (**Figure 4.3**).
5. **Viral vectors** can be constructed with recombinant DNA technology and allow gene transfer into cells. They have been used as an approach to treat diseases, particularly monogenic disorders and some cancers, and are being studied as agents to immunize against other infectious agents.

IV. VIRAL PATHOGENESIS

A. **General characteristics:** Viral pathogenesis is the process of disease production following infection. It may lead to **clinical** or **subclinical** (asymptomatic) disease. Several viral and host factors are involved.
   1. **Viral entry into a host**
      a. Viruses enter the host most often through the mucosa of the respiratory tract but may also enter through the mucosa of the gastrointestinal (GI) or genitourinary (GU) tract or via dam-aged skin.
      b. Entry can be accomplished by direct virus injection into the bloodstream via a needle or an insect bite.

2. **Asymptomatic viral disease** may also be called **subclinical infection** because no clinical symptoms are evident. It occurs with most viral infections and can stimulate humoral and cellular immunity.

3. **Clinical viral disease** results from direct or indirect viral effects (eg, viral-induced cytolysis, immunologic attack on infected cells), which lead to physiologic changes in infected tissues. It is associated with a particular **target organ** for a specific virus.
   a. Disease does not always follow infection and therefore is not an accurate indicator of viral infection; it occurs much less often than in apparent infection.
   b. It frequently depends on the size of the viral inoculum.

B. Viral aspects of pathogenesis

1. **VAPs located on the viral capsid in naked viruses or contained within the viral membrane of enveloped viruses** interact with cellular receptor sites to initiate infection.
   a. VAPs may react with specific antibodies (neutralizing antibodies) and become incapable of interaction with cellular receptor sites.
   b. pH, enzymes, and other host biochemical factors can inactivate VAPs.

2. **Viral virulence** refers to the ability of a particular viral strain to cause disease. It is a composite of all the factors that allow a virus to overcome host defense mechanisms and damage its target organ.
   a. Virulence is genetically determined.
   b. It is decreased in **attenuated strains** of virus.

● ● ● Clinical Pearl

Viral cytopathogenesis may occur as a result of viral replication such as (1) inhibition of cellular protein synthesis for preferential viral protein production, (2) alteration of cell membrane structure and increased permeability due to enveloped virus egress, (3) disruption of cellular cytoskeleton, and (4) syncytia formation or toxicity of virion components.

C. Cellular aspects of pathogenesis

1. **Cellular receptor sites** interact with VAPs to initiate infection. They help determine **cell tropism** of viruses. The presence or absence of particular sites may be determined by the differentiation stage of a cell.

2. **Cell tropism** refers to the propensity of a virus to infect and replicate in a cell. For infection to occur a cell must be susceptible to virus entry and permissive for viral replication. Tropism is largely determined by the interaction of virus attachment proteins and cellular receptor sites and the cell's ability to provide other components (eg, substrates and enzymes) essential for viral replication.

3. The **target organ** is responsible for the major clinical signs of a viral infection and is largely determined by viral virulence and cell tropism.

4. **Cellular responses to viral infection** result in clinical disease. These responses may be inapparent or may include:
   a. Cytopathic effects.
   b. Cytolysis.
   c. Inclusion body formation.
   d. Chromosomal aberrations.
   e. Transformation.
   f. Interferon (IFN) synthesis.

5. **Cytopathogenic effects** include inhibition of host-cell macromolecular biosynthesis, alterations of the plasma membrane and lysosomes, and development of **inclusion bodies** (Table 4.1).
   a. Infectious virus progeny may not be produced.
   b. Effects may aid in identification of certain viruses (eg, polykaryocyte formation by measles virus).

D. Types of infections

1. **Inapparent infections** occur when too few cells are infected to cause clinical symptoms; they are synonymous with **subclinical disease** (Figure 4.4).
   a. Sufficient antibody stimulation can cause immunity from further infections.
   b. They frequently occur when the virus inoculum is small.

Table 4.1	Viral Inclusion Bodies		
Virus	**Inclusion Site**	**Staining Properties**	**Inclusion Name**
Adenovirus	Nucleus	B	—
Cytomegalovirus	Nucleus	B	Owl's eye
Herpes simplex virus	Nucleus	A	Cowdry type A
Measles virus	Both	A	—
Poxvirus	Cytoplasm	A	Guarnieri bodies (smallpox)
			Molluscum bodies (molluscum contagiosum)
Rabies virus	Cytoplasm	A	Negri body
Reovirus	Cytoplasm	A	—
Rubella virus	Cytoplasm	A	—

A, acidophilic; B, basophilic.

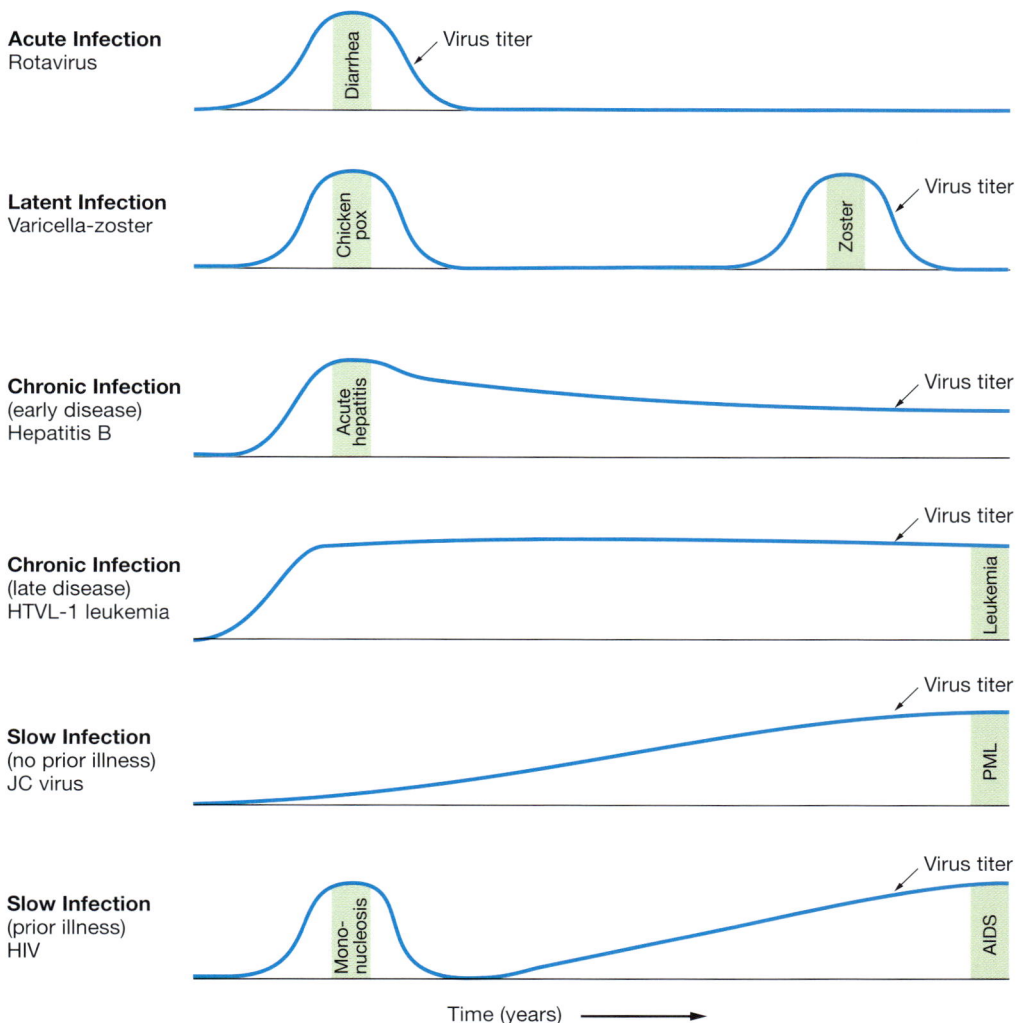

FIGURE 4.4. Patterns of viral disease. AIDS, acquired immune deficiency syndrome; HIV, human immunodeficiency virus; HTVL-1, human T-lymphotropic virus; PML, progressive multifocal leukoencephalopathy.

2. **Acute infections** occur when clinical manifestations of disease are observed for a short time (days to weeks) after a short incubation period.
   a. Recovery is associated with elimination of the virus from the body.
   b. Acute infections are classified as **localized** or **disseminated**, depending on whether the virus has traveled from its site of implantation to its target organ.
   c. **Persistent** or **latent** infections may follow acute infection.
3. **Persistent infections** are associated with the continuing presence of the infectious virus in the body for an extended, perhaps lifelong, period. For persistence to occur, the virus must not be overly cytolytic, avoid host defenses, maintain the integrity of the genome, and be able to reactivate if existing in a latent state.
   a. Clinical symptoms may or may not be present.
   b. Persistently infected individuals are known as **carriers**.
   c. Constant viral antigenic stimulation leads to high antibody titers for some antigens.
4. **Latent infections** occur when the infecting virus persists in the body in a noninfectious form that can periodically reactivate to produce infectious viruses and clinical diseases; they are synonymous with **recurrent diseases**.
   a. An antibody stimulus is produced only during the initial (**primary**) infection and during recurrent episodes.
   b. Subclinical reactivations may occur.
   c. Latent infections are difficult to detect in cells because viral antigen production is not detected and cytopathology is not observed during "silent" periods.
5. **Slow infections** have a **prolonged incubation** period lasting months or years.
   a. These infections do not cause clinical symptoms during incubation but can produce some infectious agents.
   b. They are most often associated with **chronic, progressive, fatal viral diseases of the central nervous system** (CNS), such as kuru and Creutzfeldt-Jakob disease.

E. **Patterns of acute disease**
1. **Localized disease** occurs when viral multiplication and cell damage remain localized to the site of viral entry into the body.
   a. Localized disease has a short incubation time and may cause **systemic clinical features** (eg, **fever**).
   b. Pronounced viremia (virions in the blood) does not usually occur.
   c. Sites include the **respiratory tract** (eg, influenza, rhinovirus), **alimentary tract** (eg, picornaviruses, rotaviruses), **GU tract** (eg, papillomavirus), and the **eye** (eg, adenovirus).
   d. Disease can spread over the surface of the body to other areas where it causes another localized infection (eg, picornavirus-induced conjunctivitis).
   e. The immune response that is induced is much weaker than the response induced by disseminated infections.
2. **Disseminated infections** involve the spread of a virus from its entry site to a target organ. They involve a **primary viremia** and perhaps a **secondary viremia**.
   a. Incubation time is moderate (eg, weeks), allowing more time for the host's immune system to eliminate the viral infection.
   b. The **main clinical symptoms are usually associated with infection of one target organ**, although infection of other organs may be involved.
   c. A substantial immune response is generated that frequently confers lifelong immunity to the host.
   d. **Viral dissemination** is a major feature of disseminated infections.
      (1) Viruses may travel in other cells (red blood cells and mononuclear peripheral white blood cells), the plasma, extracellular spaces, and nerve fibers.
      (2) Viruses can be prevented from disseminating by viral-specific cytotoxic cells and neutralizing antibodies.
3. **Congenital infections** are viral infections of a fetus and are caused by maternal viremia.
   a. These infections cross the placental barrier.
   b. They are serious because of the immaturity of the fetal immune system and the undifferentiated state and rapid multiplication of fetal cells.
   c. These infections may lead to **maldeveloped organs in the fetus.**

V. DNA VIRUSES

DNA viruses that have been determined to cause human disease are classified into seven families (Table 4.2). The replication of all viral DNA occurs in the nucleus except for poxviruses, which replicate entirely in the cytoplasm. Some DNA viruses can produce latent infections and all except parvoviruses can experimentally transform cells.

A. Naked DNA viruses

1. **Human adenoviruses**
   a. **Description: naked DNA viruses** with an **icosahedral nucleocapsid** composed of **hexons, pentons, and fibers.**
   b. **Classification:** are classified into more than 60 serotypes.
   c. **Genome:** contains **double-stranded DNA** that replicates asymmetrically.
   d. **Replication:** replicate in the nucleus of epithelial cells.
   e. **Clinical disease**
      (1) Causes localized infections of the eye, respiratory and GI tracts, and urinary bladder depending on serotype.
      (2) Frequently causes subclinical infections and can cause **latent infections of lymphoid tissue** (eg, **tonsils**).
   f. **Diagnosis:** may be diagnosed by virus isolation, antigen enzyme-linked immunosorbent assay (ELISA), or polymerase chain reaction (PCR) depending on the syndrome from specimens of the eyes, throat, urine, or feces.

2. **Papillomaviruses**
   a. **Description: naked viruses** with an **icosahedral capsid** and **double-stranded circular DNA**.
   b. **Classification:** exist in more than 100 different subtypes.
   c. **Replication:** replicate in epithelial cells of epithelial and mucosal tissue; may form **koilocytotic cells** (cytoplasmic vacuoles and enlarged nuclei) during replication.

Table 4.2	Virion and Nucleic Acid Structure of DNA Viruses				
Virus Family	**Prominent Examples**	**Virion Structure**	**Virion Polymerase**	**Capsid Symmetry**	**DNA Structure**
Adenoviridae	Adenoviruses	Naked	No	Icosahedral	Linear, double stranded
Herpesviridae	Herpes simplex virus	Enveloped	No	Icosahedral	Linear, double stranded
	Varicella-zoster virus				
	Epstein-Barr virus				
	Cytomegalovirus				
Poxviridae	Smallpox virus	Brick shaped, enveloped	Yes	Complex	Linear, double stranded
	Vaccinia virus				
	Molluscum contagiosum virus				
Papillomaviridae	Human papillomavirus	Naked	No	Icosahedral	Circular, double stranded
Polyomaviridae	JC virus	Naked	No	Icosahedral	Circular, double stranded
Hepadnaviridae	Hepatitis B virus	Enveloped	Yes	Icosahedral	Circular, double stranded
Parvoviridae	B19 virus	Naked	No	Icosahedral	Linear, single stranded

    d. Clinical disease
- **(1)** May cause lytic, latent, or transforming human infections depending on the host cell.
- **(2)** Types are categorized as high risk or low risk for cervical intraepithelial neoplasia (CIN).
- **(3) Types 16 and 18 are most associated with CIN** involving the **inactivation of tumor suppression proteins, p53 and p110Rb, by early viral proteins E6 and E7**, respectively.
- **(4)** Types 6 and 11 are associated with genital wart formation.

    e. Prevention
- **(1) Gardasil**, a recombinant viral protein vaccine containing types 6, 11, 16, and 18 viruslike particles, is available for protection.
- **(2) Cervarix**, a recombinant viral protein vaccine, contains types 16 and 18 viruslike particles.

> **● ● ● Clinical Pearl**
>
> For most people, low-risk human papillomavirus (HPV)-type infections are cleared within 1 or 2 years. Viral persistence of high-risk HPV types beyond 2 years of infection increases the risk of cancer development particularly in older individuals.

  3. Parvoviruses
- **a. Description: small, naked viruses** with **icosahedral capsids** containing **single-stranded DNA, with either negative- or positive-sense strand being packaged in the capsid**.
- **b. Clinical disease:** includes one human virus (**B19**) that causes disease involving cytolytic replication in erythroid precursor cells, transient aplastic crisis. Also associated with erythema infectiosum (fifth disease), acute arthritis, and fetal anemia.

  4. Polyomaviruses
- **a. Description: naked viruses** with an **icosahedral capsid** containing **double-stranded circular DNA**.
- **b. Clinical disease:** human viruses, **BK virus** and **JC virus**, which infect the kidney where they usually do not cause disease but become **latent**; when reactivated by immunosuppression, BK causes a urinary tract infection and JC travels to and replicates in oligodendrocytes to cause a neurologic disease (**progressive multifocal leukoencephalopathy**). **Merkel cell polyomavirus** infects Merkel cell skin mechanoreceptors and induces Merkel cell carcinoma.

B. Enveloped DNA viruses
  1. Hepadnaviruses have only one representative that infects humans: **hepatitis B virus** (**HBV**).
- **a. Description: icosahedral capsid containing a partially double-stranded DNA surrounded by an envelope; the virion of HBV is called the Dane particle.**
- **b. Replication:** have a **virion-associated multifunctional enzyme complex with reverse transcriptase (RT), DNA polymerase, and ribonuclease activity,** which is necessary for viral DNA replication.
- **c. Clinical disease:** can cause acute and symptomatic or asymptomatic chronic liver disease and is implicated in primary hepatocellular carcinoma; induces a cell-mediated response that is responsible for symptoms and recovery from the infection. Modulation of multiple cellular pathways influenced by the viral X protein (**HBx** [hepatitis B X]) contributes to the induction of cancer.
- **d. Diagnosis:** produce unique antigens (**HBsAg** [hepatitis B surface antigen], **a surface antigen**, and **HBcAg** [hepatitis B core antigen] and **HBeAg** [hepatitis B e antigen] **core-associated antigens**) associated with infections or their antibodies that are monitored by serologic tests to determine the source of HBV infections and the infection time course.
- **e. Treatment and prevention**
  - **(1)** Has been genetically manipulated to produce a **recombinant subunit vaccine (Recombivax HB and Engerix-B)** or used in a combination vaccine (Twinrix) for protection from hepatitis A virus (HAV) and HBV.
  - **(2)** Chronic infection may be treated with IFN-α or five RT inhibitors.

2. **Herpesviruses** are **enveloped viruses** with an **icosahedral nucleocapsid** containing **double-stranded DNA.**
    a. **Herpes simplex virus (HSV) types 1 and 2**
        (1) **Cytopathology:** can cause cell rounding and polykaryocyte formation or intranuclear inclusion bodies (**Cowdry type A inclusions**) and vesicular eruptions in infected epithelial cells.
        (2) **Replication:** produce a **viral-specific thymidine kinase** that is responsible for a thymidine salvage pathway necessary for DNA replication; it is the target of several antiherpes nucleoside analog drugs like acyclovir.
        (3) **Clinical disease**
            (a) **Latently infect neurons.**
            (b) Produce both acute and latent infections whose clinical lesions occur primarily on mucosal surfaces (lip and genitals) but can cause encephalitis and eye infections as well.
            (c) HSV-1 is considered the primary cause of oral herpes infections, and HSV-2 is considered the primary cause of genital herpes infections.
        (4) **Treatment:** Infections may be treated with antivirals that affect the viral DNA polymerase (foscarnet, trifluridine, or vidarabine) or stop DNA chain elongation (acyclovir, penciclovir, famciclovir, and valacyclovir), but **none eliminate latent infections**.
    b. **Varicella-zoster virus (VZV)**
        (1) **Cytopathology:** produces similar cytopathology to HSV and also **latently infects neurons.**
        (2) **Clinical disease:** causes vesicular skin lesions in both acute (**chickenpox**) and recurrent (**shingles**) diseases.
        (3) **Treatment and prevention:**
            (a) Infections may be treated with nucleoside analog DNA chain terminators (acyclovir, famciclovir, and valacyclovir), but latent infections are not eliminated.
            (b) An attenuated virus, the Oka strain, is used in vaccines to prevent chickenpox and diminish shingles recurrences **but is not recommended in individuals who are immunocompromised**. A recombinant **subunit vaccine is also available.**
    c. **Cytomegalovirus (CMV)**
        (1) **Cytopathology:** causes swelling of infected cells (**cytomegalic cells**) and **"owl's eye" intranuclear inclusion bodies (Cowdry type B inclusions) that do not have the same type A nuclear changes.**
        (2) **Replication:** replicates in epithelial cells of oropharynx, but **latently infects monocytes, macrophages, and lymphocytes**.
        (3) **Clinical disease**
            (a) May depress immune response during initial infection due to interaction of cells involved in cellular immunity.
            (b) Causes a **heterophile-negative mononucleosis** in contrast to Epstein-Barr virus (EBV) mononucleosis and is a potentially serious congenital infection.
            (c) Latent infections are usually reactivated to asymptomatic disease, but reactivation in individuals who are immunosuppressed can be serious (eg, giant cell pneumonia in patients with acquired immunodeficiency syndrome [AIDS]).
        (4) **Treatment:** does not produce its own thymidine kinase but does produce a protein kinase that phosphorylates **ganciclovir, a nucleoside analog** that when incorporated into viral DNA inhibits replication; **cidofovir is phosphorylated by cellular kinases** and also inhibits viral DNA replication.
    d. **Epstein-Barr virus (EBV)**
        (1) **Cytopathology:** can productively infect and abortively infect human B lymphocytes; **abortive infection induces B-cell proliferation and potential transformation. Infection of B cells causes lifelong persistence.**
        (2) **Clinical disease**
            (a) Produces several distinct antigens, including **latent membrane proteins (LMPs), nuclear antigens (EBNAs [Epstein-Barr Nuclear Antigen]), early antigens (EAs), a membrane antigen (MA), and a viral capsid antigen (VCA).**
            (b) Usually causes clinically inapparent infections but may cause **heterophile-positive infectious mononucleosis and is associated with Burkitt lymphoma and nasopharyngeal carcinoma in conjunction with c-myc translocation.**

(3) **Diagnosis:** is associated with the production of **atypical lymphocytes (Downey cells)** and **IgM (immunoglobulin M) heterophile antibodies** (antibodies detected using antigens from a source different from the one used to induce them) identified by the **mononucleosis spot test.**

e. **Human herpesviruses types 6 and 7 (HHVs 6 and 7).**
   (1) **Description: T-lymphotropic viruses** associated with roseola diseases and febrile seizures in infants.
   (2) **Clinical disease:** cause latent infections of peripheral blood lymphocytes and can reactivate during immunosuppression of patients with AIDS who have received transplants.

f. **HHV type 8 (Kaposi sarcoma–associated herpesvirus, HHVS or KSHV).**
   (1) **Pathobiology:** preferentially infect B lymphocytes and appear to be sexually transmitted.
   (2) **Genome:** contain more than 10 homologues of cellular genes (eg, cyclin D, interleukin 6, and so forth) in its genome.
   (3) **Clinical disease**
      (a) **Associated with Kaposi sarcoma, a cancer of the cells that line the lymph and blood vessels, primary effusion lymphoma, and multicentric Castleman disease.**
      (b) Linked to some AIDS-associated B-cell lymphomas.
      (c) Implicated in **multiple myeloma**.

3. **Poxviruses**
   a. **General characteristics**
      (1) **Description**
         (a) **Complex brick-shaped virion** that consists of an **outer envelope enclosing a core containing linear, double-stranded DNA** and two lateral bodies.
         (b) Have more than 100 structural polypeptides, including many enzymes and a transcriptional system associated with the virion.
      (2) **Replication:** replicate in the cytoplasm of the cell.
      (3) **Cytopathology:** produce **eosinophilic inclusion bodies called Guarnieri bodies** and membrane hemagglutinins in infected cells.
      (4) **Classification:** include **human viruses** (vaccina, variola, human Mpox [monkeypox], and molluscum contagiosum) and **animal viruses** (cowpox virus, paravaccinia virus [in cows], and orf virus [in sheep]); the animal viruses can cause highly localized occupational infections (usually of the finger).
   b. **Variola virus** causes smallpox.
   c. **Vaccinia virus** is the variant of variola virus that generally produces only a mild disease and is used as the immunogen in smallpox vaccination. It is being studied as a **possible immunizing vector** containing foreign genes for polypeptides, which would elicit neutralizing antibodies for other viruses (eg, HSV types 1 and 2).
   d. **Molluscum contagiosum virus** infects epithelial cells, where it causes a localized disease involving small, wartlike lesions on the face, arms, back, buttocks, and genitals that usually resolves spontaneously in several months; it also **causes a sexually transmitted disease** with papular lesions that can ulcerate and mimic genital herpes.
   e. **Mpox** virus is transmitted by contact with infected skin or lesions present in the mouth or on the genitals. The virus causes a characteristic blister-like rash which may be painful and may appear anywhere on the body. The infection usually resolves within 2 to 4 weeks.

VI. RNA VIRUSES

Although both naked and enveloped RNA viruses exist, they are usually discussed based on the nature of their RNA genome, which may be single stranded or double stranded. There are, therefore, four categories of RNA viruses: (1) **positive sense** (virion ssRNA can serve as mRNA), (2) **negative sense** (ssRNA complementary to the virion RNA serves as mRNA), (3) **ambisense** (virion RNA has portions of both positive-sense and negative-sense RNA), and (4) **double stranded** (virion RNA is double stranded). All of these viruses except the influenza viruses and HIV (human immunodeficiency virus) replicate entirely in the **cytoplasm** of the cell, and since cells lack cytoplasm RNA polymerase, they must code for and produce their own. All negative-sense RNA viruses are enveloped and an RNA polymerase acts as a transcriptase or replicase associated with the virion. Many RNA viruses have developed unique mechanisms to produce individual polypeptides from polycistronic RNA.

A. Positive-sense viruses (Table 4.3)

1. Caliciviruses
   a. Description: naked viruses with an **icosahedral nucleocapsid** that **contain positive-sense, single-stranded RNA**.
   b. Classification: have been classified into four genera, of which two infect humans to cause gastroenteritis; those belonging to the **Norovirus genus** (previously called *Norwalk agents*) cause epidemics of gastroenteritis associated with contaminated food and are transmitted via the fecal-oral route.

> ● ● ● **Clinical Pearl**
>
> Outbreak settings for Norovirus are more frequently experienced in restaurants, nursing facilities, and school locations than in vacation settings such as cruise ships.

Table 4.3   Virion and Nucleic Acid Structure of Positive-Sense RNA Viruses

Virus Family	Prominent Examples	Virion Structure	Virion Polymerase	Capsid Symmetry	RNA Structure
Caliciviridae	Norwalk agent	Naked	No	Icosahedral	Linear single stranded, nonsegmented
Picornaviridae	Coxsackieviruses, Echoviruses, Enteroviruses, Hepatitis A virus, Polioviruses, Rhinoviruses	Naked	No	Icosahedral	Linear, single stranded, nonsegmented
Flaviviridae	Dengue virus, Hepatitis C virus, St. Louis encephalitis virus, Yellow fever virus	Enveloped	No	Icosahedral	Linear, single stranded, nonsegmented
Togaviridae	Eastern, Western, and Venezuelan equine encephalomyelitis viruses	Enveloped	No	Icosahedral	Linear, single stranded, nonsegmented
Retroviridae	Human immunodeficiency virus, Leukemia viruses, Sarcoma viruses	Enveloped	No[a]	Helical	Linear, single stranded, nonsegmented[a]
Coronaviridae	Coronaviruses, SARS-CoV	Enveloped	No	Helical	Linear, single stranded, nonsegmented

[a]Retroviruses are diploid and have reverse transcriptase.

2. Coronaviruses
   a. Description
      (1) Enveloped viruses with a **helical nucleocapsid that contains single-stranded RNA with positive (messenger) polarity.**

(2) Have distinctive club-shaped surface projections (spike proteins) that give the appearance of a solar corona to the virion.

b. Clinical disease: Four types most frequently associated with the common cold in adults and gastroenteritis in infants. Three types, **SARS-CoV-1** (severe acute respiratory syndrome coronavirus 1), **MERS**-CoV (Middle East respiratory syndrome coronavirus), **and SARS-CoV-2, are zoonotic infections that cause severe acute respiratory syndrome.**

3. Flaviviruses

a. General characteristics

(1) Description: enveloped viruses with a **single-stranded, positive-sense RNA** and **an imperfect icosahedral symmetry.**

(2) Replication: replicate in the cytoplasm of the cell, where the RNA is translated into a large polyprotein that is subsequently cleaved (by **posttranslational cleavage**) into individual proteins.

b. Dengue virus

(1) Description: arbovirus transmitted from nonhuman primates and humans to humans by mosquitoes.

(2) Clinical disease

(a) Four serotypes exist; antibodies (called **"enhancing" antibodies**) to one serotype increase the efficiency of infection by another serotype, resulting in more serious disease.

(b) Causes characteristic skin lesions as well as fever with muscle and joint pain; is sometimes called **break bone fever.**

(c) Can cause dengue hemorrhagic fever.

(d) A vaccine, Denvaxia, is available for children ages 9 to 16 years, when they have been previously infected with dengue and living in areas where dengue is common.

c. Hepatitis C virus (HCV)

(1) Description: also known as **non-A, non-B hepatitis virus,** exists in **six genotypes** with different worldwide distribution.

(2) Clinical disease

(a) Infects the body after parenteral entry and **causes 90% of blood transfusion-associated or blood product administration-associated hepatitis.**

(b) Can cause **chronic infections** involving carrier state individuals and is **implicated in primary hepatocellular carcinoma.**

(3) Diagnosis: by ELISA serology and **molecular genotyping of circulating virions** to determine the patient's likelihood to respond to treatment with IFN-α and ribavirin since only two genotypes respond.

(4) Treatment: currently three classes of direct-acting anti-HCV drugs that function as protease and polymerase inhibitors. HCV is the only virus capable of being cured at present.

d. St. Louis encephalitis virus

(1) Description: an **arbovirus** with a mosquito vector that transfers the virus from wild birds to humans.

(2) Clinical disease: usually causes inapparent infections but may produce encephalitis.

e. Yellow fever virus

(1) Description: arbovirus that is usually transferred from primates to humans by mosquitoes.

(2) Clinical disease

(a) Causes a biphasic disease with clinical signs involving the vascular endothelium during initial virus replication and involving the liver during later replication resulting in jaundice.

(b) Can cause chronic infections; therefore, individuals with the virus are in a carrier state.

(c) Can result in a hemorrhagic disease.

(3) Diagnosis: by **eosinophilic hyaline masses called Councilman bodies** in the cytoplasm of infected liver cells.

(4) Prevention: by immunization with the **attenuated vaccine strain 17D.**

f. West Nile virus (WNV)
   (1) Description: arbovirus that is transferred from a bird reservoir (especially crows and jays) to humans by a mosquito vector; **leading cause of arboviral encephalitis in the United States.**
   (2) Clinical disease: causes an encephalitis that is most serious for those older than 50 years of age. Can also result in extremity weakness.

> ••• **Clinical Pearl**
>
> Most (70%-80%) of WNV cases are asymptomatic, and approximately 19% to 29% experience only mild symptoms. However, less than 1% of cases may experience severe neurologic complications.

4. Hepevirus (hepatitis E-like viruses)
   a. Description: naked viruses with a **single-stranded, positive-sense RNA genome,** which has been divided into **four genotypes**.
   b. Clinical disease: produces a hepatitis transmitted by the fecal-oral route but not endemic in the United States.
5. Picornaviruses
   a. General characteristics
      (1) Description: small, naked viruses with an **icosahedral nucleocapsid** that contains **single-stranded, positive-sense RNA covalently linked to a small protein** (**VPg [viral protein genome linked]** in poliovirus).
      (2) Replication: replicate in the cytoplasm of the cell, where RNA is translated into a large polyprotein that is subsequently cleaved (**posttranslational cleavage**).
      (3) Classification: classified into nine genera, currently five (**enteroviruses, hepatoviruses, kobuviruses, parechoviruses, and rhinoviruses) cause human disease.**
   b. Enteroviruses cause a variety of human diseases involving infections of the alimentary tract (are stable at **acidic pH 3-5**). Transmission can occur through direct contact with infected body secretions or feces or fomites. They include polioviruses, coxsackie A and B viruses, and echoviruses.
      (1) Coxsackie viruses
         (a) Classification: divided into two groups, depending on the type of paralysis they cause following inoculation into mice (**group A causes flaccid paralysis; group B causes spastic paralysis**).
         (b) Clinical disease: cause a variety of diseases involving enanthems and exanthems (rashes), the eye, and the meninges.
            1. Group B are cardiotrophic and can cause severe chest pain due to the infection of muscles between the ribs.
            2. Cause infections that tend to occur in summer and early fall.
            3. Are most often not identified during infections but are simply classified as enteroviral disease.
      (2) Echoviruses
         (a) Clinical disease: cause diseases similar to coxsackie viruses except not particularly associated with heart disease or chest pain; most associated with aseptic meningitis.
         (b) Diagnosis: not frequently identified during infections but are simply classified as enteroviral infections.
      (3) Enteroviruses cause diseases similar to coxsackie and echoviruses, particularly CNS and eye infections.
      (4) Polioviruses
         (a) Classification: exist in three serotypes.
         (b) Pathobiology: spread in the body by hematogenous and neural routes.
         (c) Clinical disease
            1. Replicate in the intestine where they usually produce an asymptomatic infection but can spread to the spinal cord and CNS via neural pathways.
            2. Destroy anterior horn cells of the spinal cord as a result of replication there.
            3. May cause a rare paralytic disease as a result of invasion of the CNS.

(d) Prevention: The three serotypes have been inactivated and combined in a **trivalent vaccine (Salk vaccine)**; live attenuated strains were present in the Sabin vaccine, which is no longer recommended.

c. Hepatovirus
   (1) Description: contains the **hepatitis A viruses** that replicate in hepatocytes where they cause a foodborne or waterborne hepatitis.
   (2) Treatment and prevention: may be treated prophylactically with immune human globulin or prevented by immunization with **killed virus vaccines (Havrix or VAQTA) containing formalin-inactivated virions or a combination vaccine for HAV and HBV (Twinrix).**

d. Kobuviruses are associated with a variety of clinical illnesses including diarrhea, vomiting, fever, conjunctivitis, and respiratory symptoms. The **Aichi A virus 1 species infects humans**. They have a bumpy appearance via electron microscopy and are named "kobu" which means "knob" in Japanese.

e. Parechoviruses
   (1) Description: consist of three human pathogens (HPeV-1, -2, and -3).
   (2) Clinical disease: produce **gastroenteritis** and **respiratory disease;** may occasionally cause aseptic meningitis and encephalitis.

f. Rhinoviruses
   (1) Description: exist in more than 100 serotypes; are **acid labile**.
   (2) Replication: bind to ICAM (intercellular adhesion molecule)-1 and replicate best at 33 °C/91 °F; replication may be inhibited by **pleconaril**, an experimental compound that binds to the capsid and prevents viral attachment to cells.
   (3) Clinical disease: are the leading cause of the **common cold**.

• • • Clinical Pearl

Winter colds are commonly caused by rhinoviruses while colds that occur in the summer months tend to be caused by enteroviruses.

6. Retroviruses
   a. General characteristics
      (1) Description: enveloped viruses with a polymorphic icosahedral capsid.
      (2) Genome
         (a) Contain **two identical copies of single-stranded positive-sense RNA (diploid genome)** with a host tRNA (transfer RNA) bound to the 5′ end and a viral-specified **RT enzyme complex** (RNA-dependent DNA polymerase and RNase activity), integrase enzyme, and protease enzyme.
         (b) Have three notable gene regions: **gag (structural proteins), pol (reverse transcriptase),** and **env (envelope glycoproteins),** which are flanked by **long terminal repeat sequences** in the cDNA form with regulatory functions.
         (c) Use posttranslational cleavage processes during the synthesis of *gag* and *env* gene products.
         (d) Need the host-cell transfer RNA to interact with RT before the RT complex can bind to RNA and initiate DNA synthesis.
      (3) Classification
         (a) Divided morphologically into four types (A, B, C, and D).
         (b) Classified into three groups: **lentiviruses** (HIV), **spumaviruses,** and **oncoviruses** (types B, C, and D RNA tumor viruses).
      (4) Clinical disease: cause mostly "slow" diseases of animals and various cancers, except for HIV, which causes immunosuppression due to depletion of CD4+ helper T cells. There are also limited reports of myelodysplastic syndrome (MDS).
   b. Human immunodeficiency virus type 1 and 2 (HIV-1 and -2)
      (1) Description: members of the lentivirus subfamily and exist as **lymphotropic (CXCR4) and macrophage-tropic (CCR5) strains.**

    (2) Pathobiology

        (a) Initiate infection by interaction of a viral envelope glycoprotein (gp120) with the cellular (CD4) surface receptor, which is expressed on a subset of T cells, macrophages, monocytes, and natural killer cells.

        (b) Synthesize core **proteins (p18, p24, and RT) and transregulatory proteins (*tat rev* and *nef*).**

        (c) Have **regulatory genes (TRE and *rre*).**

        (d) Infect and kill T-helper cells, resulting in depression of both humoral and cell-mediated immunity.

    (3) Clinical disease: cause immunosuppression, leading to opportunistic infections, cancers, and neurologic disorders.

    (4) Treatment: Replication may be inhibited by **seven classes of antivirals: nucleoside analogs and nonnucleoside inhibitors of RT, integrase inhibitors, protease inhibitors, capsid inhibitors, attachment inhibitors, and fusion inhibitors.**

  c. Human T-cell lymphotropic viruses (HTLV-1 and -2) belong to the oncovirus subfamily and are associated with human cancers (**adult T-cell leukemia** [**HTLV-1**], **hairy cell leukemia** [**HTLV-2**]), and a neurologic myelopathy (**tropical spastic paraparesis** [**HTLV-1**]).

7. Togavirus

  a. General characteristics

    (1) Description: enveloped viruses with an **icosahedral nucleocapsid** containing **single- stranded, positive-sense RNA;** have **hemagglutinins** associated with their envelope.

    (2) Classification: divided into four groups of which two (alphaviruses and rubiviruses) are human pathogens.

  b. Alphaviruses

    (1) Description: arboviruses with mosquito vectors and animal reservoirs.

    (2) Clinical disease

        (a) Cause encephalitis or moderate systemic disease following the bite of a mosquito that has fed on an animal viral reservoir.

        (b) Lead to more serious encephalitis than do flaviviruses.

        (c) Include **Eastern equine encephalomyelitis virus (EEEV), Western equine encephalomyelitis virus (WEEV), and Venezuelan equine encephalomyelitis virus (VEEV).**

    (3) Diagnosis: by serologic tests, usually ELISA for IgM, because virus isolation is difficult.

  c. Rubivirus—Rubella virus

    (1) Clinical disease: causes **German measles** in children and **congenital infections with serious consequences** to fetuses infected during the first 10 weeks of pregnancy.

    (2) Diagnosis: by ELISA tests for IgM and immunity determined by ELISA to IgG.

    (3) Prevention: Strain RA 27/3 has been attenuated for use in a live Rubella vaccine.

B. Negative-sense viruses (Table 4.4)

  1. Bunyavirales

    a. Description

      (1) Enveloped arboviruses with **bi- or tri-circular helical nucleocapsids**, each containing a unique piece of **single-stranded, negative-polarity RNA** (L, M, and S segments), viral nucleoprotein (NP), and transcriptase enzyme. Composed of the families of Phenuiviridae, Arenaviridae, Nairoviridae, and Hantaviridae.

      (2) They can interact with viruses that are closely related serologically to produce recombinant viruses by genetic reassortment.

    b. Replication: replicate within the cytoplasm and bud from the membranes of the Golgi apparatus.

    c. Clinical disease

      (1) Have rodent hosts and infect humans during an arthropod bite.

      (2) Cause **mosquito-borne encephalitis (California and LaCrosse encephalitis viruses), sandfly and mosquito-borne fever (sandfly fever virus and Rift Valley fever virus),**

Table 4.4	Virion and Nucleic Acid Structure of Negative-Sense RNA Viruses				
Virus Family	**Prominent Example**	**Virion Structure**	**Virion Polymerase**	**Capsid Symmetry**	**RNA Structure**
Paramyxoviridae	Mumps virus Measles virus Parainfluenza virus Respiratory syncytial virus	Enveloped	Yes	Helical	Linear, single stranded, nonsegmented
Rhabdoviridae	Rabies virus Vesicular stomatitis virus	Enveloped	Yes	Helical	Linear, single stranded, nonsegmented
Filoviridae	Ebola virus Marburg virus	Enveloped	Yes	Helical	Linear, single stranded, nonsegmented
Orthomyxoviridae	Influenza viruses	Enveloped	Yes	Helical	Linear, single stranded, eight segments
Peribunyaviridae	California encephalitis virus Hantavirus	Enveloped	Yes	Helical	Circular, single stranded, three segments
Unclassified (genus: δ virus)	Hepatitis D virus	Naked	No	Helical	Circular, single stranded

rodent-borne hemorrhagic fever (Hantaan virus), and respiratory distress syndrome (Hantavirus).

(3) **Hantavirus (Sin Nombre virus) causes an acute, potentially fatal, pulmonary syndrome** initiated by inhaling the virus contained in dried deer mouse saliva, urine, or feces.

(4) **Arenaviruses: ambisense viruses.**

   (a) **Description: enveloped viruses** with **two string-of-bead nucleocapsids, each containing a unique single-stranded, circular RNA.**

   (b) **Genome:** have two molecules (L or large, and S or small) of single-stranded, ambisense RNA.

   (c) **Replication:** replicate in the cytoplasm and **have host-cell ribosomes in their virion.**

   (d) **Clinical disease**

      1. Infect mice, rats, or both as their natural hosts; are initially passed from rodents to humans but can be transferred by direct human contact.

      2. Cause highly contagious hemorrhagic fevers (Junin, Machupo, and Lassa viruses) that are not endemic to the United States and a meningitis-like illness (**lymphocytic choriomeningitis virus**) that is endemic.

● ● ● Clinical Pearl

Arenaviruses are challenging to diagnose, as many pathogens that cause sepsis and lead to disseminated intravascular coagulation may be considered first in an early diagnosis. This may result in misdiagnosis. Arenaviruses should be considered in areas of higher geographic risk.

2. **Orthomyxoviruses (influenza)**

   a. **General characteristics**

      (1) **Description: enveloped,** spherical or filamentous viruses with **eight helical nucleocapsids** containing a unique single-stranded, **negative-sense RNA**.

(2) Components: have a **hemagglutinin (H), a neuraminidase (N), a matrix protein (M) associated with the envelope, a transcriptase (P) that is associated with the nucleocapsid, and a nucleoprotein (NP) associated with the RNA.**

(a) Influenza virus hemagglutinin
1. This **envelope glycoprotein contains a virus receptor that binds to the cellular receptor site.** Agglutinates many species of red blood cells.
2. It induces neutralizing antibodies and has fusion activity that allows the virion envelope to fuse with the host-cell plasma membranes.
3. Antigenic changes are **responsible for influenza epidemics.** Frequent minor mutations result in antigenic changes, leading to **antigenic drift**; major antigenic changes resulting from reassortment between the hemagglutinin-coding RNA segments of animal or human viruses (see Figure 4.3) cause **antigenic shift.**

(b) Influenza virus neuraminidase
1. This envelope glycoprotein removes terminal sialic acid residues from oligosaccharide chains, resulting in less viscous mucous secretions, thereby facilitating virus spread.
2. It is involved in the release of virions from infected cells.
3. It can undergo antigenic shift and drift mutations; however, epidemics do not result from these changes.
4. Its activity is **inhibited by the antivirals oseltamivir and zanamivir.**

(c) Influenza virus M2 protein This protein forms a proton channel during replication that **facilitates uncoating by acidification** and is rendered nonfunctional in influenza A virus infections by the antivirals amantadine and rimantadine.

(3) They are assembled in the cytoplasm but **have a nuclear phase since they depend on host nuclear functions**, including RNA polymerase II for cap snatching, for transcription.

b. Classification
(1) Are classified as type A, B, or C, depending on a nucleocapsid antigen; A is the only one infecting both animals and humans.
(2) Are designated by the nomenclature: virus type, species isolated from (unless human), site of isolation, strain number, year of isolation, and hemagglutinin and neuraminidase subtype; for example, A/swine/NewJersey/8/76 (H1N1) and A/Philippines/2/82 (H3N2).

c. Influenza is a localized infection of the respiratory tract that may result in **pandemics** due to reassortment of the hemagglutinin.

d. Avian flu is a contagious disease of animals caused by influenza A viruses that normally infect birds and occasionally pigs but have rarely crossed species lines to infect humans.
(1) It is caused by influenza A viruses with H5, H7, or H9 hemagglutinins.
(2) Prevention: Egg-based vaccines and an adjuvanted influenza A (H5N1) monovalent vaccine containing an inactivated reassortment strain of an H5N1 avian virus are currently licensed.

3. Paramyxoviruses
a. General characteristics
(1) Description: spherical, enveloped viruses with a **single helical nucleocapsid** containing **single-stranded, negative-sense RNA;** exist in a few antigenic types.
(2) Components: have a **hemagglutinin-neuraminidase (HN), a fusion protein (F), a matrix protein (M) associated with the envelope, and a nucleocapsid-associated transcriptase (P).**

(a) Paramyxovirus HN
1. This large surface glycoprotein has both hemagglutinating and neuraminidase activity, except in measles virus, which lacks neuraminidase activity, and in respiratory syncytial virus (RSV), in which both activities have been lost.
2. **HN is responsible for virus adsorption.**
3. It stimulates the production of neutralizing antibodies.

    (b) Paramyxovirus fusion protein
        1. This surface glycoprotein has fusion and hemolysin activities, except in RSV, in which hemolysis activity is lost.
        2. It is **responsible for virus penetration into the cell.**
    (3) Replication: replicate in the cytoplasm of the cell.
    (4) Clinical disease: causes acute and persistent infections.
    (5) Classification: divided into three genera based on chemical and biologic properties: **paramyxoviruses (parainfluenza and mumps viruses), morbilliviruses (measles virus), and pneumoviruses (RSV and metapneumovirus).**

  b. Parainfluenza viruses
    (1) Classification: exist in four serotypes.
    (2) Clinical disease: cause a **variety of fall and winter upper and lower respiratory tract illnesses; croup** (type 2 virus) is a well-known infant disease.
    (3) Diagnosis: may be diagnosed using fluorescent antibody (FA) techniques on nasopharyngeal washes or swab to detect viral antigens or direct detection of nucleic acid by PCR in a multi-pathogen respiratory panel.

  c. Mumps virus
    (1) Classification: exists in **one serotype**.
    (2) Clinical disease: often causes asymptomatic infections but can cause a generalized disease involving enlargement of the parotid glands.
    (3) Diagnosis: usually diagnosed clinically.
    (4) Prevention: Infections are inhibited by a **live attenuated vaccine containing the Jeryl Lynn strain of virus** (usually included with live attenuated measles and rubella virus strains).

  d. Measles virus
    (1) Description: exists in **one serotype**.
    (2) Components: has hemagglutinin but no neuraminidase activity (H protein rather than HN protein).
    (3) Pathobiology: transmitted via air droplets and uses CD46 molecules as its cellular receptor. It can replicate in multiple tissues.
    (4) Replication: frequently **forms giant multinucleated cells (syncytia)** as part of its replication process (called **Warthin-Finkeldey cells in nasal secretions**).
    (5) Clinical disease: causes an acute generalized disease characterized by a maculopapular rash, fever, respiratory distress, and Koplik spots on the buccal mucosa.
    (6) Prevention: Infections can be prevented by a **live attenuated measles vaccine (Moraten strain)** that is part of the trivalent (measles, mumps, and rubella) vaccine given to children.

  e. Respiratory syncytial virus (RSV)
    (1) Description: exists in **one serotype but two antigenic groups (A and B).**
    (2) Components: has attachment (G protein) and fusion (F protein) activity, no hemagglutinin or neuraminidase activity.
    (3) Replication: induces syncytia formation during replication.
    (4) Clinical disease: causes a **potentially serious respiratory tract pathogen in infants.**
    (5) Diagnosis: by enzyme immunoassay (EIA) for viral antigens in nasopharyngeal washes.
    (6) Prevention: a bivalent recombinant protein vaccine is available for adults 60 years and older (Abrysvo) and a monoclonal antibody fusion-inhibitor immunization (Nirsevimab) for children under 19 months of age.

  f. Human metapneumovirus (hMNV) causes bronchiolitis and pneumonia in infants and lower respiratory tract infections in the older adults. Similar disease course to RSV.

  g. Newcastle disease virus
    (1) Description: natural respiratory tract pathogen of birds, particularly chickens.
    (2) Clinical disease: causes an **occupational disease of poultry workers** presenting as a mild conjunctivitis without corneal involvement.

4. Rhabdoviruses
  a. General characteristics
    (1) Description: enveloped, bullet-shaped viruses with a **helical nucleocapsid** containing **single-stranded, negative-sense RNA**.
    (2) Replication: have a **virion-associated transcriptase** and replicate in the cytoplasm.

(3) Classification: include the human pathogen rabies virus and the bovine pathogen vesicular stomatitis virus.

b. Rabies virus

(1) Replication: has a virion-associated transcriptase or replicase.

(2) Cytopathology: produces specific **cytoplasmic inclusion bodies, called Negri bodies,** in infected neurons.

(3) Pathobiology

    (a) Uses acetylcholine receptors on muscle cells to initiate infection.

    (b) Has a **predilection for the hippocampus (Ammon's horn cells).**

    (c) Can travel throughout the nervous system in nerve fibers.

(4) Clinical disease

    (a) Produces disease after inoculation by an animal bite (**zoonotic disease**) or, occasionally, inhalation such as via dried bat guano.

    (b) Causes fatal disease unless the infected person previously received immunization or receives postexposure prophylaxis consisting of passive immunization with human rabies immune globulin and immunization with a vaccine.

(5) Diagnosis: identified in suspected tissues by a direct immunofluorescent test for viral antigens utilizing the nape of neck hair follicles.

(6) Treatment and prevention

    (a) Grown in human MRC-5 (medical Research Council cell strain 5) diploid cell cultures (Pitman-Moore strain of virus) before inactivation and used in active immunization.

    (b) Has been grown (Flury LEP strain) in primary chicken fibroblasts before inactivation and inclusion in a PCEC (purified chick embryo cell culture) vaccine used for post-exposure vaccination.

5. Filoviruses

a. Classification: include Marburg and Ebola viruses.

b. Description: enveloped viruses with a **helical nucleocapsid** containing **single-stranded, negative-sense RNA**.

c. Clinical disease: cause African hemorrhagic fevers, which then lead to death.

d. Reservoir: believed to be African fruit bat and enter the human population via bush meat.

e. Vaccines: rVSV-ZEBOV (approved in the United States) and Ad26.ZEBOV and MVA-BN-Filo (approved in the European Union) for Ebola; target the viral glycoprotein.

C. Double-stranded RNA viruses

1. Reoviruses

a. General characteristics

(1) Description: naked viruses with a **double-shelled (outer shell and core) icosahedral capsid containing 10, 11, or 12 segments of double-stranded RNA.**

(2) Replication: replicate in the cytoplasm; have a **core-associated transcriptase or replicase.**

(3) Classification: classified into five groups; reoviruses, orthoreoviruses, rotaviruses, orbiviruses, and coltiviruses have strains that infect humans.

b. Coltiviruses

(1) Genome: have **12 segments of double-stranded RNA.**

(2) Clinical disease

    (a) Infect Ixodid ticks, which transfer the virus to humans.

    (b) Cause mild fevers in humans.

    (c) Represented by **Colorado tick fever virus (CTFV)**, which is carried by the wood tick *Dermacentor andersoni*.

c. Orthoreoviruses

(1) Genome: have **10 segments of double-stranded RNA.**

(2) Components: have an outer shell-associated hemagglutinin (d 1) that agglutinates human or bovine erythrocytes; is the viral receptor, therefore determining tissue tropism and is the determinant for the three serotypes of reoviruses.

(3) Clinical disease: produce minor upper respiratory tract infections and GI disease but also are frequently recovered from healthy people.

(4) Diagnosis: may be diagnosed by ELISA for viral antigens in clinical specimens.

d. Rotaviruses
  (1) Genome: have **11 segments of double-stranded RNA;** virion has wheel-and-spoke morphology.
  (2) Classification: exist in at least **seven serotypes, with type A being involved in most human infections.**
  (3) Clinical disease: cause infantile diarrhea and are the most common cause of gastroenteritis in children; are frequent causes of **nosocomial infections.**
  (4) Diagnosis: diagnosed by demonstrating virus in the stool or by serologic tests, particularly ELISA.
  (5) Prevention: have been modified and genetically manipulated for preparation of live attenuated vaccines **(RotaTeq and Rotarix).**
e. Orbiviruses
  (1) Description: arboviruses, transmitted by biting flies, mosquitoes, or ticks.
  (2) Genome: contain **10 segments of double-stranded RNA.**
  (3) Classification: classified into 14 serotypes, 4 cause human disease.
  (4) Clinical disease: basically a domestic animal disease, but may cause a febrile illness and occasionally encephalitis in humans in Africa, Central America, Russia, and Eastern Europe.

D. Viroid-like agents: hepatitis D virus (δ-associated virus).
  1. Description: virus with **circular, single-stranded RNA molecules (viroid-like) and an internal core δ antigen surrounded by an HBV envelope and surface antigens.**
  2. Replication: is **defective** and can replicate only in the presence of HBV.
  3. Clinical disease: is associated with both acute and chronic hepatitis and always with HBV; causes more severe hepatitis than does HBV alone.
  4. Diagnosis: may be diagnosed serologically with an ELISA test and confirmed by RNA detection in serum.

VII. SLOW VIRAL DISEASES AND PRIONS

A. JC virus
  1. Description: a **papovavirus** that frequently infects humans but rarely produces disease unless the host is immunosuppressed.
  2. Clinical disease
    a. Has been isolated from patients with **progressive multifocal leukoencephalopathy (PML),** a rare CNS disease.
    b. Causes demyelination by infecting and killing oligodendrocytes.

B. HIV-1-associated dementia (HAD)
  1. Description: HIV has a slowly progressing disease course when left untreated. HAD is often observed in end-stage HIV disease.
  2. HIV-1-associated dementia has a disease course similar to that of Alzheimer and Parkinson diseases.
  3. Results in behavioral, cognitive, affective, motor, psychiatric disorders.

C. Human papillomavirus
  1. Description: Sexually transmitted infection that usually clears by age 30 years. High-risk subtypes may lead to persistence after initial asymptomatic infection.
  2. Clinical disease: Precancerous CIN or anal intraepithelial lesions may progress slowly from low-grade to high-grade lesions. Progression from untreated high-grade lesions to cancer can take many years.

D. Rabies virus
  1. Description: a slow zoonotic infection transferred most often by animal bite.
  2. Clinical disease: causes damage to neurons of the CNS. After transmission and initial incubation lasting 60 to 365 days after the bite, the infection progresses through three phases.

    a. Prodromal phase occurs 2 to 10 days after animal bite and results in flu-like symptoms.

    b. Acute neurologic phase results in furious encephalitic rabies or paralytic dumb rabies 2 to 7 days after prodrome.

      (1) Furious rabies results in hyperactivity and agitation. Symptoms may include hydrophobia, anxiety, insomnia, restlessness, aggressive behavior, and hallucinations.

      (2) Paralytic rabies results in lethargy and muscle weakness.

    c. Coma and death phase occurs often within a week of the onset of neurologic symptoms primarily due to respiratory failure or other complications.

E. Subacute sclerosing panencephalitis

    1. Description: a slow persistent infection related to measles.

    2. Clinical disease: causes **subacute sclerosing panencephalitis**, a rare, fatal, slowly progressive demyelinating CNS disease of teenagers and young adults; may result from improper synthesis or processing of the matrix (M) viral protein.

F. Prions

    1. Description

    a. Not viruses but are **proteinaceous material lacking nucleic acid** that may be acquired or inherited and **is identical or closely related to a 30 to 35 kDa host membrane glycoprotein (PrP^c [prion protein]).**

    b. PrP^c can undergo a change in its tertiary structure (eg, the PrP of scrapie [PrP^{sc}] that causes aggregation of itself and PrP^c on neuronal cell surfaces); the aggregates (amyloid) are released and cause slow diseases called **spongiform encephalopathies.**

    2. Clinical disease: associated with several degenerative CNS diseases (subacute spongiform virus encephalopathies): kuru and Creutzfeldt-Jakob disease of humans, scrapie of sheep, bovine spongiform encephalopathy (or mad cow disease), and transmissible encephalopathy of mink.

VIII. ONCOGENIC VIRUSES

A. General characteristics

    1. Oncogenic viruses **cause cancers** when they infect appropriate animals. To be considered a human oncogenic virus, the virus causes cancer in animals and humans; it frequently establishes persistent infections in the natural host; they are seldom complete carcinogens; they may have direct- or indirect-acting oncogenic potential; they modulate growth control pathways; viral markers are usually present in the tumor cells (eg, viral integration). They are classified as DNA or RNA tumor viruses.

    2. Pathobiology

    a. Oncogenic viruses **transform infected cells** by altering cell growth, cell-surface antigens, and biochemical processes.

    b. When they enter cells, these viruses introduce "transforming" genes or induce expression of quiescent cellular genes, which results in the **synthesis of one or more transforming proteins.**

    c. The RNA viral genome of retroviruses is converted to DNA by RT and integrated into the host-cell chromosome, forming a **provirus which may induce transformation.**

    d. HIV does not have oncogenic potential but does cause perturbation in immune surveillance for cancer and thereby increases the likelihood of tumorigenesis from other causes.

B. DNA tumor viruses

    1. General characteristics

    a. Cause **transformation** in **nonpermissive cells** (infected cells that do not support total virus replication).

    b. Classification

      (1) Human viruses include human papillomaviruses: HBV, EBV, Merkel cell polyomavirus viruses, and HHV-8.

      (2) Protein products of some DNA tumor viruses interact with cellular **tumor suppressor gene products, particularly p53 and p110Rb**, that suppress oncogene expression.

2. **Human papillomavirus** may have a strong association (types 16 and 18) or a moderate association (types 31, 33, 35, 45, 51, 52, and 56) with cervical carcinoma. HPV synthesizes an **E6 protein** that binds to cellular **p53** and **E7 protein** that binds to cellular **p110^{Rb}**.

3. **EBV** is a cofactor in the etiology of **Burkitt lymphoma** and **nasopharyngeal carcinoma.** It can immortalize and transform B lymphocytes due to specific EBNA and LMP proteins. Viral protein EBNA3C, in particular, interacts with p53 and p110Rb. c-Myc translocation in concert with viral infection.

4. **HBV** is associated with primary hepatocellular carcinoma. It synthesizes an X protein, which binds to cellular p53.

5. **Merkel cell polyomavirus** causes Merkel cell carcinoma, a small nodular tumor of neuroendocrine cells. Synthesizes an early protein called **large tumor (T) antigen,** which associates with two antioncogene proteins, p53 and p110^{Rb}; establishes and maintains **SV40-like induced transformation.**

6. **HHV-8**, Kaposi sarcoma–associated herpesvirus, has several captured oncogenes that modulate inflammatory responses. It causes Kaposi sarcoma, a cancer of skin and mucous membranes, particularly in HIV-induced immune dysfunction. It is also associated with primary effusion lymphoma and multicentric Castleman disease.

C. RNA tumor viruses

1. **HTLV-1 and -2**

   a. **Description: retroviruses** (oncovirus group). **Genome** has **virogenes** (*gag*, pol, and *env*); however, HTLV-1 and -2 lack cellular-derived oncogenes. They have low oncogenic potential.

   b. **Pathobiology:** are nondefective human retroviruses with regulatory proteins Tax and HTLV-1 bZIP factor that have demonstrated oncogenic potential. Tax interacts with p53 while HBZ interacts with Nf-κB. They transform T4 antigen-positive cells.

   c. **Clinical disease:** are associated with **human adult acute T-cell lymphocytic leukemia** and tropical spastic paraparesis (HTLV-1) and some forms of **hairy cell leukemia** (HTLV-2).

2. **HCV**

   a. **Description:** flavivirus with geographic distribution of six genotypes.

   b. **Pathobiology:** targets hepatocytes and mononuclear lymphocytes. Has several viral proteins that influence proliferation and apoptosis, genome instability, and inflammatory responses.

   c. **Clinical disease:** causes advanced hepatic fibrosis and cirrhosis and is associated with primary hepatocellular carcinoma. No oncogene identified as yet but believed to be caused by chronic inflammatory and virally induced antiapoptotic activity.

Review Test

Directions: Each of the numbered items or incomplete statements in this section is followed by answers or completions of the statement. Select the *one* lettered answer that is *best* in each case.

1. Clinical viral disease is associated with which of the following conditions?

   (A) Is most frequently due to toxin production
   (B) Usually follows virus infection
   (C) Can result without infection of host cells
   (D) Is associated with target organs in most disseminated viral infections

2. The eclipse period of a one-step viral multiplication curve is defined by which of the following time periods?

   (A) Start of uncoating and assembly of the virus
   (B) Start of the infection and the first appearance of extracellular virus
   (C) Start of the infection and the first appearance of intracellular virus
   (D) Start of the infection and uncoating of the virus

3. Which of the following best characterizes HTLVs?

   (A) Are associated with leukemias
   (B) Are defective RNA tumor viruses
   (C) Carry tyrosine protein kinase oncogenes
   (D) Synthesize early proteins that interact with p53 and Rb

4. Linear, single-stranded DNA is the genetic material of which of the following viruses?

   (A) Caliciviruses
   (B) Flaviviruses
   (C) Papillomaviruses
   (D) Parvoviruses

5. Host-cell tRNAs are involved in the genome replication of which of the following viruses?

   (A) Influenza A virus
   (B) Retroviruses
   (C) RSV
   (D) Rhinovirus

6. Which of the following RNA virus has a nuclear phase to its replication process?

   (A) Coronavirus
   (B) Rhabdovirus
   (C) Retrovirus
   (D) Togavirus

7. Negri bodies are observed with which of the following viral infections?

   (A) CMV infections
   (B) HSV infections
   (C) Rabies virus infections
   (D) Rubella virus infections

8. Persistent virus infections are characterized by which of the following?

   (A) Are usually confined to the initial site of infection
   (B) Are preceded by acute clinical disease
   (C) Elicit a poor antibody response
   (D) May involve infected carrier individuals

9. Localized viral disease is described as which of the following?

   (A) Is a major feature of congenital viral infections
   (B) Is associated with a pronounced viremia
   (C) Can be associated with carrier individuals
   (D) May have systemic clinical features such as fever

10. Lymphotropic and macrophage trophic designation is important in the pathogenesis of which of the following viruses?

    (A) CMV
    (B) HSV
    (C) HIV
    (D) JC virus

11. Dane particles are associated with which of the following hepatitis viruses?

    (A) HAV
    (B) HBV
    (C) HCV
    (D) Hepatitis E virus

12. The exchange of homologous segments of RNA between two different influenza type A viruses is termed which of the following?

    (A) Complementation
    (B) Genetic reassortment
    (C) Phenotypic masking
    (D) Phenotypic mixing

13. The monospot test is based on which of the following features?

(A) Destruction of Downey cells
(B) Heterophile antibodies
(C) Syncytia inhibition
(D) VCA antibodies

14. Disinfection of day care center play tables with 70% ethanol is least likely to affect the viability of which of the following viruses?

(A) CMV
(B) Parainfluenza virus
(C) RSV
(D) Rotavirus

15. A virus that infects and lyses progenitor erythroid cells causing aplastic crises in patients with hemolytic anemia is which of the following?

(A) California encephalitis virus
(B) EBV
(C) Parvovirus B19
(D) Yellow fever virus

16. A viral protein that is thought to induce tumors by binding to a cellular tumor suppressor protein is identified as which of the following?

(A) Hepatitis C virus protein X
(B) Hepatitis B virus e protein
(C) HIV *gag* protein
(D) Human papillomavirus E6 protein

17. Which of the following viruses have a genome of messenger (positive-sense) polarity?

(A) Adenoviruses
(B) Papovaviruses
(C) Paramyxoviruses
(D) Polioviruses

Answers and Explanations

1. **The answer is D.** [IV A] Many viral infections are asymptomatic or subclinical. Clinical disease, however, is often associated with viral replication in target organs during disseminated viral infections.

2. **The answer is C.** [Figure 4.2] The period of time between the adsorption and penetration of the virus until the first appearance of intracellular virus is the eclipse phase.

3. **The answer is A.** [VI A 6 c] HTLV-1 is associated with adult T-cell leukemia; HTLV-2 is implicated in human hairy cell leukemia.

4. **The answer is D.** [V A 3 a] Parvoviruses have linear, single-stranded DNA, while papovaviruses have circular, double-stranded DNA. Caliciviruses and flaviviruses are RNA viruses.

5. **The answer is B.** [VI A 6 a (2) (a)] Host-cell tRNAs act as primers for the synthesis of retrovirus DNA by RT.

6. **The answer is C.** [III C 4] The RT of retroviruses makes a DNA copy of the genomic RNA. This DNA must be integrated into the host-cell DNA in the nucleus for the remaining steps in the replication process to occur.

7. **The answer is C.** [VI B 4 b (2)] Negri bodies are intracytoplasmic inclusion bodies found in rabies virus-infected neurons and are important in the diagnosis of infected animals.

8. **The answer is D.** [IV D 3] Some persistent virus infections, such as serum hepatitis caused by-HBV, involve carrier individuals who may or may not have clinical signs of the disease.

9. **The answer is D.** [IV E 1] Although localized infections are not associated with pronounced viremia, they can have clinical features similar to viremic systemic infections.

10. **The answer is C.** [VI A 6 b (1)] Strains of HIV are classified as lymphotropic or macrophage trophic depending on their preferred site of latency.

11. **The answer is B.** [V B 1 a] The spherical virion of HBV is called the Dane particle.

12. **The answer is B.** [III D 4] Genetic reassortment is the name given to the process whereby homologous pieces of RNA are exchanged between two different strains of influenza viruses replicating in the cell.

13. **The answer is B.** [V B 2 d (3)] IgM antibody produced in response to most EBV infections agglutinates sheep and beef erythrocytes and forms the basis for the monospot test used in diagnosing infectious mononucleosis caused by EBV.

14. **The answer is D.** [VI D 1 a (3)] Since rotavirus is a naked virus, it is least susceptible to inactivation by 70% alcohol, a lipid solvent disrupting the envelope of the three enveloped viruses.

15. **The answer is C.** [V A 3 b] The target cells of human parvovirus B19 are progenitor erythroid cells; infections in patients with hemolytic anemia can be serious.

16. **The answer is D.** [VIII B 2] Human papillomavirus E6 protein is involved in the replication process, but it can bind to cellular tumor suppressor protein p53 and inactivate its normal cellular function, which results in cellular transformation.

17. **The answer is D.** [VI 5 b (4)]. Polioviruses contain a single-stranded positive-sense RNA genome. Adenoviruses and Papovaviruses have double-stranded genomes. Paramyxoviruses have a single-stranded negative-sense genome of opposite polarity from messenger RNA.

5

System-Based and Situational Viral Infections

In this chapter, the diseases associated with viral infections are divided into three categories: system based, location based, and situation based. The majority of the information for a specific virus is found under the system- or situation-based disease section with which it is most closely associated. Generalized symptoms of viral infection include fever, fatigue, and head and body aches. Viruses causing clinical signs and symptoms within more than one system or situation are noted in all sections, but only important aspects of virus interactions relevant to that occasion are noted. Treatment for viral infections is supportive unless noted. The viruses listed under each heading are the most prominent ones; comprehensive lists are found in virology infectious disease textbooks.

SYSTEM-BASED DISEASE

I. EYE INFECTIONS

Viruses are the most common cause of conjunctivitis. Conjunctivitis is inflammation of the membrane that covers the sclera and inside of the eyelid. These infections are usually self-limiting and resolve in 1 to 3 weeks. Listed here are the primary pathogens of viral conjunctivitis. Herpes simplex virus (HSV) and varicella zoster virus (VZV) infections are more serious. HSV can be misdiagnosed as a typical adenovirus infection.

A. Adenoviruses
   1. **Features**
      a. Up to 90% of cases are due to adenovirus infection.
      b. They are highly contagious and spread by contact with eye secretions.
      c. Risk factors for transmission are swimming pool water, living in a home with someone who is infected, or self-inoculation.
   2. **Disease**
      a. Adenoviruses are involved in respiratory tract infections but can cause a conjunctivitis known as *pinkeye*, which resolves spontaneously in a few days.
      b. Symptoms include redness, itching, and watery eyes.
      c. Pharyngoconjunctival fever also includes pharyngitis, high fever, and swollen lymph nodes.
      d. They can cause a serious **epidemic keratoconjunctivitis,** which may be transmitted by contaminated ophthalmologic instruments.
      e. Keratoconjunctivitis includes corneal inflammation.

B. Enterovirus type 70 is associated with hemorrhagic conjunctivitis.

C. Herpes simplex virus (HSV)
   1. **Features**
      a. Pseudomembranes are not present as compared to adenovirus infection.
      b. HSV eye infections have a high rate of recurrence.

   2. **Disease**

   a. **HSV** can produce **conjunctivitis** that may progress to **keratitis** involving the formation of a **dendritic ulcer**, which, if untreated, can lead to visual impairment.

   b. Beyond conjunctivitis symptoms, the infection may cause accompanying vesicular eyelid lesions.

   c. A high degree of pain is associated with HSV ocular infections.

   d. Neonatal conjunctivitis can originate from vertical transmission from mother to child via an infected birth canal.

   e. **Treatment:** topical acyclovir.

D. Varicella-Zoster Virus (VZV) is estimated to cause **conjunctivitis** in 4% of chickenpox cases; it may reactivate in the ophthalmic branch of the trigeminal nerve to cause **herpes zoster ophthalmicus.**

> ● ● ● **Clinical Pearl**
>
> Adenovirus conjunctivitis is usually observed to be bilateral, whereas HSV conjunctivitis is unilateral.

II. EAR INFECTIONS

   1. Viral upper respiratory tract infections that cause colds and pharyngitis often lead to otitis media and sinusitis. Common respiratory viruses such as **rhinovirus, respiratory syncytial virus** (**RSV**), and **adenoviruses** may cause 50% of these infections.

III. UPPER RESPIRATORY TRACT (MOUTH AND THROAT) INFECTIONS

Viral diseases included here range from infections largely confined to the mouth (herpangina) and nose and throat (colds) to systemic infections with pharyngitis as a major symptom (infectious mononucleosis). Many viruses whose prominent clinical symptoms originate farther down the respiratory tract (RSV and influenza viruses) begin their infectious process in the mouth and throat. Viruses that cause respiratory infections, in general, occur with particular seasonality (Figure 5.1).

A. Coxsackie A viruses
   1. **Features**

   a. These are members of the enterovirus genera of the Picornavirus family.

   b. Transmission risk is greatest for children younger than age 5 years.

   c. Can be transmitted by droplets and fomites.

   2. **Disease**

   a. **Herpangina** is characterized by sudden fever, sore throat, vomiting, and discrete vesiculo-papular lesions on the tongue, tonsils, and the roof of the mouth.

   b. **Hand, foot, and mouth disease** is a febrile illness producing vesicular lesions or blisters on the palate, hands, and feet. Coxsackie A 16 is the usual cause.

B. Herpes simplex viruses (HSV-1 and HSV-2)
   1. **Features**

   a. HSV-1 is spread most often by oral secretion from infections around the mouth area.

   b. Primary infection of HSV-1 occurs most often in childhood.

   c. HSV-2 is spread most often by body secretion from infections originating in the genital area.

   d. Primary HSV-2 infections occur with sexual activity.

   e. Virus latently infects neurons and may be reactivated to travel to peripheral tissue by physical or emotional stress, or immune suppression.

   2. **Disease**

   a. These viruses may cause a clinically apparent primary infection (eg, **gingivostomatitis** by HSV-1 in children and HSV-2 in young adults) or recurrent infection (eg, **cold sores**).

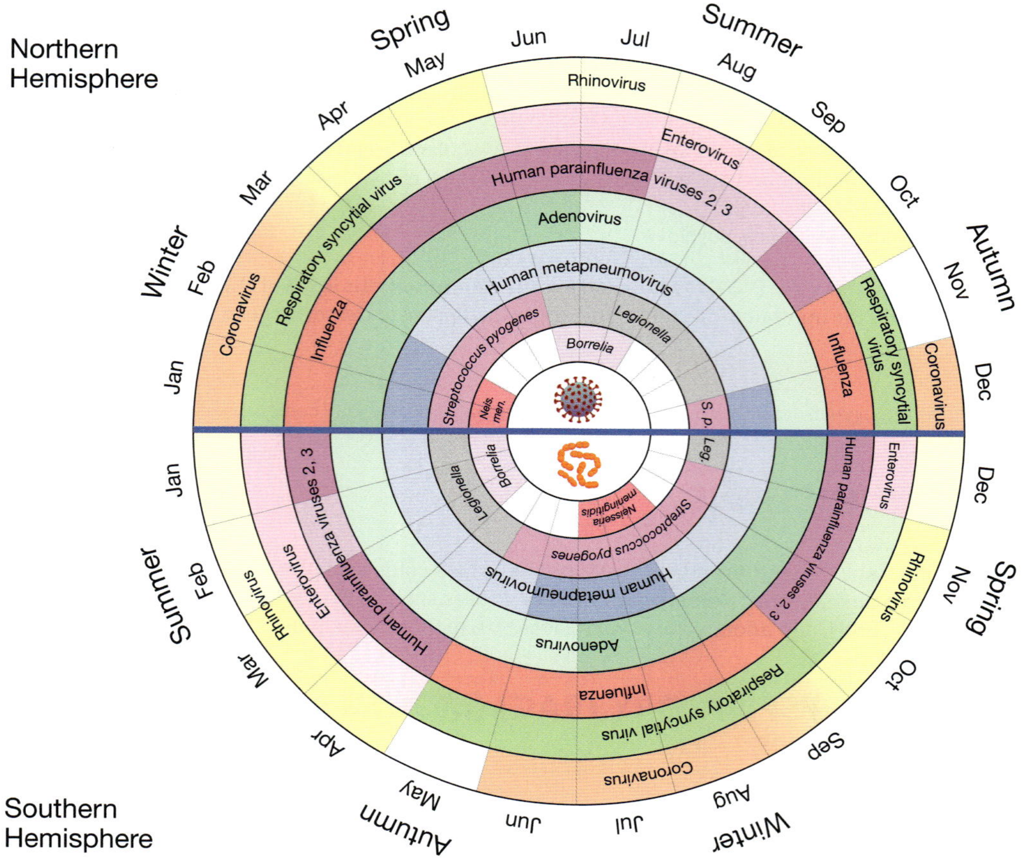

FIGURE 5.1. Examples of microbial seasonality. While respiratory viruses best exemplify the seasonal variations of waxing and waning infections, other microbes can also display seasonality influenced by environmental conditions, vector reproductive patterns, and social distancing behaviors. The darker shades of color indicate peak infection times for the microbe at the time of year in that hemisphere. The lighter shades of color indicate the background levels of infection if applicable for that time of year. (Adapted from Buensalido JAL, Valencia JCB. Rhinovirus (RV) infection (common cold). *Medscape.* Updated August 18, 2023. https://emedicine.medscape .com/article/227820-overview.)

    b. Progression to a severe, fatal encephalitis (HSV-1) or meningitis (HSV-2) can occur.

    c. **Diagnosis:** cause vesicular lesions with an erythematous base that contain cytopathology visualized by a **Tzanck smear** for rapid identification of the virus.

    d. **Treatment:** can be treated by acyclovir, penciclovir, famciclovir, or valacyclovir, but drug-resistant strains can arise; the virus is **not eliminated by treatment once latency has been established**.

C. Epstein-Barr virus (EBV)

  1. Features

    a. Human gammaherpesvirus-4.

    b. Latently infects B cells, epithelial cells, and natural killer T cells.

    c. Usually causes a clinically inapparent systemic infection but may cause infectious mononu-
cleosis and is associated with Burkitt lymphoma and nasopharyngeal carcinoma.

  2. Disease

    a. Infectious mononucleosis

      (1) This **systemic disease** of children and young adults (sometimes called the *kissing dis-ease*) is characterized by sore throat, fever, enlarged lymph nodes and spleen, and, sometimes, hepatitis.

      (2) Diagnosis

        (a) Associated with the production of atypical reactive T lymphocytes (**Downey cells**) and **immunoglobulin M (IgM) heterophile antibodies** (IgM interacts with Paul-Bunnell antigen on sheep, horse, or bovine erythrocytes, causing agglutina-tion) and may be identified by the **monospot test.**

        (b) Can also be diagnosed by serologic tests involving immunofluorescence pro-cedures on fixed EBV-producing cells or enzyme-linked immunosorbent assay (ELISA) tests.

    b. Burkitt lymphoma and nasopharyngeal carcinoma are characterized by cells that express EBV nuclear antigens (EBNAs) and latent membrane proteins (LMPs) and carry multiple copies of viral DNA.

D. Cytomegalovirus (CMV)

  1. Features

    a. Human betaherpesvirus-5.

    b. Latently infects hematopoietic progenitor cells, monocytes.

  2. Disease

    a. Usually causes asymptomatic infection in children and adults. It causes approximately 10% of mononucleosis cases that are clinically similar to those caused by EBV, except that no het-erophile antibodies are produced.

    b. Can cause congenital infections without symptoms. Possible long-term health is-sues can result, such as hearing and vision loss, seizures, developmental delays, and microcephaly.

E. Rhinoviruses

  1. Features

    a. There are more than 160 serotypes.

    b. They are highly contagious and are transmitted by respiratory droplets.

  2. Disease: These viruses are the most frequent cause of the **common cold.**

    a. Treatment and prevention

      (1) A vaccine is improbable due to the number of serotypes.

      (2) Rhinoviruses can be inhibited with **pleconaril** (not U.S. Food and Drug Administration [FDA] approved), which binds to capsid and prevents uncoating.

F. Coronaviruses

  1. Features: The viruses are considered zoonotic, infecting both humans and animals.

  2. Disease

    a. Causes 5% to 10% of colds (second to rhinoviruses; four common coronavirus types).

    b. More severe lower respiratory tract infections can occur with the severe acute respiratory syndrome—coronavirus-1 (SARS-CoV-1), SARS-CoV-2, and Middle Eastern respiratory syn-drome (MERS).

G. Adenoviruses

  1. Features

    a. They may cause latent infections of human tonsils.

    b. They have multiple subtypes that cause disease in different systems.

2. Diseases
  a. Respiratory diseases caused by adenoviruses range from acute febrile pharyngitis to **pharyngoconjunctival fever** and occasionally acute pneumonia (types 4 and 7).
  b. Adenoviruses may contaminate swimming pools and lead to pharyngoconjunctival fever.

H. Enteroviruses
  1. Features
    a. The genus is composed of over 70 antigenically distinct species.
    b. Transmission by saliva, sputum, mucus, or feces from an infected person.
  2. Diseases
    a. They generally cause mild illness.
    b. Several groups including Coxsackie viruses and echoviruses can cause **summer and autumn epidemics of pharyngitis**.
    c. Enteroviruses that are also involved in pharyngitis are not identified, although rapid diagnosis by reverse transcription-polymerase chain reaction (RT-PCR) is available.

I. Parainfluenza virus and RSV can cause mild upper respiratory tract infections similar to colds but are more noted for diseases farther down the respiratory tract.

J. Human papillomavirus (HPV) can cause **laryngeal papillomas** or warts.

> **• • • Clinical Pearl**
>
> According to the Infectious Disease Society of America guidelines, viral causes of sinusitis are likely if the symptoms seem to improve after 3 days of onset. Bacterial causes are more likely if symptoms last 10 days without improvement, get worse or have new symptoms after initially improving, or have severe symptoms including a fever for more than 3 days after onset.

IV. LOWER RESPIRATORY TRACT INFECTIONS

Many of these diseases are manifestations of upper respiratory virus progression down the respiratory tract. They include some notable childhood infections such as croup and some serious interstitial viral pneumonias that predispose in the lungs for secondary bacterial infection. Viral pneumonias are classified as atypical pneumonias. Coxsackie B virus causing pleurodynia is also included here.

A. Parainfluenza viruses
  1. Features
    a. Human parainfluenza viruses (HPIV-1 and HPIV-2) circulate in alternate years during the fall.
    b. HPIV-3 circulates in spring and early summer.
  2. Diseases
    a. Laryngotracheobronchitis, called *croup*, usually occurs in the fall in 2- to 5-year-old children and is characterized by a **distinctive "barking" cough**.
    b. Pneumonia in infants and older adults and nosocomial disease in facilities are dedicated to these groups.
    c. Diagnosis: rapidly diagnosed by detection of viral antigens in nasopharyngeal washings or swabs by immunofluorescent techniques or by nucleic acid testing in multipathogen respiratory panels.

B. Respiratory syncytial virus
  1. Features
    a. RSV is the **most important infant respiratory virus.**
  2. Diseases
    a. It causes **75% to 80% of bronchiolitis cases, 70% of which** progress to pneumonia.
    b. Serious disease occurs in premature infants, older adults, and people who are immunosuppressed.

    c. It is a frequent cause of **nosocomial infections.**

    d. Diagnosis: may be diagnosed by several laboratory techniques including immunofluorescent and enzyme immunoassay (EIA) for viral antigens in nasopharyngeal washings or swabs or by nucleic acid testing in multipathogen respiratory panels.

    e. Treatment: may be treated with **ribavirin** aerosols in severe cases; high-risk children and infants treated prophylactically with **RSV-IGIV (RespiGam) or palivizumab (Synagis). Recent subunit vaccines are available that target the viral F protein.**

C. Influenza

1. Features

    a. Influenza has an abrupt onset, usually within 1 day.

    b. It has a seasonal periodicity, usually occurring in mid-to-late fall and into winter in the northern hemisphere; peaking in December to March.

2. Disease

    a. Influenza is a localized infection of the respiratory tract with symptoms ranging from a mild rhinotracheitis to a fatal pneumonia.

        (1) In healthy individuals, influenza is usually not serious; in the older adults or in patients with a secondary bacterial pneumonia, it may cause serious complications.

        (2) It may rarely progress to encephalitis a few weeks postinfection.

        (3) It is associated with Guillain-Barré syndrome (influenza virus types A and B) and Reye syndrome (influenza virus type B).

    b. Pandemics may result due to reassortment of the hemagglutinin.

    c. Diagnosis

        (1) It can be diagnosed by EIA, direct immunofluorescence, or RT-PCR of respiratory secretions or serologically. Usually included in multipathogen respiratory panels.

        (2) The rapid influenza diagnostic test (RIDT) is a laminar flow test that is quick but frequently inaccurate.

        (3) Diagnostic algorithms for RIDT interpretation consider the time of year when virus is circulating to determine true from false results and need for confirmatory testing.

    d. Prevention: may be prevented by either an **inactivated trivalent vaccine** (whole, split, and subunit vaccines exist) or a **live attenuated trivalent vaccine** containing recent A/H_1N_1 A/H_3N_2, and B strains.

    e. Treatment: may be prevented chemoprophylactically and treated (both A and B strains) by administration of **zanamivir, oseltamivir, peramivir, or laninamivir** (viral neuraminidase inhibitors); or baloxavir marboxil **(polymerase acidic endonuclease inhibitor)**; amantadine and rimantadine (M2 ion channel inhibitors) are no longer recommended for the treatment of influenza A and are ineffective against influenza B.

D. Adenoviruses

1. Features

    a. Multiple serotypes result in different clinical presentations.

    b. The respiratory infection can spread to other organ systems.

2. Disease

    a. These viruses are associated with *acute respiratory disease* (**ARD**), a term referring to certain clinical signs, symptoms, and pathology in military recruits.

    b. Adenovirus types 4 and 7 are used in an oral bivalent vaccine that is administered to prevent ARD in the military.

E. Hantavirus (Sin Nombre virus)

1. Features

    a. Rare but most often found in Southwestern United States, Canada, and South America.

    b. It is transmitted by inhalation by infected deer mouse urine or feces to humans.

2. Disease

    a. Hantavirus starts with flulike symptoms that lead to interstitial pulmonary edema and respiratory failure (**hantavirus pulmonary syndrome**).

    b. Severe infection can lead to low blood pressure and shock.

    c. Thrombocytopenia is a common laboratory finding associated with infection.

F. Coronavirus
   1. Features: severe cases resulting in hypoxia and respiratory failure.
   2. Disease
      a. SARS coronavirus (SARS-CoV-1) causes **severe acute respiratory syndrome (SARS)** last reported in Asia in April 2004.
      b. SARS-CoV-2 is responsible for the 2020 global pandemic and causes coronavirus disease-2019 (COVID-19). Infected individuals may be asymptomatic carriers. Additional symptoms may include loss of senses of taste and smell and finger and toe tips turning blue (Raynaud phenomenon).

> **● ● ● Clinical Pearl**
>
> Postacute sequelae of COVID (PASC) are defined as persistent or new symptoms evident beyond 30 days postrecovery of the initial infection. Symptoms include loss of or change in smell or taste, malaise, fatigue, brain fog, dizziness, and gastrointestinal symptoms, among others.

      c. MERS is responsible for a severe acute respiratory infection that is transmitted zoonotically from dromedaries to humans.

G. Human metapneumovirus (hMPV)
   1. Features: often misdiagnosed as RSV.
   2. Disease
      a. Bronchiolitis and pneumonia in infants and lower respiratory tract disease in the older adults.
      b. It may also cause winter epidemics and is a possible nosocomial disease.

H. Coxsackie B virus causes **epidemic pleurodynia (Bornholm disease)** characterized by sudden onset of severe paroxysmal chest pain, fever, headache, and fatigue. It is more likely to occur in teenagers and young adults.

V. GASTROINTESTINAL INFECTIONS

Viruses have been estimated to cause **two-thirds of all infective diarrheas.** Viral gastroenteritis is the second most common viral illness after upper respiratory infections. They are clinically similar (vomiting, fever, abdominal pain, and watery diarrhea) to some bacterial gastroenteritis, but no blood or pus appears in the stool.

A. Rotaviruses
   1. Features
      a. Accounts for 50% to 80% of all cases of **viral gastroenteritis**, with more severe symptoms in **neonates and infants** and asymptomatic infections in older children and adults.
      b. There is a higher incidence of infection in the winter months in temperate climates but can be observed to occur all year in tropical climates.
   2. Disease
      a. It also causes **possible nosocomial disease** and outbreaks in day care centers.
      b. When infection occurs in malnourished children, the mortality rate is 30%.
      c. Diagnosis: usually diagnosed by EIA for rotavirus antigens in the feces or by nucleic acid detection in multipathogen panels.
      d. Prevention: have been genetically manipulated and attenuated to prepare two live, oral vaccines.
         (1) Rotarix vaccine contains attenuated subtypes G1, 3, 4, and 9 human viruses.
         (2) RotaTeq vaccine contains five reassortment viruses with WC3 bovine parent and G1, G2, G3, G4, and PL human VP7 outer protein subtypes.

B. Adenoviruses are the second most common cause of gastroenteritis in neonates and young children. They may be associated with small outbreaks.

C. Astroviruses produce a disease similar to rotaviruses, as well as adenoviruses in neonates and young children.

D. Noroviruses (Norwalk and similar viruses)
   1. **Features**
      a. **Extremely contagious and transmissible.**
      b. **It has a very quick onset and short duration.**
      c. **The virus can survive in the environment for an extended period of time.**
   2. **Disease**
      a. **Gastroenteritis associated with contaminated water or shellfish and other food in adults and school-aged children.**
      b. Infections occur most frequently in contained settings like schools, cruise ships, camps, and hospitals.
      c. Noroviruses are the cause of **winter vomiting disease**, a disease involving school and family outbreaks.

VI. LIVER INFECTION

Viruses are the major cause of infectious liver disease. The virus may be transmitted enterically, parenterally, or, in one case, by a mosquito bite. Clinically, the diseases range from asymptomatic or mild to severe acute disease to chronic disease (types B, C, and D). Types B and C viruses are associated with primary hepatocellular carcinoma (PHC). **Acute infections by these viruses cannot be distinguished from each other clinically,** but serum enzyme increases in aspartate aminotransferase (AST) and alanine aminotransferase (ALT) allow differentiation from other liver disease. Jaundice is another symptom that may be present in acute hepatitis (**Figure 5.2**). Vaccines, antivirals, and human gamma globulin preparation are available for protection or treatment of some viruses. Other viruses such as **viral hemorrhagic fevers, adenovirus, coronavirus**, HSV, CMV, EBV, **and rubella can cause acute hepatitis as part of the systemic disease.**

A. Enterically transmitted viruses
   1. **Hepatitis A virus (HAV)**
      a. **Features**
         (1) HAV does not cause chronic infection.
         (2) Infection confers lifelong immunity.
         (3) Disease severity increases with the age of infection.

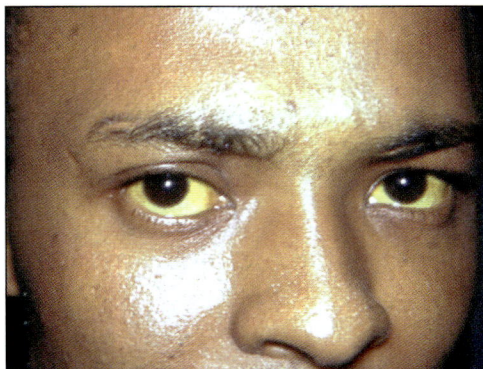

FIGURE 5.2. Jaundice of the conjunctivae and facial skin resulting from hepatitis A infection involves the yellow coloration imparted to these areas due to the deposition of the pigment bilirubin. (Photo courtesy of CDC Public Health Image Library [PHIL], image 2860.)

b. Disease

(1) HAV causes **"infectious hepatitis,"** an acute disease that is clinically milder or asymptomatic in young children.

(2) It is transmitted by close personal contact between individuals in places like homes and child day care centers and shed in the feces for 2 weeks before symptoms are apparent.

(3) Diagnosis: usually identified by EIA for HAV IgM or ELISA for HAV antigen in feces.

(4) Prevention: inactivated by formalin for inclusion in **Havrix and VAQTA vaccines** that can be used to protect children aged 12 months and above. Havrix is combined with Energix-B to form **Twinrix** for use in individuals aged 18 years and above, which protects against HAV and hepatitis B virus (HBV).

2. Hepatitis E virus (HEV)

a. Features

(1) HEV can cause a chronic infection in populations who are immunocompromised.

(2) HEV subtypes HEV-3 and HEV-4 are most often associated with chronic infection.

(3) Experiences a dose-dependent disease severity profile.

b. Disease

(1) HEV causes disease in endemic areas (not in the United States) and is transmitted by drinking fecally contaminated drinking water.

(2) It causes a clinical disease similar to HAV but is more severe in pregnant patients (15%-25% mortality rate when infected during the third trimester).

(3) Prevention: Genotype 1 recombinant protein vaccine has been effective in preventing clinical disease but is not currently available in the United States.

B. Parenterally transmitted viruses

1. Hepatitis B virus (HBV)

a. Features: The virus is able to persist in infected cells.

b. Disease

(1) HBV causes acute clinical disease previously called *serum hepatitis* in approximately 25% of infected individuals. Between 5% and 10% of HBV infections lead to chronic disease; 10% of these individuals develop cirrhosis and permanent liver damage.

(2) Progression to chronic disease is inversely related to the age of infection (~90% in infected neonates).

(3) It is transmitted by body fluids (blood, saliva, semen, vaginal secretions, and breast milk) and can be considered a **sexually transmitted disease (STD)**; it can be transmitted by asymptomatic **chronic carriers**.

(4) It is associated with the development of **primary hepatocellular carcinoma (PHC).**

(5) Serologic markers indicate the course of infection:

(a) HBeAg—infectious virus and transmissibility.

(b) IgM HBc—recent infection.

(c) IgG HBc—recovery and lifelong immunity.

(d) HBeAg and HBsAg—chronic infection if no antibodies to them are present.

(e) IgG HBs—vaccinated for HBV.

(6) Treatment and prevention

(a) Disease can be prevented by immunization with two recombinant subunit **vaccines (Recombivax HB and Engerix-B)** containing HBsAg: one **HAV/HBV combination vaccine** (**Twinrix** for those aged 18 years and above) and two **pediatric vaccines (Comvax and Pediarix).**

(b) Chronic infections can be treated with five drugs: standard and pegylated interferon-α and reverse transcriptase inhibitors (tenofovir disoproxil fumarate, entecavir, lamivudine, adefovir, and dipivoxil) to improve survival and reduce progression to PHC.

2. Hepatitis D virus (HDV)

a. Features

(1) HDV is a satellite virus, a **defective virus** that contains the **delta antigen** and requires HBV for replication.

(2) It can cause a **coinfection** (infection by both HBV and HDV in a naive individual) or a **superinfection** (HDV infection of a person chronically infected with HBV).

    b. Disease
- **(1)** Coinfection may cause a more severe acute disease than HBV alone but carries a lower risk of chronic infection.
- **(2) Superinfection may develop into a chronic infection with a high risk of severe chronic liver disease.**
- **(3) Treatment and prevention**: may be treated and prevented using the antivirals and vaccines directed against HBV.

  3. Hepatitis C virus (HCV)
- **a. Features:** HCV is a common cause of **transfusion and liver transplant–associated hepatitis** if the patient's blood and liver are not prescreened. It can also be considered an **STD** and can be transmitted at birth from an HCV-infected mother, with a transmission rate of about 5%.
- **b. Disease**
  - **(1)** Acute disease is usually mild or asymptomatic, but up to **70% of those infected develop chronic disease.** A high percentage of these individuals have asymptomatic disease that leads to cirrhosis and liver failure or PHC.
  - **(2)** RNA levels in the blood are monitored by RT-PCR techniques to diagnose chronic HCV infections and monitor response to antiviral therapy.
  - **(3) Treatment: Current treatment strategies to reach sustained virologic response toward cure of HCV infection are the direct-acting agents sofosbuvir/velpatasvir, ledipasvir/sofosbuvir, elbasvir/grazoprevir, and glecaprevir/pibrentasvir.**

> **● ● ● Clinical Pearl**
>
> Both HBV and HCV contribute to hepatocellular carcinoma, though by differing mechanisms. There is a vaccine available for HBV prevention, and HCV can be cured with direct-acting agents. In this case, it can be argued that these vaccines and direct-acting agents have anticancer effects by preventing the contributions of these viruses to liver cancer development.

C. Mosquito-transmitted virus: yellow fever virus
- **1. Features**
  - **a.** Yellow fever virus is acquired through the bite of a mosquito so is an **arboviral disease**.
  - **b.** It causes an acute disease in Africa and Central and South America.
- **2. Disease**
  - **a.** It may be an asymptomatic or a **biphasic** infection with three stages:
    - **(1)** Infection symptoms of fever, chills, myalgia, headache, general malaise, nausea, jaundice, and lower back pain last about 3 days.
    - **(2)** Remission of symptoms occurs for about 48 hours.
    - **(3)** Intoxication occurs in 20% of cases of individuals who have symptoms several days after initial onset. Symptoms of this stage are fever, vomiting, nausea, jaundice, epigastric pain, bradycardia, and hemorrhaging that may last for a week.
  - **b. Prevention:** may be prevented from causing disease by vaccination with the **live, attenuated vaccine strain 17D** of the virus.

VII. URINARY TRACT INFECTIONS

Viral urinary tract infections (UTIs) are rare, but acute and latent infections occur. Some viral systemic diseases shed virus in the urine during symptoms, for example, CMV in congenitally infected children. A number of viruses can induce kidney injury due to the immune response, such as the hepatitis viruses, human immunodeficiency virus (HIV), and hantavirus.

A. Adenoviruses cause a **hemorrhagic cystitis** with dysuria and hematuria, predominantly in young boys.

B. John Cunningham virus causes a latent infection in the kidneys, which, if reactivated in immunosuppression, can lead to progressive multifocal leukoencephalopathy.

C. BK virus
   1. **Features**: Virus-infected cells located in the urine are termed *decoy cells* as they are similar to renal carcinoma cells.
   2. **Disease**
      a. Causes asymptomatic infection early in childhood but establishes a **latent infection** in the kidney and ureter epithelium, which can reactivate during immunosuppression.
      b. Can cause a progressive kidney disease in renal transplant cases.
      c. Symptoms of active infection are pain or discomfort during urination, hematuria, pain in the lower back or stomach, and other symptoms related to spread of infection to the lungs or brain.

VIII. CARDIOVASCULAR INFECTIONS

Viruses are the most common infectious cause of myocarditis and pericarditis. Sore throats, fever, and malaise frequently precede cardiac signs and symptoms. In addition to the following viruses, several viruses causing multisystem infections such as influenza, EBV, mumps, and adenovirus can cause myocarditis as part of other infectious processes. Some arboviruses cause hemorrhagic fevers in endemic areas.

A. Coxsackie B virus is the main viral cause of acute infection **myocarditis and pericarditis**.

B. Other enteroviruses (Coxsackie A and echoviruses) are less common causes of pericarditis and myocarditis.

C. Dengue virus and several other arboviruses can cause **hemorrhagic fever**, occasionally leading to **shock syndrome.**

D. SARS-CoV-2 causes a 16-fold greater risk of myocarditis in patients with COVID-19 compared to patients without COVID-19.

IX. NERVOUS SYSTEM INFECTIONS

Viruses cause acute, latent, and slow infections of the nervous system. Some acute infections lead to acute postinfection syndromes. Acute disease varies from mild meningitis to fatal encephalitis. Blood-borne invasion is most common, although entrance to the central nervous system (CNS) via the cerebrospinal fluid (CSF) or retrograde axoplasmic flow from peripheral nerves also occurs. Viral penetration of the blood-brain barrier results in **perivascular cuffing involving sensitized T cells, B cells, and macrophages.** Meningitis and encephalitis should first be considered viral rather than bacterial disease. Arboviruses can be involved in acute disease and unconventional agents called *prions* in slow infections.

A. Aseptic meningitis: Viral (aseptic) meningitis is milder and more common than bacterial meningitis, except in children younger than age 10 years, where bacterial meningitis is more common.
   1. **Enteroviruses (Coxsackie and echoviruses)**
      a. **Features**: Infection occurs primarily in late summer and early fall.
      b. Disease
         (1) These viruses **cause 90% of aseptic meningitis**.
         (2) **Diagnosis**: may be rapidly diagnosed by RT-PCR tests for viral RNA in the CSF.
   2. **Mumps virus** causes a spring infection in unvaccinated individuals.
   3. **Lymphocytic choriomeningitis (LCM) virus** is transferred to humans through contact with urine of infected mice, guinea pigs, or hamsters **(zoonotic infection).**

4. **HSV-2** almost always causes meningitis during a primary genital infection.
5. **Human immunodeficiency virus (HIV).**
    a. **Features**
        (1) HIV infection of the brain occurs early in the disease process.
        (2) The virus infects astrocytes, microglial cells, and macrophages of the CNS.
    b. **Disease**
        (1) Causes meningitis in 5% to 10% of cases during initial infection.
        (2) Causes HIV-associated neurocognitive disorder (HAND) and HIV-associated dementia (HAD).

B. **Meningoencephalitis/encephalitis:** These diseases, if of an infectious origin, are primarily viral diseases with HSV-1, arboviruses, and rabies causing life-threatening disease. **Cerebral dysfunction occurs.** Several childhood illnesses such as measles, mumps, and chickenpox may have a meningoencephalitis component. Prognosis usually depends on the agent, but antiviral therapy is available for HSV infections and immune globulins for rabies.
    1. **Herpes simplex viruses**
        a. **Features: HSVs are alphaherpesviruses that establish latency in sensory neurons.**
        b. **Disease**
            (1) HSVs are the most common cause of severe sporadic meningoencephalitis.
            (2) They cause disease following primary infection of infants (usually HSV-2) or due to reactivation of HSV-1 following some type of immunosuppression in adults.
            (3) The infection is **localized to the temporal lobes**, so computed tomography (CT) scans and electroencephalograms (EEGs) are diagnostic aids.
            (4) **Treatment**: may be treated with high-dose, intravenous acyclovir, or with ganciclovir or foscarnet in patients who experience intolerance to acyclovir. The mortality rate is 70% in untreated patients.
    2. **Rabies virus**
        a. **Features**: The virus travels by retrograde axoplasmic flow in peripheral nerves to the brain from the site of inoculation.
        b. **Disease**
            (1) Rabies virus is usually acquired through the bite of an infected animal (**zoonotic infection**) and is always fatal if the patient is untreated or unimmunized.
            (2) It may be acquired from aerosols containing the virus.
            (3) The incubation time may last several months depending on the initial site of infection.
            (4) Rabies disease may take two forms:
                (a) Furious rabies signs are hyperactivity, hydrophobia, hallucinations, and lack of co-ordination. Disease progression to death is rapid.
                (b) Paralytic rabies has a slower disease course beginning with muscle paralysis at the site of inoculation and ending with coma and death.
            (5) **Diagnosis:** by epidemiology and clinical findings including fever, headache, muscle spasms, and convulsions.
            (6) **Prevention:** prevented by vaccination with a **killed vaccine** (**HDCV,** commercially called *Imovax-Rabies*) or treated with rabies **immunoglobulin** (**RIG,** commercially called *Imogam-Rabies*).
    3. **Arboviruses**
        a. **West Nile virus**
            (1) **Features**
                (a) West Nile virus is the **leading cause of arboviral encephalitis in the United States.**
                (b) Birds, particularly **crows and jays, are natural hosts.**
            (2) **Disease**
                (a) The virus is normally transmitted by mosquito bite but can be transferred by blood transfusions, breastfeeding, and through the placenta.
                (b) It causes asymptomatic disease in 80% of those infected, but 20% develop **West Nile fever**, and less than 1% develop **West Nile neurologic disease (WNND),** which is more likely to occur in individuals older than age 60 years.

b. Other arboviruses (St. Louis, LaCrosse, California, Eastern equine encephalitis [EEE], and Western equine encephalitis [WEE] viruses)
  (1) These viruses cause mosquito-borne infections with bird or mammal reservoirs.
  (2) Diseases vary in severity depending on the virus. (California virus infection rarely results in fatalities, while the EEE virus is estimated to have a 50% mortality rate.)

C. Poliomyelitis/poliovirus
  1. Features: The leading cause of polio worldwide is from vaccine-derived strains of the virus. Wild polio is endemic only in Afghanistan and Pakistan as of 2022.
  2. Disease
    a. Poliovirus usually causes an asymptomatic (95%) or minor upper respiratory tract (4%) infection. In rare cases, it can cause an aseptic meningitis that can progress to a paralytic disease by destroying the lower motor neurons of the spinal cord and brainstem, resulting in paralysis of the lower limbs and, occasionally, respiratory paralysis.
    b. Prevention: may be prevented by a **trivalent inactivated vaccine (Salk vaccine);** an effective World Health Organization (WHO) vaccine program has eliminated this disease from most parts of the world.

D. Transverse myelitis/human T-lymphotropic virus type 1 (HTLV-1)
  1. Features: The virus is prominent in various populations of Native Australians, those in equatorial regions of Africa, some South American countries, the Caribbean, and parts of Japan and the Middle East. The virus is also associated with development of adult T-cell leukemia/lymphoma.
  2. Disease
    a. HTLV-1 causes a disease known as *tropical spastic paraparesis* (TSP), which is a slowly progressive demyelinating upper motor neuron disease in which 30% of those infected are bedridden and 45% are unable to walk after 10 years.
    b. TSP is endemic in the Caribbean.

E. Acute postinfectious encephalomyelitis:
In this rare disease, the neurologic signs and symptoms develop late during the clinical infection or weeks after recovery. The symptoms include personality and behavioral changes, which may proceed to convulsions and coma. **Immunopathologic mechanisms** perhaps involving autoimmune reactions to CNS antigens are thought to be responsible.
  1. HIV, CMV, and EBV are frequently associated with **Guillain-Barré syndrome.**
  2. Influenza B, VZV, and adenovirus have been implicated in conjunction with salicylates in **Reye syndrome.**
  3. Various childhood viruses such as measles, mumps, rubella, and VZV have been implicated.
  4. Rabies virus vaccine has been observed to cause this disease.

F. Latent or recurrent infections:
After primary systemic infection with some viruses, the virus becomes latent in neurons and reactivates to cause disease under conditions of immunosuppression induced by drug treatment, advancing age, and so forth.
  1. Herpes simplex viruses
    a. Features: HSVs can **latently infect neurons** in the trigeminal ganglia.
    b. Disease
      (1) Reactivation to cause **fever blisters or cold sores.**
      (2) Treatment: may be treated with topical or oral acyclovir, but the **virus** is **not eliminated.**
  2. Varicella zoster virus
    a. Features: VZV reactivates from the neurons of sensory ganglia (usually in areas supplied by the trigeminal nerve and thoracic ganglion).
    b. Disease
      (1) Causes **herpes zoster or shingles** (Figure 5.3).
      (2) Postherpetic neuralgia (PHN) may occur after skin lesions of shingles have crusted.

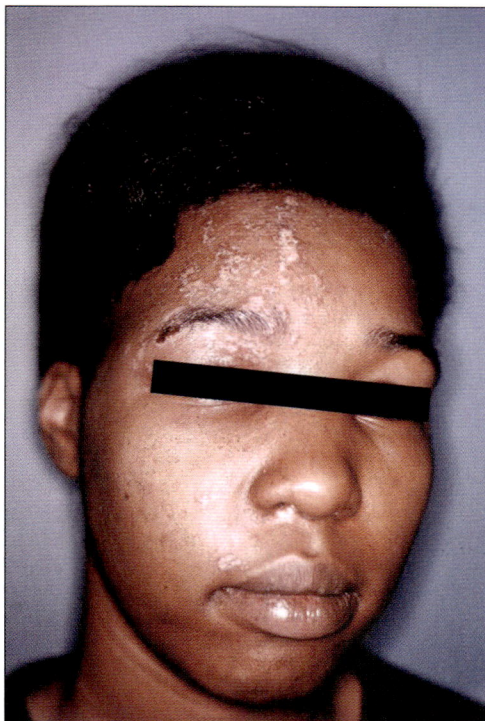

FIGURE 5.3. The lesion on this woman's face represents a shingles outbreak, due to varicella zoster virus (VZV), also known as *human herpesvirus-3* (HHV-3). The infection causes a pustulovesicular rash after lying dormant in the spinal nerve roots of an individual with chickenpox infection and then reactivating. (Photo courtesy of CDC Public Health Image Library [PHIL], image 12621.)

   (3) Treatment and prevention
      (a) Shingles may be treated with oral acyclovir and famciclovir; PHN may be treated with famciclovir.
      (b) The incidence of both diseases is decreased by immunization of the older adults (age ≥60) with **Zostavax vaccine** (containing a higher dose of live attenuated virus than childhood VZV vaccines).
      (c) Shingles may also be treated or infection prevented by **varicella zoster immune globulin (VZIG)** preparations.

G. Slow CNS infections: Two of these infections involve rare complications of common viruses, while the spongiform encephalitis involves "unconventional" infectious agents called *prions*.
   1. Measles virus can cause a rare **subacute sclerosing panencephalitis (SSPE)** that develops 1 to 10 years after apparent recovery from acute measles.
   2. JC virus
      a. Features
         (1) It is a benign latent infection of up to 90% of the adult population.
         (2) Risk for reactivation is increased in people living with HIV, patients with cancer, or those receiving chemotherapy and some immunobiologics.
      b. Disease
         (1) JC virus can reactivate to cause a rare syndrome known as ***progressive multifocal leukoencephalopathy* (PML).**
         (2) Diagnosis: may be diagnosed by PCR techniques for viral DNA in the CSF or second-generation ELISA for antibodies in serum.
   3. Kuru and variant Creutzfeldt-Jakob disease (vCJD) prions
      a. Features: They are distinguished by long incubations and lack of inflammation.
      b. Disease

(1) These prions cause progressive brain disorders involving typical spongiform histologic changes in affected areas of the brain.

(2) They are transmitted by cannibalism practices (kuru) or consumption of beef containing the prion associated with bovine spongiform encephalopathy (**vCJD**).

(3) Sporadic CJD can occur spontaneously, be inheritable, or be iatrogenically transmitted.

X. SKIN, MUCOSAL, AND SOFT TISSUE INFECTIONS

Some viruses cause acute localized infections (eg, HPV [warts]), while others produce exanthems and enanthems as part of their systemic disease process (eg, VZV [chickenpox]). The exanthems are manifested as a vesicular or maculopapular rash, which may act as diagnostic aids. Enanthems are small spots on mucous membranes. Those viruses that cause lesions in the mouth and throat were previously covered, and those that produce lesions in the genitalia are discussed under STI. Those viruses that mainly affect children are included in the childhood infections section.

A. Human papillomavirus

1. HPV causes **cutaneous warts** (common, plantar, and flat), which can be curetted or ablated by freezing with liquid nitrogen.

2. The warts or papilloma lesions contain **koilocytotic cells.**

B. Human herpesvirus-8

1. Features

a. Known as *Kaposi sarcoma–associated herpesvirus.*

b. Kaposi spots visible as red or purple skin lesions result from the virus inducing abnormal angiogenesis beneath the skin (Figure 5.4).

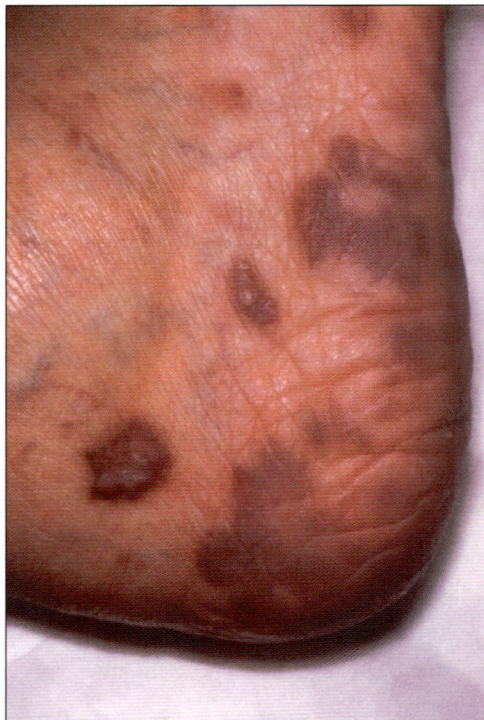

FIGURE 5.4. Kaposi sarcoma (KS) on a patient's right heel shows the characteristic bluish red cutaneous plaques arising from a cancer of the lymphatic endothelial lining. KS is a malignant tumor of the lymphatic endothelium caused by human herpesvirus-8 (HHV-8), also known as *Kaposi sarcoma–associated herpesvirus* (KSHV). (Photo courtesy of CDC Public Health Image Library [PHIL], image 14430.)

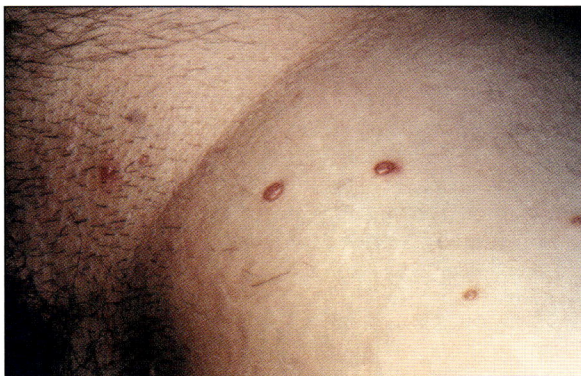

FIGURE 5.5. This patient presented to a clinical setting with pearly papules, characteristic of the viral infection, molluscum contagiosum. Though difficult to see in this view, the papules were slightly umbilicated (depressed center). (Photo courtesy of CDC Public Health Image Library [PHIL], image 16687.)

2. **Disease**
    a. **Causes intermittent fevers, night sweats, fatigue, and weight loss.**
    b. **Induces Kaposi sarcoma lesions on the face, legs, in the genital area, or in the mouth.**
    c. Also causes other conditions such as multicentric Castleman disease and primary effusion lymphoma.

C. Molluscum contagiosum virus
    1. **Features**
        a. **Has a long incubation period from weeks to months.**
        b. **It infects only keratinocytes.**
    2. **Disease**
        a. Causes water wart lesions or mollusca that typically occur in groups on the arms and face (Figure 5.5).
        b. Transmitted by skin-to-skin contact or indirectly from fomites.

D. Orf virus
    1. **Features**: The animal manifestation is pustular or scabby lesions around the mouth and nose.
    2. **Disease**
        a. This virus causes a sheep or goat disease that can be transferred to humans (**zoonotic infection**).
        b. It causes papulovesicular lesions that usually begin on the finger but can also occur on the face.

E. HSV, VZV, human herpesviruses 6 and 7, human parvoviruses, measles virus, rubella virus, Coxsackie and echoviruses, and other rash-producing viruses are covered in other sections.

SITUATION-BASED DISEASES

XI. CHILDHOOD INFECTIONS

This section describes the viruses associated with the common childhood diseases that occur in unvaccinated children. Important congenital and neonatal infections are covered later (section XII).

A. Measles (Morbillivirus)
    1. **Features**
        a. Humans are the only natural host.
        b. Measles can remain contagious in the air for several hours or on surfaces for up to 2 hours.

2. Disease

a. Measles virus causes an infection producing a **maculopapular rash** (first seen below the hairline and behind the ears) and produces a high fever, cough, coryza, conjunctivitis, and **Koplik spots** on buccal mucosa (12-24 hours before the rash) (Figure 5.6).

b. Measles may cause complications, including a postinfectious encephalitis, giant cell pneumonia, atypical measles (disease in those previously vaccinated), and, after many years, SSPE (subacute sclerosing panencephalitis).

c. **The virus is transmitted by respiratory droplets.**

d. **Temporary immunosuppression** occurs due to lymphocyte infection.

e. **Diagnosis:** can be clinically diagnosed, but laboratory confirmation of measles outbreaks and sporadic cases is needed.

    (1) Can be detected by throat swab or urine test.

    (2) Serum IgM for acute illness or quantitative RT-PCR using respiratory specimens.

f. **Prevention:** may be prevented by **vaccination with the live attenuated Enders-Edmonston strain** either by itself or in combination with attenuated strains of mumps and rubella viruses (measles, mumps, and rubella [MMR] vaccine).

B. Mumps virus

1. Features

a. Humans are the only natural hosts.

b. Mumps virus is often associated with asymptomatic disease but can cause a late winter or early spring disease.

2. Disease

a. It is characterized by sudden onset, fever, and parotitis; it is sometimes accompanied by orchitis, pancreatitis, and meningoencephalitis (50% have involvement, but only 10% have symptoms) (Figure 5.7).

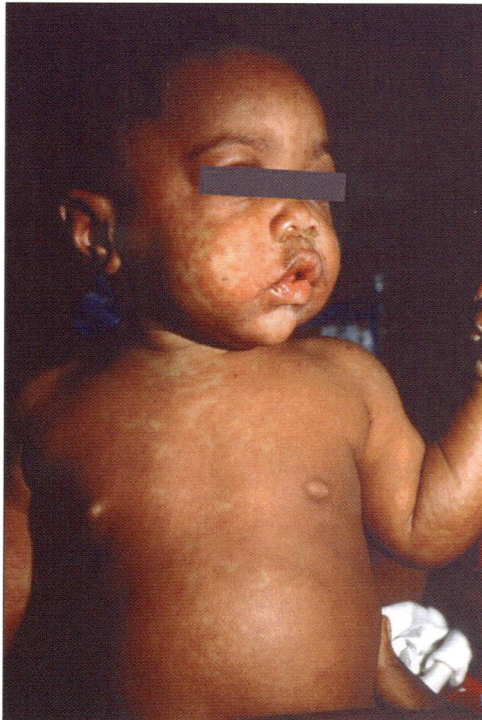

FIGURE 5.6. This photograph depicts the head, neck, and chest of an infant infected with Morbillivirus, the cause of measles, or rubeola. The characteristic rash associated with this viral infection had spread to all regions visible, involving the infant's face upper extremities, and torso. (Photo courtesy of CDC Public Health Image Library [PHIL], image 17639.)

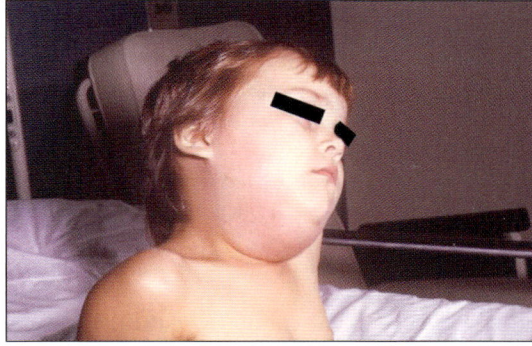

FIGURE 5.7. In this child with a mumps infection, note the characteristic swollen neck region due to an enlargement of the child's salivary glands, and in this case, swelling and tenderness of the thyroid gland. (Photo courtesy of CDC Public Health Image Library [PHIL], image 130.)

    b. Diagnosis: has a clinical diagnosis or ELISA for IgM.
    c. Prevention: Disease is prevented by vaccination with the **live attenuated Jeryl Lynn strain** or in combination with attenuated strains of measles and rubella viruses (MMR vaccine).

C. Rubella virus
    1. Features
        a. Humans are the only natural host.
        b. The virus is transmitted by respiratory droplets.
        c. Swollen posterior auricular lymph nodes and in the neck are a prominent clinical feature.
        d. Also known as *German measles.*
    2. Disease
        a. Rubella virus causes a benign disease in children, which may be subclinical or symptomatic. Symptoms include a 3- to 5-day rash consisting of macules that coalesce to a "blush," fever, malaise, and swollen neck and suboccipital lymph nodes. It causes a more severe disease in adults that may be complicated by arthralgia, arthritis, and a postinfectious encephalitis (1/5,000 cases) (**Figure 5.8**).
        b. It can produce a **severe congenital infection,** leading to severe teratogenic effects in fetuses of nonimmune mothers.
        c. Diagnosis: Infections are diagnosed by ELISA for IgM and immune status of individuals by ELISA for IgG.
        d. Prevention: Disease is prevented by vaccination with the **live, attenuated RA 27/3 strain** of the virus or in combination with attenuated strains of measles and mumps viruses (MMR vaccine).

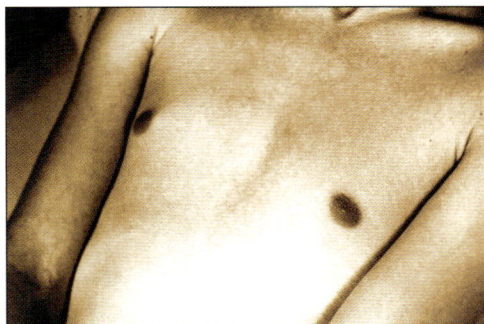

FIGURE 5.8. This macular rash over the chest and upper arms is due to a German measles viral infection, also referred to as rubella. (Photo courtesy of CDC Public Health Image Library [PHIL], image 22150.)

D. Varicella zoster virus
1. **Features**: VZV latently infects neurons.
2. **Diseases**
    a. VZV causes a disease (**chickenpox**) characterized by fever and vesicular rash on the trunk, face, and scalp, which is usually benign and self-limiting in healthy children but more severe in adults (potential for pneumonia) (Figure 5.9).
    b. The virus can reactivate to cause herpes zoster or shingles later in life.
    c. Transmission is by contact of fluid-filled blisters of an infected person or by inhalation of droplets.
    d. **Diagnosis:** diagnosed clinically. Vesicular fluid or scabs submitted for PCR evaluation are used for confirmatory testing.
    e. **Prevention:** may be prevented by **vaccination with the live, attenuated Oka strain** or treatment of individuals at high risk or who are immunosuppressed with **VZIG. A recombinant vaccine and live attenuated vaccine are available for those older than age 50 years to prevent shingles.**

E. Human parvovirus B-19
1. **Features**
    a. The virus is tropic for erythrocyte precursors in the bone marrow.
    b. The infection is more common in children.
    c. It can be transmitted by respiratory droplets.
2. **Disease**
    a. Although these infections are usually asymptomatic, this virus can cause **erythema infectiosum (fifth disease),** a biphasic illness first presenting as flulike, but progressing in several weeks to arthralgia accompanied by a **"slapped cheek" rash,** which first appears on the face and then spreads to the arms and legs (Figure 5.10).

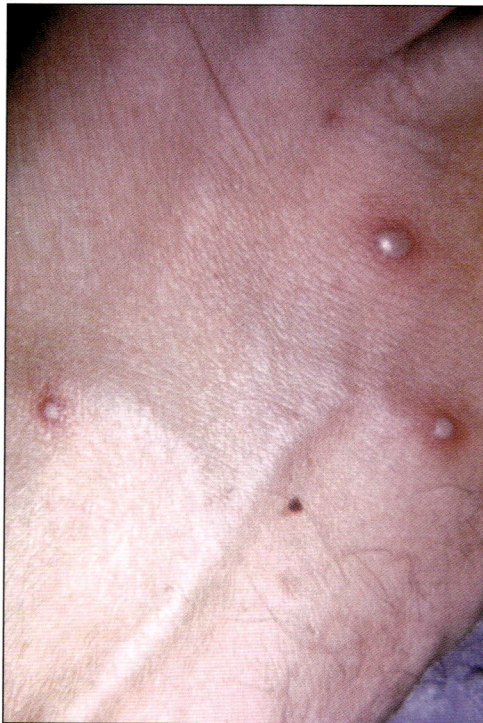

FIGURE 5.9. This close-up view of a maculopapular rash on the dorsum of the right foot was determined to be a case of chickenpox, caused by the varicella zoster virus (VZV), also known as *human herpesvirus-3* (HHV-3). These vesicles are in the eruptive stage, consisting of fluid-filled blisters. (Photo courtesy of CDC Public Health Image Library [PHIL], image 21,502.)

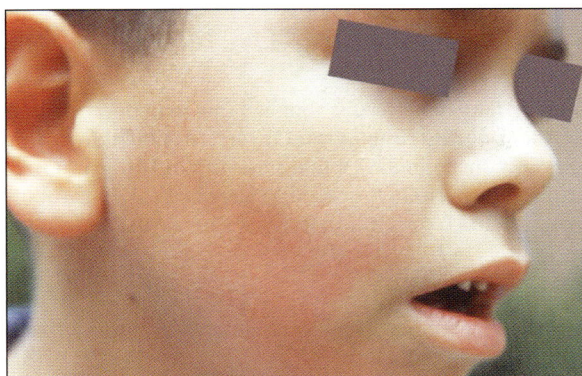

FIGURE 5.10. Erythema infectiosum, or fifth disease, is caused by the human parvovirus B-19. (Photo courtesy of CDC Public Health Image Library [PHIL], image 4509.)

    b. It may cause **aplastic crises** in individuals suffering from chronic hemolytic anemia.

    c. Diagnosis: may be diagnosed by ELISA for IgM.

F. Human herpesviruses 6 and 7 cause a benign disease in young children called *exanthem subitum (roseola),* which is characterized by a rapid onset fever and an immune-mediated generalized rash.

G. Mpox virus

    1. Features

        a. It is considered a **zoonotic** infection as it was discovered in monkey research colonies and can infect small mammals. The animal reservoir is unknown.

        b. The virus is usually reported in areas of central and western Africa.

        c. In 2022, a **worldwide outbreak** of Mpox clade II virus occurred, which is less severe than clade I.

        d. While generally not considered a sexually transmitted infection, the virus can be transmitted during sex and intimate contact.

        e. Most cases in the 2022 outbreak have occurred in men who have sex with men.

    2. Disease

        a. Symptoms of infection may include swollen lymph nodes, headache, fever, chills, muscle and body aches.

        b. The virus causes a rash that may blister and then scab over. These may be itchy or painful.

        c. The rash is often observed on the hands, feet, trunk, face, and/or in the genital area (**Figure 5.11**).

        d. More severe disease, including death, can occur in individuals who are immuno-compromised.

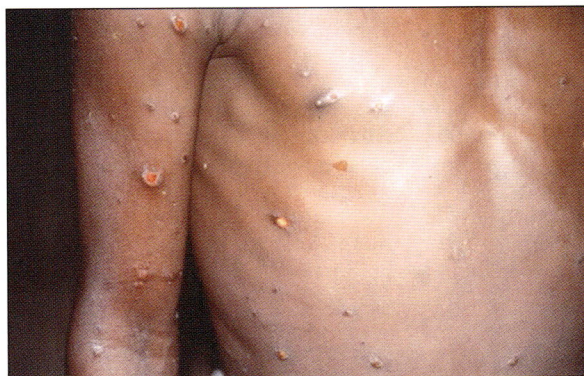

FIGURE 5.11. This image was taken during a 1997 investigation into an outbreak of Mpox in the Democratic Republic of the Congo, formerly Zaire. Pictured here are the right arm and torso of a patient displaying a number of lesions due to an active case of Mpox. Note how this rash resembles smallpox. (Photo courtesy of CDC Public Health Image Library [PHIL], image 12779. PHIL images 12745 through 12784 depict the story of this investigation.)

XII. CONGENITAL AND NEONATAL INFECTIONS

Several viruses can infect the fetus with results that vary from inconsequential effects to death. **Disease is frequently dependent on the time of fetal infection.** Infection during the first 5 months of pregnancy may have serious consequences. Other viruses like HSV can infect infants during travel through an infected birth canal (perinatal) or shortly after birth (HBV). All of the following viruses, except HBV, can cross the placenta (congenital). Primary disease in children and adults has been discussed previously.

A. Rubella virus
   1. Rubella virus causes a 90% chance of multiple **defects in fetuses** infected during the first 10 weeks of pregnancy.
   2. It causes some reversible effects such as hepatitis and meningoencephalitis in the neonate, but permanent auditory and other CNS-related problems are common.
   3. There is no treatment, and a baby infected during the first 3 months is likely to be severely affected.

B. Cytomegalovirus
   1. CMV causes the **most common congenital infection** that almost always accompanies a primary infection in a pregnant patient.
   2. Infections are usually asymptomatic at birth, but approximately 25% will develop deafness and neurologic problems.
   3. CMV can infect neonates during delivery through an infected birth canal or via breastfeeding, but infants usually remain healthy.

C. Parvovirus B-19 can infect both mother and fetus during epidemics, but the outcome is good for both, unless the infection of the fetus occurs during the first 20 weeks of pregnancy, when a severe anemia resulting in death can occur.

D. Varicella zoster virus
   1. VZV can cause deformities in fetuses exposed during weeks 13 to 20 of pregnancy, but administration of VZIG to the mother offers protection.
   2. VZV may have a 40% mortality rate in neonates born to mothers with an active chickenpox infection at the time of birth; VZIG given to the newborn can help minimize the effect of VZV infection.

E. Herpes simplex virus
   1. HSV can be transferred to the fetus transplacentally from the mother. It results in severe disease with high mortality; treatment with acyclovir is helpful.
   2. Transmission at the time of delivery can cause a serious disseminated disease, and intravenous acyclovir should be administered.

F. Human immunodeficiency virus
   1. HIV may be transmitted transplacentally, during vaginal birth, or after birth through breast milk of an HIV-infected mother. Maternal treatment during pregnancy reduces transmission during birth and transplacentally by almost 99%. Females with HIV are advised not to breastfeed.
   2. It can be diagnosed in newborns by detecting HIV RNA in the blood.

G. HBV can be transmitted by fluids including breast milk to infants born to chronically infected mothers (HBeAg$^-$ in 10%-25% and HBeAg$^+$ in 90%). It usually causes an asymptomatic disease, with a high probability of becoming a chronic infection.

XIII. SEXUALLY TRANSMITTED INFECTIONS

HIV, HSV-1, HSV-2, and HPV are the main viruses emphasized in this section. Although not known for their genital signs and symptoms, HIV and HBV are well known as *STIs*. Both HSV and HPV are associated with distinctive genital lesions. HBV and CMV may be acquired through sexual contact but have no genital signs or symptoms. The diseases associated with these viruses are described elsewhere in this chapter.

A. Human immunodeficiency virus
1. **Features**
   a. Has a long (years) **latency period.**
   b. **Kills CD4$^+$ T cells causing immunosuppression.**
2. **Diseases**
   a. HIV causes an **asymptomatic or infectious mononucleosis-like primary infection** that progresses to acquired immunodeficiency syndrome **(AIDS)-related complex (ARC) disease and finally AIDS.**
   b. It may be transmitted intrauterinely, perinatally, or through breast milk.
   c. It can be inhibited by several classes of antivirals:
      (1) Inhibitors of reverse transcriptase (both nucleoside analogs and nonnucleosides).
      (2) Viral protease inhibitors.
      (3) Fusion inhibitors.
      (4) Capsid inhibitors.
      (5) CCR5 antagonists.
3. **Treatment**
   a. Treated with **highly active antiretroviral therapy (HAART)**, a combination of two nucleoside analogs and a protease inhibitor.
   b. Long-acting injectables are available.
   c. HIV sequencing of genetic mutations is done to identify optimal therapy regimens.

B. Herpes simplex viruses
1. **Features**
   a. **HSV-1 is predominantly orally transmitted.**
   b. **HSV-2 is predominantly transmitted by sexual contact.**
2. **Diseases**
   a. HSV causes the most common infections that lead to genital ulcers (**Figure 5.12**).
   b. Mild meningitis may be associated with the genital disease and frequently leads to **latent infections with recurrent disease.**

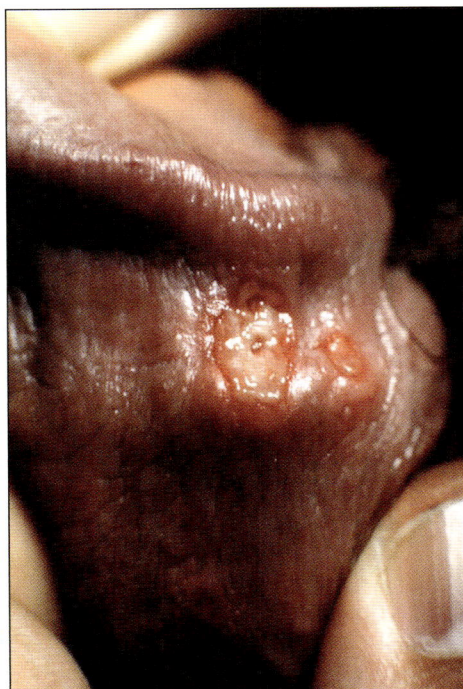

FIGURE 5.12. This outbreak of herpes genitalis manifested as blistering on the underside of the penile shaft, just proximal to the corona of the glans, due to herpes simplex virus-2 (HSV-2), otherwise referred to as genital herpes. Sexually transmitted HSV-2 typically causes one or more blisters to form on or around the genitals or rectum, which break, leaving tender ulcers that may take 2 to 4 weeks to heal. (Photo courtesy of CDC Public Health Image Library [PHIL], image 15822.)

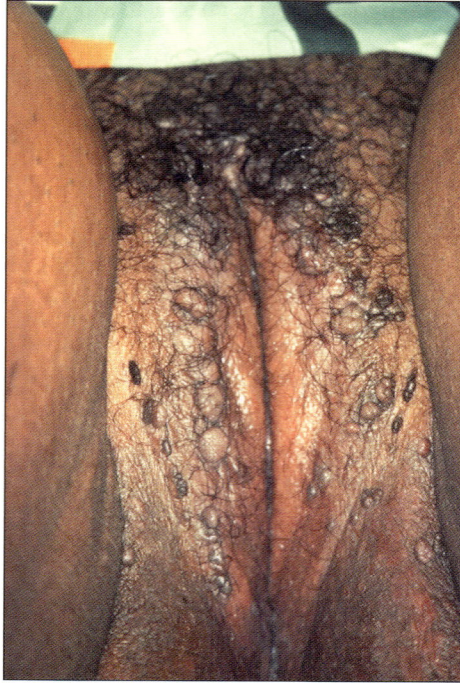

FIGURE 5.13. This close view of the exterior vaginal region of a female patient's perineum reveals the presence of numerous genital warts, located primarily on the labia majora, which were long-standing and remained after repeated attempts to remove them. (Photo courtesy of CDC Public Health Image Library [PHIL], image 17418.)

     c. Treatment: can be treated with oral acyclovir, valacyclovir, or famciclovir to shorten disease associated with primary infection and recurrences, but **antiviral-resistant strains** can emerge during prolonged therapy, and the virus is never eliminated from the infected ganglion by antiviral treatment.

C. Human papillomavirus
  1. Features: There are low- and high-risk types defined originally by their contribution to cervical neoplasia.
  2. Disease
    a. Several strains of HPV cause **venereal warts, the most common STI** (Figure 5.13).
    b. Some types (most commonly 16 and 18) are *also* associated with cervical dysplasia and **cervical intraepithelial neoplasia** (**CIN**).
    c. Treatment and prevention
     (1) Genital warts may be treated with podophyllin or cryotherapy.
     (2) A recombinant quadrivalent vaccine (Gardasil) containing virus-like particles of types 6, 11, 16, and 18, the causes of 90% of genital warts and 70% of CIN, and Cervarix, a bivalent vaccine containing L1 proteins from type 16 and 18 viruses, is available.

D. HBV. Although it does not produce genital signs or symptoms, HBV is considered an STI (see VI B 1 for clinical diseases).

XIV. POSTINFECTIOUS DISEASE

A number of viruses are associated with postinfectious disorders. Most have been mentioned in the nervous system section. They include VZV; measles, influenza, and mumps viruses (meningoencephalitis); CMV (Guillain-Barré syndrome); influenza B; and VZV (Reye syndrome). Possible mechanisms include persistent low-grade infection, autoantibodies, and immune complexes.

A. EBV sometimes causes **erythema multiforme** following virus infection of toddlers.

B. HSV can cause **erythema multiforme** during recurrences of cold sores.

XV. ORGAN TRANSPLANT–ASSOCIATED DISEASES

Two mechanisms are involved in initiating these infections: the virus in the transplanted organ and reactivation of the virus during immunosuppressive therapy of the patient.

A. HBV can cause chronic asymptomatic infections involving the pancreas and the liver, and a donor should be serologically monitored for this virus before being deemed acceptable.

B. CMV can be reactive in patients with AIDS and other immune-suppressed conditions to cause a life-threatening pneumonitis.

XVI. ARBOVIRAL AND ZOONOTIC DISEASES

A. The majority of important **arboviral diseases** have been discussed: **West Nile virus** and **encephalitis viruses** in the nervous system and **yellow fever virus** in the gastrointestinal system.

B. The **four important zoonotic infections—hantavirus, rabies virus, LCM virus, and orf virus—** have been discussed in the respiratory, nervous, and skin sections, respectively.

C. Dengue virus features
1. Transmitted by a **mosquito bite** in the **Caribbean or Southeast Asia.**
2. There are four virus types.
3. **Primary infection produces neutralizing antibodies, but a secondary viral infection of a different type will be enhanced by the antibodies produced in the primary infection.**
4. Disease
    a. It causes **"breakbone fever"** consisting of high fever, headache, rash, and back and bone pain.
    b. It is particularly dangerous in children where reinfection by a different serotype can result in a severe hemorrhagic fever and can lead to a **fatal dengue shock syndrome**.
    c. **The Dengvaxia dengue vaccine is recommended for children aged 9 to 16 years with a previously laboratory-confirmed dengue infection.**
    d. **The vaccine protects against all four dengue types.**

Directions: Each of the numbered items or incomplete statements in this section is followed by answers or completions of the statement. Select the *one* lettered answer that is *best* in each case.

1. An 8-year-old boy is brought to your office by his mother. He has had a slight fever and a sore throat for the past 2 days. He has eight ulcerative lesions in his mouth, three vesicular lesions on his left hand, and five similar lesions on his right foot. Which of the following viruses is the most probable cause of his disease?

(A) Coxsackie A virus
(B) Human herpesvirus-6
(C) HSV
(D) HPV

2. A 16-year-old male presents at your office with a sore throat, fever, and enlarged lymph nodes. His tonsils are enlarged, his pharynx is inflamed, and splenomegaly is observed. He reports severe fatigue. Confirmation of the causative agent is best done by observing which of the following?

(A) Positive Tzanck smear
(B) IgM heterophile antibodies
(C) Koilocytotic cells
(D) RT-PCR for enterovirus

3. A 32-year-old pregnant woman presents to her obstetrician for a prenatal visit at 10 weeks of gestation. She is currently well and reports no significant illness during this pregnancy. The physician counsels that patient on the importance of screening for congenital infections. What is the most common cause of congenital infections leading to fetal malformations?

(A) CMV
(B) HSV
(C) Parvovirus
(D) Rubella virus

4. A 23-year-old medical student on the Caribbean island of Dominica presents at the Student Health Clinic with an increasingly severe headache and back and bone pain. Yesterday, they were nauseated and vomited several times during the night. They have a 39.5 °C/103 °F fever, which appeared suddenly, and a generalized rash that blanches under pressure. They have been hiking in the rainforest 1 week earlier and were particularly bothered by mosquitoes at that time. Which of the following agents is causing their symptoms?

(A) Dengue virus
(B) LCM virus
(C) West Nile virus
(D) Yellow fever virus

5. A 4-year-old girl is brought to a rural clinic office by her mother who states the child has a runny nose, barking cough, and sore throat. An examination indicates respiration is labored. None of her three siblings is sick. Which of the following viruses is the most probable cause of her symptoms?

(A) Adenovirus
(B) Influenza virus
(C) Parainfluenza virus
(D) RSV

6. Which of the following individuals is most at risk to develop chronic liver disease?

(A) A 1-month-old infant infected with HBV
(B) A 22-year-old coinfected with HBV and HDV
(C) A 26-year-old alcoholic intravenous drug abuser infected with HBV
(D) A 30-year-old infected with yellow fever virus

7. A 64-year-old man living on a farm in southern Minnesota was brought to the emergency department on July 15 by his brother. The brother said the man had a 2-day history of fever, headache, and some vomiting, but today, he appeared confused. He is confused by some of the simple questions asked him during his examination. His spinal tap is clear with 75% polymorphonuclear neutrophils (PMNs), and a head CT is normal. Which of the following viruses is most likely the cause of his symptoms?

(A) California encephalitis virus
(B) Enterovirus
(C) HSV
(D) West Nile virus

8. A mother brings her 18-month-old son to your office. She was called by her day care center who reported he had vomited twice during the morning and had diarrhea as well. She noted he had a slight fever the past 2 days and had not been very hungry. Which of the following agents is most likely the cause of his illness?

(A) Adenovirus
(B) Astrovirus
(C) Norovirus
(D) Rotavirus

9. A 62-year-old patient with end-stage liver disease is evaluated for liver transplantation. When a donor becomes available, for which of the following viruses should they be monitored and determined to be serologically negative?

(A) CMV
(B) EBV
(C) HBV
(D) HEV

10. On September 17, a 22-year-old male college student appeared at the Student Health Clinic reporting moderate headache, nausea, and vomiting. His temperature was 38.5 °C/101 °F, and his physical examination showed stiffness in the neck. What is the most likely viral cause of the symptoms?

(A) CMV
(B) Enterovirus
(C) EBV
(D) HSV-1

11. A 28-year-old woman presents to the clinic with symptoms consistent with a recent viral infection of fever, fatigue, general malaise, and swollen lymph nodes. A complete blood count identified a low CD4$^+$ T-cell count. Knowing the mutational genotype of which of the following viruses would be important for initiating treatment?

(A) HBV
(B) HIV
(C) HPV
(D) HSV

12. A 40-year-old man presents to the urgent care clinic with fever, cough, and sore throat for the past 3 days. He mentions other family members in the house with similar symptoms. A rapid influenza test confirms influenza A infection. Which of the following medications is a neuraminidase inhibitor commonly used for influenza treatment?

(A) Acyclovir
(B) Amantadine
(C) Oseltamivir
(D) Ribavirin

Answers and Explanations

1. **The answer is A.** [III A 2 b] Coxsackie A virus causes hand, foot, and mouth disease, which is characterized by vesicular lesions in the mouth and extremities.

2. **The answer is B.** [III C 2 a (2) (a)] This boy's symptoms are consistent with infectious mononucleosis caused by EBV. During its pathogenesis, this virus produces an IgM heterophile antibody that is the basis for the monospot test.

3. **The answer is A.** [XII B 1] CMV is the most common cause of congenital infections that can lead to various symptoms in the newborn.

4. **The answer is A.** [XVI C] Dengue virus, which is transmitted by mosquito bites, is present in the Caribbean and causes "breakbone fever," which is consistent with these symptoms.

5. **The answer is C.** [IV A 2 a] The child's symptoms are those found with croup caused by parainfluenza virus.

6. **The answer is A.** [VI B 1 b (2)] The potential for chronic liver disease following HBV infection is inversely proportional to the age of infection. The probability is over 90% with neonates.

7. **The answer is D.** [IX B 3 a] The symptoms are most consistent with WNND, a rare complication of West Nile virus infections.

8. **The answer is D.** [V A] Rotaviruses are the most likely cause of infant gastroenteritis.

9. **The answer is C.** [VI B 3 a] Donors for liver transplants are serologically monitored for evidence of previous HBV and HCV infections since they can be asymptomatic yet transfer the virus to the liver recipients.

10. **The answer is B.** [IX A 1 b (1)] Enteroviral meningitis, for which there is only supportive treatment, is frequently seen in late summer or early fall.

11. **The answer is B.** [XIII A 3 c] As part of a new diagnosis of HIV infection, patient virus is submitted for next-generation sequencing to establish if any relevant therapy resistance mutations are present that could impact first-line antiretroviral therapy (ART). Genotyping is not needed for the other viruses relevant to therapy decisions.

12. **The answer is C.** [IV C 2 e] Oseltamivir is an example for a currently recommended neuraminidase inhibitor. Acyclovir is used as treatment for symptoms of herpesviruses. Ribavirin is approved for the treatment of HCV and pediatric RSV.

6

Mycology

I. FUNGAL STRUCTURE

A. **Fungi are eukaryotic organisms,** so they have similarities to human cells. **Differences targeted by antifungals include:**
   1. Fungal cells have **cell walls** (CWs).
      a. Fungal CWs **protect cells from osmotic shock, determine cell shapes,** and have components that **are antigenic**.
      b. Fungal CWs are primarily composed of **complex carbohydrates** such as **chitin, along with glucans and mannose-proteins.** The **CW glucan** (not found in humans) serves an **antifungal target for echinocandins like caspofungin**.
   2. **Ergosterol** is the dominant **fungal membrane sterol** (rather than human cholesterol) **targeted by imidazoles, triazoles, and polyenes antifungals.**

B. **Types** of fungi include **molds, mushrooms,** and **yeasts**.
   1. **Hyphae** are **filamentous cells of molds** (also known as the **filamentous fungi**) and **mushrooms.** Hyphae grow at the tips (apical growth).
      a. **Septae**, or septations, are **cross walls of hyphae** that occur in the hyphae of most disease-causing fungi. They are referred to as septate hyphae (**Figure 6.1**).
      b. **Nonseptate** or **aseptate hyphae lack regularly occurring cross walls.** These cells are multinucleate and are also called **coenocytic.** They often are quite variable in width with broad branching angles (**Figure 6.2**).
      c. Hyphae may be **dematiaceous (dark-colored)** or **hyaline (colorless).**
      d. Fluffy surface masses of hyphae and their "hidden" growth into tissue or laboratory medium are called **mycelia**.
   2. **Yeasts** are **single-celled fungi,** generally round to oval-shaped (**Figure 6.3**). They reproduce by **budding** (blastoconidia).
   3. **Pseudohyphae** (hyphae with sausage-like constrictions at septations) are formed by certain yeasts when they elongate but remain attached to each other. *Candida albicans* is notable for its development into **pseudohyphae and true hyphae** when it invades tissues (**Figure 6.4**).
   4. **Dimorphic fungi** are fungi capable of converting from a **yeast or yeast-like form to a filamentous form** and vice versa.

> **• • • Clinical Pearl**
>
> Overall, very few fungi are dimorphic; however, this ability is relatively common among fungi of medical importance, especially in terms of systemic fungal infections.

      a. Environmental conditions such as temperature and nutrient availability trigger this conversion.
      b. They exist in a **yeast or yeast-like form in a human host** and as **filamentous forms in the environment**, following the saying **"Yeastie beasties in body heat; mold in the cold."**

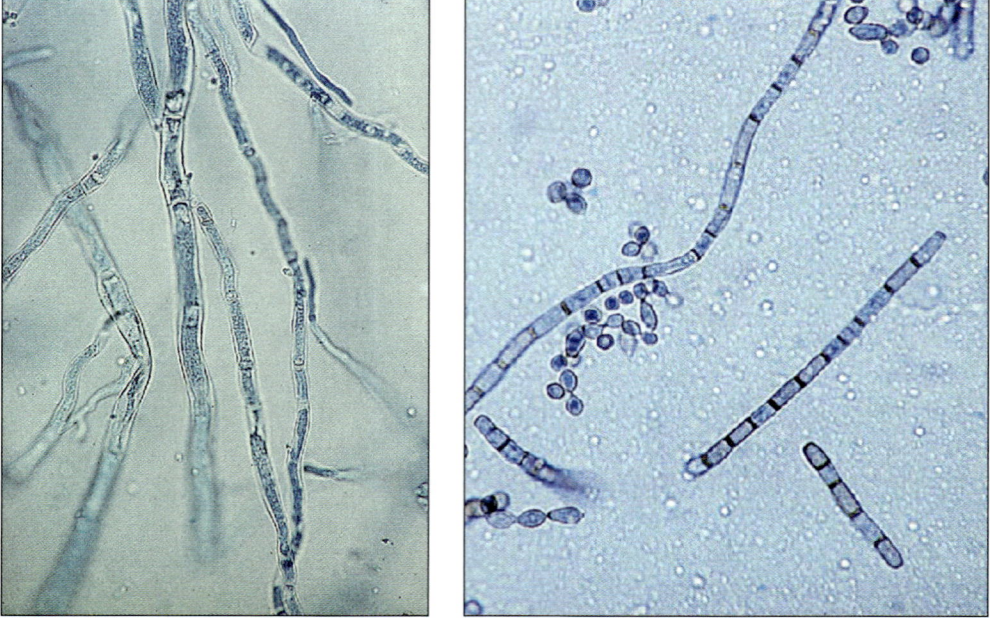

FIGURE 6.1. Microscopic examples of fungi with septate hyphae. (Courtesy of Glenn D. Roberts, PhD, Mayo Clinic, Rochester, MN.)

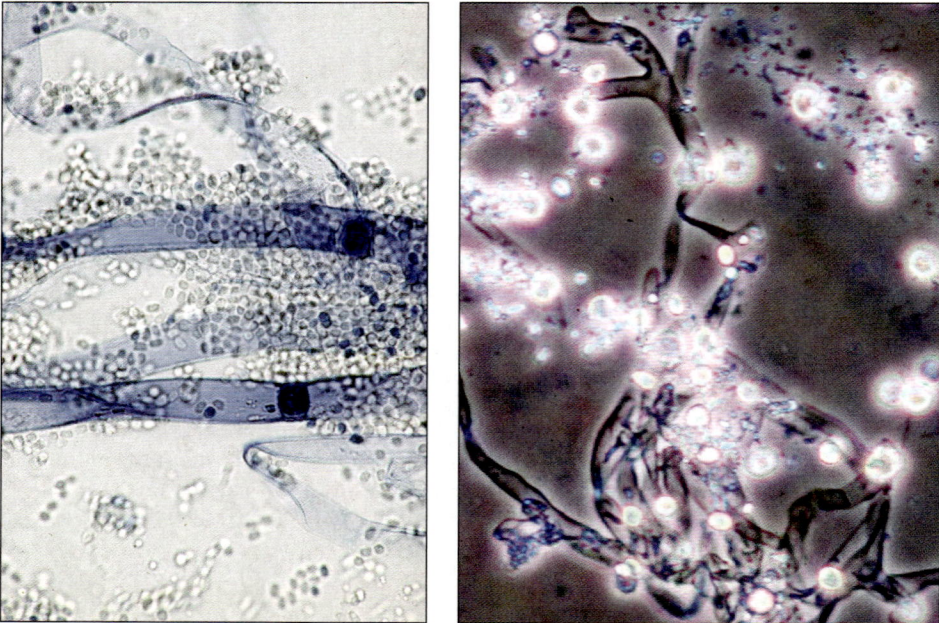

FIGURE 6.2. Microscopic examples of fungi with nonseptate hyphae. (Courtesy of Glenn D. Roberts, PhD, Mayo Clinic, Rochester, MN.)

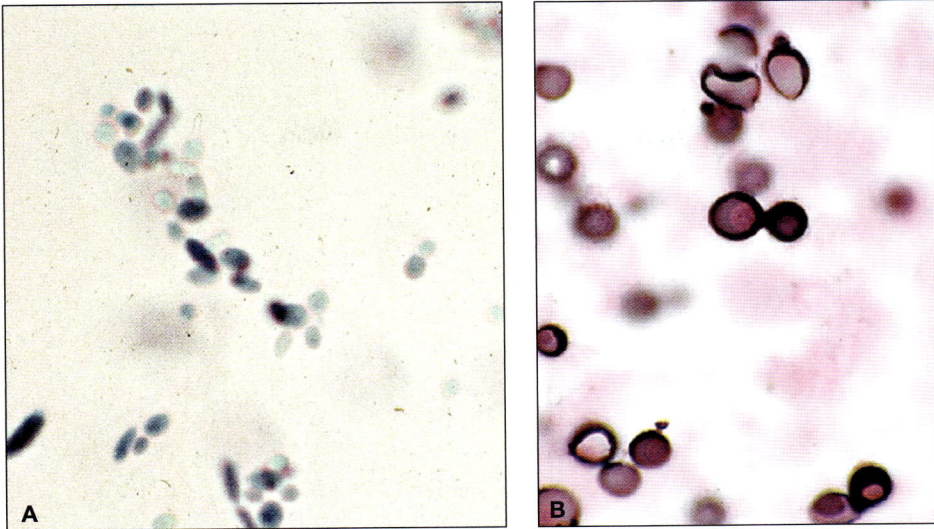

FIGURE 6.3. Budding yeasts. A. Budding yeasts stained with lactophenol blue. B. Budding yeasts stained with silver stain. This fungus is *Cryptococcus neoformans*, but the capsule cannot be clearly seen with the silver stain. (Courtesy of Glenn D. Roberts, PhD, Mayo Clinic, Rochester, MN.)

    c. Among the major pathogens are ***Blastomyces, Histoplasma, Coccidioides,*** and ***Sporothrix*** in the United States, and *Paracoccidioides* in South and Central America. For comparison of *Blastomyces'* two forms, refer to Figure 6.5.

• • • Clinical Pearl

Only one fungal species of medical importance produces a capsule, and that is *Cryptococcus neoformans*.

    5. Fungal spores are formed either asexually or by a sexual process involving nuclear fusion and meiosis. Fungal morphology, including spores, may be used in identification.
        a. Conidia are **asexual spores** of filamentous fungi (molds) or mushrooms (Figure 6.6A).
        b. Blastoconidia are new **yeast "buds"** (Figure 6.6B).
        c. Arthroconidia are **formed by laying down joints** in hyphae followed by fragmentation of the hyphal strand (Figure 6.6C).

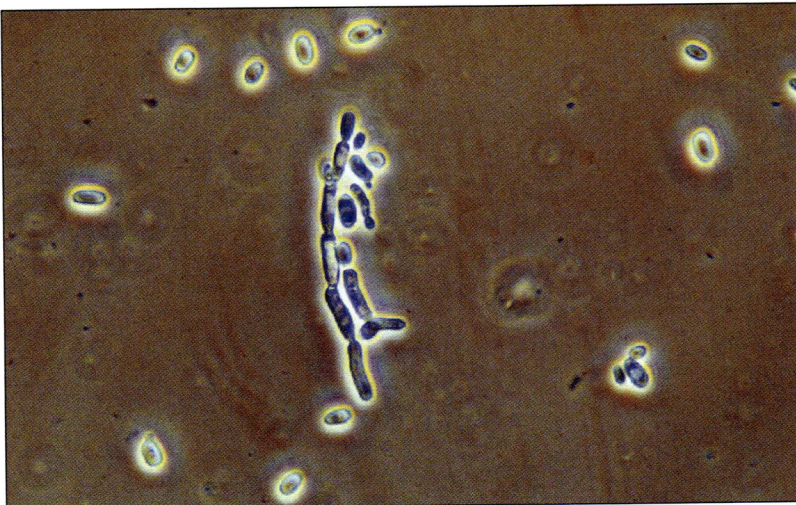

FIGURE 6.4. Pseudohyphae. When yeasts like *Candida albicans* bud but do not separate and instead continue to elongate, the result is pseudohyphae. Note the sausage-like constrictions between the cells. (Courtesy of Glenn D. Roberts, PhD, Mayo Clinic, Rochester, MN.)

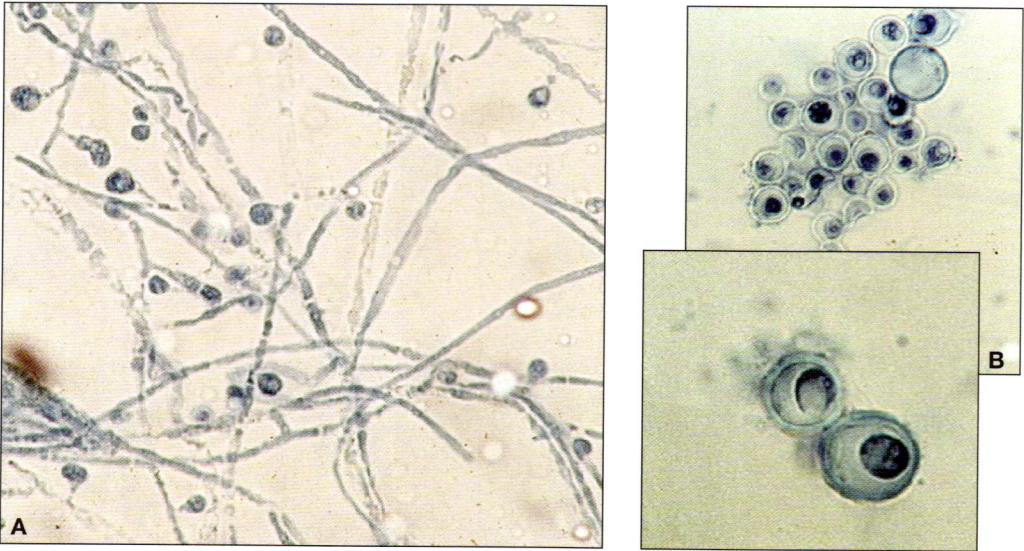

FIGURE 6.5. *Blastomyces* is a dimorphic fungus. Shown here are its hyphal and yeast forms. A. Hyphal form: This photo shows the environmental hyphae and conidia of *Blastomyces dermatitidis*. B. Yeast form: Note the large yeasts of *Blastomyces'* with thick cell walls and the broad base between the mother cell and the bud (as seen in the inset). This is the form of the fungi seen in tissues during infection. (Courtesy of Glenn D. Roberts, PhD, Mayo Clinic, Rochester, MN.)

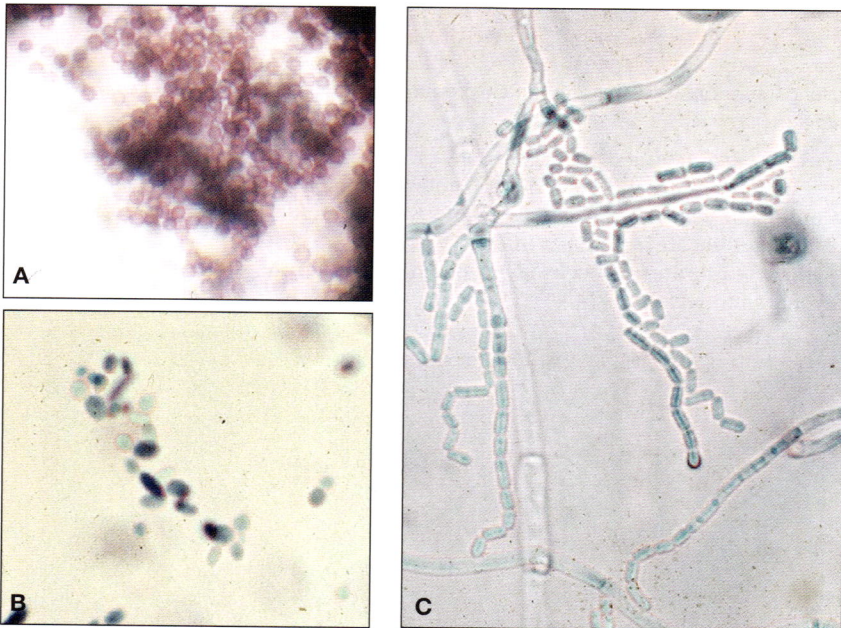

FIGURE 6.6. Common spore types. A. **Conidia**. B. **Blastoconidia**, commonly called buds. C. Strands of hyphae breaking up into **arthroconidia**. Arthroconidia may be seen when dermatophytes grow on the skin, where they often reproduce with minimal branching and produce arthroconidia. Distinctive barrel-shaped conidia may also be produced by *Coccidioides immitis* (see Figure 6.3A). (Courtesy of Glenn D. Roberts, PhD, Mayo Clinic, Rochester, MN.)

II. FUNGAL GROWTH AND REPLICATION

Fungal nutrition: Fungi require preformed organic compounds derived from their environment.

1. **Saprobes** live on **dead organic material.** Some are opportunistic, causing disease if traumatically implanted into tissue.
2. **Commensal colonizers** generally **live in harmony with humans,** deriving their nutrition from compounds on body surfaces. Some are **opportunists,** because under certain conditions (eg, reduced immune responsiveness), they may invade tissue or vasculature and cause disease.
3. **Pathogens** infect the healthy but cause more severe disease in the compromised hosts. The damage to living cells provides nutrition. Most are also environmental saprobes.

III. FUNGAL GROUPS

Fungi can be divided into **groups:**

A. Zygomycetes (phycomycetes) are **nonseptate fungi.** Common genera are *Mucor* and *Rhizopus.* (Most fungi have cross walls.)

B. Dermatophytes consists of three genera of **filamentous fungi that cause cutaneous infections:** *Trichophyton*, *Epidermophyton*, and *Microsporum.*

C. Dimorphic fungi found in the United States include *Histoplasma*, *Blastomyces*, *Coccidioides*, and *Sporothrix*.

D. Dematiaceous fungi are **darkly pigmented fungi.**

IV. ANTIFUNGAL DRUGS

Fungi have **ergosterol** as their dominant membrane sterol; humans have cholesterol. **In ergosterol synthesis, squalene is converted to lanosterol, which is converted to ergosterol. Human cells have no CWs and do not synthesize glucans.** Because fungi are eukaryotic and their ribosomes and many pathways resemble those of humans, drugs that inhibit ribosomal function or inhibit common pathways cannot be used. Instead, unique fungal pathways have to be targeted.

A. Polyene antifungals
   1. **General characteristics**
      a. Polyenes **bind to ergosterol** in fungal membranes, creating ion channels that **lead to leakage** and cell death.
      b. Because polyenes also bind to cholesterol (but with less affinity than ergosterol), they are quite toxic. The toxicity is reduced by the use of liposomal formulations.
      c. They have poor gastrointestinal absorption.
   2. **Amphotericin B (AMB)**
      a. AMB is administered intravenously (IV) for serious fungal infections and is the drug of choice for most life-threatening fungal infections. Lipid formulations have reduced toxicity.
      b. Resistance is infrequent, but there is some reduced AMB sensitivity among certain *Candida* species. Resistance is associated with lower membrane levels of ergosterol.
   3. **Nystatin** is used topically, intravaginally, or orally to treat *Candida* overgrowth or infections of cutaneous or mucosal surfaces.

B. 5-Fluorocytosine (5-FC, flucytosine)

1. 5-FC is an **antimetabolite** converted in fungal cells to 5-fluorodeoxyuridylic acid monophosphate, which competes with uracil, **causing miscoding and disruption of RNA, protein, and DNA synthesis.**

2. Because **resistance develops quickly** when used alone, 5-FC is used **in combination with amphotericin B or fluconazole** for cryptococcal meningitis.

C. Imidazole drugs are azole drugs with two nitrogens in the azole ring. They inhibit lanosterol 14-α-demethylase, thereby interfering with ergosterol synthesis (fungal membrane lipid).

1. **Ketoconazole** may be orally administered but is used only in non–life-threatening fungal infections.

2. **Miconazole** is used topically against dermatophytes and *Candida* spp. infections.

D. Triazoles are azole drugs with three nitrogens in the azole ring. They have better systemic activity than the imidazoles.

1. **Fluconazole**
   a. Fluconazole has excellent oral bioavailability.
   b. It is used for systemic infections, most commonly with *Candida* and *Coccidioides,* and as maintenance therapy after cryptococcal meningitis.
   c. It is used in combination with other drugs in specific situations for specific fungi.

2. **Itraconazole**
   a. This lipophilic imidazole drug is administered orally.
   b. It is used for the treatment of mucocutaneous *Candida* infections, non–life-threatening *Aspergillus* infections, moderate to severe histoplasmosis or blastomycosis, and sporotrichosis.

3. **Voriconazole**
   a. This drug has a **broad spectrum of activity**, with the exception of the nonseptate fungi (Zygomycetes); however, it may be effective against other fungi that have developed AMB resistance.
   b. It is a **primary drug for the treatment of invasive aspergillosis**, serving as an alternative to AMB.

4. **Posaconazole** is an azole licensed for the treatment of Zygomycetes (nonseptate fungi) infections.

E. Griseofulvin is a **fungistatic** CW synthesis inhibitor that is active against fungi with chitin in their CWs. It inhibits protein assembly, which interferes with cell division by blocking microtubule assembly.

F. Echinocandins inhibit fungal glucan synthesis, leading to a weakened CW and cell lysis.

1. Echinocandins include caspofungin, micafungin, and anidulafungin.

2. They are effective against *Aspergillus* spp., *Candida* spp., *Pneumocystis jirovecii*, and a variety of other fungi.

G. Topical antifungals (including imidazoles, allylamines: terbinafine and naftifine, tolnaftate, and many others) may be used for dermatophytes and mucosal yeast infections.

Review Test

Directions: Each of the numbered items in this section is followed by answer choices. Select the *one best* lettered answer for each question.

1. What is a mass of fungal filaments called?

(A) Hyphae
(B) Mycelium
(C) Pseudohyphae
(D) Septum
(E) Yeast

2. What is the correct term for a filamentous fungus subunit?

(A) Coenocyte
(B) Hypha
(C) Mycelium
(D) Septum
(E) Yeast

3. To treat a patient with a life-threatening fungal infection, which of the following antifungal drug causes pore formation in the fungal membrane and kills the cells?

(A) AMB
(B) Griseofulvin
(C) Ketoconazole
(D) Miconazole
(E) Nystatin

4. Which of the following drugs inhibits ergosterol synthesis, is important in treating *Candida fungemia*, and is used orally to suppress relapses of cryptococcal meningitis in patients with acquired immunodeficiency syndrome (AIDS)?

(A) AMB
(B) Echinocandins
(C) Fluconazole
(D) Griseofulvin
(E) Nystatin

5. Which of the following is a polyene antifungal agent used for many life-threatening fungal infections?

(A) AMB
(B) Griseofulvin
(C) Itraconazole
(D) Miconazole
(E) Nystatin

6. Which of the following terms best describes a fungal cross wall?

(A) Coenocyte
(B) Hypha
(C) Mycelium
(D) Septum
(E) Yeast

7. Which of the following cellular features differentiates fungal cells from human cells?

(A) 80S ribosomes
(B) Enzymes that allow them to use carbon dioxide as their sole carbon source
(C) Ergosterol as the major membrane sterol
(D) Presence of chloroplasts
(E) Presence of an endoplasmic reticulum

Answers and Explanations

1. **The answer is B.** [I B 1 d] A mycelium is a mass of hyphae (fungal filaments).

2. **The answer is B.** [I B 1] The fungal subunit, called a hypha, is a filamentous structure with or without cross walls (septae).

3. **The answer is A.** [IV A 2] Although both AMB and nystatin are polyenes, only AMB is used systemically. The imidazoles inhibit ergosterol synthesis, and griseofulvin, which localizes in keratinized tissues, inhibits the growth of dermatophytes by disrupting microtubule assembly.

4. **The answer is D.** [IV D 1] Fluconazole is an imidazole; all imidazoles inhibit ergosterol synthesis. Fluconazole has become the mainstay in the treatment of serious *Candida* infections and it also used to prevent relapse of fungal central nervous system (CNS) infections in compromised patients. AMB and nystatin both bind to ergosterol and create membrane pores, causing cell leakage and death. Echinocandins inhibit the fungal CW synthesis. Griseofulvin is not used against *Candida*, as it may make the infection worse.

5. **The answer is A.** [IV A 2] AMB, a polyene, is the most effective treatment for many life-threatening fungal infections. Nystatin, also a polyene, is used topically or orally but is not absorbed.

6. **The answer is D.** [I B 1 a] The cross wall of a hypha is called a septum or septation.

7. **The answer is C.** [I A 2] Ergosterol is the major fungus membrane sterol, and its presence is important in the chemotherapy of fungal infections. For example, AMB binds to ergosterol, producing pores that leak out cellular contents, killing the fungus. Imidazole drugs inhibit the synthesis of ergosterol. Both fungi and humans have 80S ribosomes and endoplasmic reticulum. Fungi are heterotrophic rather than autotrophic, meaning they cannot use carbon dioxide as their carbon source; instead, fungi break down organic carbon compounds. Fungi are also not photosynthetic.

7

System-Based and Situational Fungal Infections

I. OVERVIEW OF FUNGAL DISEASES

A. Fungal allergies are common. Molds may grow on *any* damp organic surface, and their spores are constantly in the air. These spores (and, in some cases, volatile fungal metabolites) play a role in conditions such as sick building syndrome, allergies, farmer's lung, silo worker's disease, and allergic bronchopulmonary aspergillosis and can become a major problem following flooding.

B. Mycotoxicoses may result from ingestion of fungal-contaminated foods (eg, St Anthony fire from ergot-contaminated rye bread or aflatoxin [a carcinogen]-contaminated peanuts) or the ingestion of psychotropic (*Psilocybe*) or toxic (*Amanita*) mushrooms.

C. Fungal infections (mycoses)
   1. Mycoses range from superficial to systemic infections that may be rapidly fatal (especially in compromised individuals).
   2. Mycoses are increasing in prevalence as a result of increased use of antibiotics, corticosteroids, and cytotoxic drugs, as well as world-wide environmental changes.
   3. Mycoses are commonly classified as superficial, cutaneous, mucocutaneous, subcutaneous, and systemic infections. Systemic infections are subdivided into those caused by pathogenic or opportunistic fungi.

Table 7.1 summarizes common or serious major fungal diseases in the United States.

Table 7.1 Common or Serious Major Fungal Infections in the United States		
Type	**Disease**	**Causative Organism**
Superficial mycoses	Tinea nigra	Dematiaceous fungi
	Pityriasis versicolor	*Malassezia furfur*
Cutaneous mycoses	Tinea or ringworm	Dermatophytes: *Trichophyton, Epidermophyton, Microsporum*
Mucocutaneous mycoses	Candidiasis	*Candida albicans, Candida* spp.
Subcutaneous mycoses	Sporotrichosis	*Sporothrix schenckii*
Systemic mycoses	Coccidioidomycosis	*Coccidioides immitis*
	Histoplasmosis	*Histoplasma capsulatum*
	Blastomycosis	*Blastomyces dermatitidis*

(continued)

Table 7.1	Common or Serious Major Fungal Infections in the United States (*continued*)	
Type	**Disease**	**Causative Organism**
Opportunistic mycoses	Cryptococcal meningitis	*Cryptococcus neoformans*
	Aspergillosis	*Aspergillus fumigatus, Aspergillus* spp.
	Zygomycosis (phycomycosis)	*Mucor, Absidia, Rhizopus, Rhizomucor*
	Candidiasis, systemic and local	*Candida albicans* and other *Candida* spp. that have greater drug resistance (ie, to fluconazole)
	Pneumocystis pneumonitis/ pneumonia	*Pneumocystis jirovecii* (aka, *Pneumocystis carinii*)

II. SUPERFICIAL SKIN INFECTIONS

> **● ● ● Clinical Pearl**
>
> Very few fungal species are components of the normal skin flora; the exceptions are *Malassezia furfur* and *Candida* spp.

A. General aspects of superficial mycoses
1. Fungi grow on the surface of the skin and do not penetrate the stratum corneum of the epidermis.

B. Pityriasis (tinea) versicolor
1. Fungal overgrowth disrupts melanin synthesis and manifests as **hypopigmented or hyperpigmented skin patches,** usually on the trunk of the body. There is usually little to no immune response.
2. **Epidemiology:** It is caused by overgrowth of the lipophilic fungus *M. furfur*, which is part of the normal flora.
3. **Diagnosis** is by a potassium hydroxide **(KOH) wet mount** of skin scales, with short, curved, septate hyphae and yeast-like cells (spaghetti and meatballs appearance).

C. Tinea nigra
1. A superficial infection on the palmar or plantar surfaces causing benign, **flat, dark, melanoma-like macules.**
2. Caused by a **dematiaceous** (darkly pigmented) **fungus** (*Hortaea werneckii* or *Exophiala werneckii*) that produces melanin, which colors the skin.
3. **Diagnosis** is by a **KOH wet mount** of skin scales with black, two-celled oval yeast.

III. CUTANEOUS MYCOSES

A. General aspects of cutaneous mycoses
1. **Cutaneous mycoses may be caused by any of the dermatophytes or, less frequently, by** *Candida* **spp.** The **dermatophytes** are a homogeneous group of **filamentous fungi** with **three genera,** *Epidermophyton, Microsporum,* **and** *Trichophyton.* Most cutaneous infections are dermatophytic, and **dermatophytes do not disseminate.** *Candida* **infections are more frequently mucocutaneous or occur in skin folds, and they can sometimes disseminate (see section IV on Mucocutaneous Candidiasis).**
2. Skin, hair, or nails may be affected; infections are classified by the area of the body involved.
3. Dermatophytic infections are generally not life-threatening, even in compromised hosts.
4. **Epidemiology**
   a. Diseases acquired from animals (**zoophilic**) tend to cause lesions that are **inflammatory.** Common zoophilic species include *Microsporum canis* and *Trichophyton rubrum.*
   b. Diseases acquired from humans (**anthropophilic**) tend to cause lesions that are **less inflammatory.** Common anthropophilic species include *Epidermophyton floccosum* and *Microsporum audouinii.*

5. **Diagnosis** is often by microscopic examination of skin, hair, or nail material mounted on a slide in 10% KOH. **Dermatophytes can be visualized as relatively unbranched hyphae, sometimes with arthroconidia (see Figure 6.6C).** Selection of areas to sample in *Microsporum* **spp**. infections may be aided by the use of a **Wood (ultraviolet [UV]) lamp** (other dermatophytes do not fluoresce with a Wood lamp).
6. **Treatment**
   a. These are often treated empirically. Lesions may become superinfected with bacteria (often presents as pus) that also must be treated.
   b. These diseases often require treatment with oral drugs if hair (and hair follicles) are involved.
   c. **ID reaction:** New **sterile lesions** may arise during treatment. This **hypersensitive state,** known as the **dermatophytid (or "id") reaction, occurs in response to circulating fungal antigens** and indicates treatment response.

Table 7.2 lists the tissues most commonly infected with each genus of dermatophytes.

Table 7.2	Tissues Commonly Infected by Dermatophytes and *Candida*			
Tissue Infected				
Group	**Genus**	**Hair**	**Skin**	**Nails**
Dermatophytes	*Trichophyton*	Yes	Yes	Yes
	Epidermophyton	—	Yes	Yes
	Microsporum	Yes	Yes	—
Yeast	*Candida*	—	Yes	Yes

Cutaneous mycoses are classified by the area of the body involved:

B. Tinea capitis (ringworm of the scalp, skin, or hair; Figure 7.1)
   1. **Anthropophilic tinea capitis**
      a. Occurs in **prepubescent children** and is epidemic, spread by headgear, combs, and so on.
      b. Caused by *M. audouinii.*
      c. It is usually noninflammatory and produces **gray** patches of hair.
   2. **Zoophilic tinea capitis** (nonepidemic)
      a. Transmitted by **pets or farm animals**.
      b. It is most commonly caused by *M. canis* or by *Trichophyton mentagrophytes.*
      c. It is **inflammatory**, often with boggy tender areas (kerion); it may also cause **temporary alopecia** and **keloids.**
   3. **Black-dot tinea capitis**
      a. This chronic infection occurs in **adults** and is characterized by **hair breakage, followed by filling of the follicles with dark conidia.**
      b. Caused by *Trichophyton tonsurans.*

C. Tinea barbae (ringworm of the beard, neck, or face; see Figure 7.1)
   1. This infection is an **acute or chronic folliculitis,** most commonly caused by *Trichophyton verrucosum.*
   2. It may produce pustular or dry, scaly lesions.

D. Tinea corporis (ringworm of the body; see Figure 7.1)
   1. This **dermatophytic infection affects glabrous skin** and is commonly caused by *T. rubrum, T. mentagrophytes,* or *M. canis.*
   2. It is characterized by **annular lesions** with an active border that may be pustular or vesicular.

E. Tinea cruris (ringworm of the groin)
   1. This **acute or chronic fungal infection** is commonly called "jock itch."
   2. It is often accompanied by athlete's foot/nail infections, which also must be treated.
   3. It is caused by *E. floccosum, T. rubrum, T. mentagrophytes,* or yeasts like *Candida.*

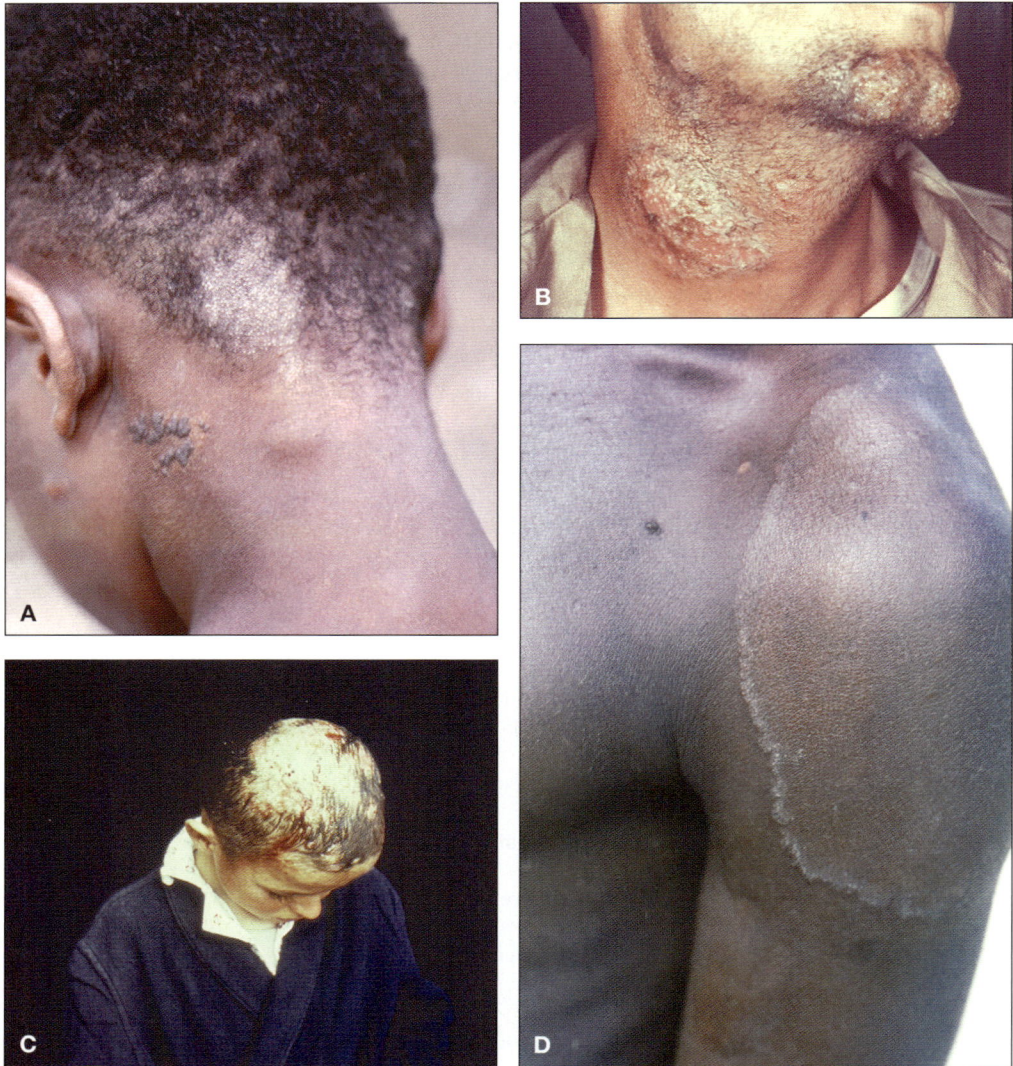

FIGURE 7.1. A. Tinea capitis (ringworm of the scalp, skin, or hair). This patient's neck reveals a cutaneous scalp lesion diagnosed as tinea capitis, caused by the dermatophytic fungal organism, *Trichophyton rubrum*. B. Tinea barbae (ringworm of the beard, neck, or face). This patient presented with a dermatophytic fungal infection in the bearded region of his neck that was diagnosed as a case of tinea barbae, caused by *Trichophyton mentagrophytes*. C. This photograph highlights the scalp of a young male who exhibits symptoms of a cutaneous fungal infection known as favus, a form of tinea capitis, which had infected the scalp skin and hair follicles. Note the thinning of the hair in the area of the infection. This cutaneous illness is caused by a fungal organism known as a dermatophyte. D. Tinea corporis (ringworm of the body). This patient's left shoulder displays a cutaneous lesion diagnosed as a ringworm, or tinea corporis, caused by *T. rubrum*. (Photos courtesy of CDC Public Health Image Library [PHIL], images 2284, 7655, 22843, and 17381, respectively.)

F. Tinea pedis (ringworm of feet)
  1. This acute to chronic **fungal infection** is commonly called "athlete's foot."
  2. It is most commonly caused by *T. rubrum*, *T. mentagrophytes*, or *E. floccosum*.
  3. There are three common clinical presentations:
     a. Chronic intertriginous tinea pedis (usually white macerated tissue between the toes).
     b. Chronic dry, scaly tinea pedis (hyperkeratotic scales on the heels, soles, or sides of the feet).
     c. Vesicular tinea pedis (vesicles and pustules).

G. Favus (tinea favosa) (see Figure 7.1)
1. It is a **highly contagious** and severe form of **tinea capitis with scutula** (crust) **formation** and **permanent hair loss** caused by scarring. **Prophylaxis** of all close contacts is needed.
2. It is caused by ***Trichophyton schoenleinii***.
3. Favus occurs in both children and adults.

IV. MUCOCUTANEOUS CANDIDIASIS/*CANDIDA ALBICANS* (AND OTHER SPECIES)

A. General characteristics of mucocutaneous candidiasis
1. *Candida* **spp.** are part of the **normal flora** of the skin, mucous membranes, and gastrointestinal (GI) tract.
2. Most *Candida* **spp.** are **yeast on body surfaces.** Normal colonization must be distinguished from infection (when fungi overgrow or invade the tissues).
3. *Candida albicans* in infected tissues grows as **pseudohyphae, true hyphae, blastoconidia,** and **yeast** forms but is still referred to as a yeast.
4. **Diagnosis** of these infections is usually by a KOH mount of the discharge and visualization by microscopy (Figure 7.2). A **germ tube test** may also be performed by growth in serum.

B. Oral thrush is a yeast infection of the oral mucocutaneous membranes.
1. It manifests as white curd-like patches in the oral cavity.
2. At-risk populations include premature infants, infants on antibiotics, individuals with asthma who do not use spacers with inhalers, individuals who are immunosuppressed and on long-term antibiotics, and individuals who have acquired immunodeficiency syndrome (AIDS). In patients who have immunosuppression, the infection may extend through the GI tract, causing a painful gastritis.

C. Vulvovaginitis or vaginal thrush is a yeast infection of the vagina.
1. It manifests with a thick yellow-white discharge, a burning sensation, curd-like patches on the vaginal mucosa, and inflammation of the peritoneum.
2. Predisposing factors include diabetes, antibiotic therapy, oral contraceptive use, and pregnancy.

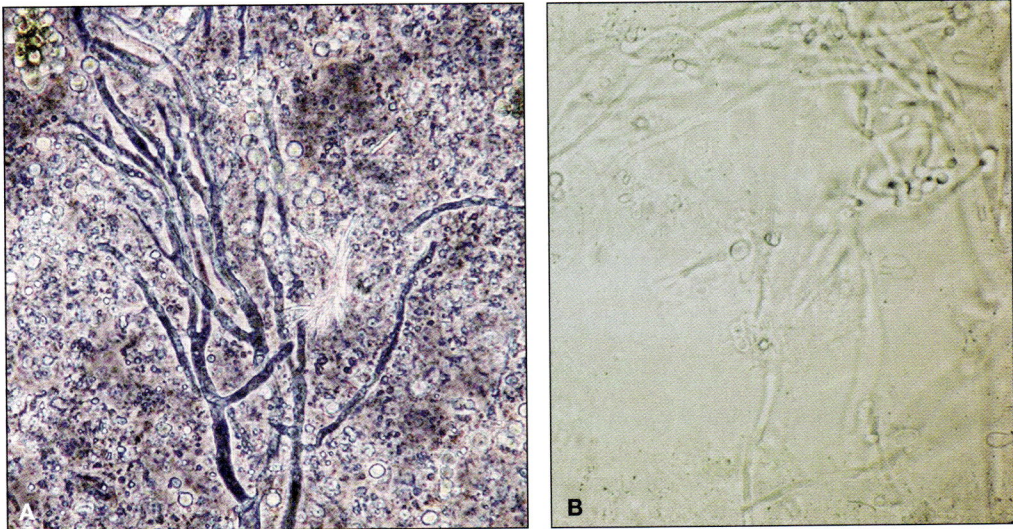

FIGURE 7.2. Wet mounts. A. Dichotomously branching hyphae released by tissue by KOH (potassium hydroxide) digestion. (Courtesy of Glenn D. Roberts, PhD, Mayo Clinic, Rochester, MN.) B. Wet mount of mucosal scrapings for vaginitis showing pseudohyphae and some yeasts.

D. **Cutaneous candidiasis** involves the nails (a predisposing factor is prolonged use of false nails), skin folds (often in infants or individuals who are obese), or the groin (and the penis).
  1. Lesions may be eczematoid or vesicular and pustular, and often manifest as visible, creamy growth.
  2. Infection is predisposed by moist conditions.

V. SUBCUTANEOUS MYCOSES

These mycoses begin with **traumatic implantation** of fungi but **remain localized in the cutaneous or subcutaneous tissues.** These infections tend to be chronic and develop slowly; most are relatively **uncommon in the United States except for sporotrichosis.**

A. **Sporotrichosis** (also known as "rose gardener's disease") is caused by the **dimorphic** fungus *Sporothrix schenckii.*
  1. At **37 °C,** *S. schenckii* grows as **cigar-shaped to oval, budding yeasts;** at 25 °C, it grows as sporulating hyphae with a "rosette" pattern of conidia.
  2. *S. schenckii* is found in or on **plant materials** such as roses, plum trees, or sphagnum moss and is **traumatically introduced** by florist's wires, splinters, or thorns from roses or plum trees into subcutaneous tissues. Infections are most commonly seen in gardeners, florists, and agriculture workers.
  3. This fungal disease is generally not painful. When it spreads along the lymphatics (lymphocutaneous sporotrichosis), it produces a chain of lesions on the extremities, with the older lesions ulcerating and the newer ones becoming nodular.
  4. **Diagnosis:** Clinical diagnosis may be confirmed by culture.
  5. **Treatment:** Itraconazole is the preferred treatment.

B. **Eumycotic mycetoma** (also known as "Madura foot")
  1. **Eumycotic mycetoma** is characterized by (1) swelling (**tumefaction**), (2) **sinus tracts** erupting through the skin (if not treated), and (3) presence of "sulfur" **granules** (microcolonies) in the exudate.
  2. Fungal causative agents are *Pseudallescheria boydii* and *Madurella* spp., which are filamentous true fungi found in soil or on vegetation.
  3. Infections are most common in **rural, agricultural workers** in tropical low-income countries.

C. **Chromoblastomycosis**
  1. **Chromoblastomycosis** is caused by **dematiaceous (dark) fungi.** These fungi are seen in tissues as pigmented (often copper colored), spherical yeast called **Medlar bodies**.
  2. **Colored lesions** start out scaly and become raised, **cauliflower-like** warty nodules.
  3. Infections are most common in the tropics.

VI. SYSTEMIC MYCOSES

> ● ● ● **Clinical Pearl**
>
> The geographic location in the United States can be very helpful for a presumptive diagnosis of a systemic fungal infection, as all the fungi are dimorphic.

A. **General characteristics of systemic mycoses.** In the United States, the three dimorphic fungal pathogens are *Histoplasma, Coccidioides,* and *Blastomyces* **spp.**
  1. During the saprobic phase, these fungi are filamentous, grow in specific environments, and produce **airborne spores** that may be inhaled into alveoli, initiating infection.
  2. These **pathogens** are acquired in **specific geographic regions.** Dust-containing spores can travel on cars or archaeological artifacts and infect individuals with naïve immune systems outside the endemic zone.

3. These fungi have true **virulence factors** and can cause disease in healthy individuals. The outcomes of infection largely depend on immune status of the host, the inhaled dose, and the strain of fungal pathogen.

4. They cause a spectrum of diseases in three basic forms:

  a. Acute self-limited pneumonia, from asymptomatic to severe but generally self-resolving, occurs in healthy people. However, some organisms may survive in granulomas and can reactivate if the immune system becomes compromised.

  b. Chronic disease (generally pulmonary) generally occurs in individuals who are debilitated.

  c. Disseminated infection may occur in individuals who are immunocompromised or when a large spore dose is able to overwhelm the immune system.

B. Histoplasmosis and *Histoplasma capsulatum* (Figure 7.3)

1. *Histoplasma* are **thermally dimorphic, facultative intracellular fungal pathogens** (with no capsule).

2. Epidemiology

  a. The organisms are endemic to the **river plains of the Ohio, Missouri, and Mississippi Rivers** in the United States, the St Lawrence Seaway of the United States and Canada, and Central and South America, Africa, Asia, and Australia.

  b. They are found in **soil enriched with bat or bird guano** as hyphae with **distinctive tuberculate macroconidia** and nondescript **microconidia.** The small size of the microconidia allows them to enter the alveoli to start infection. Bat caves, old chicken coops, starling roosts, etc, have high levels of spores.

3. Pathogenesis

  a. Inhaled conidia convert to yeast cells that are phagocytosed but can survive and replicate in the phagocytic cells, including circulating monocytes.

  b. The yeast forms interfere with phagocytic killing. Glucan in the cell wall appears to play a role in the fungus killing the phagocytic cells, aiding in its spread.

  c. *H. capsulatum* **has no capsule,** so it is misnamed. In stained smears, the cytoplasm shrinks away from the cell wall, leaving a clear space resembling a capsule.

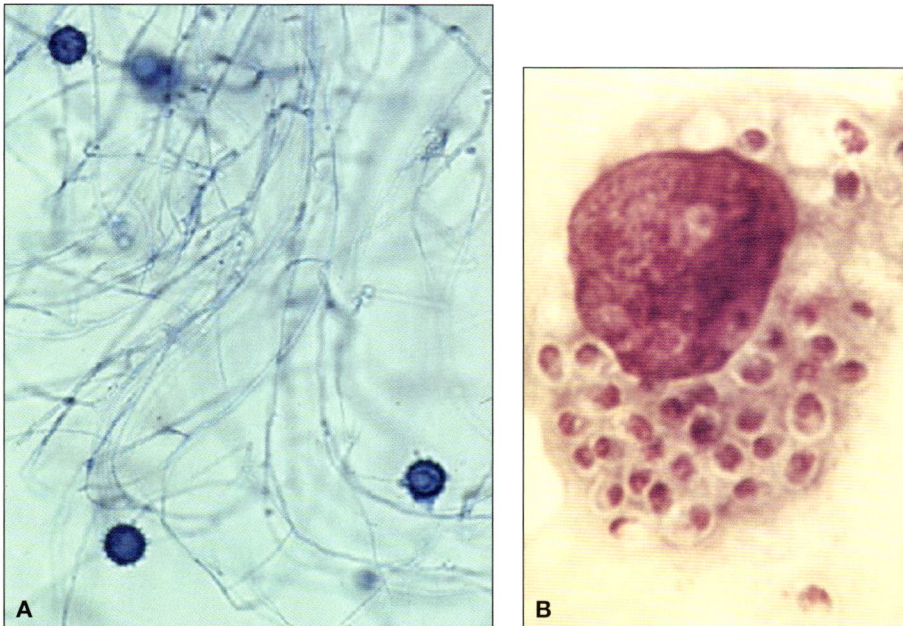

FIGURE 7.3. *Histoplasma capsulatum.* A. *H. capsulatum* showing hyphae and tuberculate macroconidia characteristically found in bird feces– or bat feces–enriched soils of the Ohio, Missouri, and Mississippi River plains in the United States. (Courtesy of Glenn D. Roberts PhD, Mayo Clinic.) B. *H. capsulatum* in a single histiocyte (enlarged). Each phagocytic cell can have hundreds of the tiny intracellular yeast. Note the prominent presence of the histiocyte nucleus that distinguishes it from a spherule. (Spherules also have a cell wall.) (Courtesy of CDC Public Health Image Library/Dr T. McClenan.)

4. Clinical presentation

- **a.** **Acute histoplasmosis** ranges from subclinical to severe pneumonia but tends to self-resolve. Infected polymorphonuclear neutrophils (PMNs) circulate in the blood, so **thick blood smears and blood cultures are useful for diagnosis,** even in an infection limited to lungs. Hilar lymphadenopathy and splenomegaly are often prominent. A Th1 response and granuloma formation are critical to resolution, although some viable organisms may remain in granulomas.
- **b.** **Disseminated histoplasmosis** may occur in individuals with heavy spore exposure, underlying immune cell defects (eg, patients with AIDS, T-cell deficits, or lymphoma), and children under the age of 1 who appear to have a defect in dendritic cell function. Symptoms include **mucocutaneous lesions** and Addison disease (in approximately 50% of fulminant cases).

C. Blastomycosis and *Blastomyces dermatitidis* (Figure 7.4)

1. *Blastomyces* are **thermally dimorphic fungi**.
2. **Epidemiology**
   - **a.** The organisms are found in *Histoplasma* **endemic areas, particularly in the southeastern US seacoast** (excluding Florida) and extending north through Minnesota into Canada.
   - **b.** These organisms are **filamentous fungi with small conidia in rotting organic material, including wood.**
   - **c.** Conidia are inhaled into alveoli, where they convert into *Blastomyces'* **large, budding yeasts with thick walls and broad bases on buds.**
3. **Pathogenesis:** The organisms are found in **tissues as large yeast cells with a double refractile wall and broad-based buds.** Strains shedding high levels of cell wall glycoprotein WI-1 are not recognized by macrophages; these strains continue to replicate, likely triggering a Th2 response.
4. **Clinical presentation**
   - **a.** **Acute pulmonary blastomycosis** may not self-resolve; therefore, even acute infections are treated with itraconazole.
   - **b.** **Chronic pulmonary blastomycosis** (coin lesions) may be misdiagnosed as carcinoma.
   - **c.** **Disseminated blastomycosis** may have bone and skin lesions. The latter can be useful for rapid diagnosis by demonstrating **broad-based, budding yeasts in KOH** mounts of scrapings from the active edges of a **skin lesion.**

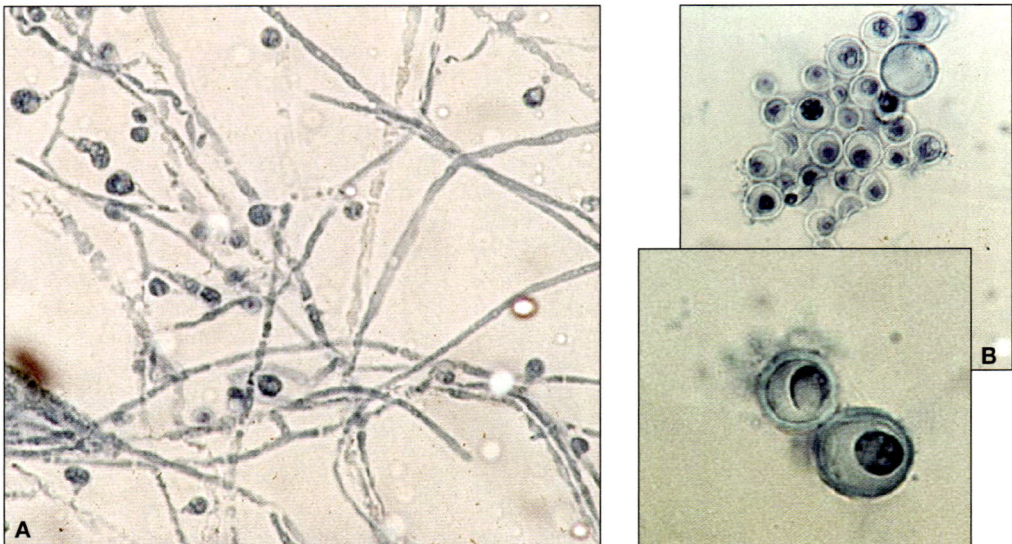

FIGURE 7.4. *Blastomyces dermatitidis*. A. *B. dermatitidis* hyphae and conidia characteristically found in highly organic soil (often with rotting wood) in an endemic area. (Courtesy of Glenn D. Roberts, PhD, Mayo Clinic.) B. The distinctive *B. dermatitidis* budding yeast. Note the thick cell wall and the broad base between the mother cell and the blastoconidium (bud). One budding pair has been enlarged in the inset for detail. (Courtesy of Glenn D. Roberts, PhD, Mayo Clinic.)

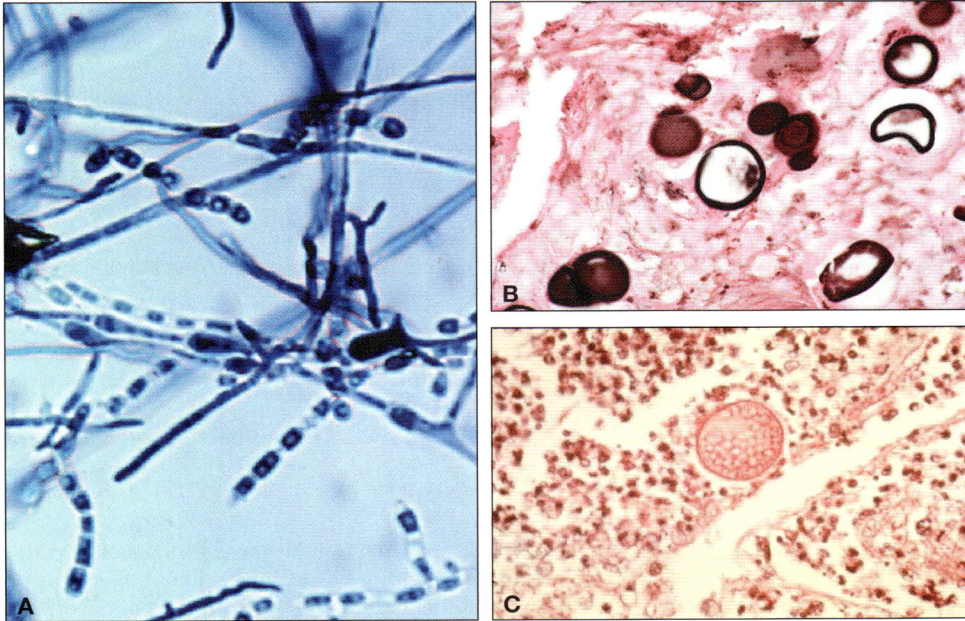

FIGURE 7.5. *Coccidioides immitis.* A. *C. immitis* hyphae and arthroconidia, which are the forms found in the southwestern United States. (Courtesy of Glenn D. Roberts, PhD, Mayo Clinic.) B. *C. immitis* spherules (some of them empty) from lung tissue, stained with silver stain. (Courtesy of Glenn D. Roberts, PhD, Mayo Clinic.) C. *C. immitis* single spherule in tissue showing endospores inside the spherule. (Courtesy of CDC Public Health Image Library/ Dr Lucille K. Georg.)

D. Coccidioidomycosis (also known as Valley Fever) and *Coccidioides immitis* (Figure 7.5)

1. *C. immitis* are **thermally dimorphic pathogens.**
2. **Epidemiology**
   a. The organism is endemic to California's **San Joaquin Valley** and the **Lower Sonoran Desert in the southwestern United States and Mexico.**
   b. **Arthroconidia** are found in alkaline desert sand. When inhaled, they resist phagocytosis due to their extremely hydrophobic nature.
   c. In the lungs, inhaled arthroconidia develop into larger spherical, walled structures called **spherules** with internal **endospores.**
3. **Clinical presentation**
   a. **Acute, self-limiting coccidioidomycosis** is similar to acute histoplasmosis, except that erythema nodosum or multiforme are more likely. Persons with AIDS and pregnant women in the third trimester, appear to be more at risk of dissemination. Itraconazole or fluconazole is used to treat individuals at high risk of dissemination.
   b. **Chronic coccidioidomycosis** does not self-resolve.
   c. **Disseminated coccidioidomycosis** occurs under conditions of reduced cell-mediated immunity and high complement-fixing antibody (Th2 response). The clinical presentation is similar to disseminated histoplasmosis, with dissemination frequently observed in the meninges and mucous membranes.

VII. OPPORTUNISTIC MYCOSES

A. General characteristics of opportunistic mycoses

1. Caused by endogenous or ubiquitous organisms of low virulence causing infection in debilitated or individuals who are immunocompromised.
2. Infections range from uncomfortable/painful mucous membrane or cutaneous infections in individuals who are mildly immunocompromised to serious disseminated infections in individuals who are severely immunocompromised.

3. They are most commonly caused by fungi of the genera *Candida, Cryptococcus, Aspergillus, Pneumocystis, Rhizopus, Mucor,* and *Pneumocystis.* However, any fungus may cause an opportunistic infection if a patient is immunocompromised.

4. Incidence is increasing as the number of individuals who are immunocompromised increases.

B. Candidiases are the most common opportunists.

1. *Candida* spp. may cause mucocutaneous infections (see IV B) or more serious infections involving the bronchi or lungs, GI tract, bloodstream, urinary tract, and, less commonly, the heart or meninges.

2. The most common cause is *C. albicans*, but the incidence of infections due to other species of *Candida* is increasing.

3. Predisposed individuals include the very young or very old, those with wasting or nutritional diseases, those who are pregnant or immunosuppressed, and those with diabetes, a history of long-term antibiotic and steroid use, indwelling catheters, or AIDS. Areas with excessive moisture, such as skin folds, are also susceptible.

4. Systemic candidiases are generally treated with fluconazole, lipid-based amphotericin B, or caspofungin.

5. Clinical presentation

   a. Oral thrush (see IV B).

   b. Candidemias or blood-borne infections most commonly occur in patients with indwelling catheters or GI tract overgrowth and minor bowel defects; these infections present as fever, macronodular skin lesions, and endophthalmitis, leading to **endocarditis** or **cerebromeningitis.**

   c. Bronchopulmonary infection may occur in patients with chronic lung disease; it usually manifests as persistent cough.

C. *M. furfur* **septicemia** occurs primarily in premature neonates on intravenous lipid emulsions and usually resolves if lipid supplements are stopped.

D. Cryptococcal meningitis/meningoencephalitis and *Cryptococcus neoformans*

1. *C. neoformans* is a **yeast** (not dimorphic) that possesses an **antigenic polysaccharide capsule.** It is found in weathered pigeon droppings.

2. Central nervous system (CNS) disease most commonly occurs in patients with Hodgkin lymphoma, diabetes, AIDS (where it is the dominant meningitis), leukemias, or leukocyte enzyme deficiency diseases.

3. Clinical presentation: Initial symptoms include headache of increasing severity, usually with fever, followed by typical signs of meningitis and sometimes personality changes.

4. Diagnosis is by cerebrospinal fluid (CSF) latex particle agglutination test for *Cryptococcus*, **India ink** wet mount, and culture following lysis of white blood cells in CSF.

5. Treatment involves amphotericin B plus 5-fluorocytosine or fluconazole.

E. Aspergilloses are a variety of infections and allergic diseases that are caused *by Aspergillus fumigatus* and other species of *Aspergillus.*

1. *A. fumigatus* is a **ubiquitous filamentous fungus** whose airborne spores (conidia) are constantly in the air.

2. Aspergilli have characteristic **septate hyphae branching dichotomously at acute angles** (ie, **monomorphic**).

3. Clinical presentation

   a. Allergic bronchopulmonary aspergillosis is an allergic disease where the organism colonizes the mucous plugs formed in the lungs but does not invade lung tissue. Diagnosis is by high titers of immunoglobulin E (IgE) to *Aspergillus.*

   b. Aspergilloma (fungus ball) is a roughly spherical growth of *Aspergillus* in a preexisting lung cavity; growth does not invade the lung tissues. It presents clinically as recurrent hemoptysis and is diagnosed by radiology ("air sign" shift with a change in the position of the patient).

   c. **Invasive aspergillosis** is most common in patients with severe neutropenia, starting in the lungs or spreading from sinus colonization. It requires aggressive treatment with voriconazole or lipid formulation of amphotericin B.

F. **Rhinocerebral zygomycoses** (also called **phycomycoses** or **mucormycoses**) are infections caused by **nonseptate fungi** (phylum Zygomycota, genera *Rhizopus, Absidia, Mucor,* and *Rhizomucor*).
1. Occurs in individuals with **acidotic diabetes or leukemia;** it is **highly invasive,** having a predilection for **invading blood vessels and the brain** and causing rapid decline or death.
2. **Clinical presentation includes facial swelling,** blood-tinged exudate in the turbinates and eyes, **mental lethargy,** blindness, and fixated pupils.
3. **Diagnosis** must be rapid, usually by a KOH mount of necrotic tissue or exudates from the eye, ear, or nose.
4. **Treatment** must be rapid! It consists of (1) control of diabetes, (2) surgical debridement, and (3) aggressive treatment with amphotericin B or posaconazole.

G. *Pneumocystis* **pneumonitis/pneumonia (PCP)** is an infection caused by ***Pneumocystis jiroveci*** (formerly *Pneumocystis carinii*).
1. *P. jiroveci* is an **obligate fungal organism** of humans (cannot be grown in vitro) that is extracellular, growing on the surfactant layer over the alveolar epithelium. **Trophozoites** and larger **cysts** are seen in the alveoli by **methenamine-silver** or calcofluor white stain of tissue.
2. **Clinical presentation**
   a. **Interstitial plasma cell pneumonitis** occurs in malnourished infants, transplant patients, patients on antineoplastic chemotherapy, and patients on corticosteroid therapy. Radiographs show a patchy, diffuse appearance, sometimes referred to as **ground-glass** opacities.
   PCP causes morbidity and mortality when $CD4^+$ counts decrease to less than $200/mm^3$ (ie, AIDS), unless prevented with prophylaxis. Unlike pneumonitis, PCP lacks plasma cells in the alveolar spaces. The organism causes a decline in partial pressure of oxygen (pO_2) that is out of proportion to radiologic appearance. Radiographs show a characteristic **ground-glass** opacities.
3. **Diagnosis** by microscopy of biopsy specimen or alveolar fluids (Giemsa, specific fluorescent antibody, toluidine blue, methenamine-silver, or calcofluor stains). Presence of serum antibodies is not a useful indicator of infection because almost all healthy individuals and who are immunocompromised have antibodies to *Pneumocystis,* suggesting exposure is common.
4. **Treatment** prophylactically with trimethoprim-sulfamethoxazole or trimethoprim and dapsone.

> **• • • Clinical Pearl**
>
> There are many methods to visualize fungi microscopically. Routinely used are the differential stains calcofluor white stain, Gomori methenamine-silver stain, and periodic acid-Schiff stain. Calcofluor white stains fungi blue, Gomori methenamine-silver stains fungi black, and periodic acid-Schiff stains fungi a pink or red color.

VIII. TABLES FOR SELF-TESTING

These tables present fungal infections in a format useful for solving case-history questions on the United States Medical Licensing Examination (USMLE). For optimal use, cover the last column, which has the answers, and use these tables to test yourself the first time you use them.

A. Table 7.3 summarizes superficial, cutaneous, mucocutaneous, subcutaneous, and allergic fungal diseases in healthy individuals.

B. Table 7.4 summarizes systemic infections in immunocompetent patients.

C. Table 7.5 summarizes opportunistic infections in patients who are immunocompromised.

Table 7.3	Symptoms and Test Findings for Diagnosis of Fungal Diseases in Generally Healthy Patients With Superficial, Cutaneous, Mucocutaneous, Subcutaneous, or Allergic Fungal Diseases	
Presenting Symptoms	**Test Findings[a]**	**Fungal Agent/Disease**
Scattered small hypo- or hyperpigmented areas of skin, generally on the trunk	KOH: yeast-like cells and short, curved, septate hyphae	*Malassezia furfur*/pityriasis versicolor
Cutaneous lesions with various degrees of inflammation; lesions spread from the periphery and may be spread by scratching	KOH: hyphae and arthroconidia	Dermatophytes: *Epidermophyton, Trichophyton, Microsporum*/tineas
	KOH: pseudohyphae and yeasts	*Candida albicans* and *Candida* spp./candidiasis
Mucocutaneous lesion (vaginitis or diaper rash)	KOH: pseudohyphae and yeast	*Candida albicans* and *Candida* spp./candidiasis
Subcutaneous lesions following lymph nodes or solitary nodule	KOH: sparse cigar-shaped yeast in tissue (37 °C)	*Sporothrix schenckii*/sporotrichosis
	Hyphae and conidia at 25 °C	
Colorful subcutaneous lesions, often pedunculated	KOH: dark, yeast-like cells with planar septations (sclerotic bodies) in giant cells	*Fonsecaea pedrosoi* and related forms/chromoblastomycosis
Subcutaneous swelling with sinus tracts and granules in exudate	Granules that are microcolonies of fungus	*Pseudallescheria boydii*/eumycotic mycetoma
Chronic cough; reduced lung capacity; mucous plugs in bronchus	High IgE levels against *Aspergillus*	*Aspergillus* spp./allergic bronchopulmonary aspergillosis

[a]KOH: Examination of skin scrapings or other tissue mounted in and cleared with potassium hydroxide (KOH) and examined microscopically.

Table 7.4	Symptoms and Test Findings/Clues for Diagnosis of Fungal Diseases in Generally Healthy Individuals With Systemic Symptoms	
Presenting Symptoms	**Test Findings/Clues**	**Fungal Agent/Disease**
Acute pulmonary disease (cough, fever, night sweats) not responsive to antibacterials	Environmental form or 25 °C culture: hyphae with microconidia and large tuberculate macroconidia	*Histoplasma capsulatum*/histoplasmosis
	Tissue form (37 °C): small, intracellular yeast	
	Risk factor: Exposure to dusty environments such as bat-infested attics or caves, old chicken coops, construction in the Great Plains around the Ohio, Mississippi, and Missouri riverbeds	
	Environmental form or 25 °C culture: hyphae with microconidia	*Blastomyces dermatitidis*/blastomycosis
	Tissue form (37 °C): large, budding yeast with double retractile wall	
	Risk factor: Exposure to dust/soil containing rotting organic material/wood in the Great Plains around the Ohio, Mississippi, and Missouri riverbeds plus southeastern seaboard of the United States and up through Minnesota to Canada	

Table 7.4	Symptoms and Test Findings/Clues for Diagnosis of Fungal Diseases in Generally Healthy Individuals With Systemic Symptoms (*continued*)		
Presenting Symptoms	**Test Findings/Clues**	**Fungal Agent/Disease**
	Environmental form (25 °C): hyphae with arthroconidia	*Coccidioides immitis/* coccidioidomycosis
	Tissue form (37 °C): spherules with endospores	
	Risk factor: Exposure to blowing sand with arthroconidia in the southwestern United States (sand storms, dirt biking, rodeos)	
Chronic pulmonary disease (cough, fever, night sweats, weight loss, protracted)	Same as for all three acute pulmonary diseases but with long-term symptoms and elevated sedimentation rate	Same as above
Disseminated disease (extrapulmonary sites such as skin, mucous membrane lesions, brain)	Same as for acute pulmonary disease but with poor immune response as demonstrated	Same as above

Table 7.5	Symptoms and Underlying Conditions Associated With Opportunistic Mycoses	
Symptoms	**Common Underlying Condition**	**Fungal Disease**
Vaginitis (erythema and pain)	Antibiotic use; pregnancy, diabetes, AIDS	*Candida* vaginitis
Facial swelling; lethargy; red exudate from eyes and nares; necrotic tissue	Ketoacidotic diabetes, leukemia	Rhinocerebral mucormycosis
Fever without pulmonary symptoms	Neonates with IV lipid supplements	Fungemia: *Malassezia*
	Indwelling IV catheters	Fungemia: *Candida*
Fever; pain on urination	Urinary catheter	Urinary candidiasis
Difficulty in swallowing	AIDS	Esophageal candidiasis
Meningeal symptoms	AIDS	Cryptococcal meningitis, *Histoplasma* or coccidioidal meningitis, *Candida* cerebritis
	Severe neutropenia	*Aspergillus* central nervous system infection
	Hodgkin lymphoma; diabetes	Cryptococcal meningitis (chronic)
Pulmonary symptoms	Patient who is immunocompromised, particularly if neutropenic	Invasive *Aspergillosis*
	AIDS	*Pneumocystis* pneumonia (PCP), histoplasmosis, coccidioidomycosis
	Urban unhoused, suffering from alcohol use disorder	Sporotrichosis (pulmonary)

(*continued*)

Table 7.5	Symptoms and Underlying Conditions Associated With Opportunistic Mycoses (*continued*)	
Symptoms	**Common Underlying Condition**	**Fungal Disease**
Cough without upper respiratory symptoms, hemoptysis	Previous lung damage, especially cavities	Aspergilloma (fungus balls)
Endocarditis	Intravenous drug user	*Candida* or *Aspergillus* endocarditis
Enteritis (often with anal pruritus)	Antibiotic use	*Candida* enteritis
Whitish covering in mouth	Premature infants, children on antibiotics	*Candida* thrush
Corners of mouth sore	Older adults suffering from malnourishment	Perlèche
Sore gums	Dentures	Denture stomatitis
Skin lesions; endophthalmitis	Indwelling catheter	Candidemia

Review Test

Directions: Select the *one* lettered answer that is *best* in each case. Commit to and write down your answers before checking the answers and explanations. Each of the numbered items in this section is followed by answers with explanations, in the following section.

1. A 48-year-old woman presents to her physician with a subcutaneous lesion on her hand. She is a florist and she thinks the wound resulted from a jab she received while making a sphagnum moss-wire frame for a floral wreath. The nodule has ulcerated and not healed despite the use of antibacterial cream, and a new nodule is forming above the original lesion. What is the most appropriate treatment for this infection?

(A) Cortisone cream
(B) Miconazole cream
(C) Oral griseofulvin
(D) Oral itraconazole or potassium iodide
(E) Penicillin

2. A sample from the nodule described in the case in question 1 is removed and prepared for microscopy. What would be expected to be visualized under the microscope?

(A) Cigar-shaped to oval yeasts
(B) Long, branching hyphae with acute angles
(C) Lots of hyphae
(D) Yeasts with broad-based buds
(E) Yeast with multiple buds (mariner's wheel)

3. A 28-year-old presents with paranasal swelling and bloody exudate from both their eyes and nares. Upon examination, the individual is found to be nearly comatose. Necrotic tissue in the nasal turbinates is collected and visualized by microscopy. Nonseptate hyphae consistent with *Rhizopus, Mucor,* or *Absidia* (phylum Zygomycota, class Phycomycetes) are observed. What is the most likely underlying condition compromising this patient, leading to this infection?

(A) AIDS
(B) B-cell defects
(C) Chronic sinusitis
(D) Ketoacidotic diabetes
(E) Neutropenia

4. A 19-year-old presents to the clinic with a circular, itchy, inflamed skin lesion that is slightly raised. The lesion is on the individual's left side, where his dog sleeps next to him. His dog has had some localized areas of hair loss. The patient has no systemic symptoms. What would be expected to be found in a KOH preparation of this patient's skin scrapings?

(A) Budding yeasts with some pseudohyphae and true hyphae
(B) Clusters of yeast-like cells and short, curved septate hyphae
(C) Filariform larvae
(D) Hyphae with little branching, possibly with some hyphae breaking up into arthroconidia
(E) Large budding yeast cells with broad bases on the buds and thick cell walls

5. A 73-year-old woman is brought to the emergency department with severe shortness of breath. She is found to be severely neutropenic and diagnosed with pneumonia. A sample of bronchial alveolar fluid is visualized by microscopy and shows dichotomously branching (generally with acute angles) septate hyphae. What is the most likely causative agent?

(A) *Aspergillus*
(B) *Candida*
(C) *Cryptococcus*
(D) *Malassezia*
(E) *Rhizopus*

6. A 15-year-old girl is brought to the emergency department by her guardian with severe shortness of breath. Her guardians report that the girl, a dirt-bike rider, is visiting southern California for the first time. She is diagnosed with pneumonia. The causative organism has an environmental form that consists of hyphae that break up into arthroconidia, which become airborne. What is the agent?

(A) *A. fumigatus*
(B) *B. dermatitidis*
(C) *C. immitis*
(D) *H. capsulatum*
(E) *S. schenckii*

7. A 23-year-old presents to the clinic with splotchy hypopigmentation on the chest and back with only slight itchiness. What is most likely to be seen on a KOH mount of a skin scraping?

(A) Cigar-shaped yeasts
(B) Clusters of round fungal cells with short, curved, septate hyphae
(C) Darkly pigmented, round cells with sharp interior septations
(D) Filaments with lots of arthroconidia
(E) Yeasts, pseudohyphae, and true hyphae

8. A 19-year-old man presents to the clinic with a dry, scaly, erythematous penis. Skin scales were collected and stained with calcofluor white. Microscopy reveals fluorescent blue-white yeasts and a few pseudohyphae. What is the most likely causative agent of this dermatophyte look-alike?

(A) *Candida*
(B) *Malassezia*
(C) *Microsporum*
(D) *Trichophyton*
(E) *Trichosporon*

9. A 43-year-old presents to the clinic with a swollen face and extremely poor dental hygiene, including the loss of an adult tooth, which appears to be the focus of the current infection. Social history indicates that the patient is a recent immigrant from rural Brazil. There are two open ulcers on the outside of the swollen cheek. Small yellow "grains" are seen in one of the ulcers. Gram stain of a sample from the ulcer shows purple-staining fine filaments. What is the most likely disease that this patient is presenting with?

(A) Actinomycotic mycetoma
(B) Chromomycosis
(C) Eumycotic mycetoma
(D) Paracoccidioidomycosis
(E) Sporotrichosis

10. A 22-year-old man presents to the clinic with a large, raised, colored, cauliflower-like ankle lesion. He states he is a recent immigrant from a remote area in a tropical country with no access to medical care and is now working with a group of migrant crop harvesters. A tissue biopsy is performed and reveals darkly pigmented, yeast-like sclerotic bodies. Which of the following is the most likely diagnosis?

(A) Actinomycotic mycetoma
(B) Chromoblastomycosis
(C) Eumycotic mycetoma
(D) Sporotrichosis
(E) Tinea nigra

11. A premature neonate is brought to the physician 4 days after birth with a white coating on her buccal mucosa extending onto her lips. She immediately cries out when the area is touched. What is the most likely causative agent?

(A) *Actinomyces*
(B) *Aspergillus*
(C) *Candida*
(D) *Fusobacterium*
(E) *Microsporum*

12. Which of the following stains allows differentiation of fungi from human tissue by staining the fungi a pink-red color?

(A) Calcofluor white stain
(B) Gomori methenamine-silver stain
(C) Hematoxylin and eosin stain
(D) Periodic acid-Schiff stain

13. An 8-year-old boy is brought to the clinic at the end of July with a fever, cough, and lower respiratory symptoms (but no upper respiratory tract symptoms). He has been ill for 4 days. His parents state that he is normally healthy and that they are from Florida but visiting friends on a farm in Iowa for the month of July. The boy's chest sounds are consistent with pneumonia, so a chest radiograph is obtained. The radiograph shows small, patchy infiltrates with hilar adenopathy. A blood smear shows small, nondescript yeast forms inside monocytic cells. What is the most likely causative agent?

(A) *A. fumigatus*
(B) *B. dermatitidis*
(C) *C. immitis*
(D) *H. capsulatum*
(E) *P. jiroveci*

14. A logger undergoing chemotherapy for a cancer diagnosis develops pneumonia and skin lesions. Biopsy of the skin lesions demonstrates the presence of large yeasts with thick cell walls and broad-based buds. What is the most likely causative agent?

(A) *A. fumigatus*
(B) *B. dermatitidis*
(C) *C. immitis*
(D) *H. capsulatum*
(E) *S. schenckii*

15. A 33-year-old man presents to the clinic with a stiff neck and a severe headache for the past several days. His medical history indicates a diagnosis of human immunodeficiency virus (HIV) infection about a decade prior. He states that he does not take the anti-HIV medication that had been prescribed due to the cost. His headache was initially lessened by analgesics, but the analgesics are no longer effective. His current $CD4^+$ count is $180/mm^3$. He is not on any prophylactic drugs. What is the most likely causative agent?

(A) *Aspergillus*
(B) *Candida*
(C) *Cryptococcus*
(D) *Malassezia*
(E) *Sporothrix*

Answers and Explanations

1. **The answer is D.** [V A 5] This is a classic case of lymphocutaneous sporotrichosis in which a gardener or florist is infected via a puncture wound. The drug of choice is either itraconazole or potassium iodide (administered orally in milk). Topical antifungals are not effective, and the cortisone cream would probably enhance the spread of the disease. Griseofulvin localizes in the keratinized tissues and would not halt the subcutaneous spread of this infection. Penicillin would have no effect because *Sporothrix* is not a bacterium.

2. **The answer is A.** [V A 1] This is a classic case of lymphocutaneous sporotrichosis. *S. schenckii* is dimorphic; the tissue form comprises cigar-shaped yeasts, but they are hard to find by histology.

3. **The answer is D.** [Table 7.5] Zygomycota are aseptate fungi that cause serious infections, primarily in patients with diabetic ketoacidosis and cancer. Fungal infections common in patients with AIDS include *Candida* infections (ranging from oral thrush early to fungemias later), cryptococcal meningitis, and disseminated histoplasmosis and coccidioidomycosis. Patients with severe neutropenia are most likely to have invasive *Aspergillus* infections.

4. **The answer is D.** [III D] The case is ringworm acquired from a dog. In tissue, any of the dermatophytes would show hyphae and arthroconidia. Pityriasis versicolor would have clusters of yeasts with short, septate, curved hyphae (spaghetti and meatballs appearance). A filariform larvae would only be characteristic of dog hookworm, which is usually acquired from walking barefoot where there are dog feces. It would not be acquired from sleeping with the dog and would not cause hair loss in the dog. Choice D describes *Candida,* which does not fit the case. Choice E would describe *Blastomycosis,* which is highly unlikely.

5. **The answer is A.** [VII E 3 c] *Aspergillus* spores are commonly airborne. Invasive infections with *Aspergillus* are controlled by phagocytic cells. In severe neutropenia, risk of infection is high.

6. **The answer is C.** [VI D] *C. immitis* is found in desert sand, primarily as arthroconidia and hyphae.

7. **The answer is B.** [II B 2] *M. furfur* is seen in tissues as clusters of round fungal cells with short, curved septate hyphae (spaghetti and meatballs appearance) and is the causative agent of pityriasis or tinea versicolor; *M. furfur* overgrowth causes pigmentation disturbances.

8. **The answer is A.** [IV A, D] *Candida* may cause skin infections that resemble some dermatophytic infections. The patient described in the question has *Candida* balanitis. In tinea cruris, the penis is not usually involved.

9. **The answer is A.** [Chapter 2, III B 9] The disease syndrome is lumpy jaw, which is a form of mycetoma. The location of the lesions and presenting signs seen in this patient suggest actinomycotic mycetoma, a bacterial infection caused by the *Actinomyces* part of the gingival crevices flora. (Students: You needed a nonfungal question!) Yeasts will also stain gram-positive. Remember that *Actinomyces* is a gram-positive anaerobic bacterium that is not acid-fast.

10. **The answer is B.** [Table 7.3; V C 1] The finding of dematiaceous (dark), yeast-like sclerotic bodies that have sharp planar division lines, and the clinical presentation are both characteristic of chromoblastomycosis. Tinea nigra would show dematiaceous hyphae in flat palmar or plantar lesions.

11. **The answer is C.** [IV B] The disease described is thrush, caused by *Candida.*

12. **The answer is D.** [VII G 4] Calcofluor white stain, Gomori methenamine-silver stain, and periodic acid-Schiff stain are all differential stains, but only the periodic acid-Schiff stain turns fungi a pink-red color. The hematoxylin and eosin stain turns fungi a pink-red color also but does not differentiate between the fungi and human tissue, so it is not a correct answer.

13. **The answer is D.** [VI B 2 a] *Histoplasma* and *Blastomyces* are both endemic in Iowa (central United States bordering the Mississippi River), but only *Histoplasma* fits the description of a facultative intracellular parasite circulating in the reticuloendothelial system.

14. **The answer is B.** [VI C 2 b] *Blastomyces* has a double refractile wall and buds with a broad base of attachment to the mother cell. The environmental association appears to be rotting wood.

15. **The answer is C.** [VII D] *Cryptococcus,* an encapsulated yeast, is the major causative agent of meningitis in patients with AIDS.

8

Parasitology

I. CHARACTERISTICS OF PARASITES AND THEIR HOSTS

A. **Symbiotic relationships** between microbes and hosts may be of these three types:
1. **Mutualistic:** having benefits to both the microbe and the host.
2. **Commensalistic**: having benefits to the microbe but with no benefits or ill effects to the host.
3. **Parasitic**: having benefits to the microbe but deleterious to the host.

B. **Parasites**
1. **Ectoparasites** live on the skin or hair (eg, lice); **endoparasites** live in the host. The rest of the chapter covers human endoparasites.
2. They may be **obligate parasites (entirely dependent on the host)** or **facultative parasites** (free living or associated with the host).
3. They rival malnutrition as the major cause of morbidity and mortality worldwide.
4. Parasites may be present in a host as a commensal organism. Factors such as a low-protein diet may favor virulence and growth of organisms, such as *Entamoeba histolytica*. Parasite numbers also influence the severity and progression of disease. Any decrease in immune functioning (particularly cell mediated) is likely to cause both increased susceptibility to infection and more severe infections.

C. **Hosts** may be one of these types:
1. A host in which either eggs (usually ingested) or very early larval forms develop into larval or intermediate parasite stages is by convention called an ***intermediate host***.
2. A host in which the larval stages infect and mature into the sexually mature adult parasites is called a ***definitive host***.
3. A **reservoir host** is any host essential to parasite survival and a focus for spreading to other hosts (eg, pigs [swine] for the pig roundworm *Trichinella spiralis*).
4. A host may be **accidental where the parasite is able to exist without the host** in which it is found.
5. A host may be **obligatory** in so far as part or all of the parasite's life cycle must occur in that specific host.

D. **Vectors** are living transmitters of disease and are classified as one of the following:
1. **Mechanical vectors** are nonessential to the life cycle of the pathogen (eg, flies who track *Chlamydia trachomatis* from one child's eye to another).
2. **Biologic vectors**, by contrast, serve as the site of some developmental events in the life cycle of the parasite, such as mosquitoes in malaria.

E. **Pathogenesis:** Parasites may cause disease by a single or multiple mechanisms.
1. Many parasites cause nutritional deficiencies by competing with the host for nutrients (eg, hookworms).

2. Many parasites cause tissue damage by:
   a. Toxin production, such as with apicomplexan *Plasmodium falciparum.*
   b. Mechanical damage or obstruction, such as tapeworm *Taenia* species.
3. Some parasites evade the host's immune response by creating antigenic variation (eg, protozoa, blood worm infections).
4. Some parasites alter immune function such as switching a Th1 response for a Th2 immune response or altering cytokine profiles, such as *Leishmania* species.
5. Some parasites can cause allergic or autoimmune reactions, such as *Toxoplasma gondii.*
6. Many parasites cause inflammation (eg, *E. histolytica*).
7. Parasites may disrupt normal microbiota.

> **• • • Clinical Pearl**
>
> Parasitic infections often have geographic distributions. Knowledge of the patient's travel history/residence or exposure to vectors in particular geographic regions can be crucial for diagnosis and prevention.

II. PROTOZOAN PARASITES

A. General characteristics: Protozoan parasites are single-celled animals and, therefore, have no multicellular stages, such as larvae. There are often two distinctive forms:
   1. **Trophozoites** are the actively motile invasive forms, which are delicate and do not survive long outside the body; if ingested, they rarely withstand normal stomach acid, so they are generally considered noninfectious.
   2. **Cysts** are sturdy resting stages and the most common infective form in fecal-oral spread as they survive at least a while in the environment and pass through normal stomach acid.

B. Amoebae move by **pseudopods created by streaming protoplasm** and include *Entamoeba, Acanthamoeba,* and *Naegleria.*

C. Flagellates move by the action of **flagella** and include *Giardia, Trichomonas, Trypanosoma,* and *Leishmania.*
   1. *Giardia* and *Trichomonas* have simple trophozoites that replicate by longitudinal binary fission and cysts.
   2. *Trypanosoma* and *Leishmania* **species** are **hemoflagellates** that infect blood and tissues. They have life cycles involving several forms:
      a. **Trypomastigotes** are free living, elongated, flagellated forms with an undulating membrane. They are seen extracellularly in blood in *Trypanosoma* infections.
      b. **Amastigotes** are "oval" cells that do not have a flagellum or an undulating membrane. They are seen in infected tissue (eg, heart tissue infected with *Trypanosoma cruzi*) or macrophages (*Leishmania*).

D. *Ciliates* move by the action of **cilia.** ***Balantidium coli,*** a rare cause of dysentery, is the only human ciliate of note.

E. Apicomplexa (also called *sporozoa* or *coccidia*) are intracellular protozoans with complex life cycles involving more than one host, a gliding ("tractor") motility, and an apical organelle complex that allows them to be taken up by host cells. They include *Plasmodium, Toxoplasma, Cryptosporidium, Cyclospora, Isopora,* and *Babesia.*

III. HELMINTHS (WORMS)

A. Trematodes are the **flatworms** (**Platyhelminthes**), informally called *flukes.* Depending on the fluke, **human acquisition requires either being in water or ingestion of the parasites found in or on aquatic plants, fish, or crabs.**

1. **Flukes** have complex life cycles involving two or three sequential hosts (depending on the fluke) but always **involving water and mollusks.**
2. **Adult flukes** develop in **vertebrate hosts, including humans.** Adult flukes:
   a. Are **flat** and **fleshy.**
   b. Are **hermaphroditic, except for the genus** *Schistosoma*, which has separate males and females; thus, there is the schistosome and nonschistosomal fluke division.
   c. **Lay eggs** in the vertebrate host; the eggs pass outside.
3. **If fluke eggs land in water,** they develop a motile **early larval form,** which, when released, enters the **first intermediate host (aquatic snails or clams) by ingestion or invasion.** They increase in number and are released from the first host as **cercaria,** the second motile-stage larvae form.
4. The **cercaria of the schistosomes invades the skin of people in water.** For the other trematodes (depending on which one), the late larval **cercaria either encyst on aquatic plants or infect crabs or fish.** Humans are accidentally infected by nonschistosomal flukes through the **ingestion of plants, crabs, or fish.**

B. Cestodes are **flatworms** (**Platyhelminthes**), informally called ***tapeworms.***
   1. **Adult tapeworms** develop in their definitive host.
      a. The **adult tapeworm** has the following **parts**
         (1) **Scolex (head)**, a knobby structure with suckers or a sucking groove **used to adhere to the vertebrate host's small intestinal mucosa.**
         (2) **Neck, which produces the segments, or proglottids, producing the worm.**
         (3) **Proglottids,** which mature as they move away from the scolex. **Each proglottid is hermaphroditic**, with both male and female reproductive organs developing in each section (proglottid) and **mature eggs produced in the most distal proglottids.**
      b. **Adult cestodes (tapeworms) inhabit the small intestines of** humans or their other **vertebrate definitive host.** Lacking a gastrointestinal (GI) tract, they absorb nutrients from the host's GI tract.
   2. **Eggs from proglottids are released in the feces from the vertebrate definitive host** and may contaminate soil or food.
      a. **Ingested eggs** develop into invasive larval forms that migrate through tissues and **may cause serious** diseases, such as **neurocysticercosis**.
      b. **Hosts ingesting the larvae,** generally in undercooked fish or meat, **develop intestinal tapeworms, which generally cause mild disease.**
      c. **Cysticercosis does not occur from eating undercooked fish or meat.**
   3. **Cestode infections**
      a. **When humans are the definitive host, the presence of the adult tapeworm in the small intestine** does not cause major symptoms, but it may affect nutrition. Human adult tapeworms include *Taenia saginata* (beef), *Taenia solium* (pork flatworm), *Diphyllobothrium latum* (broad fish tapeworm found in fish in some lakes in cold regions, such as Canada and Alaska), *Hymenolepis nana* (humans and rodents), and *Dipylidium caninum* (dogs and cats).
      b. When humans serve as the intermediate host, more serious disease results. Symptoms depend on the **migration of the larval forms.** Diseases include cysticercosis (*T. solium*), sparganosis (*D. latum*), unilocular hydatid cyst disease (*Echinococcus granulosus*), and alveolar hydatid cyst disease (*Echinococcus multilocularis*).
      c. Infection can be diagnosed by demonstration of eggs or proglottids in the feces or cysticerci in tissues.

C. Nematodes are the **roundworms** (Table 8.1).
   1. Nematodes have **round, unsegmented adult bodies covered by a tough cuticle.**
   2. **Nematodes have multiple larval stages:**
      a. **Filariform larvae** are the infective form.
      b. **Rhabditiform larvae** are noninfective and are the diagnostic form.

Table 8.1	Roundworm Mnemonic							
N	**E**	**M**	**A²**	**T³**	**O**	**D**	**E**	**S**
Necator (hookworm) [the United States]	_Enterobius_ (pinworm)	Mosquito borne: _Wuchereria_ and _Brugia_	A^2: _Ascaris_ and _Ancylostoma_	T^3: _Trichuris_, _Trichinella_, and _Toxocara_	_Onchocerca_ (river blindness)	_Dracunculus_ (guinea worm, nearly eradicated)	_Eye worm_ (_Loa loa_)	_Strongyloides_ (threadworm)

3. **Transmission** can occur in several ways:
    a. **Ingestion of eggs** (_Enterobius_, _Ascaris_, _Trichuris_, and _Toxocara_).
    b. **Ingestion of larvae** in undercooked game or pork (_Trichinella_) (Table 8.2).
    c. **Direct invasion** of skin by larval forms in soil contaminated with feces (_Necator_, _Ancylostoma_, and _Strongyloides_).
    d. **Larvae transmission via insect bite** (_Wuchereria_, _Loa_, _Mansonella_, and _Onchocerca_).

● ● ● Clinical Pearl

Eosinophilia is a common finding in many parasitic infections. Elevated eosinophil levels in the blood may suggest a parasitic etiology and prompt further investigation.

Table 8.2	Roundworm Infection by Ingestion of Eggs Mnemonic	
E	**A**	**T³**
Enterobius	_Ascaris_	_Trichuris_, _Toxocara_, and _Trichinella_

Directions: Select the one lettered answer that is best in each case. Commit to and write down your answers before checking the answers and explanations. Each of the numbered items in this section is followed by answers with explanations, in the following section.

1. A 35-year-old traveler recently returned from a tropical region and presents with abdominal pain, diarrhea, and weight loss. Stool examination reveals the presence of cysts identified as *E. histolytica*. Which of the following best describes the relationship between *E. histolytica* and its host?

(A) Commensalistic
(B) Mutualistic
(C) Parasitic
(D) Symbiotic

2. A 45-year-old patient presents with eosinophilia, abdominal pain, and diarrhea. Stool examination reveals the presence of large, multicellular worms with a thick, segmented body. The patient reports consumption of contaminated undercooked pork. Which of the following best describes the type of parasite and its human host?

(A) Commensal parasite in a commensal host
(B) Ectoparasite in a definitive host
(C) Ectoparasite in an intermediate host
(D) Endoparasite in a definitive host
(E) Endoparasite in an intermediate host

3. A medical student is creating flash cards to prepare for an examination. While going over lectures on parasites, the student categorizes parasites as either protozoa or helminths. Which of the following characteristics best distinguishes protozoans from worms?

(A) Mating process
(B) Mechanism of pathogenesis
(C) Method of transmission
(D) Multicellularity

4. A 24-year-old man presents with fever, malaise, and abdominal pain. He recently returned from a trip to sub-Saharan Africa. Physical examination reveals hepatosplenomegaly and tender lymph nodes. Laboratory investigations show elevated eosinophil count and liver function tests. Microscopic examination of a fecal sample reveals rhabditiform larvae. Which of the following mechanisms best describes how helminths contribute to the pathogenesis in this patient?

(A) Antitoxin production
(B) Enhance host microbiome
(C) Increasing macronutrients
(D) Inhibition of inflammation
(E) Mechanical tissue damage

5. A parasitologist is preparing a presentation for students about the features of different groups of protozoan parasites. Which of the following characteristics best distinguishes ciliates from amoebae, apicomplexans, and flagellates?

(A) Arthropod vector
(B) Formation of cysts
(C) Induce pathogenesis
(D) Type of locomotion
(E) Multicellular life stage

Answers and Explanations

1. **The answer is C.** [I A] Parasitic relationships are characterized by one organism benefiting at the expense of the host. Commensalistic relationships are characterized by one organism benefiting, but the host receiving no benefit or harm. Mutualistic relationships are characterized by both the organism and the host receiving benefits. Symbiotic relationships are a broader characterization that encompasses all the various relationships between different species living together.

2. **The answer is D.** [III B 3] The description matches a worm endoparasite that requires a pig intermediate host for its life cycle with a human as the definitive host. Ectoparasites live on the outside of their host. A commensal relationship is not occurring here as the patient is experiencing symptoms.

3. **The answer is D.** [II A] Protozoans are unicellular organisms, while helminths are multicellular. Some protozoans as do helminths have sexual reproductive cycles. Both protozoans and helminths have examples of causing disease by tissue damage among other ways. Some protozoans as with many helminths can be transmitted via similar methods like ingestion.

4. **The answer is E.** [I E] Worm infections can cause tissue damage by mechanical means. Parasites in general can cause host pathology by disturbing the balance between the host and microbiome, causing nutrient deficiencies, increasing inflammation, and producing toxins.

5. **The answer is D.** [II B–E] Ciliates move by short hairlike structures called *cilia*. Flagellates move by flagella. Amoebae move by projecting pseudopods. Apicomplexans move by a tractor motility.

9

System-Based and Situational Parasitic Infections

Although parasitic diseases still have a tremendous impact on health worldwide, the level of sanitation, temperate climate in most areas, and reasonably good housing conditions in the United States limit their impact in this country. This review focuses on parasitic diseases common in the United States or commonly seen in travelers in the United States. The diseases are presented in a series of tables. Each table is organized to facilitate self-testing to check your preparedness for the United States Medical Licensing Examination (USMLE) case-based questions. Symptoms are presented first. Your first task is to identify the causative agent based on the information presented. As you progress from the first left cell toward the right, your choices should narrow. Small images are incorporated into the tables; they are not to scale.

To use these tables for self-testing or later review, use two cover sheets, one to cover all subsequent rows and a second top sheet to move left to right on the row you are testing yourself on, starting with only the left cell revealed. On the top sheet, you may want to jot down the column headings, which are basically the most commonly asked USMLE questions, to make sure you can answer them for each of the organisms. See Tables 9.1 to 9.3 as well as Figures 9.1 and 9.2.

> • • • **Clinical Pearl**
>
> It is important to understand the geographic distribution of the high-yield parasites. This can provide clues to exposure and transmission risk factors such as fecal-oral, vector-borne, and ingestion of contaminated food and water to assist in the diagnosis of different infections.

Table 9.1 Central Nervous System, Eye, Blood, and Tissue (Including Skin) Parasites

Signs/Symptoms/Case Details	Infective Form/Transmission	Diagnostic Form	Diseases/Treatment	Species/Type
Fever, auras (often odor), severe headache, rapid progression to coma and death; generally occurs during summer in the southern United States in healthy young children	Amoeba acquired through cribriform plate from jumping or swimming in warm water swimming holes (environmental amoeba)	Trophozoites (sluglike amoebae) and smooth-walled cysts in CSF	Primary amoebic meningoencephalitis; Poor prognosis; amphotericin B	Naegleria/free-living amoebae
Altered mental status with chronic onset in patients who are debilitated or immunocompromised	Possibly transmitted in cyst-contaminated dust; probably enters through lungs or eyes (majority of infected individuals wear contact lenses); environmental organism	Trophozoites (below) and wrinkled cysts in CSF[a]	Granulomatous amoebic encephalitis; BSB	Acanthamoeba/free-living amoebae
Neonate with fever, pneumonitis, and hepatosplenomegaly, or infant or young child with active chorioretinitis, encephalomyelitis, hydrocephaly, or microcephaly	Congenital transmission of tachyzoites across placenta if mother's primary infection occurs during pregnancy; maternal antibody from prior infection protects fetus	Clinical diagnosis; Intracerebral calcifications; PCR on amniotic fluid; PCR on neonatal urine	Toxoplasmosis; BSB	Toxoplasma gondii/protozoan parasite
Keratitis with severe ocular pain but a mild inflammatory response; corneal infection leading to ulceration may require both trauma (from contacts) and exposure (contaminated contact solution or dust); often a chronic onset; may lead to loss of eyesight.	Cysts in environment; home-made contact saline solution has been implicated in some cases; almost all patients are contact wearers.	Motile trophozoites (amoeba) or cysts in corneal scraping; stain with calcofluor white and fluoresce	Keratitis; BSB	Acanthamoeba/free-living amoebae

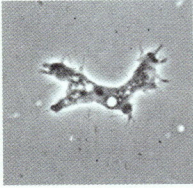

(continued)

Table 9.1 Central Nervous System, Eye, Blood, and Tissue (Including Skin) Parasites (continued)

Signs/Symptoms/Case Details	Infective Form/Transmission	Diagnostic Form	Diseases/Treatment	Species/Type
Patient with posterior cervical lymph node enlargement, irregular fevers, rigors, headache, night sweats; patients eventually develop stupor; travel to Africa.	Bite of tsetse fly carrying trypomastigotes	Flagellated trypomastigotes with undulating membrane in blood or CSF; hypergammaglobulinemia[b] 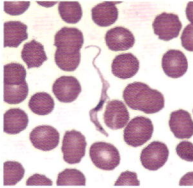	African sleeping sickness; organisms not cleared due to antigenic variation BSB	Trypanosoma brucei/hemoflagellate noted for antigenic variation
Heart failure; autopsy reveals greatly enlarged heart; travel or residence in poor areas of South America.	Defecating reduviid bug bites a person and deposits feces with trypomastigotes; bite itches; scratching inoculates organism into bite.	Amastigotes (no undulating membrane nor flagella) in heart tissue; trypomastigotes in blood early 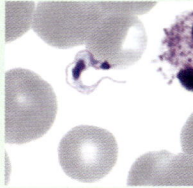	Chagas disease[c] BSB	Trypanosoma cruzi/hemoflagellates often C or U shaped
Patients with compromised T-cell function; fever with lymphadenopathy and pneumonia; often changes in mental status (calcified lesions seen on CNS imaging); chorioretinitis (Symptoms in healthy adults resemble mononucleosis)	Ingestion of infective oocysts from cat feces or contaminated undercooked meat. Excreted form becomes an infective oocyst in ~2 d; may also be reactivated in AIDS.	Serologic diagnosis; the distinctive crescent-shaped replicating tachyzoites and cysts are seldom seen. Immunofluorescence staining more sensitive 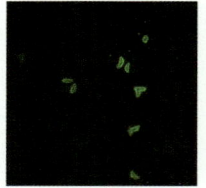	Toxoplasmosis Prophylaxis is TMP-SMT for Pneumocystis. Treatment is BSB.[d]	T. gondii/protozoan parasite Once infected, humans remain infected unless treated. T. gondii reactivates with immunosuppression, but not with pregnancy (see Figure 9.1).

Signs/Symptoms/Case Details	Infective Form/Transmission	Diagnostic Form	Diseases/Treatment	Species/Type
Influenza-like prodrome followed by recurring intense paroxysms[e] (chills [rigors for 10-15 min] followed by a hot phase for several hours ending with profuse sweating); patterns depend on species; anemia[f]	Anopheles mosquito bite bearing sporozoites; associated with travel to endemic area, except in cases of rare "airport malaria," in which an individual who resides near an international airport is bitten by a mosquito	Hematocrit is low and urine often dark. Merozoites in red blood cells	Malaria	Plasmodium spp./ Apicomplexa (see life cycle in Figure 9.2) See species features compared in Table 9.2.
Subcutaneous nodules, dermatitis: wrinkled skin and eye infection Central America and Africa	Larvae-infected black fly bite (Simulium) near running water	Microfilariae are seen on skin examination (adults develop in nodules and migrate around).	Surgical removal of nodules and ivermectin	Onchocerca volvulus/ river blindness
Fever, lymphangitis, and lymphadenitis; recurring fevers; limb or scrotal elephantiasis	Mosquitoes transmitting filarial worms	Often a clinical diagnosis in endemic areas; microfilaria in blood	Filarial worms BSB	Wuchereria and Brugia
Calabar swellings with some pain and pruritus; migrating; may cross conjunctiva Western central Africa	Mango fly (Chrysops) transmit infective filariae	Eosinophilia and symptoms	Loiasis; little damage; surgical removal; ivermectin	Loa loa/African eye worms[g]

BSB, beyond the scope of book; CNS, central nervous system; CSF, cerebrospinal fluid; PCR, polymerase chain reaction; TMP-SMT, trimethoprim/sulfamethoxazole.

[a]Trophozoites of Acanthamoeba spp. from culture. (Courtesy of Centers for Disease Control DPDx Parasite Image Library.)

[b]T. brucei sp. in thin blood smears stained with Wright-Giemsa. (Courtesy of Centers for Disease Control DPDx Parasite Image Library.)

[c]Trypanosoma cruzi trypomastigote in a thin blood smear stained with Giemsa. (Courtesy of Centers for Disease Control DPDx Parasite Image Library.)

[d]Formalin-fixed T. gondii tachyzoites stained by immunofluorescence assay (IFA). This is a positive reaction (tachyzoites + human antibodies to Toxoplasma + Fluorescein isothiocyanate (FITC)-labeled antihuman immunoglobulin G = fluorescence.) (Courtesy of Centers for Disease Control DPDx Parasite Image Library.)

[e]Paroxysms are caused by the release of toxic hemoglobin metabolites when merozoites lyse red cells. Anemia is caused by the loss of red blood cells. Cerebral malaria (Plasmodium falciparum) is due to adherence of infected erythrocytes in cerebral venules and the effects of metabolic byproducts in the CNS.

[f]A parasite called Babesia microti primarily causes disease in cattle and may cause anemia with malaria-like symptoms in humans (babesiosis). Because it is **transmitted by the Ixodes tick, coinfections with Borrelia burgdorferi or Anaplasma** may occur. Babesiosis is diagnosed by the presence of multiple ringlike forms in the red blood cells.

[g]L. loa African eye worm stained with fluorescent antibody. (Courtesy of Centers for Disease Control Public Health Image Library.)

Table 9.2   Malaria

Species[a]	Disease	Diagnosis (Giemsa Stained)[b]	Treatment
Plasmodium vivax	Tertian malaria	Oval-shaped host cells with Schüffner granules and ragged cell wall are seen on thick and thin blood examination.	Chloroquine phosphate, then primaquine
Plasmodium malariae	Quartan malaria[c]	Bar and band forms; rosette schizonts	Chloroquine
Plasmodium falciparum	Malignant tertian malaria[d]	Multiple ring forms and crescents (gametocytes) → schizonts rare in peripheral blood[e]	Chloroquine; chloroquine-resistant strains are treated with quinine sulfate with doxycycline; complicated falciparum malaria with quinidine sulfate.[f]

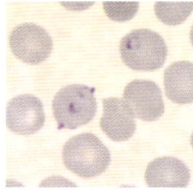

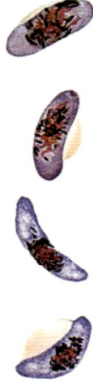

All *Plasmodia* have two distinct hosts. A vertebrate (human or cattle) is the intermediate host where the asexual phase of the parasite's life cycle (schizogony) takes place in the liver and red blood cells. The *Anopheles* mosquito is the definitive host and is the site of the sexual phase of the parasite's life cycle (sporogony). (See Figure 9.2 for the life cycle.)

[a]*Plasmodium ovale* (rare) causes benign tertian (ovale) malaria. Transmission, diagnosis, and treatment are similar to those for *P. vivax*. **Both *P. ovale* and *P. vivax* form hypnozoites (or sleeping forms) in the liver** that may not progress to merozoite production until months later (and like other liver forms are not sensitive to chloroquine). This recurrence of symptoms is called *relapse* from *liver* forms.

[b]Immunofluorescent antibodies and agarose DNA gels and probes are now used in identification instead of morphology.

[c]Recurrence of *P. malariae* symptoms, called *recrudescence*, may result from a persistent low level of parasites in the red blood cells.

[d]*P. falciparum*–infected red blood cells adhere to the endothelium of peripheral capillaries, resulting in "sludging." Severe anemia results from multiple infections of both immature and mature red blood cells. The severe disease that results constitutes a medical emergency.

[e]Multiply infected red blood cells with appliqué forms in thin blood smears. (Courtesy of Centers for Disease Control DPDx Parasite Image Library.)

[f]Left two are mature macrogametocytes (female); right two are mature microgametocytes (male). (Courtesy of Centers for Disease Control DPDx Parasite Image Library.)

Table 9.3 Gastrointestinal and Urogenital Parasitic Infections

Species/Type	Diseases/Treatment	Diagnostic Form	Infective Form/Transmission	Signs/Symptoms/Case Details
Entamoeba histolytica/amoebae[a] 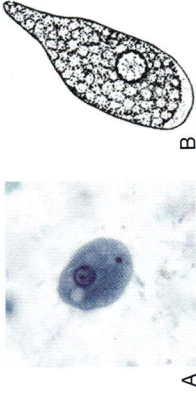 A B	Amoebic dysentery Metronidazole followed by paromomycin or iodoquinol	Cysts and motile trophozoites with wagon-wheel-like nuclei and ingested WBCs/RBCs are seen in stools; serologic testing	Fecal-oral by water, fresh fruits, and vegetables; nonmotile cysts are infective stage.	Dysentery; inverted flask-shaped ulcers of large intestine with extraintestinal abscesses (particularly liver) common
Giardia lamblia/flagellate[b] 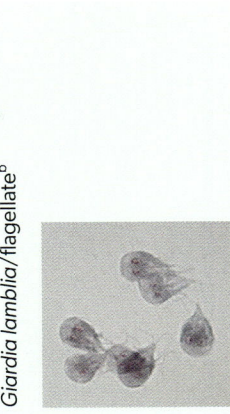	Giardiasis Tinidazole or nitazoxanide	Pyriform flagellated trophozoites with ventral sucking disk may not be seen; cysts found in stool Fecal antigen test is more sensitive.	Quadrinucleate cysts Fecal (eg, human, beaver, muskrat) by water, food, oral-anal intercourse, daycare centers	Diarrhea with malabsorption; starts watery and then, as more and more trophozoites attach through their ventral sucking disk, the malabsorption gets worse and diarrhea more "fatty"; severe pain on ingestion of dairy is common.
Cryptosporidium spp./Apicomplexa protozoan[c]	Cryptosporidiosis No good treatment in AIDS, except antiretroviral therapy	Acid-fast oocysts in stool Biopsy: dots (cysts) in intestinal glands 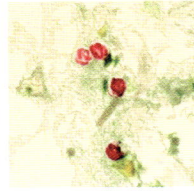	Chlorine-resistant cysts are found in up to 85% of U.S. surface water removed during water treatment by flocculation or filtration; patients with AIDS should boil or filter water.	Transient diarrhea in healthy persons; severe diarrhea in persons who are immunocompromised

(continued)

Table 9.3 Gastrointestinal and Urogenital Parasitic Infections (*continued*)

Signs/Symptoms/Case Details	Infective Form/Transmission	Diagnostic Form	Diseases/Treatment	Species/Type
Vitamin B_{12} anemia in genetically predisposed; mild abdominal discomfort	Ingestion of late larvae (still viable) in smoked, pickled, undercooked, or raw fish from cold water lake regions such as Scandinavia or Canada[d]	Proglottids (left) and eggs in stool Proglottids wider than long ("broad" fish tapeworm); worm up to several meters long	Intestinal tapeworm: Vitamin B_{12} anemia results if the organism attaches in the proximal portion of the jejunum in genetically predisposed individuals.	*Diphyllobothrium latum*/cestode (tapeworm) 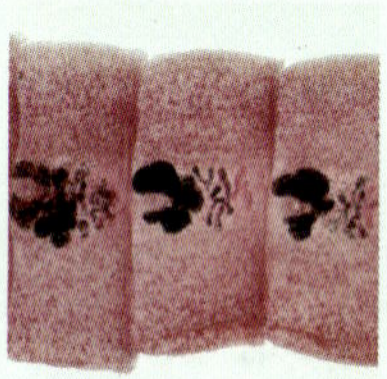
Perianal itching; sometimes with vaginitis; generally found in children[e]	Eggs from bed linens and clothes are spread by air currents and stay viable for several days. Reinfection by contaminated fingers is common.	Scotch tape mount; eggs (below) and 2- to 5-mm-long roundworms that are no >0.5 mm in diameter 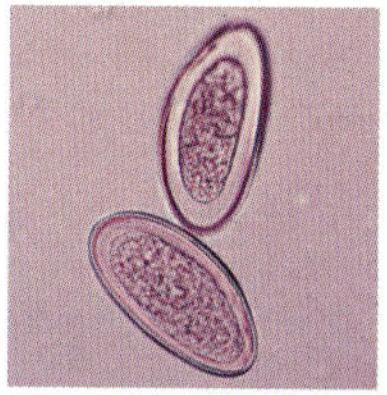	Pinworms Albendazole or mebendazole	*Enterobius vermicularis*/(pinworm); the most common roundworm in the United States
Pneumonitis early; GI symptoms may be absent or a writhing sensation may be felt; anesthetics, fever, and drugs may induce adult worms to migrate to places such as the bile ducts or pancreas; intestinal blockage may occur in children with heavy worm burden.	Ingestion of egg-contaminated feces; larvae exit GI tract into tissues and reach lymphatics and then lungs; larvae are coughed up and swallowed and then mature into adults in small intestines where they mate.	Bile-stained knobby eggs (right) or 6- to 12-inch-long roundworms seen on radiograph or cholangiogram; serologic test shows some cross-reaction with *Trichuris.*	Ascariasis Supportive therapy during pneumonitis; surgery for ectopic migrations Albendazole or mebendazole	*Ascaris lumbricoides*/(roundworm; egg shown below)[f] 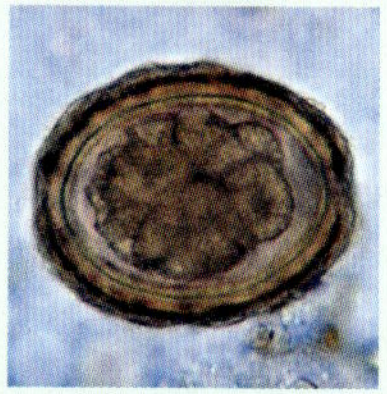

Signs/Symptoms/Case Details	Infective Form/Transmission	Diagnostic Form	Diseases/Treatment	Species/Type
Generally asymptomatic but symptoms, when present, may be severe abdominal pain with bloody diarrhea, appendicitis, and rectal prolapse from strain to defecate.	Ingestion of eggs (eg, use of human feces as vegetable fertilizer; contaminated food and water)	Microscopic detection of barrel-shaped eggs with bipolar plugs (below)	Trichuriasis Albendazole[9]	*Trichuris trichiura*/nematode (roundworm)
Diarrhea, vomiting, abdominal pain, iron deficiency anemia following ground itch at site of entry of parasite	Filariform larvae in soil penetrate intact skin of bare feet (shoes reduce transmission); larvae travel from skin to circulation to lungs, then ascend to epiglottis and are swallowed; adult worms attach to and mature in the small intestine.	Non-bile-staining segmented eggs in stool; possible occult blood in stools; no need to identify genus	Hookworm infection Albendazole or mebendazole	*Necator americanus* (New World hookworm); *Ancylostoma duodenale* (Old World hookworm)/nematodes
Skin pruritus, mild pneumonitis; asymptomatic to severe diarrhea with malabsorption	Filariform larvae penetrate intact **skin** of bare feet; free-living cycle occurs outside host; larvae migrate from skin to blood to lung to small intestine; adults lay eggs; larvae may hatch in GI tract, facilitating reinfection without exiting body (**autoinfection**).	Larvae in stool; serologic testing[h]	Strongyloidiasis Ivermectin	*Strongyloides stercoralis*/nematodes Because of auto- or reinfection, infections may last decades outside endemic area

(continued)

Table 9.3	Gastrointestinal and Urogenital Parasitic Infections (continued)			
Signs/Symptoms/Case Details	Infective Form/Transmission	Diagnostic Form	Diseases/Treatment	Species/Type
Infections are commonly asymptomatic but may cause gastritis, fever, and muscle aches; high hemorrhages eosinophilia; splinter.	Consumption of encysted larvae in **undercooked meat** (bear, pork, horse meat)	Eosinophilia with classic symptoms; serology; later, calcifications in muscle	Trichinosis	*Trichinella spiralis*/pork roundworm
Transient reaction and itching at skin site of infection; mild infections may be asymptomatic; may cause generalized malaise, fever, urticaria, abdominal pain with diarrhea or dysentery.	Cercaria from infected snails enter water and penetrate intact skin of individuals swimming or standing in water. **Adults are shown here.** [i] 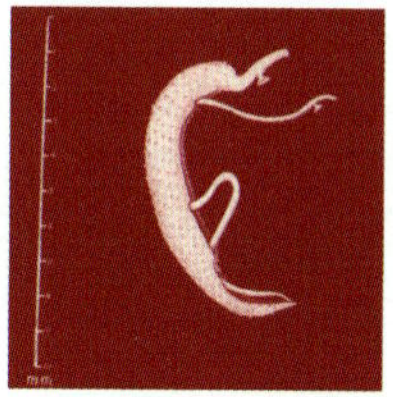	Eggs with lateral spine in feces [j] 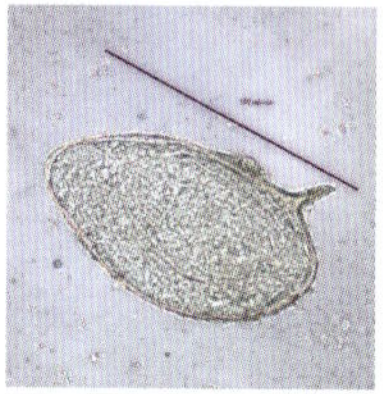	Intestinal schistosomiasis Praziquantel	*Schistosoma mansoni*/nematodes Mating pairs are found in vasculature; male is flat and fleshy and folds around the more cylindrical female in copulating pairs.
Transient reaction and itching at skin site of infection; mild infections may be asymptomatic; may cause generalized malaise, fever, urticaria, abdominal pain with blood in urine at end of micturition, and dysuria.	Cercaria from infected snails enter water and penetrate intact skin of individuals swimming or standing in water.	Eggs with terminal spine in urine	Vesicular schistosomiasis Praziquantel	*Schistosoma haematobium*/mating pairs are found in vasculature; male is flat and fleshy but folded around the more cylindrical female in copulating pairs.

Signs/Symptoms/Case Details	Infective Form/Transmission	Diagnostic Form	Diseases/Treatment	Species/Type
Asymptomatic or may cause symptoms of vaginitis with discharge associated with burning or itching, or, in males, urethral discharge	Sexual contact; transmitted via trophozoites (below)[k]	Motile trophozoites with undulating membrane, tuft of four polar flagella, and axostyle "tail"; excessive neutrophils in methylene blue wet mount; motility is jerky and nondirectional.	Trichomoniasis Metronidazole or tinidazole.	*Trichomonas vaginalis*/flagellates

GI, gastrointestinal; RBCs, red blood cells; WBCs, white blood cells.

[a]**(A)** *Entamoeba coli* trophozoite stained with trichrome. Occasionally, the cytoplasm contains ingested bacteria (as seen in the photo), yeasts, or other materials. **(B)** Line drawing of an *E. histolytica/Entamoeba dispar* trophozoite. (Courtesy of Centers for Disease Control DPDx Parasite Image Library.)

[b]*Giardia intestinalis* in in vitro culture, from a quality control slide. (Image contributed by the Oregon State Public Health Laboratory.)

[c]*Cryptosporidium parvum* oocysts stained using the modified acid-fast method. (Courtesy of Centers for Disease Control Public Health Image Library.)

[d]Carmine-stained proglottids of *D. latum*, showing rosette-shaped ovaries. (Courtesy of Centers for Disease Control DPDx Parasite Image Library.)

[e]Eggs of *E. vermicularis* in a wet mount. (Courtesy of Centers for Disease Control DPDx Parasite Image Library.)

[f]*Ascaris* fertilized egg in a wet mount with embryo in a more advanced stage of development. (Courtesy of Centers for Disease Control DPDx Parasite Image Library.)

[g]Egg of *Trichuris trichiura* in an iodine-stained wet mount. (Courtesy of Centers for Disease Control DPDx Parasite Image Library.)

[h]Free-living adult male *S. stercoralis*. Arrow points to spicule found in males. (Courtesy of Centers for Disease Control DPDx Parasite Image Library.)

[i]Adults of *S. mansoni*. The thin female resides in the gynecophoral canal of the thicker male. Note the tuberculate exterior of the male. (Courtesy of Centers for Disease Control DPDx Parasite Image Library.)

[j]Eggs of *S. mansoni* in unstained wet mounts. (Image contributed by the Wisconsin State Laboratory of Hygiene. Courtesy of Centers for Disease Control DPDx Parasite Image Library.)

[k]Two trophozoites of *T. vaginalis* obtained from in vitro culture stained with Giemsa. (Courtesy of Centers for Disease Control DPDx Parasite Image Library.)

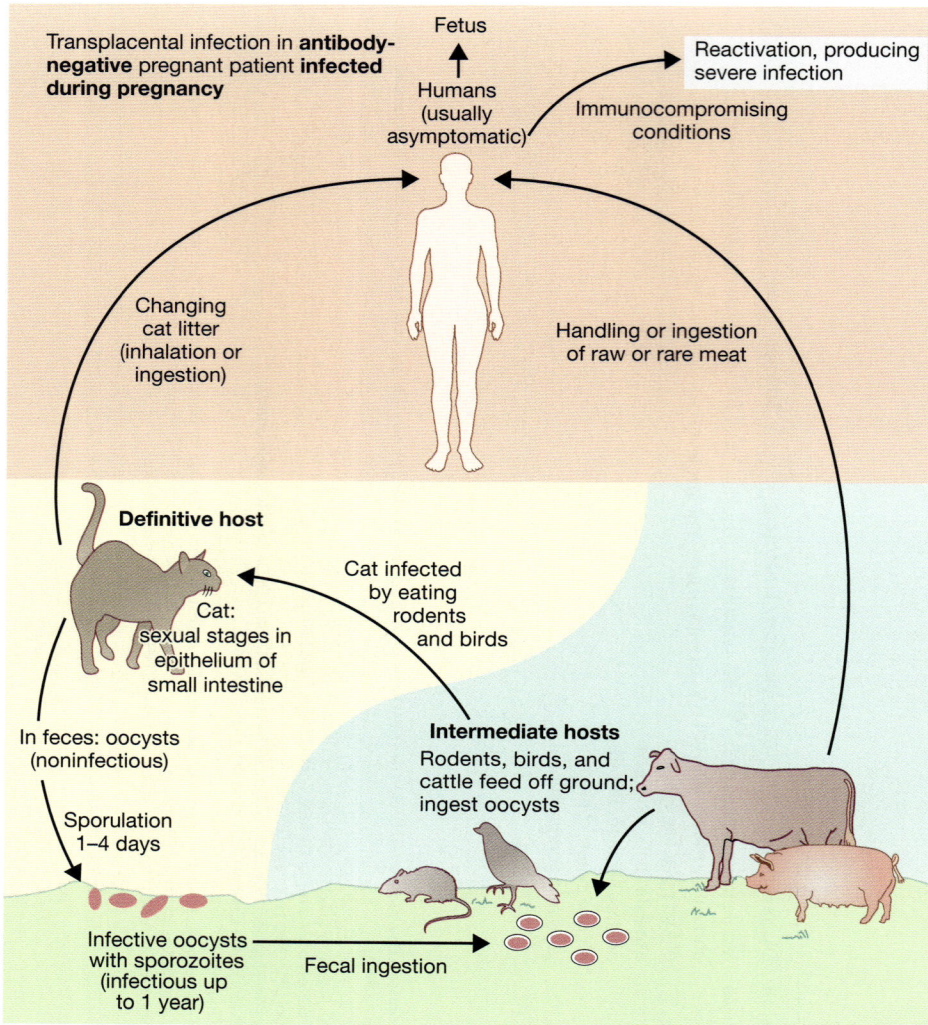

FIGURE 9.1. Toxoplasmosis life cycle. This illustration shows how widely distributed *Toxoplasma* is in nature and how humans can be infected and the populations that are impacted. (Modified from Engelberg NC, DiRita V, Dermody TS. *Schaechter's Mechanisms of Microbial Disease.* 5th ed. Wolters Kluwer Health/Lippincott Williams & Wilkins; 2013.)

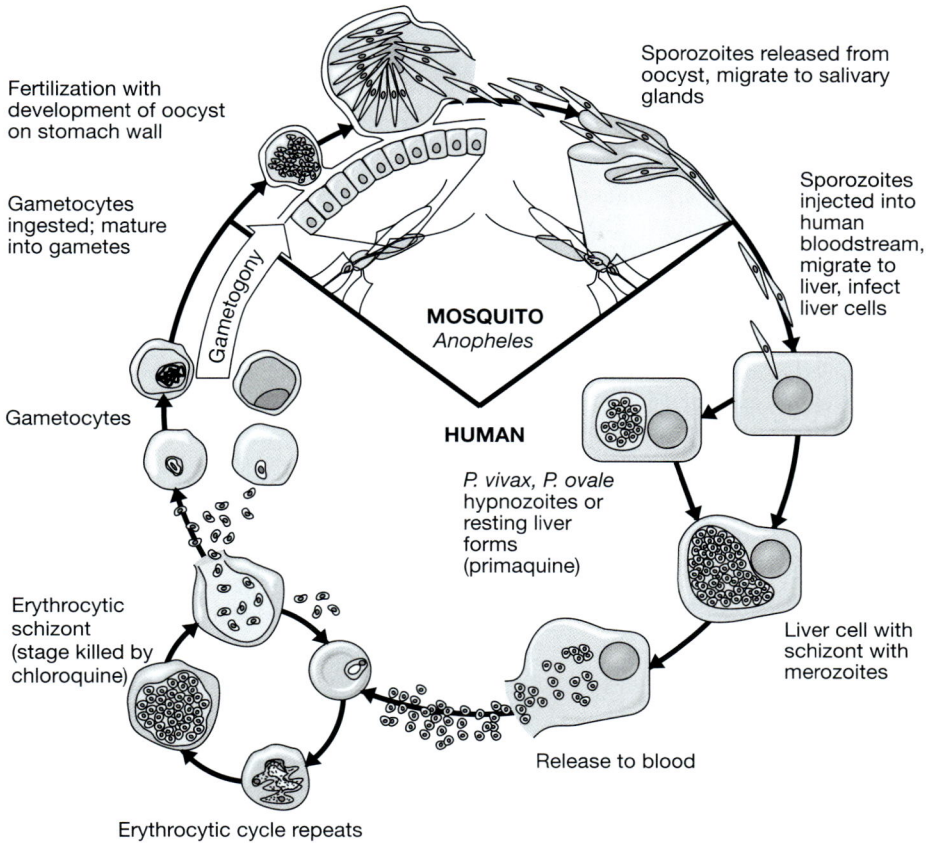

Fertilization with development of oocyst on stomach wall

Sporozoites released from oocyst, migrate to salivary glands

Gametocytes ingested; mature into gametes

Gametogony

Sporozoites injected into human bloodstream, migrate to liver, infect liver cells

MOSQUITO
Anopheles

Gametocytes

HUMAN

P. vivax, P. ovale hypnozoites or resting liver forms (primaquine)

Erythrocytic schizont (stage killed by chloroquine)

Liver cell with schizont with merozoites

Release to blood

Erythrocytic cycle repeats

FIGURE 9.2. The general life cycle of the *Plasmodium* species that causes malaria. (Reprinted with permission from Hawley L. *High-Yield Microbiology and Infectious Diseases.* Lippincott Williams & Wilkins; 2007:159.)

Review Test

Directions: Select the one lettered answer that is best in each case. Commit to and write down your answers before checking the answers and explanations. Each of the numbered items in this section is followed by answers with explanations, in the following section.

1. A biology graduate student who recently visited a tropical region of Africa presents with a new visual impairment and the sensation that something is moving in her eye. She tells you that she is concerned because she had been warned about eye disease transmitted by black flies. When in Africa, she was in a river area, and, despite her best efforts, she received a lot of black fly bites. She also has some subcutaneous nodules. If her infection was acquired by black fly bite, which of the following organisms is the most likely causative agent?

(A) *Ancylostoma braziliense*
(B) *Dracunculus medinensis*
(C) *Loa loa*
(D) *Onchocerca volvulus*
(E) *Wuchereria bancrofti*

2. A U.S. woman had a compound leg fracture pinned and set in Mexico and has returned to the U.S. 3 days later. Social history reveals she imports food from Mexico and spends several months per year in rural Mexico. She now has signs of acute appendicitis and is taken to surgery in Houston. When her appendix is removed, it is found to contain a light-colored, 20.5-cm-long roundworm as well as bile-stained, knobby eggs consistent with *Ascaris*. By which of the following mechanisms did she acquire this infection?

(A) Ingestion of food contaminated with the eggs
(B) Ingestion of water containing filariform larvae
(C) Inhalation of dust carrying the cysts
(D) Skin penetration by filariform larvae
(E) Skin penetration by rhabditiform larvae

3. A patient whose major source of protein is smoked and cooked fish develops what appears to be pernicious anemia. Which of the following parasites is noted for causing a lookalike vitamin B_{12} anemia in certain genetically predisposed infected individuals?

(A) *Dipylidium caninum*
(B) *Diphyllobothrium latum*
(C) *Echinococcus granulosus*
(D) *Hymenolepis nana*
(E) *Taenia solium*

4. Which of the following protozoans is free living and acquisition does not generally indicate fecal contamination?

(A) *Acanthamoeba*
(B) *Dientamoeba fragilis*
(C) *Entamoeba histolytica*
(D) *Entamoeba coli*
(E) *Giardia*

5. A 26-year-old woman with uncomplicated malaria who was treated initially with chloroquine now has relapsed. Which of the following is the reason for a chloroquine-treated case of *Plasmodium vivax* relapsing?

(A) Chloroquine is not one of the drugs of choice.
(B) *P. vivax* has a persistent erythrocytic stage.
(C) *P. vivax* has a persistent exoerythrocytic stage (hypnozoite).
(D) *P. vivax* has a significant level of chloroquine resistance.

6. A 38-year-old man presents to a clinic with a 3-month history of low-grade fever, splenomegaly, and weight loss. He recently traveled to a region endemic for *Leishmania donovani*. Blood smears demonstrate the presence of *L. donovani* amastigotes within macrophages. Which of the following is how *L. donovani* is transmitted?

(A) *Anopheles* mosquito bite
(B) Black fly bite
(C) *Culex* mosquito bite
(D) Sandfly bite
(E) Skin penetration by trauma

7. A 23-year-old woman returns from a recent trip to sub-Saharan Africa. She presents with symptoms of dysuria, hematuria, and pain in the lower abdomen. Urinalysis reveals microscopic hematuria and the presence of red blood cells with terminal spines. The attending physician believes her to be infected with *Schistosoma haematobium*. By which of the following mechanisms is *S. haematobium* transmitted?

(A) Handling aquatic birds
(B) Ingestion of raw or undercooked snail, frog, or snake
(C) Invasion of filariform larvae from soil
(D) Standing or swimming in contaminated water
(E) Tsetse fly bite

8. An untreated patient with acquired immunodeficiency syndrome (AIDS) (CD4$^+$ count of 180 cells/mm^3) from southern California has developed a progressively severe headache and mental confusion, along with ataxia and retinochoroiditis. Focal lesions are present on a computed tomographic scan of their brain. No mucocutaneous lesions are found. They have been living under a bridge for the past 2 years. Their level of immunoglobulin G (IgG) to the infectious agent is high. What is the most likely explanation for how this current infection started?

(A) Earlier exposure to pigeons
(B) Earlier exposure to desert sand
(C) Reactivation of bradyzoites in cysts from an earlier infection
(D) Recent exposure to cat feces
(E) Recent exposure to bats

9. A 48-year-old man presents to his primary care physician with symptoms of vague abdominal discomfort and occasional nausea. He recently immigrated from a rural farming community in a developing country. On further questioning, the patient mentioned that he consumes undercooked pork regularly. Which of the following organisms is the tapeworm acquired from eating undercooked pork?

(A) *Dipylidium* spp.
(B) *E. granulosus*
(C) *Taenia saginata*
(D) *Taenia solium*
(E) *Trichinella spiralis*

10. What roundworm is most likely to be transmitted by ingestion of food or water contaminated with feces?

(A) *Ascaris lumbricoides*
(B) *Enterobius vermicularis*
(C) *Necator americanus*
(D) *Taenia saginata*
(E) *Toxocara canis*

11. What roundworm is transmitted by filariform larvae that are found in the soil and penetrate the skin?

(A) *D. medinensis*
(B) *E. vermicularis*
(C) *S. stercoralis*
(D) *T. saginata*
(E) *T. canis*

12. How is *Clonorchis sinensis* (Chinese liver fluke) most likely transmitted to humans?

(A) Fish ingestion
(B) Mango fly (*Chrysops*)
(C) Mosquito bite
(D) Rare beef ingestion
(E) Swimming or water contact

13. A 48-year-old subsistence farmer from rural Brazil dies of heart failure. His autopsy shows a greatly enlarged heart. What was the vector for the most likely infectious agent that may have been responsible for his death?

(A) *Ixodes* tick
(B) Mosquito
(C) Reduviid bug
(D) Sandfly
(E) Tsetse fly

14. A 16-year-old man who recently returned from camping in Canada presents with fatty diarrhea and acute abdominal pain following many meals. How does the most likely agent cause the diarrhea?

(A) Coinfection with bacteria
(B) Enterotoxin production
(C) Suction disk attachment
(D) Tissue invasion leading to an inflammatory response and prostaglandin production

15. Which of the following protozoans is transmitted primarily by the motile trophozoite form?

(A) *Balantidium coli*
(B) *Entamoeba histolytica*
(C) *Giardia lamblia*
(D) *Taenia solium*
(E) *Trichomonas vaginalis*

1. **The answer is D.** [Table 9.1] *O. volvulus* causes river blindness and is transmitted by the bite of a black fly. The patient may be able to detect movement of the parasite in the eye.

2. **The answer is A.** [Table 9.3] Fertilized *Ascaris* eggs released in feces may contaminate food or water, which is then consumed. *Ascaris* does not attach to the intestine but maintains its position by mobility. The worm may become hypermotile (eg, during febrile periods, anesthetic use, or antibiotic use) and may migrate into the appendix or bile duct.

3. **The answer is B.** [Table 9.3] *Diphyllobothrium* is the tapeworm associated with anemia. It is transmitted in fish found in cool lake regions.

4. **The answer is A.** [Table 9.1] *Acanthamoeba* is a free-living organism with a sturdy cyst stage that is found in dust. A common way of acquiring *Acanthamoeba* infections in the United States is through homemade saline solutions for soft contact lenses. *Giardia* may be from animal contamination of water (rather than human) but is still not probably truly free living.

5. **The answer is C.** [Table 9.2, Figure 9.2] Both *Plasmodium ovale* and *P. vivax* may have resting liver forms, which are very slow to develop into schizonts with merozoites and proceed onto the chloroquine-sensitive erythrocytic stages after treatment is over. (It is not *over* with *P. ovale* or *P. vivax* unless you also treat it with primaquine phosphate, which kills the liver stages.) (Papua, New Guinea, and Indonesia now have chloroquine-resistant *P. vivax*.)

6. **The answer is D.** [Chapter 8, II C 2 b] All *Leishmania* are transmitted by sandflies.

7. **The answer is D.** [Table 9.3] All schistosomes are transmitted by skin penetration from standing or swimming in contaminated water. Remember that snails are intermediate hosts.

8. **The answer is C.** [Table 9.1, Figure 9.1] The most likely disease in this case is encephalitis with focal lesions. Because the patient has high levels of IgG, the current infection is likely a reactivation of an earlier infection; therefore, recent exposures (choices D and E) can be eliminated. Exposure to pigeons suggests cryptococcosis, which is often a reactivational infection. However, in cryptococcosis, antibody levels are rarely monitored, and there is no mention of India ink stain or capsular polysaccharide in the cerebrospinal fluid, which are the major diagnostic methods. In addition, based on the patient's symptoms, the infection is more likely to be encephalitis rather than meningitis or meningoencephalitis; also, retinochoroiditis is usually not present in cryptococcosis. The retinochoroiditis and lack of mucocutaneous lesions make infection with *Coccidioides* less likely. Reactivation of toxoplasmosis is most likely.

9. **The answer is D.** [Chapter 8, III B 3 b] *T. spiralis* is the pork roundworm, and *T. solium* is the pork tapeworm. *D. caninum* is the common tapeworm of both cats and dogs. It may be transmitted by ingestion of fleas harboring cysticercoid larvae. Transmission to humans usually occurs when crushed fleas harboring the disease are transmitted from a pet when it licks a child's mouth.

10. **The answer is A.** [Table 9.3] *A. lumbricoides* is transmitted via the fecal-oral route. *Enterobius* is most likely transmitted via contaminated hands, clothing, or bedding. *Necator* enters by skin penetration. *Taenia* is not a roundworm. *Toxocara* is most commonly acquired from eating fecally contaminated dirt or soil.

11. **The answer is C.** [Table 9.3] *S. stercoralis* is a type of hookworm (also a roundworm). The filariform larvae of *S. stercoralis* are acquired when walking barefoot or sitting on the ground. *D. medinensis* (the guinea worm) is acquired by drinking water with copepods containing the larvae. Filtration of all drinking water through clean sari silk or T-shirt material has reduced the incidence of new cases dramatically and may allow its eradication. (For those who are infected with *D. medinensis*, adults in subcutaneous nodules are slowly removed by rolling them out on a pencil.) *T. canis* and *Toxocara cati* are acquired most commonly by pica, the ingestion of inert material; in this case, dirt or sand with animal feces. *T. saginata* is a flatworm. *Enterobius* (pinworm) eggs are ingested.

12. **The answer is A.** [Chapter 8, III A] Raw, undercooked, smoked, or pickled freshwater fish are the most common route of transmission of *C. sinensis*. You should be able to answer this question from the general information in the preceding chapter without any specifics. The question told you it was a fluke, and so you know that water was involved in transmission; however, it is not a *Schistosoma* sp., so it has to be ingestion of aquatic plant or animal; in this case, it is fish.

13. **The answer is C.** [Table 9.1] The case of the Brazilian farmer is a classic description of heart failure from chronic Chagas disease, which is caused by *Trypanosoma cruzi*. *T. cruzi* is transmitted by reduviid bugs (cone-nose bugs or kissing bugs) that defecate as they bite. Scratching the bite spreads the trypanosome into the bite site, initiating the infection.

14. **The answer is C.** [Table 9.3] In this case, *G. lamblia* is the causative agent. *G. lamblia* is carried by muskrats and beavers, which is why it can be picked up in pristine northern lakes, such as those found in Canada. Attachment of numerous *Giardia* via their ventral sucking disks in the duodenal-jejunal area leads to malabsorption diarrhea and temporary lactose intolerance.

15. **The answer is E.** [Chapter 8, II A 2] Protozoans transmitted by the fecal-oral route are transmitted in the cyst form, which survives stomach acid. Only the sexually transmitted *T. vaginalis* is transmitted in the motile form. *T. solium* is not a protozoan, but a flatworm.

10

Immunology

I. OVERVIEW

A. Host defense mechanisms (Figure 10.1)

A collection of physiologic strategies is used to police tissues for parasites such as bacteria and non-compliant self-tissue such as cancer. The immune system is responsible for identifying self-tissue and nonself-tissue and to discern between normal and noncompliant tissue. Strategies include the following:

1. Innate immunity.
   a. Physical barriers.
   b. Inflammation.
   c. Cellular defenses.
   d. Chemical defenses.
2. Adaptive immunity.
   a. Cell-mediated immunity (CMI).
   b. Humoral immunity.

B. Concerns in medicine

1. Vulnerability to infection.
2. Cancer.

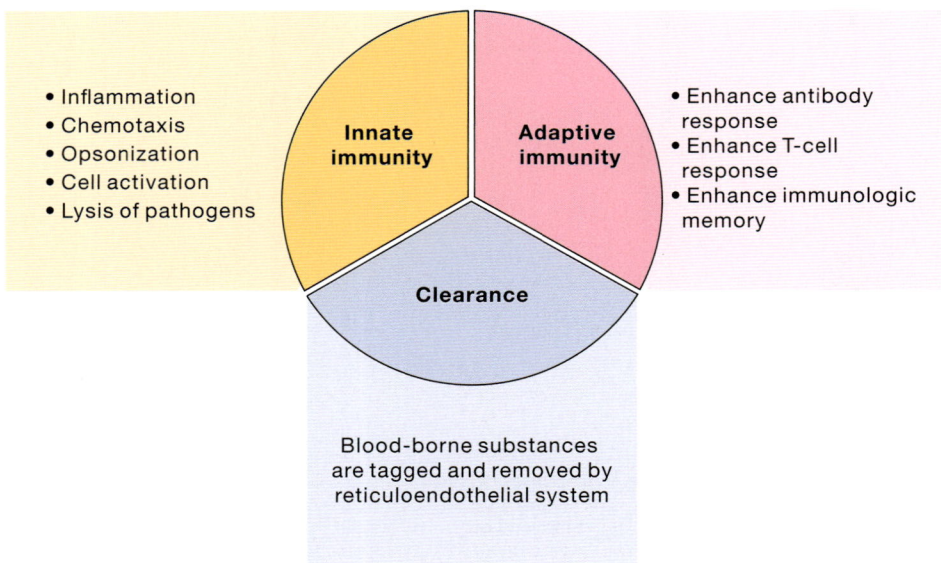

- Inflammation
- Chemotaxis
- Opsonization
- Cell activation
- Lysis of pathogens

Innate immunity

Adaptive immunity

- Enhance antibody response
- Enhance T-cell response
- Enhance immunologic memory

Clearance

Blood-borne substances are tagged and removed by reticuloendothelial system

FIGURE 10.1. Overview of host defenses.

3. Hypersensitivity.
4. Autoimmunity.
5. Complications to tissue transplantation and blood transfusions.

II. NONSPECIFIC BARRIERS

Nonspecific barriers (Figure 10.2) are composed of epithelium and demarcated zones of immunity; for instance, inside versus outside, mucosal versus interstitial, exocrine (salivary and sebaceous glands), urogenital and kidney, respiratory region, synovia of articulating joints, blood-brain barrier, eye, germ line, and placenta.

A. Stratum corneum
1. Demarcation of tissues from the extracorporeal environment.
2. Effective protection; trauma and infections are rare events; examples are lacerations, punctures, bites or nonsterile needles, antigens, solvents, ultraviolet (UV) light, detergents, microorganisms, toxins, and nanoparticles.
3. Cornified epithelium produced as the terminally differentiated keratinocytes in the stratified squamous epithelium.
4. Composed of keratin filaments in the cells with a barrier of insoluble protein matrix and highly cross-linked.
5. Desquamation of skin, sloughs off, carries bacteria approximately every 2 weeks.
6. Hair follicles, sebaceous glands, and sudoriferous glands flush the surface.
7. Common antigen-driven skin diseases include psoriasis and atopic dermatitis.
8. Skin surface area is 1.5 to 2.0 m^2.

B. Tight junctions
1. Composed of epithelial proteins, occludins, claudins, and junctional adhesion molecules.
2. Provides a tight seal at the blood-brain barrier and intestinal barrier.
3. Provides a route for Langerhans cells to capture antigen.
4. Intraepithelial T lymphocytes release interferon (IFN)-γ, interleukin (IL)-4, and IL-10 to disrupt the junction.

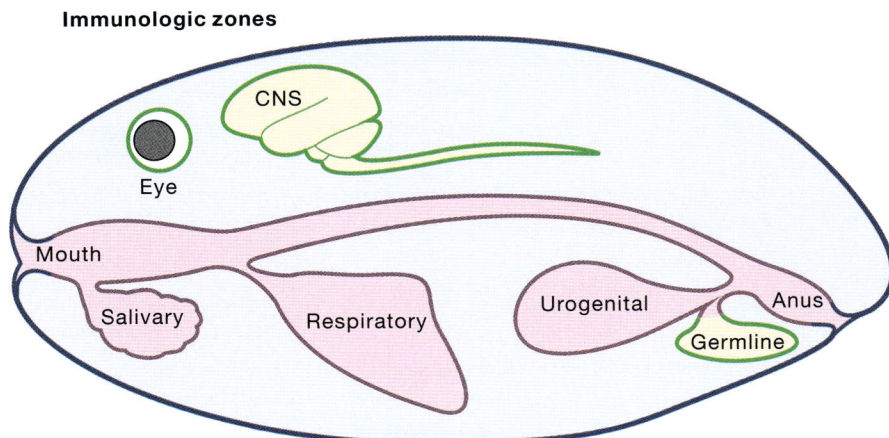

FIGURE 10.2. Zones for different immune responses. (1) **Skin** is the first line of defense, a rugged impermeable barrier shown as a blue solid line. (2) The **circulatory system** flushes the muscular and organelle tissue. (3) **Mucosal membranes** regulate material transfers into and out of the body. These barriers are specialized to separate physiologic functions and are continuously flushed clean with mucopolysaccharides, noted in purple. (4) **Barrier membranes** incorporate tight junctions to rigorously regulate the select material transfers to provide tissue-specific protection, as shown in green. CNS, central nervous system.

5. Antigen-driven tight junction diseases include:
- **a.** Skin: pemphigus vulgaris and pemphigus foliaceus.
- **b.** Gastrointestinal (GI)/mucosal: inflammatory bowel disease, celiac disease, autoimmune bullous disease of oral mucosa, Crohn disease, and ulcerative colitis.

C. Mucous layer
1. Demarcation between tissues and systemic environment.
2. Dynamic protection using viscous fluid flow mixed with a highly enriched mat of microflora; for example, oral or enteric bacteria.
3. Mucosal surface area: intestine approximately 300 m^2, lung 70 m^2, and total 400 m^2.
4. The acid mantle is a thin barrier to penetration by bacteria and viruses. Drastic pH alters the luminal environment from saliva pH of 6.2 to 7.4, stomach pH of 1.5 to 3.5, small intestine at pH 6 for duodenum gradually increasing to pH 7.4 in the ileum, and large intestine ranging from 5.7 in cecum to pH 6.7 in the rectum.
5. Intestinal mucosa is colonized by less than 10^{14} luminal bacteria from more than 500 species.
6. The largest pool of macrophages located in the intestinal wall accompanied by natural killer (NK) T cells to manage bacterial stasis to the intestinal lumina.
7. Approximately 70% of all lymphocytes are located within the lamina propria.

III. INFLAMMATION AND SOLUBLE FACTORS

This is a coordinated rapid response of innate immunity dependent on the circulatory system (cardiovascular and lymphatic systems). The system is based on a homeostatic equilibrium that rapidly responds to disturbances and utilizes complement and clotting to tag and trap foreign substances, vasodilation and extravasation to flush sites of infections, the **reticuloendothelial system** to remove debris, and a chemical identification system of **pattern recognition receptors (PRRs)**. These receptors identify pathogen-associated molecular patterns (**PAMPs**) and damage-associated molecular patterns (**DAMPs**).

A. Antimicrobial proteins (Table 10.1)
1. A collection of peptides between 12 and 60 amino acids.
2. Almost all have a net positive charge that disrupts membrane integrity.
3. Many of the antimicrobial proteins are stored in neutrophils.

Table 10.1   List of Antibacterial Compounds

Peptide	Site	Properties	Examples
Collectins	Extracellular	Collage-like domain	Mannan-binding protein, lung surfactant A, lung surfactant B
Defensins	Extracellular—vernix caseosa, amniotic fluid	Cysteine-rich cationic proteins	Neutrophils—α-defensin, release during phagocytosis
	Intracellular		Paneth cells—α-defensin
			Epithelial cells—constitutively release α- and β-defensin
Cathelicidins	Lysosomes of PMN and macrophage	Cationic peptide, release by elastase	LL-37 (leucine-leucine 37-amino acids long)
Saposin	CTL, NK cells	Acts on sphingolipids	Granulysin
Mucins	Saliva	Highly glycosidic proteins	MUC7
Histatins	Saliva	Histidine rich	Histatin-1, 3, 5
Thrombocidins	Blood	Derived from platelets	Platelet factor 4

CTL, cytotoxic T lymphocyte; MUC7, mucin 7; NK, natural killer; PMN, polymorphonuclear.

B. Role of eicosanoids in inflammation (Figure 10.3)

1. Prostaglandins, thromboxanes, leukotrienes, and lipoxins are membrane-derived lipids.
2. Act as potent paracrine and autocrine signals.
3. Phospholipase A2 releases arachidonic acid from membrane phospholipids, which are central to produce the eicosanoid.
4. These lipids are produced on demand.
5. These agents regulate vascular tone and smooth muscle contraction.
6. Eicosanoids are primarily responsible for four signs of inflammation: **calor (heat), rubor (redness), dolor (pain),** and **tumor (swelling).**
7. Eicosanoids play a significant role in anaphylaxis and asthma.

C. Effects on vasculature (Table 10.2)

1. Conduit for fluid and nutrient exchange.
   a. Barrier to tissues built on endothelial cells interlocked together to form tubes.
   b. Blood passes through vascular channels lined with endothelium interlocked with tight junctions and wrapped with smooth muscle.
   c. Lymphatics are loosely connected endothelial cells that allow fluid entry driven by Starling pressure.
   d. **Vascular dilation** occurs immediately and rapidly when stimulated by histamine, bradykinin, and prostaglandins.
   e. Dilation leads to permeability and exudation.
   f. Vasoconstriction results from smooth muscle contraction.
   g. Restricted flow permits clotting and contains pathogen locally, thus preventing systemic dissemination.
   h. Mast cells regulate vascular tone by producing vasoactive substances.
   i. Leukotrienes stimulate smooth muscle activity.
   j. Cytokines (CCL8 [C-C motif ligand 8]) recruit neutrophil entry to a trauma site by **extravasation** (Figure 10.4).

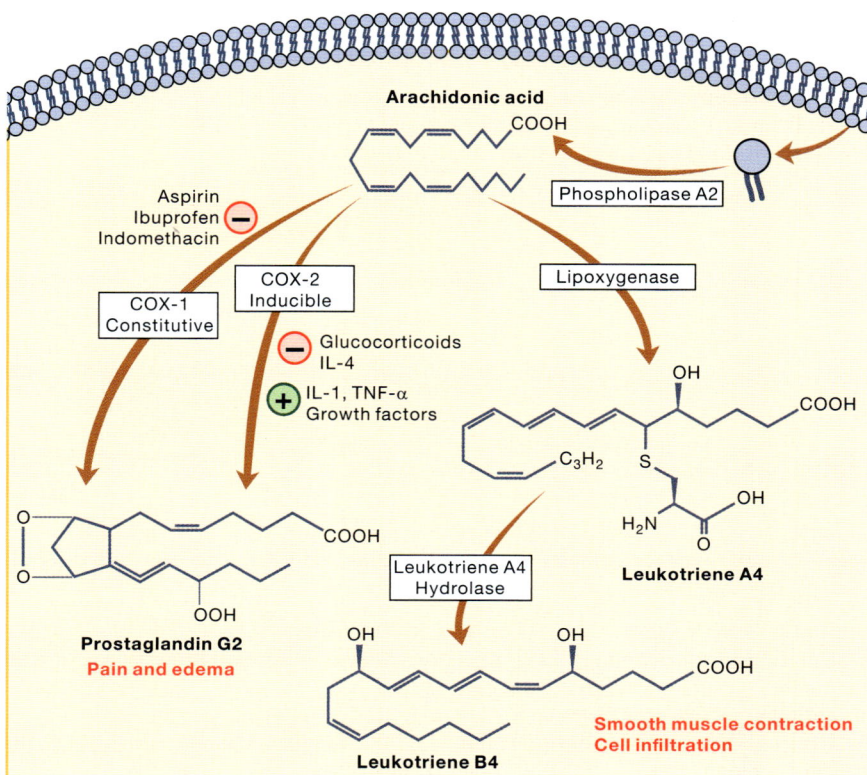

FIGURE 10.3. Production of eicosanoids. COX, cyclooxygenase; IL, interleukin; TNF, tumor necrosis factor.

Table 10.2	Types of Inflammation	
Type	**Characteristic**	**Examples**
Acute	Exudative inflammation—excessive fluid	Examples: ankle sprain, bacterial cellulitis
	Suppurative or purulent—neutrophils	
	Fibrinous	
	Serous—clear fluid	
	Hemorrhagic—vascular damage	
	Neurogenic—Lewis triple response	
	Flush: capillary dilation	
	Flare: arteriolar dilation	
	Wheal: exudation, edema	
Subacute	Neutrophil infiltration to a lesser degree than acute	Examples: de Quervain thyroiditis, subacute bacterial endocarditis
	Lymphocytes, monocytes, macrophages more prominent	
	Less severe tissue damage than acute	
	Symptoms persist for longer duration.	
	Transition to anti-inflammatory cytokines and tissue healing	
Chronic	Persistent presence of noxious stimuli	Examples: inflammatory bowel disease, chronic hepatitis, rheumatoid arthritis
	Interferes with wound healing	
	Normal wound healing process	
	Mononuclear infiltration and elimination of pathogen	
	Tissue destruction	
	Resolution by regenerating tissue of fibrosis	
	Tissue injury due to free radical oxygen, proteases, and tissue plasmin activator (tPA)	
	Fibrosis caused by cytokines, predominately transforming growth factor (TGF)-β, but also platelet-derived, fibroblast, and vascular endothelial growth factors	
	Common causes of chronic inflammation: Lyme, tuberculosis (TB), syphilis, viral hepatitis	
	Granulomatous inflammation	
Type IV hypersensitivity	Attempt to physically isolate the pathogen within macrophage	Examples: TB, leprosy, syphilitic gumma, foreign bodies, fungal infections, silicosis, sarcoidosis
	Large nucleated foam cells form as a syncytium of macrophage.	

D. Complement (Figure 10.5; Tables 10.3 and 10.4)
  1. Family of serum proteins (>30 types) produced by the liver.
  2. These proteins are functionally integrated; once triggered, they follow a cascade of reactions to instantaneously attack foreign substances.
  3. The complement proteins reside in the circulation in a homeostatic state.
  4. Any disturbance to this equilibrium causes a rapid and efficient shift in the local environment to the appearance of a series of highly reactive compounds.

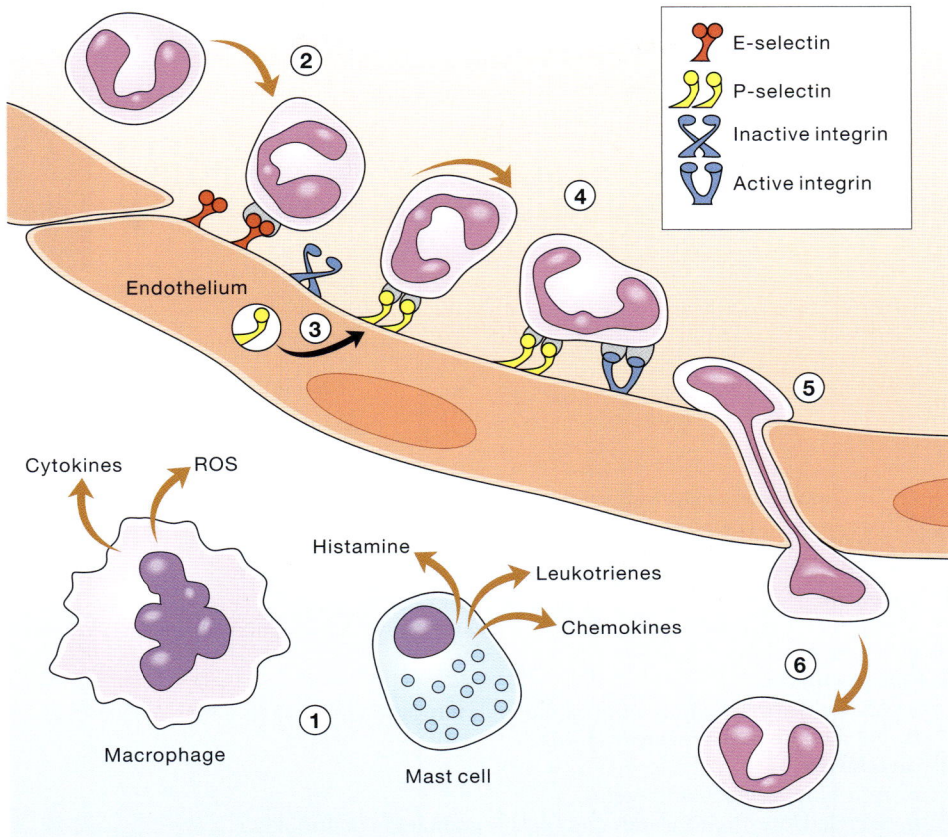

FIGURE 10.4. Leukocyte extravasation across postcapillary walls. Steps: (1) Recognition of pathogen-associated molecular pattern (PAMP), mast cell release of chemokines to recruit neutrophils, histamine, and leukotriene to promote inflammation; resident macrophage begins phagocytosis and cytolysis. (2) Neutrophil attaches to the endothelium using E-selectin; rolling action starts. (3) Weibel-Palade body exocytoses, presenting P-selectin to the surface. (4) Integrin activation and neutrophil stop moving. (5) Neutrophil crosses the endothelial barrier. (6) Neutrophil enters the site of inflammation. ROS, reactive oxygen species.

5. Recognition activates a sequence of caspases that generate **anaphylatoxin**, **opsonin,** and a **membrane attack complex** (**MAC**). These three activities facilitate macrophage clearance of the foreign objects.
6. Complement receptors on the follicular dendritic cell (FDC) in draining lymph nodes collect debris for display and screening by mature B and T cells in germinal centers.
7. Deficiencies lead to bacterial infections. Loss of C3 function leads to general bacterial infections. Loss of C5, C6, C7, C8, or C9 leads to susceptibility to meningitis (ie, *Neisseria meningitidis*). Loss of C1 inhibitor impacts complement fixation, clotting, and kinin pathways (ie, bradykinin), leading to edema.

E. Acute phase reaction
1. The liver will compensate for shifts in protein content in the plasma.
2. A fast-acting, nonspecific response by hepatocytes during disturbances in homeostasis, including trauma, infection, neoplastic growth, and immune hypersensitivities.
3. Hepatocytes change protein secretion in response to the cytokines IL-1, IL-6, and tumor necrosis factor (TNF)-α release by macrophages located at the inflammatory site.
4. Proteins such as C-reactive protein, serum amyloid, ceruloplasmin, complement factor-3, haptoglobin, fibrinogen, and α1-antitrypsin increase in secretion.
5. Proteins such as albumin and transferrin decrease secretion.

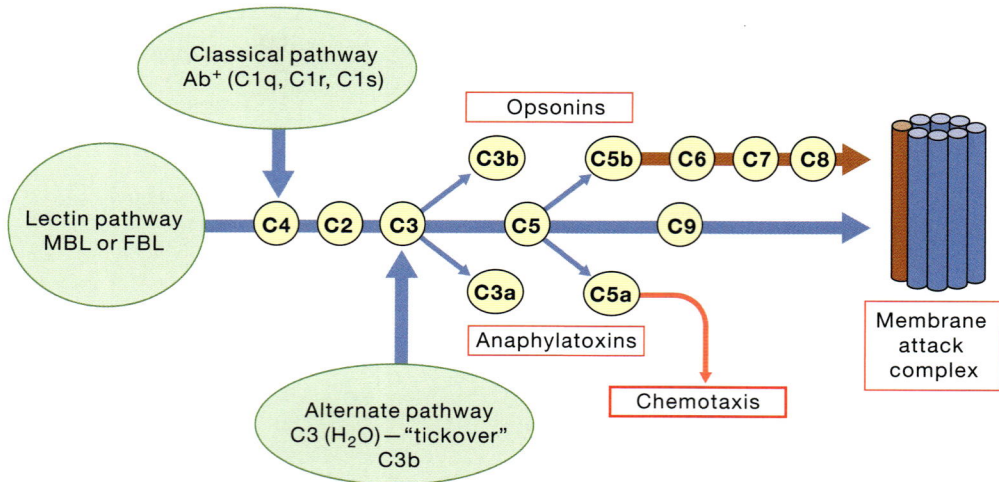

FIGURE 10.5. Overview of complement activity. FBL, fucose-binding lectin; MBL, mannose-binding lectin.

F. Secreted enzymes and proteins with immune function

1. **Lysozyme**
   a. An enzyme that hydrolyzes polysaccharides of polysaccharides found on bacterial cell surfaces.
   b. Found in saliva.

2. **Phospholipase**
   a. An enzyme that hydrolyzes phospholipids into fatty acids and lipophilic substances.
   b. Initiates the release of **eicosanoids.**

3. **Lactoferrin**
   a. Iron-binding globular protein.
   b. Secreted by exocrine glands and specific granules in neutrophils.
   c. Upon degranulation, virtually all serum lactoferrin originates from neutrophils.
   d. Acts to deprive bacteria of a source of iron.

Table 10.3	List of Complement Receptors			
Receptor	CD	Complement Ligand	Function	Cell Type
CR1	CD35	C3b, C4b, iC3b	Phagocytosis	Macrophages, monocytes
			Erythrocyte transport of immune complexes	Polymorphonuclear (PMNs) cells, erythrocytes, B cells, follicular dendritic cells (FDCs)
CR2	CD21	C3d, iC3b, C3dg	B-cell coreceptor	B cells, FDCs
CR3	CD11b/CD18	iC3b	Phagocytosis	Macrophages, monocytes, PMNs, FDCs
CR4	CD11c/CD18	iC3b	Phagocytosis	Macrophages, monocytes, PMNs, DCs
C5a	CD88	C5a	Degranulation cellularity	Endothelial cells, phagocytes
C3a		C3a	Degranulation cellularity	Endothelial cells, mast cells, phagocytes

CD, clusters of differentiation; DC, dendritic cell.

Table 10.4	Important Antibacterial Actions by Serum Complement
Function	**Components**
Recognition	Classic pathway
	Natural antibodies to carbohydrate
	Complement-fixing antibodies from adaptive immunity
	Lectin pathway
	Sugar-binding proteins are ficolins and mannose-binding lectin.
	Bacterial surfaces have high density of mannose.
	Spontaneous pathway
	Nonspecific
	Requires host proteins to prevent self-recognitions
Convertase	A serine endoprotease that converts the quiescent proprotein complement into a highly reactive form
	C3 convertase
	C5 convertase
Anaphylatoxin	Potent stimulator of phagocytosis
	C3a
	C4a
	C5a
Opsonins	Coat targets for receptor-mediated phagocytosis
	C3b—directs macrophage phagocytosis
	C5b—directs formation of membrane attack complex
Permeabilization	Membranes attack complex C5b through C9.

4. **Lactoperoxidase**
   a. A bactericidal oxidoreductase.
   b. Secreted from mucosal glands, including salivary and mammary glands.
   c. Catalyzes oxidation and the production of water using hydrogen peroxide as the electron donor.
5. **Myeloperoxidase**
   a. A bactericidal oxidoreductase.
   b. Expressed in neutrophils.
   c. Stored in azurophilic granules.
   d. Secreted following activation.
   e. Catalyzes chloride ion oxidation using hydrogen peroxide to form hypochlorous acid.
   f. The catalytic cofactor is a heme moiety that gives the green color to purulent pus.
6. **Xanthine oxidoreductase**
   a. An oxidoreductase that produces hydrogen peroxide and water from the conversion of hypoxanthine to xanthine, which is further broken down to uric acid and an additional hydrogen peroxide.
   b. Converts aliphatic compounds to aliphatic alcohol and two superoxide radicals of oxygen.
   c. Xanthine oxidoreductase is widely expressed in tissues and is a major constituent of fat globules in breast milk.

IV. MEDIATORS OF INFLAMMATION AND IMMUNITY (Table 10.5)

A. Chemokines

1. Are defined as small peptides (8,000-16,000 Da) that are released by injury and are active at very low concentrations (10^{-8} to 10^{-11} M). They exhibit approximately 30% to 50% amino acid sequence homology.

Table 10.5	Chemokines, Cytokines, and Interferons and Their Actions	
Cytokine	**Major Cell Source**	**Major Immunologic Action**
IL-1 (α, β)	Macrophages Endothelial cells Dendritic cells Langerhans cells	Stimulates interleukin (IL)-2 receptor emergence in T cells Enhances B-cell activation Induces fever, acute phase reactants, and IL-6 Increases nonspecific resistance Inhibited by an endogenous IL-1 receptor antagonist
IL-2	T_h1 cells	T-cell growth factor Activates natural killer (NK) and B cells
IL-3	T cells	Stimulates hematopoiesis
IL-4	T cells	Stimulates B-cell synthesis of immunoglobulin (Ig)E Downregulation of interferon (IFN)-γ
IL-5	T cells	Stimulates growth and differentiation of eosinophils B-cell growth factor Enhances IgA synthesis
IL-6	Monocytes T cells Endothelial cells	Induces acute phase reactants, fever, and late B-cell differentiation
IL-7	Bone marrow	Stimulates pre-B and pre-T cells
IL-8	Monocytes Endothelial cells Lymphocytes Fibroblasts	Chemotactic factor for neutrophils and T cells
IL-9	T_h cells	T-cell mitogen
IL-10	T_h2 cells	Anti-inflammatory; inhibits IFN-γ synthesis by T_h1 cells Suppresses other cytokine synthesis
IL-11	Bone marrow	Stimulates hematopoiesis Enhances acute phase protein synthesis

Table 10.5   Chemokines, Cytokines, and Interferons and Their Actions (*continued*)

Cytokine	Major Cell Source	Major Immunologic Action
IL-12	Macrophages B cells	Promotes T_h1 differentiation and IFN-γ synthesis Stimulates NK cells and CD8$^+$ T cells to cytolysis Acts synergistically with IL-2
IL-13	T_h2 cells	Inhibits inflammatory cytokines (IL-1, IL-6, IL-8, IL-10, monocyte chemoattractant protein)
IL-15	T cells	T-cell mitogen Enhances growth of intestinal epithelium
IL-16	CD8$^+$ T cells Eosinophils	Increases class II major histocompatibility complex (MHC), chemotaxis, and CD4$^+$ T-cell cytokines Decreases antigen-induced proliferation
IL-17	T_h17 cells, γδ T cells, NK cells	Increases the inflammatory response, involved in allergic asthma
IL-18	Activated macrophages	Increases IFN-γ production and NK cell action
IL-19	Monocytes, macrophages, B cells, stimulated epithelial cells, keratinocytes, vascular smooth cells	Can induce proinflammatory or anti-inflammatory activity; stimulates neutrophil cell expansion
IL-20	T cells, B cells, NK cells, monocytes, macrophages, and dendritic cells	Proinflammatory, role in skin inflammation and autoimmune responses
IL-21	T cells, NK cells	Inhibits bone marrow dendritic cells, IL-6, and IL-1β
IL-22	Lymphocytes	Epithelial homeostasis
IL-23	Macrophages, various cells	Proinflammatory, development and differentiation of T_h17 cells
IL-24	CD4$^+$ T cells, NK cells, mast cells	Antitumor effects
IL-25	T_h2 cells, bone marrow mast cells, alveolar macrophages	Induces production of Il-4, IL-4, IL-13
IL-26	T_h1, T_h17, memory CD4$^+$ cells	Promotes immune sensing of bacterial DNA; causes direct lysis of bacterial membranes; has proinflammatory activity
IL-27	Antigen-presenting cells (APCs)	Synergize with IL-12 to promote IFN-γ production by CD4, CD8 T cells and NK cells, promotes T_h1 differentiation
IL-28	Virus-infected cells, dendritic cells, Treg cells	Antiviral activities
IL-29	Macrophages, dendritic cells	Involved in clearance of skin infections

(continued)

Table 10.5	Chemokines, Cytokines, and Interferons and Their Actions (*continued*)	
Cytokine	**Major Cell Source**	**Major Immunologic Action**
IL-30	Macrophages, monocytes, dendritic cells	Anti-inflammatory, suppresses IL-17A production
IL-31	CD4$^+$ T cells, eosinophils	Proinflammatory, pruritus
IL-32	Monocytes, T cells, NK cells	Proinflammatory, angiogenesis, IL-2 production in bone marrow
IL-33	Epithelial cells, endothelial cells	Proinflammatory alarmin
IL-34	Monocytes, macrophages, Treg cells, dendritic cells	Anti-inflammatory, myeloid cell proliferation
IL-35	Treg cells, B cells	Inhibits T$_h$1 and T$_h$17 cell proliferation, Treg polarization
IL-36	Monocytes, macrophages, CD4$^+$ cells	Proinflammatory T$_h$1 responses
IL-37	Monocytes, NK cells, B cells, epithelial cells	Anti-inflammatory in skin
IL-39	Macrophages, B cells, dendritic cells	Proinflammatory
IL-40	B cells	B-cell development and homeostasis
TNF-α	Macrophages	Cytotoxic for tumors
	T cells	Causes cachexia
	B cells	Mediates bacterial shock
	Large granular lymphocytes	
TNF-β	T cells	Cytotoxic for tumors
Transforming growth factor-β	Almost all normal cell types	Inhibits proliferation of both T and B cells
		Reduces cytokine receptors
		Potent chemotactic agent for leukocytes
		Mediates inflammation and tissue repair

CD, clusters of differentiation; TNF, tumor necrosis factor.

2. Function by transmitting signals through seven transmembrane, rhodopsin-like receptors, which activate and attract leukocytes to sites with tissue damage.
3. Are classified into two subcategories based on the sequence of two pairs of the amino acid cysteine.
    a. C-X-C chemokines (α) have their first two cysteines separated by one amino acid. Most attract neutrophils; the most potent include IL-8, platelet factor 4, IFN-γ, inducible protein 10, and macrophage activation factors.
    b. C-C chemokines (β) have two adjacent cysteine residues. Most attract monocytes and T lymphocytes, while a few attract eosinophils, basophils, and NK cells via macrophage chemotactic proteins (MCPs), macrophage inflammatory proteins (MIPs), and RANTES (regulated on activation of normal T cells, expressed, and secreted).

B. Cytokines
1. Are intracellular signaling proteins acting locally in a paracrine or autocrine manner by binding to high-affinity receptors.
2. Have frequently overlapping functions, as a single activity can be caused by multiple cytokines, and multiple activities can be caused by a single cytokine (pleiotropism).

3. Lymphokines are cytokines that are produced by lymphocytes; monokines are cytokines produced by monocytes or macrophages.
4. IL-1, IL-6, and TNF-α induce MCP and IL-8 and the acute phase response and are endogenous pyrogens.
5. Transforming growth factor (TGF)-β is a potent wound healing and immunosuppressive agent inhibiting IL-2 effects and proliferation of many cell types. It also promotes the switching of B cells to immunoglobulin A (IgA) synthesis.
6. Cytokine receptors on cells can have circulating forms, consisting of only the extracytoplasmic portion of the receptor, which can combine with and block the cytokine in serum before it reaches its cellular target.

> ● ● ● **Clinical Pearl**
>
> Imbalances in cytokine production can contribute to inflammatory diseases or immunodeficiency.

C. Interferons

1. IFNs are host-coded proteins, or glycoproteins, produced in and secreted from virus-infected cells in response to virus infection, synthetic nucleotides, and foreign cells.
2. IFNs bind to cell surface receptors and induce antiviral proteins, including a protein kinase and 2′,5′A synthetase (which synthesizes an oligoadenylic acid), leading to the destruction of viral messenger RNA (mRNA).
3. They are host specific, but not viral specific.
4. Three groups or families are recognized: IFN-α, IFN-β, and IFN-γ.
5. IFN-α (Intron-A) is licensed for the treatment of chronic hepatitis B virus (HBV) and hepatitis C virus (HCV) infections and can produce adverse effects at high doses or with chronic therapy.
6. They have toxic side effects, including bone marrow suppression.

V. INNATE IMMUNITY

A cellular response by leukocytes targets pathogens decorated with chemical indicators (ie, complement and antibody) derived from inflammation or adaptive immunity. Effector cells of innate immunity (Figure 10.6) are often referred to as **granulocytes** due to their laden appearance with secretory

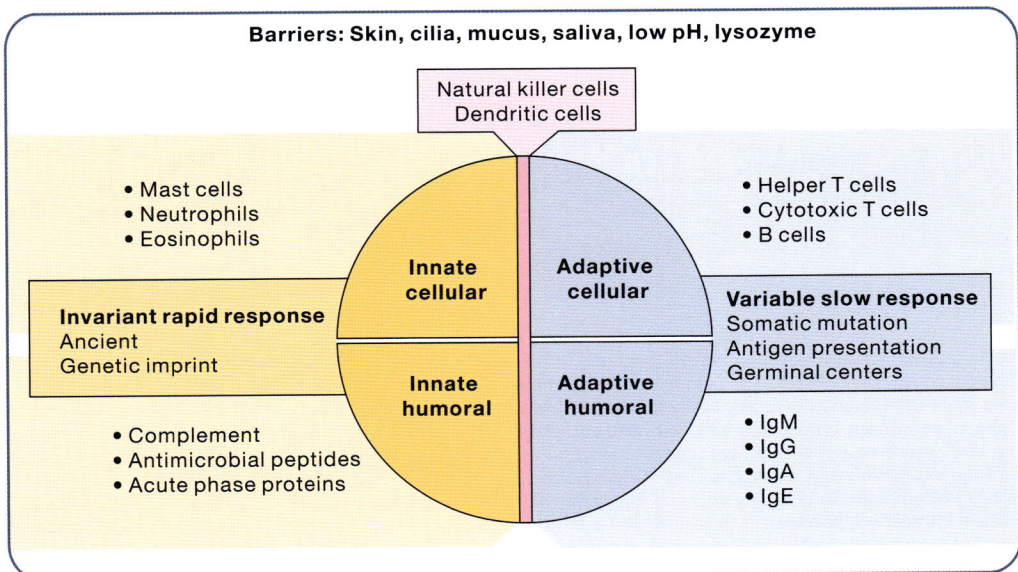

FIGURE 10.6. Integrated immune system. Ig, immunoglobulin.

vesicles, or **polymorphonuclear (PMN) cells** due to their distinctively shaped nuclei. PMN cells attracted to the chemical indicators deliver a cytolytic attack or **cytolysis** using chemical warfare.

1. Free radicals of oxygen (O_2^-, H_2O_2, OH^-, and $^1O_2$) and nitrogen (NO).
2. Antibacterial peptides (defensins and cathelicidins).
3. Apoptosis-inducing peptides (granzymes).

A. Innate immune response (Figure 10.7)

1. A sequence of events beginning with recognition of infection by either PAMPs or DAMPs stimulating leukocytes, such as mast cells and macrophages.

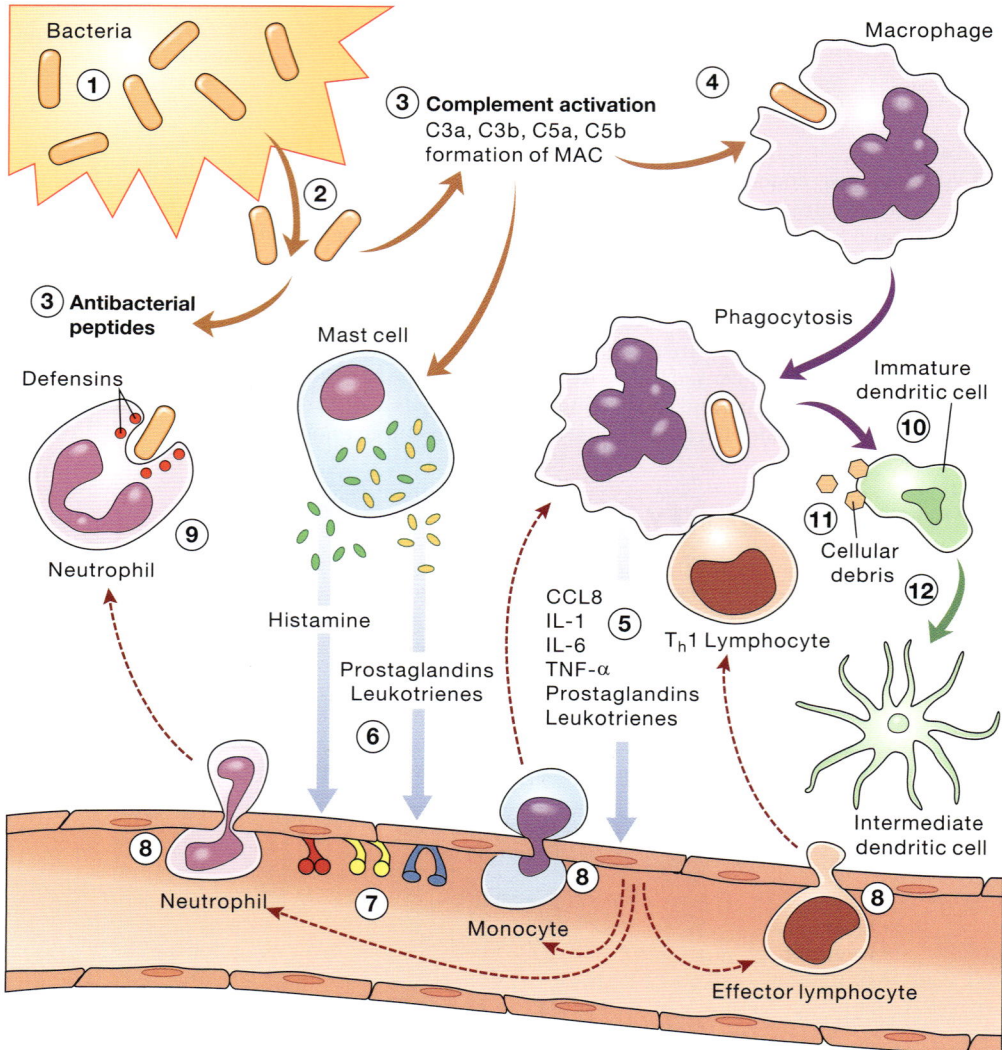

FIGURE 10.7. Sequence of innate immune responses to injury. (1) Tissue damage releases damage-associated molecular patterns (DAMPs). (2) Pathogen (bacterial or helminth) gains entry while presenting pathogen-associated molecular patterns (PAMPs). (3) Complement and antibacterial peptides begin an immediate response. (4) Resident macrophage and mast cells are activated by C3a, C5a, PAMPs, and DAMPs. (5) Macrophage releases cytokines to recruit neutrophils, dendritic cells, and additional macrophages. (6) Mast cell initiates structural changes of the vasculature, vasodilatation/vasoconstriction, and relaxation of the tight junctions to facilitate extravasation. (7) Selectin expression is increased; Weibel-Palade bodies expel contents. (8) Cellular extravasation begins. (9) Neutrophils begin massive phagocytosis and cytolysis. (10) Dendritic cells scavenge debris from the wound site. (11) PAMPs stimulate dendritic cells to mature and egress the wound site by following lymphatic flow. (12) Mature antigen-expressing dendritic cells take residence in the paracortex of the lymph node to begin the adaptive immune response. CCL8, C-C motif ligand 8; IL, interleukin; MAC, membrane attack complex; TNF, tumor necrosis factor.

2. Chemokines recruit additional leukocytes.
3. Cytokines elicit specific physiologic responses.
4. Growth factors called colony-stimulating factors induce **hematopoiesis.**
5. Bone marrow replenishes circulating leukocytes.
6. Leukocytes extravasate into the site of inflammation or park in special niches, such as draining lymph nodes.
7. Leukocytes are generally short-lived and die by apoptosis as the inflammation resolves.

B. Cell adhesion molecules

Immune cells interact with surface molecules on vascular epithelia to direct movement and to recruit cells to the sites of trauma. Two systems provide cell recognition, selectins and integrins.

1. **Selectins**
   a. Initiate cell-to-cell contact.
   b. Weak interaction, allows for the rolling effect.
   c. Must overcome shear force.
   d. **Structure**: N-terminus out, calcium-lectin, linked by complement-binding elements to a single membrane–spanning domain surface protease that downregulates L-selectin binding or shedding.
   e. Smallest family of adhesion molecules.
   f. Three types:
      (1) **L-selectin**
         (a) Found on most leukocytes.
         (b) Necessary for lymphocyte entry into immune organs, steady-state process.
         (c) Directs secondary tethering of neutrophils.
         (d) Binding partners are E-selectin and cutaneous lymphocyte antigen (CLA).
      (2) **E-selectin** found on endothelial cells:
         (a) Induced by IL-1β, TNF-α, TNF-β, and lipopolysaccharide (LPS).
         (b) NF-κB regulation, a proinflammatory transcription factor.
         (c) Downregulated by internalization and routed to lysosome.
      (3) **P-selectin** found on endothelial and platelets:
         (a) Prepackaged in **Weibel-Palade bodies**.
         (b) Rapid surface expression induced by histamine, thrombin, and oxygen radicals.
         (c) Rapid downregulation by internalization but recycled from endosomes to secretory granules.
         (d) Expression induced by TNF-α and LPS.

2. **Integrins**
   a. Chemokines emanating from inflammatory site induce tighter contact to stop leukocyte rolling.
   b. Chemokines are immobilized to proteoglycans.
   c. Other, platelet-activating factor.
   d. Chemokine induces allosteric effects to activate.

C. Pattern recognition receptors (*Commotus ingenio*) (Table 10.6)

1. An invariant recognition mechanism that detects specific and unique molecular patterns associated with pathogens and inflammation.
2. PRRs are ancient and genetically imprinted into the host.
3. Recognition molecules target molecular patterns that are also invariant and absolutely necessary for pathogen survival.
4. Target signals emanating from a pathogen are called **PAMPs**; target signals emanating from inflammation and damaged host tissue are **DAMPs**.
5. PRRs are cellular bound or soluble and provide surveillance information to early responders for inflammation (mast cells, neutrophils, macrophage, and myeloid-derived dendritic cells [mDCs]) and B cells.
6. Major receptor types screen for PAMPs/DAMPs (Table 10.6).

Table 10.6	List of Selected Pattern Recognition Receptors		
Pattern Recognition Receptor	Subcellular Location	Ligand	Cell Types
TLR-1	Cell surface	Lipoprotein	Monocytes, macrophages, dendritic cells, B cells
TLR-2	Cell surface	Glycolipid, lipoteichoic acid, HSP-70	Monocytes, macrophages, dendritic cells, mast cells
TLR-3	Intracellular compartment	dsRNA, polyI:C	Dendritic cells
TLR-4	Cell surface	Lipopolysaccharide, HSP, fibrinogen	Monocytes, macrophages, dendritic cells, mast cells, B cells
TLR-5	Cell surface	Flagellin	Monocytes, macrophages, and dendritic cells
TLR-6	Cell surface	Diacyl lipopeptides	Monocytes, macrophages, mast cells, B cells
TLR-7	Intracellular compartment	ssRNA	Monocytes, macrophages, plasmacytoid cells, B cells
TLR-8	Intracellular compartment	ssRNA	Monocytes, macrophages, dendritic cells, mast cells
TLR-9	Intracellular compartment	Unmethylated CpG DNA	Monocytes, macrophages, dendritic cells, B cells
TLR-10	Intracellular compartment	Unknown	
TLR-11	Intracellular compartment	Profilin	Monocytes, macrophages in nonhuman mammals
TLR-12	Intracellular compartment	Unknown	In nonhuman mammals
TLR-13	Intracellular compartment	Bacterial RNA	Monocytes, macrophages, dendritic cells in nonhuman mammals
AIM2-like receptor	Cytoplasm	dsDNA	Hematopoietic cells
C-lectin receptor	Cell surface	Mannose, galactose	Macrophages, dendritic cells
NOD-like receptor	Cytoplasm	Peptidoglycan, muramyl dipeptide	Primarily in phagocytes including macrophages and neutrophils and epithelial cells
Receptor for advanced glycation end products	Cell surface	Various DAMPs, advanced glycation end products	Endothelial cells
RIG-I–like receptor	Cytoplasm	dsRNA	Immune and nonimmune cells
Stimulator of interferon genes	ER membrane	Bacterial cyclic dinucleotides	Cells with intracellular pathogens, T cells, dendritic cells, and macrophages

AIM2, absent in melanoma; DAMPs, damage-associated molecular patterns; dsRNA, double-stranded RNA; ER, endoplasmic reticulum; HSP, heat shock protein; NOD, nucleotide-binding oligomerization domain; polyI:C, polyinosinic-polycytidylic acid; ssRNA, single-stranded RNA; TLR, Toll-like receptor; RIG-I, retinoic acid-inducible gene-1.

D. Leukocytes

1. **Neutrophils** are the most abundant leukocytes in circulation having multilobed nuclei and are "neutral" to staining. Neutrophils drive the active killing of invading bacteria by phagocytosis and cytolysis (**Figure 10.8**).
   a. Most abundant leukocyte, 60% of circulating leukocytes.
   b. Cells in circulation have a short lifespan of hours to days:
      (1) Approximately 6 hours in circulation.
      (2) Longer lived in spleen.
   c. Occupy a temporary niche at the surface of vascular lumen.
      (1) Tethered by a transient interaction between CD62L on the neutrophil and CD34 on the vascular wall, which causes rolling along the surface (marginalization).
      (2) Released in the presence of glucocorticoids, causing a temporary spike in circulating neutrophils.
      (3) Release is driven by a surface metalloprotease, ADAM-8.
   d. First responders to the inflammatory site.
   e. Neutrophils are recruited to the injury site by chemotaxis CCL8 (aka, IL-8), C5a, and LTB_4.
   f. Principal function is phagocytosis.
      (1) Targets material labeled by C3b, IgG, or collectins.
      (2) Process is triggered by the anaphylatoxins C3a, C4a, and C5a.
   g. Kills internalized bacteria using antibacterial peptides, digestion by hydrolytic enzymes, and oxidation by free radicals (**Figure 10.9**).

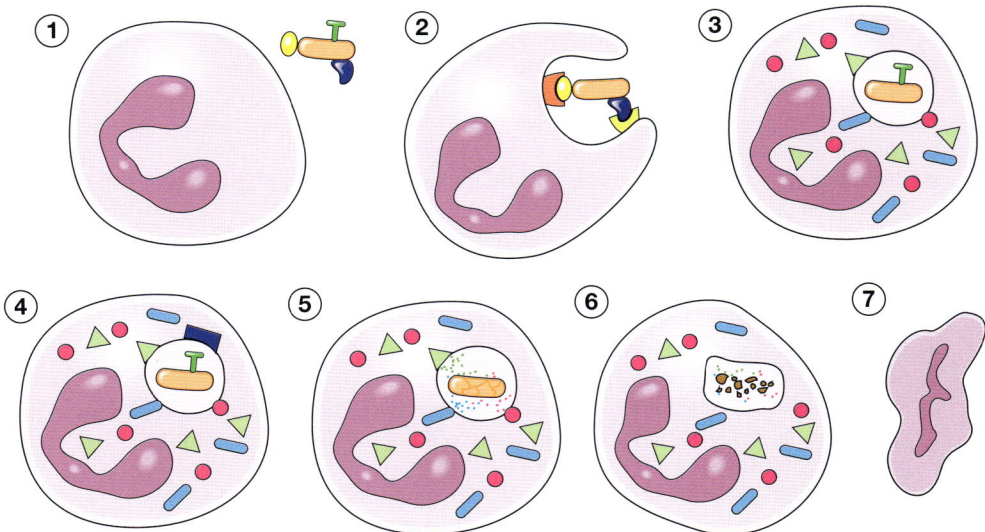

FIGURE 10.8. Neutrophil clearance of pathogen. (1) Complement fixation; C3a (yellow), C3b (dark blue), and MAC (green) are positioned on bacterium. (2) Fixed bacterium binds to complement receptors (C3a receptor, red; C3b receptor, yellow) and is phagocytosed. (3) Granules fuse to the phagosome (azurophilic granules, blue; specific granules, green; gelatinase granules, red). (4) NADPH (nicotinamide adenine dinucleotide phosphate) oxidase (dark blue rectangle). Myeloperoxidase is activated. (5) Granules deliver antibacterial substances (ie, defensins, lysosomes). (6) Bacteria are killed. (7) Neutrophil dies.

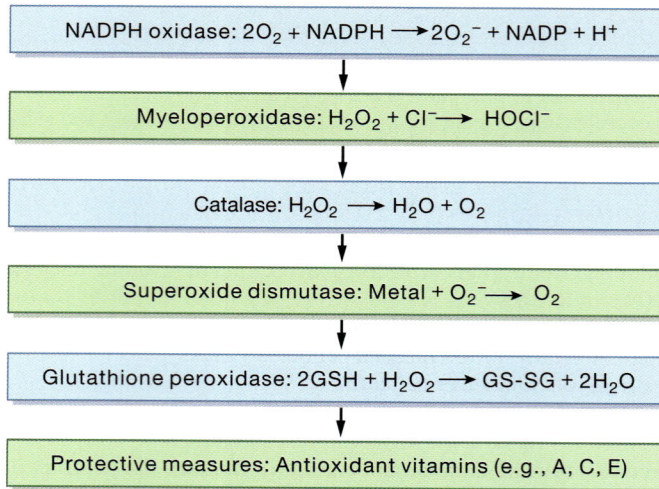

$$\text{NADPH oxidase: } 2O_2 + NADPH \longrightarrow 2O_2^- + NADP + H^+$$

$$\text{Myeloperoxidase: } H_2O_2 + Cl^- \longrightarrow HOCl^-$$

$$\text{Catalase: } H_2O_2 \longrightarrow H_2O + O_2$$

$$\text{Superoxide dismutase: Metal} + O_2^- \longrightarrow O_2$$

$$\text{Glutathione peroxidase: } 2GSH + H_2O_2 \longrightarrow GS\text{-}SG + 2H_2O$$

$$\text{Protective measures: Antioxidant vitamins (e.g., A, C, E)}$$

FIGURE 10.9. Steps in cytolysis by oxidative burst.

   h. The neutrophil has three types of secretory granules:
   (1) Azurophilic (defensins, myeloperoxidase, lysozyme).
   (2) Specifics (lactoferrin, lysozyme).
   (3) Gelatinase (acetyltransferase, gelatinase, lysozyme).
   i. Dies by apoptosis to release degraded materials.
   j. Accumulating debris constitutes pus; the greenish, purulent property comes from myeloperoxidase.
2. Basophils are innate effector cells with a multilobed nucleus and stain a dark purplish blue due to the presence of the basic dye methylene blue.
   a. Low abundance, 1% circulating leukocytes.
   b. Short-lived (hours to days) in circulation.
   c. Temporary residence in the lymph node.
   d. Directs T helper (T_h) cell differentiation.
   e. Plays an active defense role toward allergens with protease activity.
   f. Basophils release histamine, leukotrienes, and prostaglandins and are a source for heparin, platelet-activating factor, and IL-4.
   g. Basophils express Fc receptors for IgE and major histocompatibility complex (MHC) class II for antigen presentation to T_h2 cells.
   h. Basophils complete their development in the bone marrow before entering the circulation.
   i. Enhance humoral memory.
3. Eosinophils are innate effector cells that stain red with the acidic dye eosin; they have a multilobed nucleus and numerous secretory vesicles.
   a. Bone marrow is induced by IL-5 to release eosinophils.
   b. About 2% to 5% of circulating leukocytes.
   c. Secretory vesicles called *granules* contain destructive proteins, including acid phosphatase, eosinophil peroxidase, major basic protein, eosinophil cationic protein, RNase, DNase, lipase, and plasminogen.
   d. Capable of phagocytosis or degranulation to release specific effector proteins.
   e. Perform cytolysis to flood the inflammatory site with high levels of effector proteins.
   f. Secrete leukotrienes and prostaglandins.
   g. Express Fc receptors for IgG and IgE, and MHC class II, giving them the ability to activate $CD4^+$ T cells.
   h. Direct **cell-mediated cellular cytotoxicity (CMCC)**:
   (1) Delivers toxic free radicals and proteases to the parasite.
   (2) Collateral host tissue damage often results from the release of these cytotoxic agents.
   i. Defense to large extracellular parasites.
   j. Mediators of allergic inflammation.

4. Mast cells are tissue-resident myeloid cells.
   a. Ubiquitously placed in the body, including behind the blood-brain barrier.
   b. Do not ordinarily circulate.
   c. May proliferate, differentiate, and mature in the tissues.
   d. Long-lived and found throughout the body, including the brain; they are particularly enriched at the boundaries to the environment where encounters with pathogens are likely.
   e. Process trauma signals and release injury-specific mediators, including histamine, serine proteases, and serotonin.
   f. Perform similar functions compared to macrophage, including phagocytosis and antigen presentation.
   g. Principal function of mast cells is to act as a sentinel for disturbances and to regulate inflammatory and adaptive immune responses.
   h. Control vascular integrity and initiate neutrophil recruitment.
   i. Express specialized receptors for IgE called Fcε; a sensory mechanism for **reagenic** molecules.
   j. Source for histamine, heparin proteoglycan, and serine proteases tryptase and chymase.
   k. Release reactive lipids such as thromboxane, prostaglandin D2, leukotriene, and platelet-activating factors to permit neutrophil and macrophage intrusion.
   l. Function as sensors for trauma screening for DAMPs and PAMPs.
5. Macrophages are tissue-resident myeloid cells.
   a. Recruited to the inflammatory site to complete the clearance of debris and orchestrate wound healing.
   b. **Monocytes** in circulation replenish tissue-resident macrophages.
   c. Monocytes constitute 5% of circulating leukocytes.
   d. Kill internalized bacteria using antibacterial peptides, digestion by hydrolytic enzymes, and oxidation by free radicals.
   e. Expression of microbial peptides using MHC class II and phospholipids by CD1.
   f. Sequester bacteria by forming granulomas.
   g. Names for tissue-resident macrophages are Kupffer cells (liver), histiocytes (dermis), alveolar macrophage (lung), microglia (brain), and osteoclasts (bone).
   h. Two functional states:
      (1) M1 responds to bacteria and inhibits cancer growth.
      (2) M2 supports angiogenesis, suppresses immunity, and promotes cancer growth.
6. Dendritic cells
   Resident **immature mDCs** continuously collect samplings from the interstitial fluids and are responsible for recognition of nonself-antigen. Mature mDC takes residence in secondary immune organs.
   a. Immature mDC
      (1) Continuously process antigen for presentation to naive T_h cells.
      (2) Antigen is internalized by endocytosis and processed in lysosome and inserted into MHC class II molecules.
      (3) Exposure to PAMP induces maturation of the mDC.
      (4) mDC migrates to the lymph node.
   b. Mature mDC
      (1) Reduces endocytosis activity.
      (2) Increases MHC class II antigen expression.
      (3) Increases expression of coreceptors CD80/88.
      (4) Potential to release IL-12 depending on the identity of triggering PAMP.

E. The complement complex (C) is an important component of both innate and adaptive immunity.
   1. It comprises nine major factors (C1-C9), most of which are proenzymes present in normal serum and not increased by antigenic stimulation. It is effective via three pathways:
      a. The **classic pathway** results in lysis of microbial or mammalian cells to which IgM or a doublet of IgG1, IgG2, or IgG3 antibody has been bound to the membrane, followed by sequential "fixation" of C to the antigen-antibody complex.
         (1) C1qrs is bound initially via C1q, resulting in enzymatic cleavage and fragmentation of C4 and C2.

(2) C4b and C2a bind to the cell surface as C4b2a, becoming a C3 convertase that cleaves C3 into fragments C3a and C3b.

(3) C3b complexes with C4b2a to become a C5 convertase, which cleaves C5 into C5a and C5b.

(4) C5b combines with C6 and C7 and inserts into the cell membrane.

(5) C8 and C9 combine with the C5b,6,7 complex to form the **MAC** (membrane attack complex), resulting in increased permeability, changes in osmotic pressure, and cell lysis.

b. The **alternate pathway** is activated by cell walls of certain gram-negative and gram-positive bacteria, viruses, yeasts, and aggregated IgA.

(1) It acts independent of antibody or C1, C4, or C2.

(2) It is initiated by cell wall absorption of small amounts of C3b existing in normal serum.

(3) Binding of a serum protein, factor B, follows, which serves as a substrate for an enzyme, factor D. The resulting complex, C3bBb, is stabilized by properdin and has C3 convertase activity, which generates additional C3b.

(4) A complex, C3bBbC3b, forms, which becomes a C5 convertase, leading to the further reactions resulting in the MAC.

c. The **mannan-binding lectin pathway** follows the binding by an acute phase protein, mannose-binding lectin (MBL), onto mannose residues on the cell walls of certain bacteria, fungi, and viruses.

(1) This complex acts similar to C1 and thus follows the classic pathway, forming C3 and C5 convertases that result in cell lysis via MAC.

(2) It is an adjunct to innate immunity, independent of antibody.

2. Complement-induced chemotaxis and opsonization.

a. Fragments C3a and C5a are potent vasodilating and chemotactic adjuncts, adding cells and cytokines to the inflammatory response.

b. The binding of fragment C3b to microorganisms promotes their opsonization via a C3b receptor on phagocytic cells.

VI. ANTIBODIES

A. **Definition:** Antibodies are mucoproteins that are found mainly in the γ-globulin fraction of serum on electrophoresis. When injected into animals, human immunoglobulin, being foreign, becomes antigenic. The resulting antihuman antibodies are grouped into five classes: **IgG, IgA, IgM, IgE, and IgD**.

> **• • • Clinical Pearl**
>
> IgM is associated with early infection, while IgG provides long-term immunity. Measuring antibody titer or concentration of a particular antibody in the serum can provide evidence of past or present infection. This is not to be confused with measuring the pathogen, such as in viral titer that determines the concentration of virus particles in a unit volume.

B. **Structure**

1. The basic structural unit for each class is a four-chain protein with two heavy (H) and two light (L) chain polypeptides linked by disulfide bonds (Figure 10.10).

a. A differing, short amino acid sequence, specific for each of the H chains, permits differentiation into the five classes. These H-chain differences are called *isotypes* and are designated by the Greek letters gamma (γ), alpha (α), mu (μ), epsilon (ε), and delta (δ). Isotypes are genetic variations that all humans possess.

b. All five classes have an amino acid sequence in common on the L chains. Thus, they can be classified together as immunoglobulins. In addition, two isotypes, designated kappa (κ) and lambda (λ), exist for all five classes.

C. **Domains**

1. Both H and L chains are divided into constant region domains, designated CH and CL, and variable region domains, designated VH and VL.

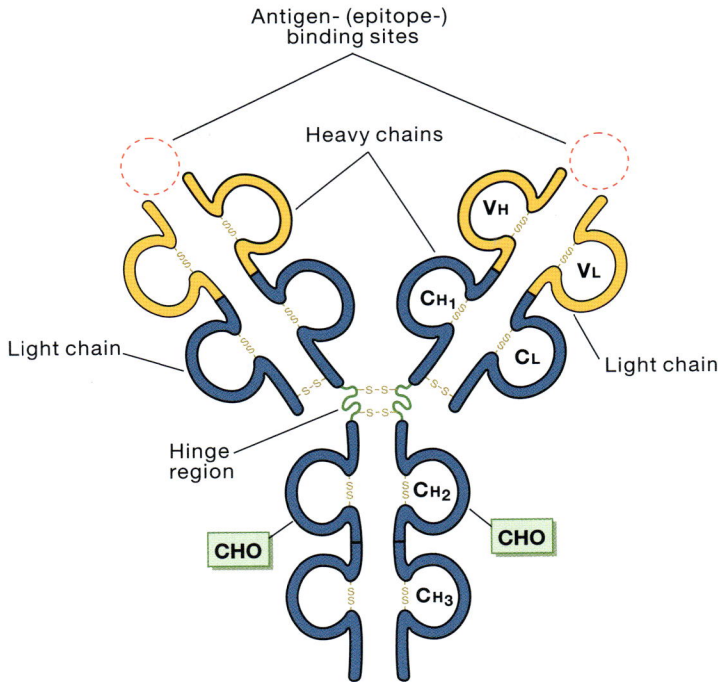

FIGURE 10.10. The basic four-peptide structure of immunoglobulins (Ig) is illustrated by this IgG pattern. Three heavy-chain constant region domains (CH_1, CH_2, CH_3) and one light-chain constant domain (CL) are shown in dark blue. The variable regions of both the light and heavy chains (VL and VH, respectively; in orange) associate to form the specific epitope-binding site. Several of the most critical disulfide bonds are shown ($-ss-$). CHO indicates where the carbohydrate is attached. (Redrawn with permission from Eisen HN. *General Immunology.* Lippincott-Raven;1990:48.)

   a. The amino acid sequence in the constant regions of both the H and L chains is similar for all antibody molecules within each class.
   b. The amino acid sequence of the variable regions on both H and L chains varies with the epitope toward which the particular antibody is directed.
   2. Amino acids that show marked differences between antibodies of different specificities form a **hypervariable region** within each variable region.
   3. The hypervariable regions of both the H and L chains associate to form two epitope-binding regions known as the antibody **idiotype.**
   4. A **hinge region** also exists between the CH_1 and CH_2 domains, permitting flexibility in the movement of the two antigen-binding sites.

D. Monoclonal antibodies: Most antigenic preparations give rise to a mixture of antibodies. However, antibodies of a single specificity are highly desirable for many purposes, including specific diagnostic tests and immunotherapy.
   1. Monoclonal antibodies can be made routinely by fusing splenic B cells from an immunized animal with malignant (immortal) plasma cells, forming a hybridoma.
   2. The B-cell hybridoma secreting the desired antibody can be isolated from the others by reactivity with the antigen of concern, then cloned and expanded in tissue culture, resulting in large amounts of antibody of a single specificity.

E. Immunotoxins
   1. Monoclonal antibodies can also be constructed using a murine antibody with the Fab domain specific for a cancer antigen; the Fc domain is removed and displaced by the toxin of choice.
   2. Such antibodies bind specifically to the cancer cell antigen via the mouse Fab hypervariable region, thereby focusing the lethal toxin on only the designated target cell.

VII. PROPERTIES OF ANTIBODIES

A. Immunoglobulin G

1. **Structural properties** (Table 10.7)
   a. IgG is composed of two L chains (each with a molecular weight of 22,000 Da) and two H chains (each with a molecular weight of 53,000 Da). The total molecular weight is 150,000 Da.
   b. The structural designation is ($\gamma 2\kappa 2$) or ($\gamma 2\lambda 2$), with the γ marker indicating the IgG H-chain isotype and the κ marker or λ marker indicating the L-chain isotype.
   c. Four **subclasses** exist: $\lambda 1$, $\lambda 2$, $\lambda 3$, and $\lambda 4$. These subclasses are differentiated by slight changes in the amino acid sequences on the H chain.
   d. **Enzymatic cleavage** (Figure 10.11)
      (1) **Papain** splits IgG into three fragments:
         (a) Two of these fragments, **Fab** (fragment, antigen binding), are similar, with each containing only one of the reactive sites for the epitope. Because Fab is monovalent, it can bind to (but cannot enter into) lattice formation and precipitate or agglutinate antigen.
         (b) A third fragment (**Fc**, crystallizable) activates complement, controls catabolism of IgG, fixes IgG to tissues or cells via an Fc receptor, and mediates placental transfer of antibody.
      (2) **Pepsin** splits behind the disulfide bond, joining the two H chains, permitting the two Fab fragments to remain joined. Consequently, this fragment is termed **F(ab′)2.**
         (a) Because F(ab′)2 is bivalent, it is capable of lattice formation and thus facilitates the removal of antigens.
         (b) F(ab′)2 is removed more rapidly from the circulation than the intact IgG.
         (c) The Fc fragment is extensively degraded.

2. **Functional properties** (Table 10.8)
   a. IgG has the highest serum concentration of all immunoglobulins (700-1,500 mg%) and a serum half-life of 18 to 25 days.

Table 10.7 Structural Properties of Human Immunoglobulins

Property	IgG	IgM	IgA	IgE	IgD
H-chain isotype	γ	μ	α	ϵ	δ
H-chain subclass	$\gamma_1, \gamma_2, \gamma_3, \gamma_4$	—	α_1, α_2	—	—
L-chain isotype	κ or λ	κ or λ	κ or λ	κ or λ	κ or λ
Associated chains	—	J chain	J chain, SP	—	—
Structural designation	$\gamma_2\kappa_2$ or $\gamma_2\lambda_2$	$(\mu_2\lambda_2)_5$ or $(\mu_2\lambda_2)_5$	**Serum:** $\alpha\kappa_2$ or $\alpha\gamma_2$ **Mucosa:** $(\alpha_2\kappa_2)_2$ J, SP or $(\alpha_2\gamma_2)_2$ J, SP	$\epsilon_2\kappa_2$ or $\epsilon_2\lambda_2$	$\delta_2\kappa_2$ or $\delta_2\lambda_2$
Percentage carbohydrate	4	15	10	18	18
Molecular weight (Da)	150,000	**Monomer:** 180,000 **Pentamer:** 950,000	**Monomer:** 160,000 **Dimer:** 318,000 **Dimer** and **SP:** 380,000	188,000	184,000

Ig, immunoglobulin; J, J chain; SP, secretory piece.
From Johnson A, Clarke B. *High-Yield Immunology.* 2nd ed. Lippincott Williams & Wilkins; 2006:15.

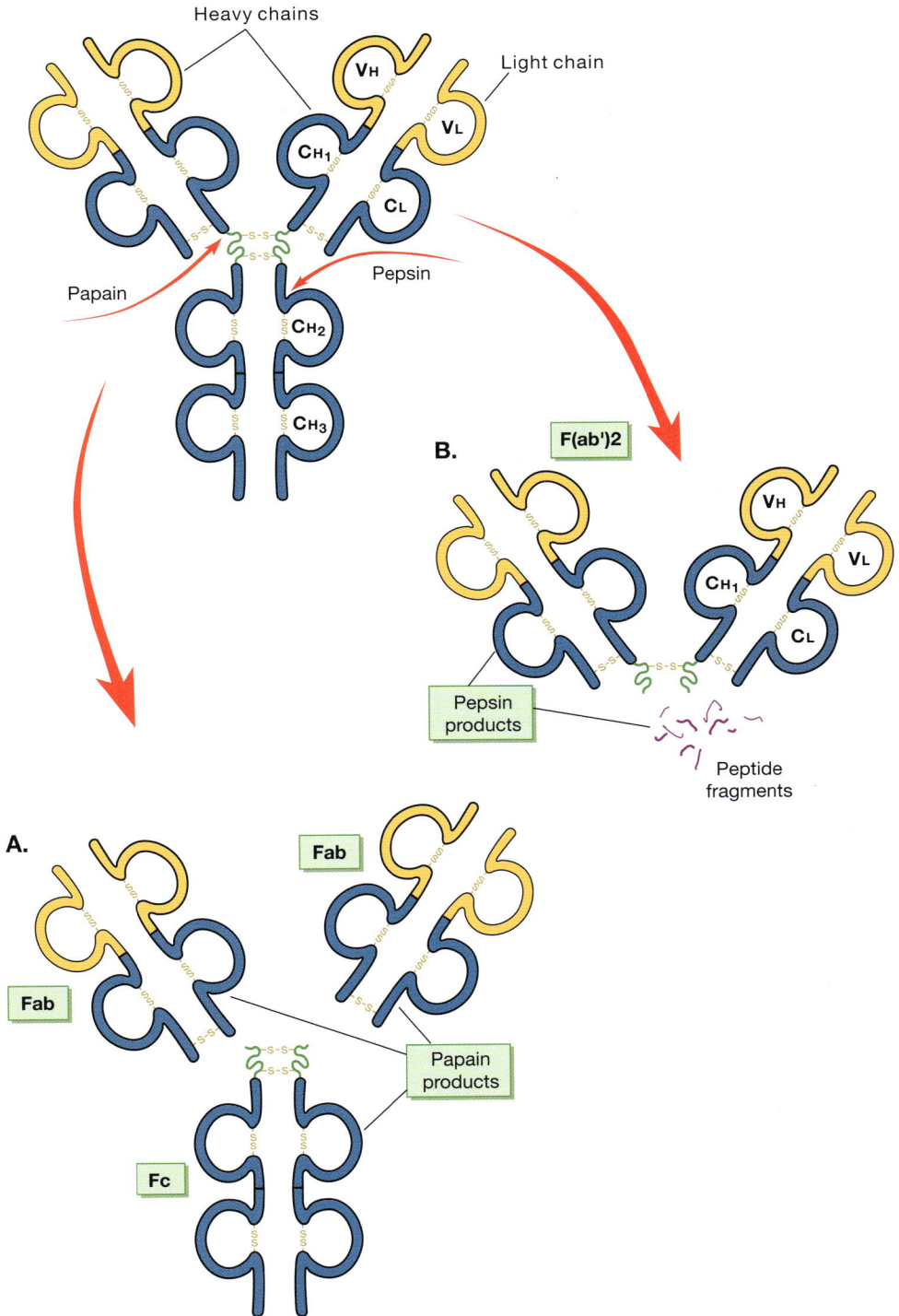

FIGURE 10.11. Enzymatic cleavage of immunoglobulin G by pepsin and papain. A. Papain cleavage results in two unlinked antigen-binding (Fab) fragments with the disulfide bonds (–*ss*–) remaining with the crystallizable (Fc) fragment. Because the fragments are univalent, they cannot precipitate or agglutinate antigens. B. Pepsin cleavage results in retention of the disulfide bonds with the two Fab fragments linked as F(ab')2. The Fc portion is degraded. CH$_1$, CH$_2$, CH$_3$, and one light-chain constant domain CL (blue), heavy-chain constant region domains; VL, VH (orange), variable region of light and heavy chains, respectively. (Redrawn with permission from Abbas AK, Lichtman AH, Jober JS. *Cellular and Molecular Immunology*. 3rd ed. W.B. Saunders; 1997:50.)

Table 10.8	Functional Properties of Human Immunoglobulins									
	IgG					**IgA**			
Property	**γ1**	**γ2**	**γ3**	**γ4**	**IgM**	**α1**	**α2**	**IgE**	**IgD**
Average serum concentration (mg%)	900	300	100	50	150	300	50	0.03	3
Serum half-life (days)	23	23	8	23	5	5	5	3	2.5
Activates complement	+	±	++	−	+++	−	−	−	−
Binds to Fc receptor	+	±	++	+	+	−	−	+	−
Crosses placenta	+	±	+	+	−	−	−	−	−

Ig, immunoglobulin.
From Johnson A, Clarke B. *High-Yield Immunology*. 2nd ed. Lippincott Williams & Wilkins; 2006:17.

   b. IgG adheres to cells that possess a receptor for the Fc fragment from IgG (Fcγ).
   c. IgG fixes complement, a series of enzymes resulting in cell lysis.
   d. IgG mediates placental passage of maternal antibody to the fetus.

B. Immunoglobulin M
   1. Structural properties (see Table 10.7)
   a. IgM exists in two structural forms:
      (1) A monomer is synthesized by B cells, retained on its membrane, and is designated μ2κ2 or μ2λ2.
         (a) It serves as the B-cell receptor specific for a single antigenic epitope.
         (b) The hypervariable region of the monomer differs for each B-cell clone.
      (2) Secreted IgM exists as a pentamer (ie, five monomeric IgM molecules joined together by a J chain; Figure 10.12). The IgM pentamer is designated (μ2κ2)5 or (μ2λ2)5.
         (a) The pentamer is secreted following antigen and cytokine activation of B cells, with the hypervariable regions on the pentamer the same as those on the membrane-bound monomeric receptor.
         (b) Of the 10 possible epitope-binding sites on the pentamer, five are of high affinity and five are of low affinity.
   b. Molecular weight: IgM has four constant domains on the H and L chains (in contrast with the three found on IgG, IgA, and IgD); therefore, its pentamer form has the highest molecular weight of the immunoglobulins, approximately 1 million.
   2. Functional properties (see Table 10.8): IgM, the earliest antibody to appear after antigenic stimulus, fixes complement avidly.

C. Immunoglobulin A
   1. Structural properties (see Table 10.7)
   a. IgA exists in three forms: a **monomer,** a **dimer** (in which a J chain joins two monomers), and a **dimer plus** a secretory piece (Figure 10.13A).
      (1) The dimer is transported across respiratory and intestinal mucosal barriers into the lumen by the secretory piece, which is a receptor for the IgA Fc region (FcαR) on the mucosal epithelium.
      (2) The secretory piece also protects IgA from proteolysis.
   b. The structural designation is (α2κ2) or (α2λ2) as the monomer and (α2κ2)2 or (α2λ2)2 as the dimer.
   c. Two subclasses exist: α1 and α2.
   2. Functional properties (see Table 10.8)

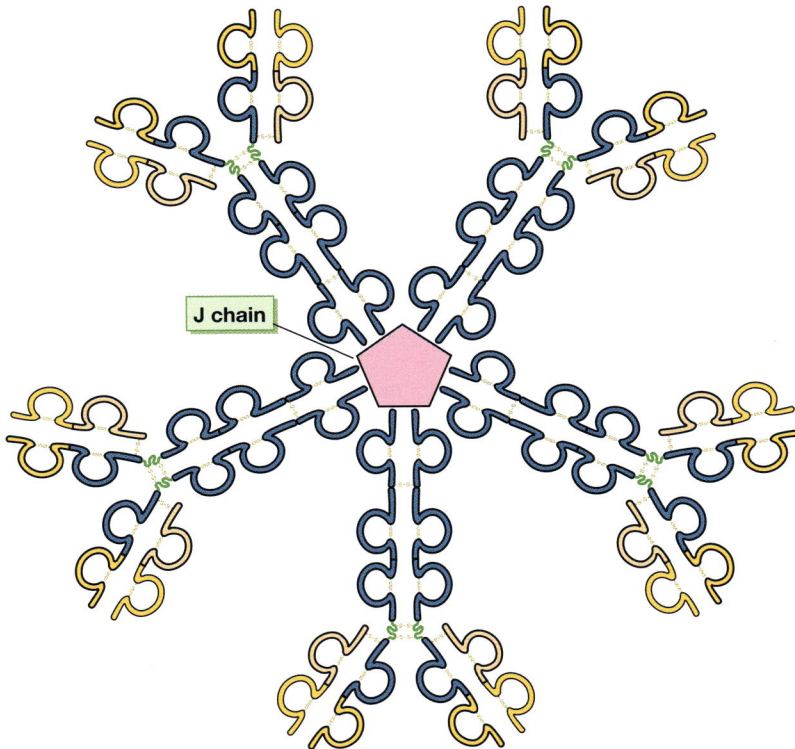

FIGURE 10.12. Immunoglobulin M pentamer. (Modified with permission from Abbas AK, Lichtman AH, Jober JS. *Cellular and Molecular Immunology*. 3rd ed. W.B. Saunders; 1997:48.)

  a. IgA is found in high concentrations in secretions; in serum, IgA exists mainly as a dimer with a half-life of 5 days.
  b. IgA is located in and protects mucosal tissues, saliva, tears, and colostrum by blocking bacteria, viruses, and toxins from binding to host cells.

D. Immunoglobulin E
 1. Structural properties (see Table 10.7)
  a. IgE has four constant domains (Figure 10.13B) and a carbohydrate content of 18%, resulting in a molecular weight of 188,000 Da.
  b. The structural designation for IgE is ε2κ2 or ε2λ2.
  c. The IgE molecule is unstable at 56C and is called *reagin*.
  d. IL-4 mediates the B-cell switch to IgE production.
 2. Functional properties (see Table 10.8)
  a. IgE has an extremely low serum concentration and half-life because its Fc region binds avidly to mast cells and basophils.
  b. IgE adheres to tissue-bound mast cells and circulating basophils via Fcε receptors on these cells. The binding of antigens to these IgE-sensitized cells triggers the release of vasoactive amines (mainly histamine), resulting in atopic disease characterized by hives (a local reaction) and anaphylaxis (a systemic reaction).
  c. IgE does not cross the placenta or fix complement by the conventional pathway.
  d. The binding of IgE to IL-5–activated eosinophils results in the elimination of parasitic helminths.
  e. Both total and allergen-specific IgE can be quantified.

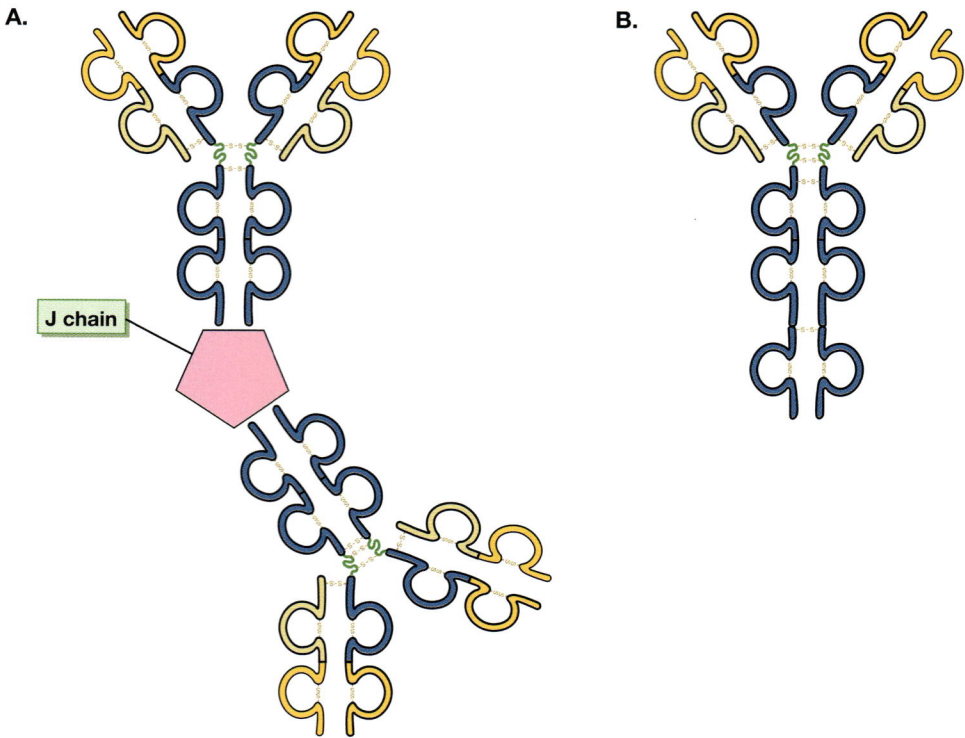

FIGURE 10.13. A. Immunoglobulin A dimer. B. Immunoglobulin E. Note the four C domains. (Modified with permission from Abbas AK, Lichtman AH, Jober JS. *Cellular and Molecular Immunology.* 3rd ed. W.B. Saunders; 1997:48.)

E. Immunoglobulin D

1. **Structural properties** (see Table 10.7). The structural formula for IgD is $\delta\kappa2$ or $\delta\lambda2$.
2. **Functional properties** (see Table 10.8)
   a. IgD is found on the B-cell membranes of 15% of newborns and again on adult peripheral blood lymphocytes in conjunction with IgM; serum levels are very low. The serum half-life is 2 to 3 days.
   b. IgD is a receptor on B-cell membranes for antigens.

VIII. IMMUNOGENETICS

A. Genetic control of immunoglobulin chain synthesis

1. **Genetic diversity:** Human antibodies exhibit an enormous range $(10^8\text{-}10^{15})$ of specificities. The genetic basis for this remarkable diversity involves several factors.
   a. **Different genes** code for the variable and constant region of the H and L chains.
   b. **Rearrangement** of the variable region and constant region genes occurs during differentiation within the genome, such that any one of the many different variable region genes can be linked to a single constant region gene, thus conserving DNA.
   c. An additional gene sequence, the **joining segment,** linking the VL gene to the CL region gene, is required during the formation of the L chain (Figure 10.14).
   d. During the formation of the H chain, an additional gene sequence, the **diversity segment,** also is required to link the VH gene to the J gene. These genes are then fused with the CH gene (Figure 10.15).

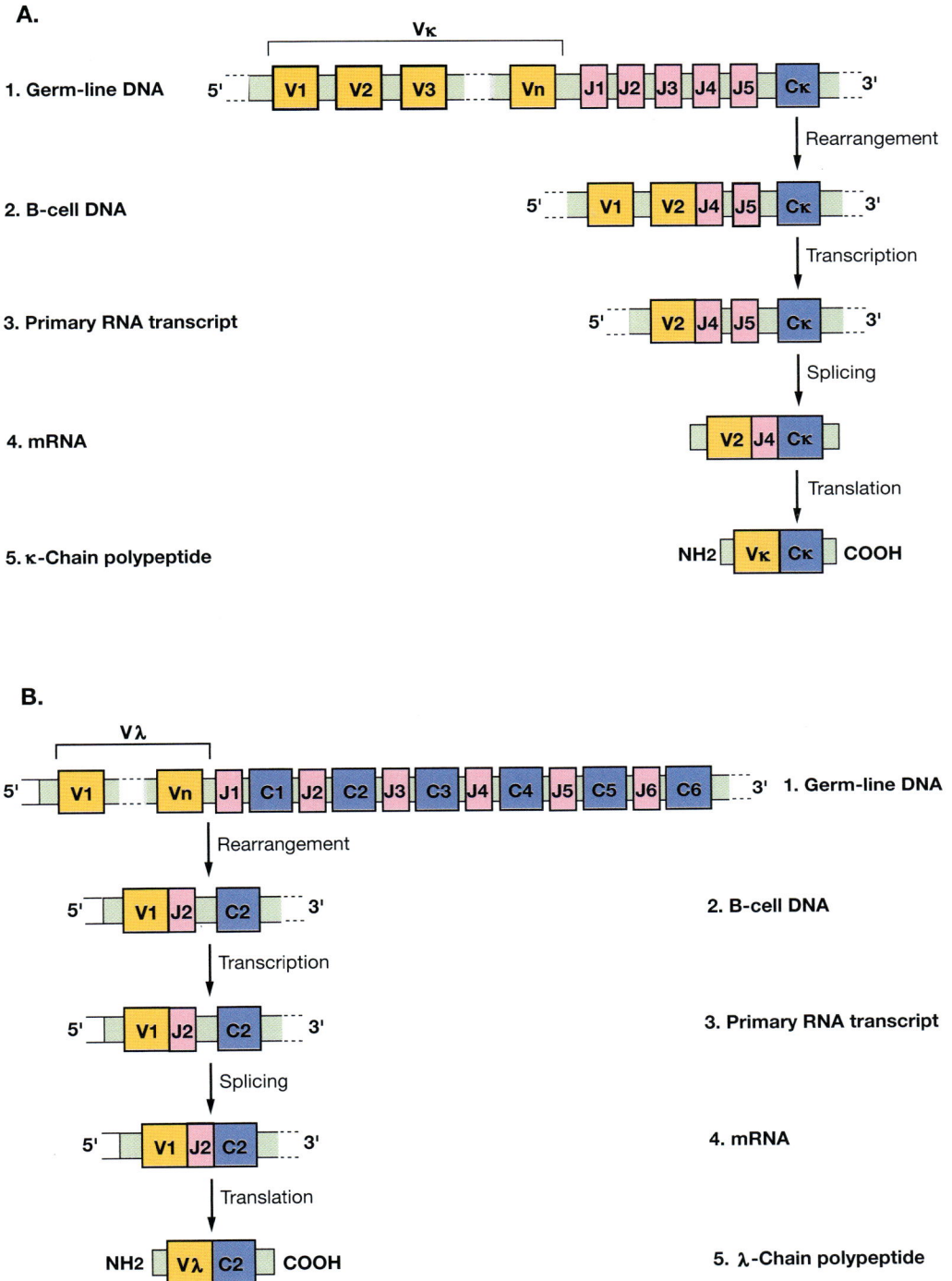

FIGURE 10.14. A. Kappa (κ) light (L)-chain synthesis. From the pool of multiple variable (V) region genes on chromosome 2 in the germ line DNA (1), one V region is joined to a joining (J) region gene, resulting in B-cell DNA (2). Following removal of introns by recombinases, the primary RNA is transcribed (3), resulting in messenger RNA (mRNA) (4) and in the κ L-chain polypeptide (5). (Redrawn with permission from Benjamini E. *Immunology: A Short Course.* 4th ed. Wiley-Liss; 2000:121.) B. Lambda (λ) L-chain synthesis. Rearrangement and synthesis of the λ, L-chain genes occurs in an identical manner on chromosome 22, except for the availability of up to six Cλ exons for union to the VJ combined region. This availability results in several subtypes.

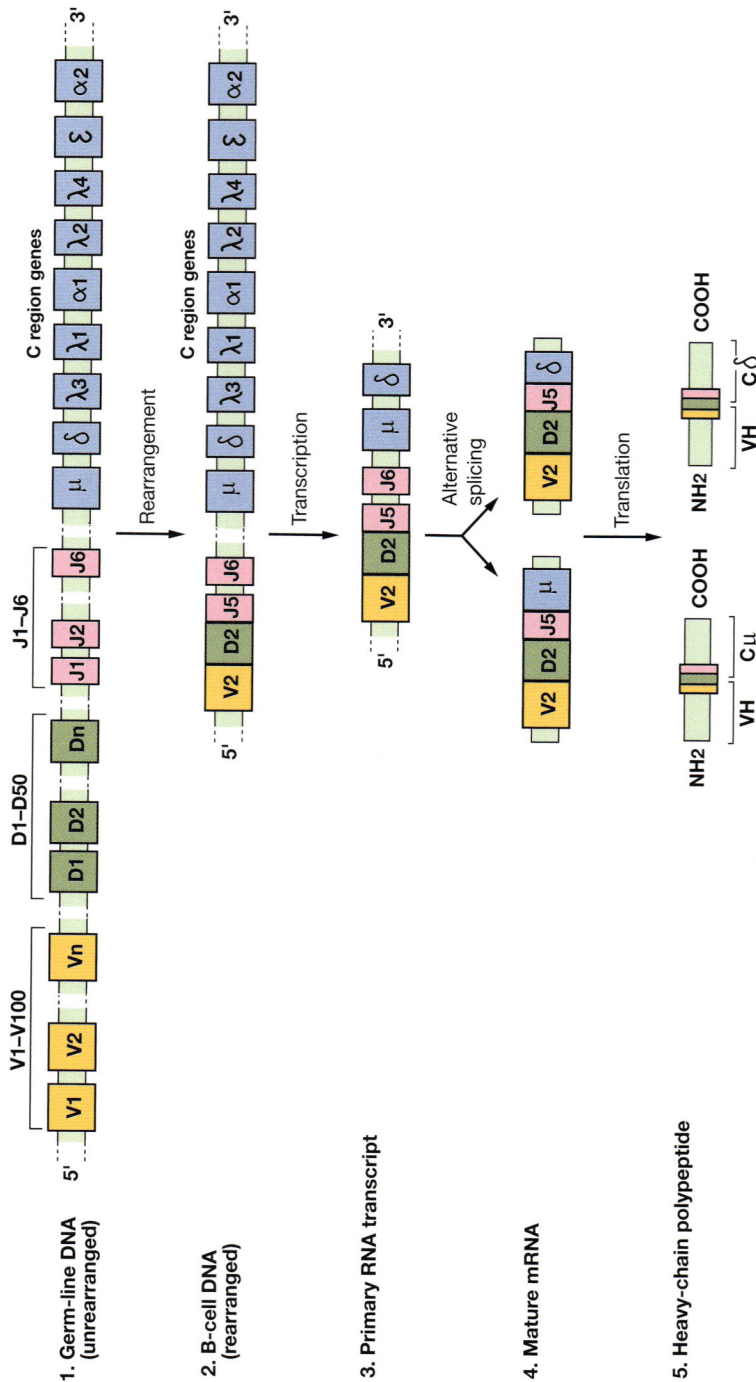

FIGURE 10.15. Heavy (H)-chain synthesis. (1) The variable region of the H chain is coded by three different gene complexes present on chromosome 14: variable (V) region genes, diversity (D) genes, and the joining (J) region genes. The constant (C) region gene complex harbors the genes controlling all of the immunoglobulin (Ig) classes. (2) During rearrangement, a J region gene links to a D region gene and then this complex links with a V region gene. The VDJ complex links to the μ or δ region genes. (3) A primary RNA transcript of the VDJ μδ complex is made; after splicing, messenger RNAs (mRNAs) for a VDJ μ and a VDJ δ appear. (4) H chains of both IgM and IgD result after translation of the mRNAs. (5) These H chains combine with light (L) chains and deposit on the B-cell membrane as the antigen receptors. Following antigen and cytokine stimulus, the IgM antibody is secreted (not illustrated). (Redrawn with permission from Benjamini E. *Immunology: A Short Course.* 4th ed. Wiley-Liss; 2000:123.)

232

e. A later rearrangement of **class genes** in the CH region dictates H-chain class switching from μ and δ to $\gamma3$, $\gamma1$, $\alpha1$, $\gamma2$, $\gamma4$, ϵ, and $\alpha2$, which is mediated by T-cell cytokines (IL-4, IL-13, IFN-γ, TGF-β).

2. Random selection by each B cell from the variety of V, D, and J germline genes available results in a large number of structural possibilities for the VL and VH epitope-binding regions of the immunoglobulins. This random selection is primarily responsible for the vast diversity of antibodies.

3. Allelic exclusion occurs since only one of the two parental alleles is expressed by a single B cell, resulting in a single H-chain isotype and L-chain subtype receptor capable of reacting with only one antigenic epitope.

B. Genetic control of human leukocyte antigens (HLAs)

HLAs control discrimination between self- and nonself-antigen presentation to T cells, but only to the same HLA type since **self-MHC (major histocompatibility complex) restriction** occurs.

C. Classes of HLAs

1. HLAs are organized into three MHC classes of molecules (Table 10.9).

a. Class I HLAs are glycoproteins that are found on the **membranes of most nucleated cells.**

(1) They are encoded by three gene regions: A, B, and C.

(2) They are linked to the **cytotoxic T (T_c) cell** through the **CD8** molecule and present peptidic epitopes to specific T_c receptors (class I restriction). A single class I molecule can bind several different epitopes.

(3) Two chains form the class I molecular structure; the α chain has three external domains, a transmembrane segment, and a cytoplasmic tail, while the β_2-microglobulin is an invariant protein.

(4) The peptide-binding site, found between domains $\alpha1$ and $\alpha2$, binds peptides containing 8 to 10 amino acids.

b. Class II HLAs are glycoproteins that are found on the **membranes of dendritic cells, macrophages, activated T cells, and B cells.**

(1) They are encoded by three gene regions: **DP, DQ**, and **DR**.

(2) They are linked to the T_h cell through the **CD4** molecule and present peptidic epitopes to specific T_h cell receptors (class II restriction). A single class II molecule can bind several different epitopes.

(3) Two chains, α and β, form the class II molecular structure. Each chain has two domains plus a transmembrane segment and a cytoplasmic tail (Figure 10.16).

(4) The peptide-binding site is formed by juxtaposition of the $\alpha1$ and $\beta1$ domains and binds peptides containing 13 to 18 amino acids.

c. Class III HLAs control certain serum proteins, including several complement components and TNFs. Class III molecules are encoded by three gene regions: C4, C2, and BF.

Table 10.9	Human Leukocyte Antigen (HLA) Classes						
MHC Class		I			II		III
Region	B	C	A	DP	DQ	DR	C4, C2, BF
Gene products	HLA-B	HLA-C	HLA-A	DP $\alpha\beta$	DQ $\alpha\beta$	DR $\alpha\beta$	C′ proteins TNF-α, TNF-β

MHC, major histocompatibility complex; TNF, tumor necrosis factor.
From Johnson A, Clarke B. *High-Yield Immunology*. 2nd ed. Lippincott Williams & Wilkins; 2006:23.

Class I HLA molecule   Class II HLA molecule

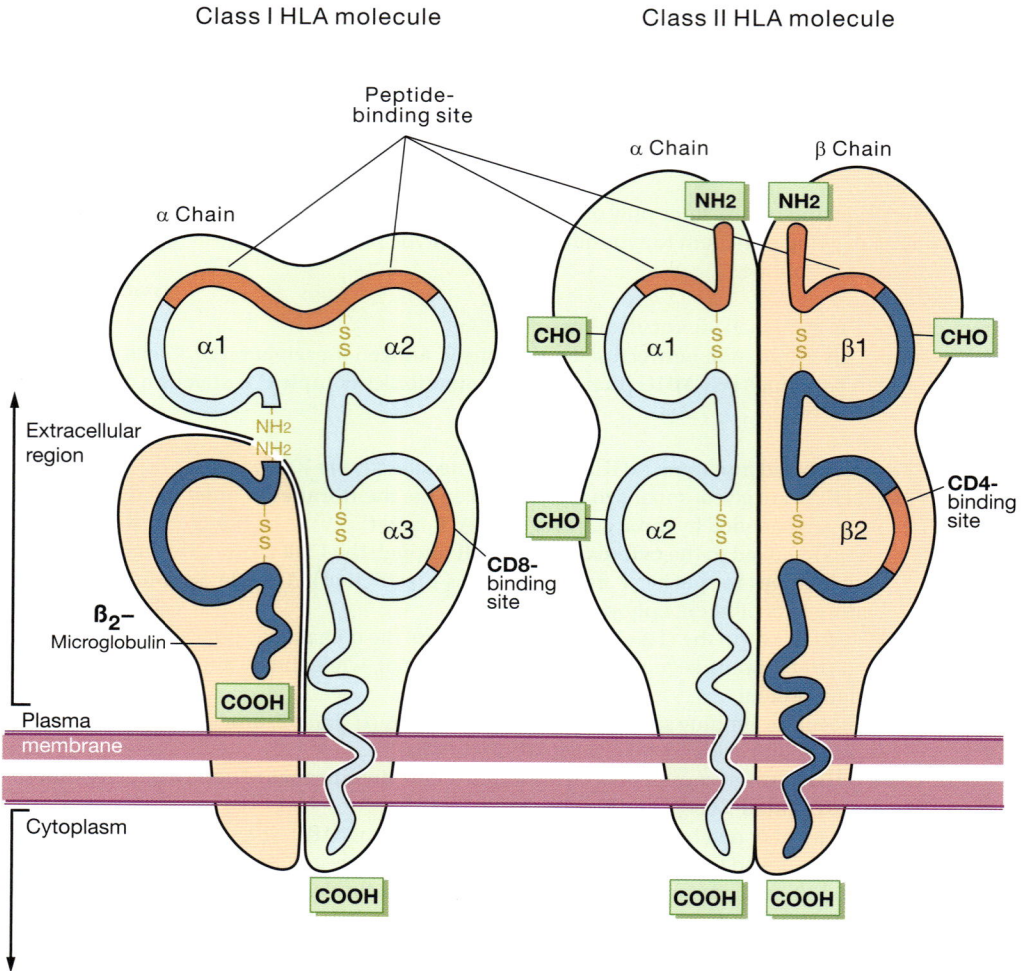

FIGURE 10.16. Structure of class I and class II human leukocyte antigen (HLA) molecules. –ss–, disulfide bond. (Redrawn with permission from Stites DP, Terr AI, Parslow TG. *Medical Immunology.* 9th ed. Appleton & Lange; 1997:86.)

    d. Polymorphism
      (1) Many **alleles** of classes I and II are present at each locus on chromosome 6 and are the major obstacles to organ transplantation.
      (2) Haplotypes from both parents are inherited and expressed codominantly.

D. Genetic control of the T-cell antigenic receptor (TCR [T-cell receptor])
  1. The TCR is a dimer of either α and β chains (~95%) or γ and δ chains (~5%).
  2. TCRs do not respond to soluble antigens, in contrast to the monomeric IgM antigen receptor on the B-cell membrane.
  3. TCRs recognize antigenic epitopes only as peptidic fragments bound to either class I or class II HLA molecules on an antigen-presenting cell (APC).
  4. The coreceptors, CD4 or CD8, determine whether humoral or cell-mediated immunity occurs.
    a. Binding of CD4 to a class II HLA molecule on an APC results in HI.
    b. Binding of CD8 to a class I HLA molecule on an APC results in CMI.
  5. Union of the specific TCR and coreceptor with the peptide-HLA membrane complex is associated with signal transduction into the cytoplasm by a complex of proteins, collectively designated **CD3**.

E. Genetic diversity: Achieved among the TCRs through gene rearrangements similar to those of immunoglobulins (Figure 10.17).

1. Recombination-activating genes (RAG-1 and RAG-2) are required for both heavy- and light-chain rearrangements in both early B-cell and T-cell antigen receptor expression, which mediates the somatic recombination of V and J or V, D, and J genes.

2. The phenomenon of allelic exclusion controls the genetic expression of TCRs.

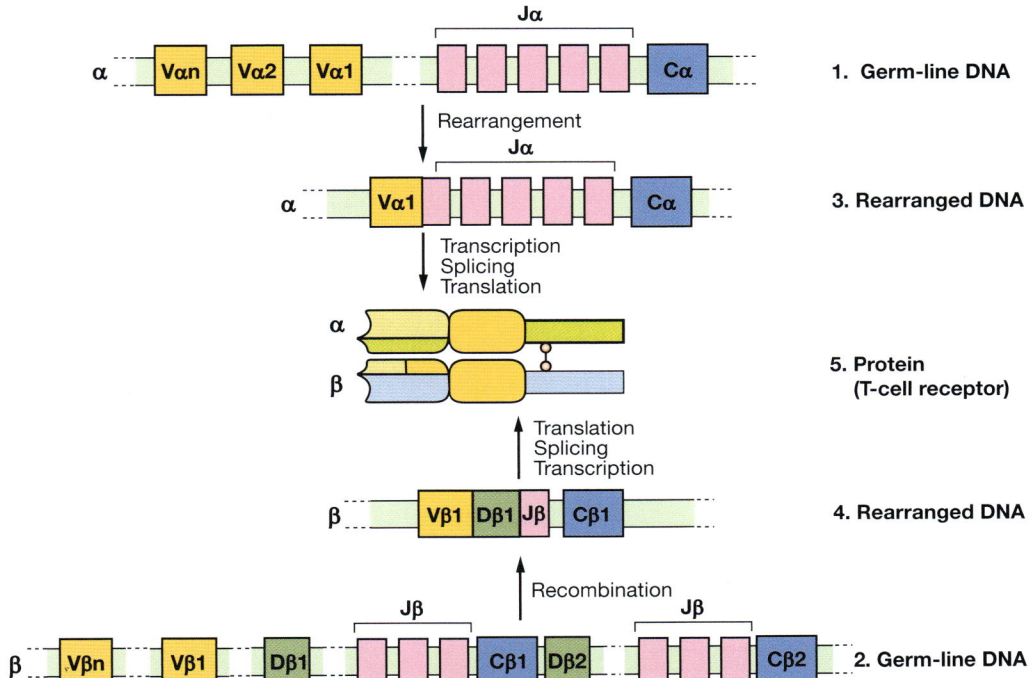

FIGURE 10.17. Synthesis of the human $\alpha\beta$ T-cell receptor (TCR) genes. Synthesis of the $\gamma\delta$ chains is thought to follow a similar pattern. (1) Multiple variable (V) region genes and joining (J) region genes occur at the TCRα locus on chromosome 14. (2) Similarly, multiple (V) region, diversity (D) segment, and J region genes occur at the TCRβ locus on chromosome 7. (3) During the rearrangement of α-chain genes, a randomly selected V gene is joined to a J gene and the exon is transcribed, combined with a constant (Cα) region gene, and translated. (4) Similarly, the β-chain exon is formed by the random linkage of a V region gene, first to a D region gene and a J region gene, and then to a Cβ gene. (Redrawn with permission from Janeway CA, Travers Jr. *Immunobiology: The Immune System in Health and Disease.* Garland Publishing; 1997:4.35.)

IX. ADAPTIVE IMMUNITY

The **adaptive immune system** (Figures 10.18-10.20) is a collection of specialized leukocytes called **lymphocytes**. Each cell expresses multiple copies of the same antigen receptors. These receptors are highly specific to a single target referred to as an **antigen**. Lymphocytes are generally long-lived and itinerant, continuously trafficking between specialized niches (immune organs) and peripheral tissues while patrolling for non–self-substances.

A. Primary immune organs are sites for the development of lymphocytes and provide the development of the lymphocyte antigen receptor.

1. Bone marrow is the site for progenitor stem cell development for both T and B cells.

a. Progenitor T-cell stem cells are produced during adolescence and transferred to the thymus.

b. Progenitor B-cell stem cells differentiate into **mature B cells** (express functional surface IgM antigen receptor and IgD).

c. Mature B cells enter the circulation and traffic between different secondary immune tissues.

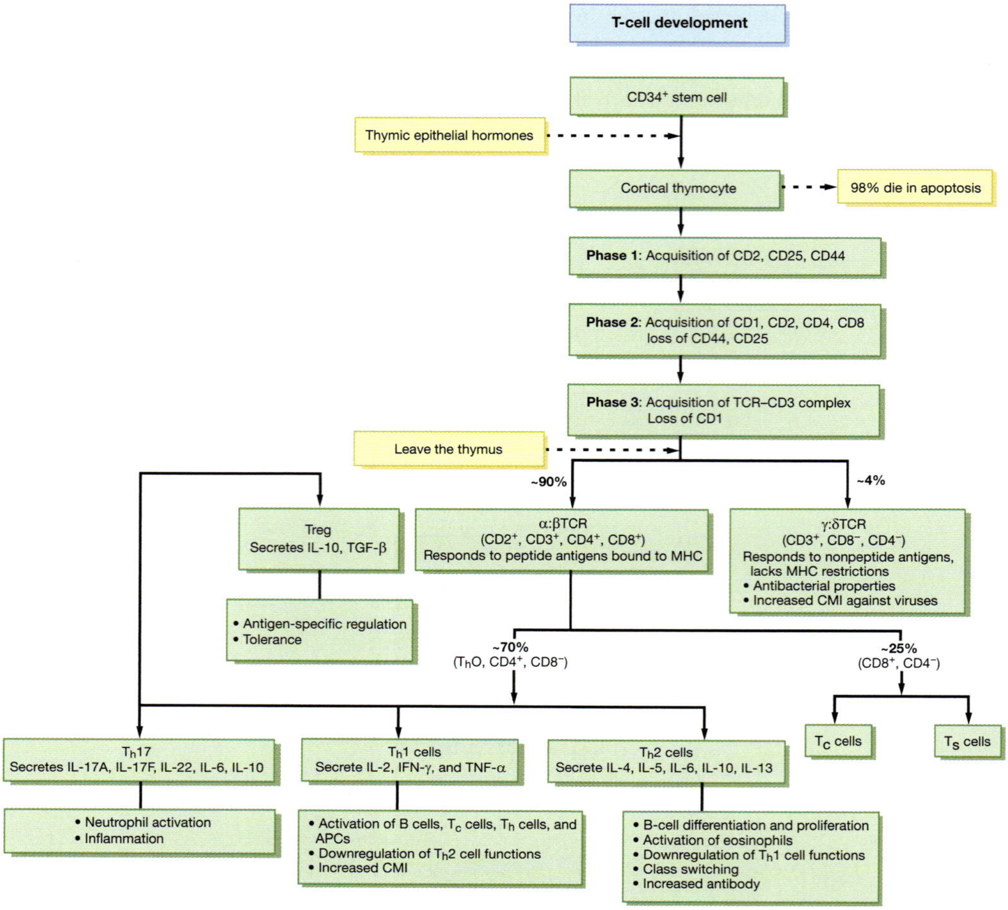

FIGURE 10.18. T-cell development. Stem cells from bone marrow bearing a CD34 marker migrate to the fetal thymus, where they become cortical thymocytes under the influence of epithelial hormones. Most of the cortical thymocytes die; the surviving 1% to 2% pass through three phases of development, during which they acquire and lose specific membrane markers (clusters of differentiation [CD]). During the final phase, which takes place in the medulla, the thymocytes acquire the T-cell antigenic receptor (TCR) and the CD3 signaling complex, and they lose the CD1 marker and leave the thymus. The T cells can have one of two types of TCR (α:βTCR or γ:δTCR); the types are differentiated according to the amino acids in the two peptide chains that form the receptor. The α:βTCR T cells respond to peptide antigens bound to the major histocompatibility complex (MHC), while the γ:δTCR cells respond to nonpeptide antigens. There are two populations of α:βTCR T cells: T_h1 cells and T_h2 cells. These cells secrete different cytokines and therefore have different functions. APC, antigen-presenting cell; CMI, cell-mediated immunity; IFN, interferon; IL, interleukin; T_c, cytotoxic T; TGF, transforming growth factor; T_h, helper T; TNF, tumor necrosis factor; T_s, suppressor T.

2. **Thymus** is the site for progenitor T-cell stem cell differentiation into mature T cells.
   a. **T_h cells** express the coreceptor CD4 and recognize the antigen displayed on MHC class II molecules.
   b. **T_c cells** express the coreceptor CD8 and recognize the antigen displays on MHC class I molecules.
   c. **Regulatory T (Treg) cells** express the coreceptor CD4, high-affinity IL-2 cytokine receptor subunit CD25, and recognize the antigen displayed on MHC class II molecules. They also display FoxP3, which is unique to Treg cells.
3. Development of the antigen receptor:
   a. Immature lymphocytes rearrange genes within the immunoglobulin gene loci (B cells) or the TCR loci (T cells) to assemble a unique antigen receptor.
   b. **RAGs** direct the reassortment of immunoglobulin genes to produce an enormous variety of possible antigen receptors.

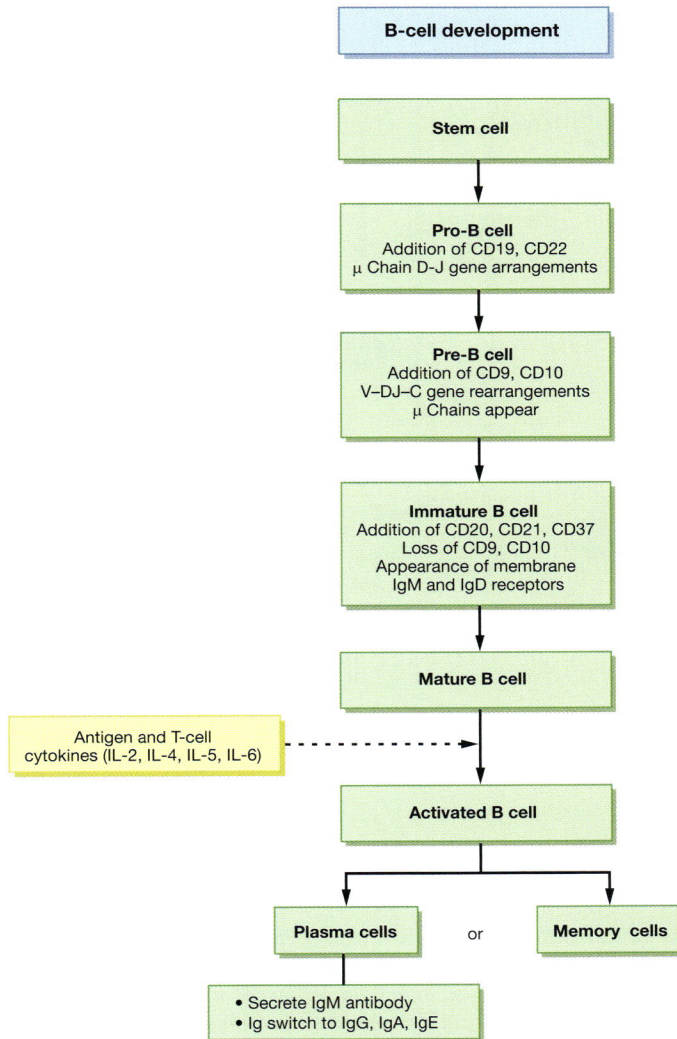

FIGURE 10.19. B-cell development. Stem cells differentiate in the bone marrow and pass through several stages of development before becoming mature B cells. Random selection by each B cell from a variety of germ line genes results in a large number of possible structures for the epitope-binding regions of the immunoglobulins. At the pro–B-cell stage, a joining (J) region gene links with a diversity (D) segment gene and then the VDJ complex links to the IA constant (C) region gene. At the immature B-cell stage, the appearance of membrane IgM and IgD receptors defines B-cell clones. Activation of the mature B cells by antigen and T-cell cytokines leads to differentiation and division of the B cells and synthesis of antibody. CD, cluster of differentiation; Ig, immunoglobulin; IL, interleukin.

    c. Positive selection screens for functional antigen receptors.

    d. The final rearrangements must pass **negative selection**, to eliminate receptors that recognize host-specific antigens.

    e. Failures to eliminate self-reactive antigen receptors result in autoreactive cells, a basis for **autoimmunity.**

    f. Mature, antigen naive lymphocytes emerge and circulate.

  4. An **anticipatory response** provides antigen receptors for a large variety of encounters.

    a. An enormous number of cells are produced, each with an antigen receptor capable of recognizing a separate and unique antigen.

    b. The immune system attempts to produce a repertoire of lymphocytes capable of recognizing new and novel antigens that the host may encounter during a lifetime.

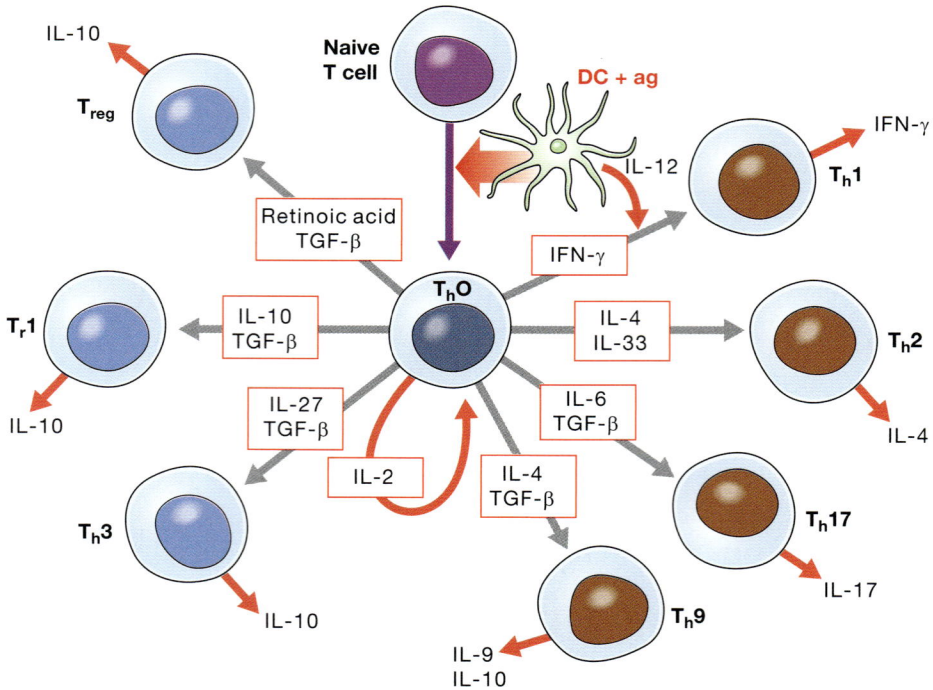

FIGURE 10.20. Family of helper T (T$_h$) cells. Red indicates agents that stimulate activation and differentiation. ag, antigen; DC, dendritic cell; IFN, interferon; IL, interleukin; TGF, transforming growth factor; Treg, regulatory T; T$_r$1, regulatory 1 T that does not express FoxP3 and occurs outside the thymus.

B. Secondary immune tissue

Secondary immune organs provide a niche for mature B and T cells to be educated to respond to a specific antigen.

1. A crossroads for itinerant naive mature T cells to enter a compartment and screen for cognate antigen recognized by the TCR.

2. Naive lymphocytes, never exposed to antigen, enter secondary immune organs.
   a. Entry to the lymph node occurs at the **high endothelial venule.**
   b. Naive T cells express CD62L that recognizes CD34 on the endothelial wall.
   c. T cell enters by **extravasation**.
   d. Naive T cells express CD62L, antigen-educated lymphocytes express CD44.
   e. Niche provides space for APCs (mDC) to display an antigen recovered from inflammatory sites.

3. Selected T cells proceed through a phase of proliferation and differentiation to specialize for an adaptive response.

4. Differentiated T cells then guide responses as humoral (antibody) or cell mediated (cell-mediated cytotoxicity).

5. **Germinal center** establishes niches for B cells to expand antibody diversity and specificity (Figure 10.21).
   a. **Somatic hypermutation** provides a means to produce an enormous diversity of antibodies.
      (1) Series of point mutations that randomly alter the amino acid sequence in the **paratope** of immunoglobulins.
      (2) Deamination of cytosine to uracil driven by **activation-induced (cytidine) deaminase** (**AID**).
      (3) Uracil is removed by **uracil-DNA glycosylase.**
      (4) Error-prone DNA polymerase repairs the gap.
   b. The B cell is capable of editing the immunoglobulin to make higher affinity interactions with an antigen.

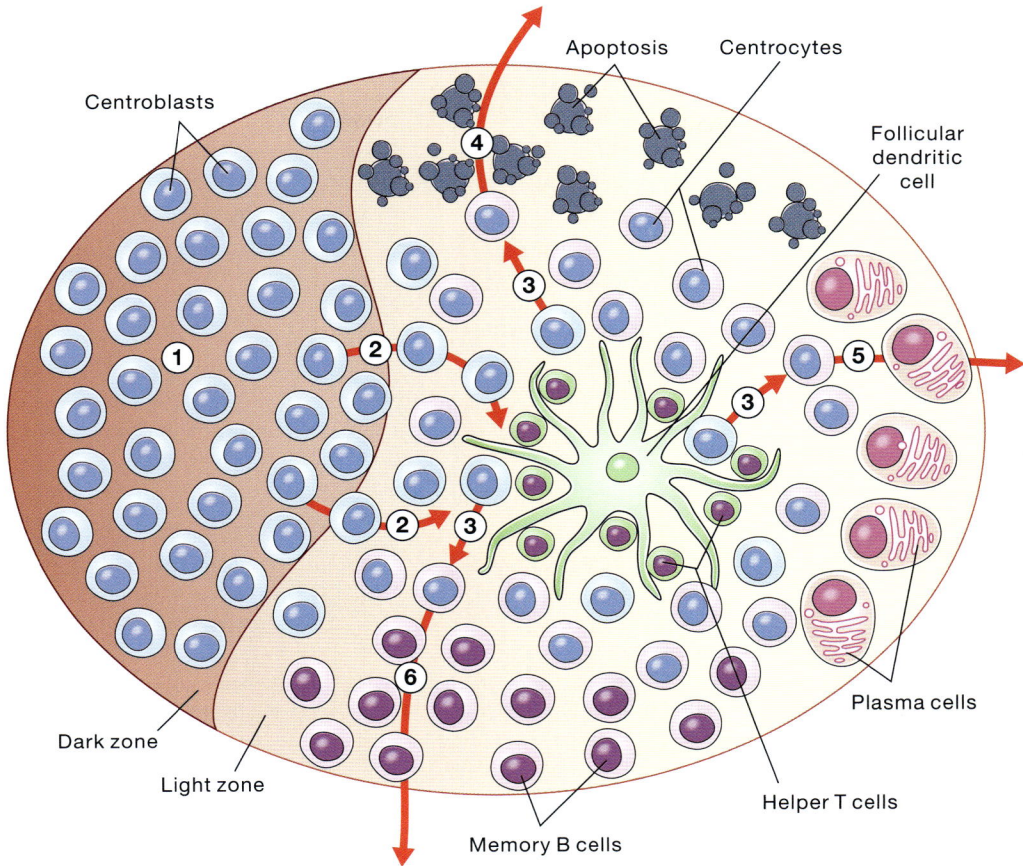

FIGURE 10.21. Germinal center. Centroblasts (light blue) (1) are reconstructing immunoglobulin specificity by somatic hypermutation within the dark zone. The **centroblasts** then migrate toward **follicular dendritic cells** (2) to become **centrocytes** (light purple) (3) and begin immunoglobulin class under the guidance of T-cell cytokines. Cells that fail to maintain a high affinity for antigens are removed by apoptosis (4). Cells retaining high-affinity progress on to become **plasma cells** (light pink) (5) or **memory B cells** (dark purple) (6).

    c. Germinal center forms, consisting of an outer mantle composed of transient lymphocytes; dark zone contains centrocytes; and light zone contains centroblasts.
    d. The dark zone is a site of active proliferation and somatic hypermutation.
    e. Epithelial-derived **FDCs** bind complement-bound antigens.
    f. FDCs collect antigens originating from the inflammatory site.
    g. B and T cells collect around the FDC screening for antigens.
    h. The B cell (centrocyte) and T cells remain associated with the antigen on the FDC.
    i. The B cell shifts antigen recognition by somatic hypermutation until the association with the FDC is lost or the T cell intervenes.
    j. Centrocytes proceed through **affinity maturation**, while somatic hypermutation is sustained by T-cell intervention.
    k. The B cell can also change isotype to enhance antibody function within different tissues; for example, IgG in the circulation and IgA in mucosal tissues.
    l. Isotype switching is driven by neighboring T cells (Figure 10.22).

C. Lymphocytes (Table 10.10)
    1. αβ **T-cell receptor** is found on thymus-derived T cells and recognizes peptides presented by MHC class II molecules.
    2. γδ **T-cell receptor** is found on mucosal epithelial T cells and can recognize free peptides; it does not need antigen presentation.

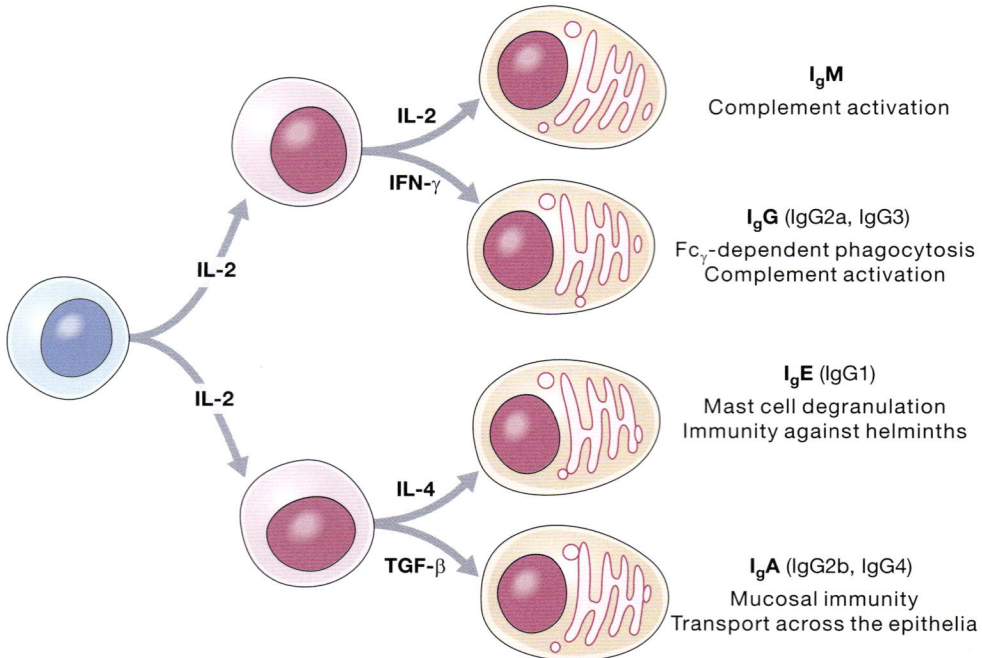

FIGURE 10.22. Immunoglobulin class switching. Centrocytes (light blue) expressing immunoglobulin (Ig)M can switch immunoglobulin secretion based on T-cell intervention with cytokines. IFN, interferon; IL, interleukin; TGF, transforming growth factor.

3. Antibodies are produced by B cells.
   a. B-1 cells are found in mucosal areas and produce antibodies to polysaccharides. B-1 cell immunoglobulins have a limited repertoire to different antigens.
   b. B-2 cells are produced in germinal centers and have the ability of immunoglobulin gene re-arrangements, somatic hypermutation, and class switching. B-2 cell immunoglobulins have a virtual limitless repertoire of antigen recognition ability. B-2 cells differentiate into plasma cells to produce large quantities of antibody.
4. mDCs activate T cells.
   a. Immature dendritic cells accumulate and identify antigens as foreign substances at a site of inflammation; exposure to PAMP induces maturation and directs migration to the draining lymph node.
   b. Mature dendritic cells present antigen to T_h **cells** using the MHC class II in specialized niches, such as the lymph nodes.
   c. Mature dendritic cells take residence in the lymph node adjacent to mature naive T cells in the paracortex.
   d. mDCs present antigens and interrogate naive T cells, express costimulatory molecule CD80/86, and increase surface display of MHC class II–bound antigen.
   e. Antigen-specific T cells begin development and clonal expansion.
   f. Naive B cells bind antigen percolating in draining lymph fluids; antigen is internalized and expressed on MHC class II.
   g. Specific T cells recognize presented antigens and stimulate B-cell activation.
5. Specialized lymphocyte:
   a. Generally localized to mucosal boundaries and express a low copy number of antigen receptors.
   b. B-1 cells secrete antibody specific for bacterial carbohydrates and LPSs.
   c. Marginal zone B cells are located in the spleen to produce antibodies to polysaccharides.
   d. ($\gamma\delta$) T cells expressing an alternative TCR are located in the boundary areas of gut mucosa and epithelia.

Table 10.10 List of T-Cell Subsets

Cell	Symbol	Function	Secretory Cytokines
Naive T-Cell CD4$^+$ or CD8$^+$	T_h0	Quiescent, progenitor, must be activated by dendritic cell	None
Activated helper T cell	T_h0^a	Activated progenitor, receptive to cytokine control	Interleukin (IL)-2
Helper T1	T_h1	Intracellular bacteria and virus	Interferon (IFN)-γ, LTα
Helper T2	T_h2	Extracellular parasites	IL-4, IL-5, IL-13, IL-25
Helper T9	T_h9	Immunity to helminths	IL-9, IL-10
Helper T17	T_h17	Extracellular bacteria and fungi, mucosae	IL-21, IL-17a, IL-17f, IL-22
Natural regulatory T CD4$^+$CD25$^+$	Treg	Tolerance, regulation, and homeostasis	Transforming growth factor (TGF)-β
Regulatory 1 T CD4$^+$CD25$^-$	T_r1	Suppress naive and memory T cells, inducible	IL-10
Anergic T CD4$^+$CD25$^-$	T_h3	Mucosal immunity, inducible	TGF-β
Suppressor T CD8$^+$CD28$^-$	T_s	Regulation, mucosal immunity	IL-10, TGF-β upregulates immunoglobulin-like transcript (ILT)3 on monocytes
Cytotoxic T-cell CD8$^+$	T_c	Cell-mediated immunity	Perforin granzyme
(γδ)T	(γδ)T	Mucosal, respiratory tract	IFN-γ, tumor necrosis factor (TNF)-α, IL-4
Natural killer T cell	NKT	Detect glycolipid antigen presented by CD1	IFN-γ, TGF-α, IL-4
Natural killer cell	NK	Cytotoxic T-cell screens for missing MHC class I, antiviral activity	Perforin, granzyme

MHC, major histocompatibility complex.

    e. NK cells search for host cells with aberrant expression of **MHC class I** surface molecules and execute target cells by cell-mediated cytotoxicity.
       (1) NK cells recognize target cells based on antibody labeling, complement labeling, and screening for low MHC class I expression.
       (2) NK cells express receptors for complement (C3b, C3a, and C5a) and IgG and IgA.
       (3) NK cells engage a target cell through lectin activity or recognition of labeling with antibody or complement.
       (4) NK cell engagement activates a cytolytic mechanism.
       (5) NK receptor screens for the absence of MHC class I using an inhibitory receptor. MHC engagement to the killer inhibitory receptor (KIR) deactivates the NK cell.
       (6) The NK cell kills target cells by inducing apoptosis if the KIR is not triggered.
       (7) Target cell death by apoptosis is driven by granule exocytosis or TNF pathway.
    f. NK T cells share properties with NK and T cells.
       (1) Displays a (αβ) TCR.
       (2) Recognizes glycolipids displayed by CD1.
       (3) Displays a killer cell lectin receptor NK1.1.
       (4) Produces IFN-γ.
    g. Plasmacytoid cells
       (1) Low abundant leukocyte (<1% circulating leukocytes).
       (2) Lymphocyte derived.
       (3) Do not express classical complement receptors.

(4) Do not express CD14, as it is not responsive to LPS.

(5) Expresses toll-like receptor 7 to detect single-stranded RNA (ssRNA).

(6) Expresses toll-like receptor 9 to detect CpG.

(7) Produces large amounts of IFN-α and IFN-β.

(8) Important to viral infections.

X. RESPONSE TO ANTIGEN

A. Fate of antigen (or vaccine)

1. If antigen entry is intravenous (Figure 10.23), it is phagocytized or pinocytosed in the spleen; if entry is other than intravenous, it traffics to the lymph node, draining the site of entry. They are processed at these sites by APCs, monocytes, macrophages, and dendritic cells.

2. Exogenous protein antigens enter the APC from the extracellular environment by pinocytosis and are processed in acidic endosomal vacuoles. The resulting peptides bind to the cleft in **MHC class II** molecules and are transported to the cell membrane where they can be presented to **CD4$^+$ T cells** to activate B cells for antibody synthesis.

3. Viruses and intracellular parasitic antigens are synthesized endogenously within the APC cytoplasm and endoplasmic reticulum and processed to peptides by proteasomes. The peptides bind to the cleft in **MHC class I** molecules and migrate to the APC membrane, where they are presented to **CD8$^+$ T cells** to initiate CMI (Figure 10.24).

   a. CMI is directed mainly against intracellular-dwelling microorganisms and aberrant, endogenous cells (eg, cancer cells) (see Figure 10.23).

   b. Antibody is not involved, except in antibody-dependent cellular cytotoxic (ADCC) reactions. In the latter, the effector cell is linked to the target cell by an antibody bridge, with the Fab portion binding to the specific membrane antigen on the target cell and the Fc portion binding to the Fc receptor on an activated effector cell.

B. Activation of T cells is initiated when the specific CD4 or CD8$^+$ TCR binds to the appropriate APC peptide-HLA complex (Figure 10.25).

1. T-cell adhesion molecules CD28, CD2, and lymphocyte function–associated antigen (LFA)-1 strengthen the binding.

   a. CD28 binds to B7.1 on the APC and increases IL-2 synthesis.

   b. CD2 binds to LFA-3.

   c. CTLA-4 binds to B7.2, which serves to downregulate IL-2 synthesis following activation.

2. An activation signal is transduced by the CD3 complex composed of three polypeptides—γ, δ, and ε—and two zeta chains.

C. T$_h$ cell response pathways: T$_h$ cells are classified into two subtypes (T$_h$1 and T$_h$2) based on the cytokines they secrete, which determine the functions they affect.

1. The **T$_h$1 cell** induces CMI following binding to the peptide-**class II MHC** by transforming, differentiating, and dividing logarithmically and secretes:

   a. IL-2, which is necessary for T- and B-cell transformation.

   b. IFN-γ, which enhances CMI by activating macrophages and NK cells. It also triggers HLA presentation by endothelial cells and can suppress antibody formation by downregulating IL-4 synthesis.

   c. TNF-α, which activates macrophages and synergizes with IL-1 in inducing and stimulating the acute phase response.

   d. IL-12 and IL-18 from dendritic cells and macrophages aid the transition of macrophages, T$_c$ cells, and NK cells to CMI.

2. The **T$_h$2 cell** induces activation of B cells and HI following binding to the peptide-**class II MHC** and stimulation by IL-2. It transforms, differentiates, and divides logarithmically while secreting for IL-4, IL-5, IL-10, and IL-13.

   a. IL-4 is essential for the development of antibody synthesis by stimulating B-cell differentiation. It is necessary for IgE production and downregulates IFN-γ by T$_h$1 cells and thus can suppress CMI.

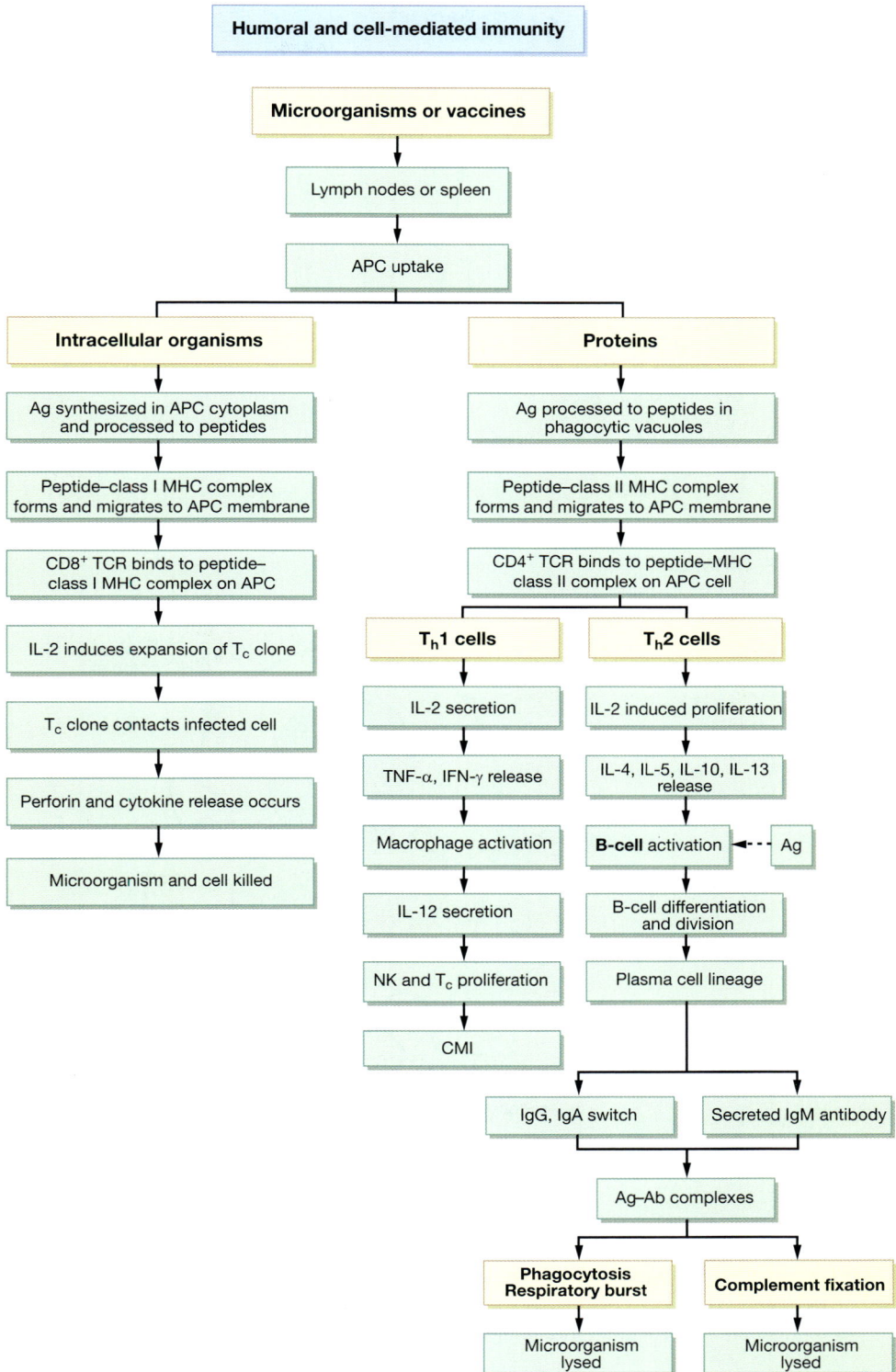

FIGURE 10.23. Humoral and cell-mediated immunity. Ag-Ab, antigen-antibody; APC, antigen-presenting cell; CD, cluster of differentiation; CMI, cell-mediated immunity; IFN, interferon; Ig, immunoglobulin; IL, interleukin; MHC, major histocompatibility complex; NK, natural killer; T_c, cytotoxic T cells; TCR, T-cell receptor; T_h, helper T cells; TNF, tumor necrosis factor.

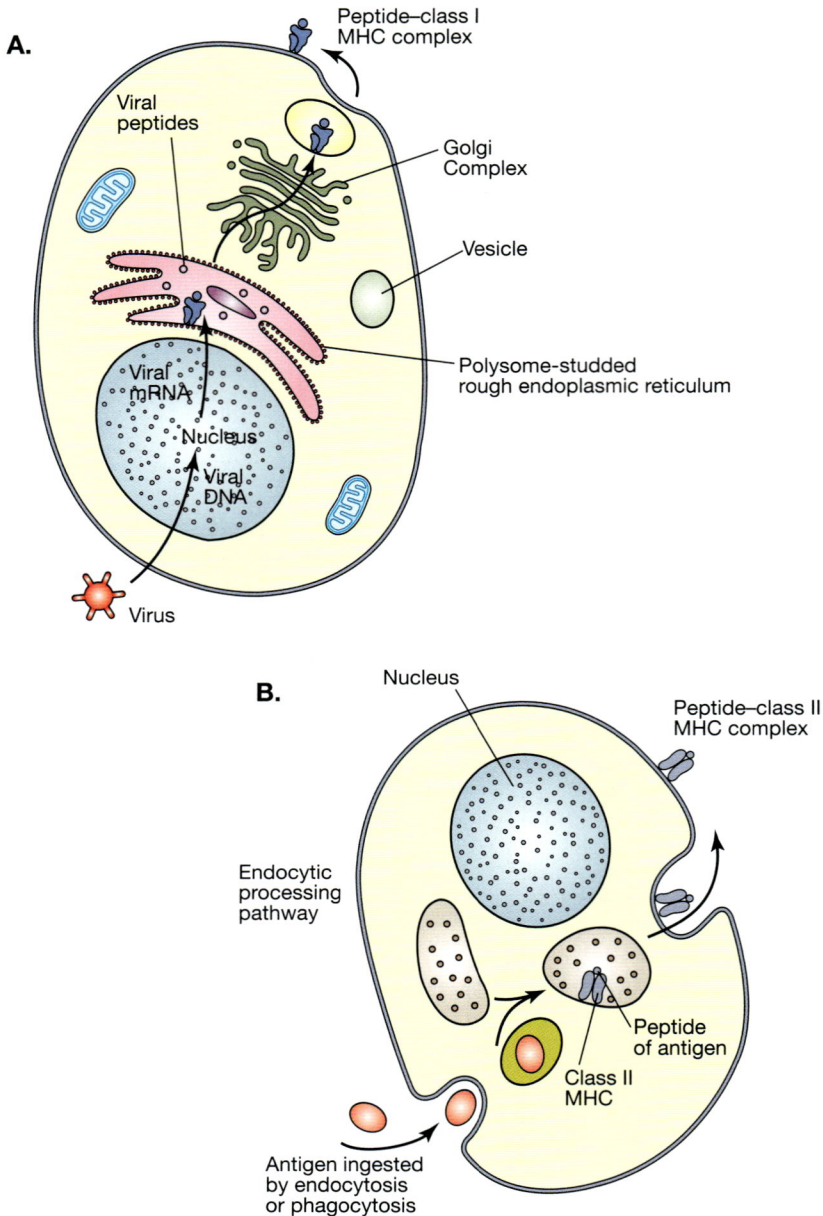

A.

Peptide–class I
MHC complex

Viral
peptides

Golgi
Complex

Vesicle

Polysome-studded
rough endoplasmic reticulum

Viral
mRNA

Nucleus

Viral
DNA

Virus

B.

Nucleus

Peptide–class II
MHC complex

Endocytic
processing
pathway

Peptide
of antigen

Class II
MHC

Antigen ingested
by endocytosis
or phagocytosis

FIGURE 10.24. Antigen processing of (A) intracellular organisms and (B) exogenous proteins. MHC, major histo-compatibility complex. (Redrawn from Kuby J. *Immunology.* 3rd ed. W.H. Freeman; 1997.)

   b. IL-5 functions synergistically with IL-4 and IL-2 to aid B-cell differentiation. It stimulates growth and differentiation of eosinophils and facilitates IgA synthesis.
   c. IL-10, like IL-4, inhibits T_h1 release of IFN-γ and IL-2, thus reducing macrophage activation by IFN-γ.
   d. IL-13 mimics IL-4 actions, inhibiting T_h1 cytokine release.

D. B-cell response is initiated by antigen selecting the clone of B cells with the membrane-bound IgM antigen receptor that is specific for the antigen epitope.
   1. Binding of antigen, along with stimuli from the T-cell cytokines IL-2 and IL-4, triggers differentiation of that B-cell clone into a large blast cell, and logarithmic division occurs.

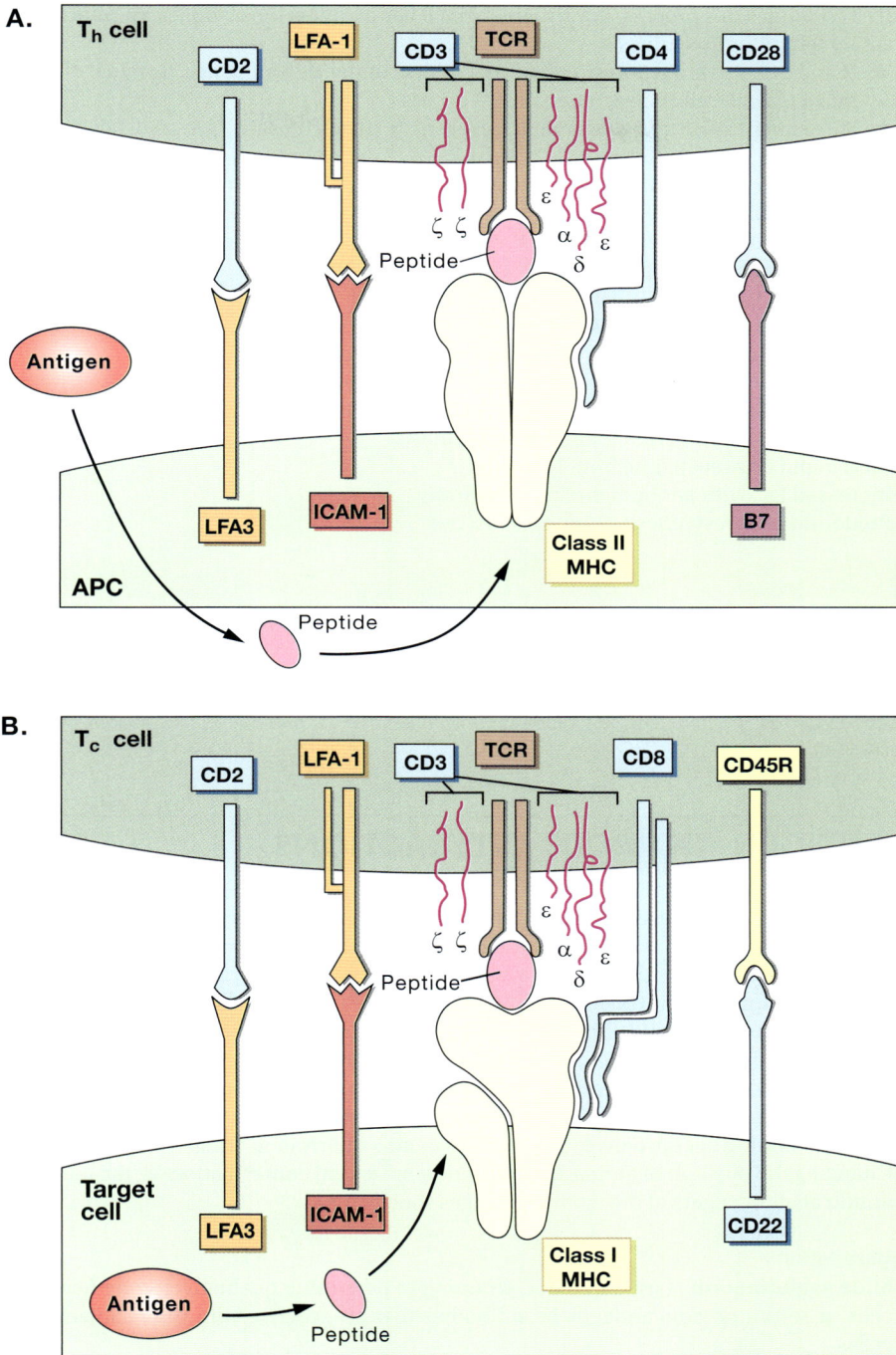

FIGURE 10.25. A. Activation of CD4$^+$ helper (T$_h$) cells. The specific T-cell antigenic receptor (α:βTCR or γ:δTCR) binds to the peptide-class II major histocompatibility complex (MHC) by the antigen-presenting cell (APC). The CD4 molecule links to the MHC. An activation signal is transduced by the TCR-CD3 complex, which is composed of three polypeptides (α, δ, ε) and two ζ chains. Accessory T-cell adhesion molecules (eg, CD2, leukocyte function–associated antigen-1 [ILFA-1], and CD28) facilitate adherence of the T$_h$ cell to the APC and influence interleukin-2 synthesis. B. Activation of CD8$^+$ cytotoxic T (T$_c$) cells. CD, clusters of differentiation; ICAM, intracellular adhesion molecule; LFA, lymphocyte function–associated antigen; TCR, T-cell receptor. (Redrawn from Kuby J. *Immunology.* 3rd ed. W.H. Freeman; 1997.)

2. IL-5 continues this process, during which the B cell acquires the cytoplasmic "machinery" necessary for antibody synthesis.
   a. H and L chains are synthesized and assembled; under IL-6 influence, terminal differentiation into a plasma cell and secretion of IgM occurs.
   b. Subsequent gene rearrangements result in a switch to IgG, IgA, and IgE synthesis and secretion.
      (1) IL-4 and IFN-γ influence the switch to IgG; TGF-β influences the switch to IgA; and IL-4 influences the switch to IgE.
      (2) The binding of CD40 on the B cell to its ligand on the T_h cell (CD40L) is necessary for switching to occur.

E. Memory cells of all classes are generated independently of the plasma cell lineage. They migrate to various lymphoid tissues, where they have an extended survival.

F. A secondary response to the same antigen can result in the following:
   1. A shorter induction period for antibody synthesis.
   2. More rapid class switching from IgM to IgG.
   3. Increased IgG with antibodies of higher affinity.
   4. Predominant IgA synthesis in mucosal tissues.

• • • Clinical Pearl

Senescence is the age-related decline in immune response, which contributes to the age-related risks often associated with infections and cancer development. Mechanistically, the production of naive T cells declines due to the age-related changes in the thymus. There are reductions in the diversity and functions of B- and T-cell populations as well as in overall cell replication capacity due to shortening of telomeres. Reduced cytotoxicity of NK cells, low-grade chronic inflammation, and a reduced response to vaccines are also seen.

XI. ANTIGEN-ANTIBODY INTERACTIONS

A. Antigens, antibodies, antigen-antibody reactivity, cytokines, drugs, and cells can be detected in vitro or in vivo, and some even in the nanogram and picogram range.
   1. The union of antigen with antibody is very sensitive, specific, and firm, but reversible; multiple short-range forces are involved.
   2. Binding occurs in seconds but is not visible until a lattice forms, which occurs more slowly. Since antibodies are bivalent, they form the lattice through cross-linkages (Figure 10.26). The composition of the lattice depends on the ratio of antigen to antibody.
   3. Affinity measures the binding energy between an antibody and a univalent epitope; **avidity** is the total binding energy between an antibody and a multivalent antigen.
   4. Changing the position of atoms, double bonds, structural conformation, or the composition of amino acids or sugars of the epitope changes specificity.

B. Agglutination
   1. Slide agglutination is used in blood grouping to determine qualitatively whether the donor's cells or serum possess antigens or antibodies that are reactive with the recipient's serum or cells.
      a. Major crossmatch uses the donor's cells plus the recipient's serum to determine whether anti-red blood cell (RBC) antibodies are present in the recipient's serum. Rapid clumping of the donor's cells will occur in vivo if antidonor RBC antibodies are present.
      b. Minor crossmatch uses the donor's serum plus the recipient's cells. Agglutination of the recipient's cells occurs if anti-RBC antibodies are present in the donor's serum. However, a transfusion reaction under these conditions would be much less severe than one associated with a major crossmatch because the amount of antibodies transfused in the donor's serum is minimal relative to the number of RBCs in the recipient.

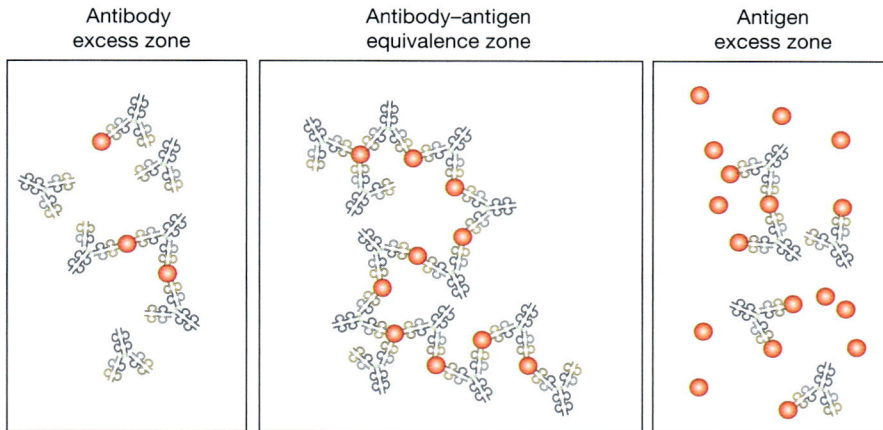

FIGURE 10.26. The size of antigen-antibody (ag-ab) complexes is determined by the ratio of antigen to antibody. In vivo, larger complexes (in antibody excess and at equivalence) are phagocytosed; smaller complexes (in antigen excess) escape and lodge in blood vessels and behind the renal basement membrane, causing vasculitis and glomerulonephritis. Antigen is depicted in red.

2. **Coombs direct test** involves the detection of **weak or nonagglutinating anti-Rh (Rhesus factor D antigen) antibody** by adding antihuman immunoglobulin **directly to the infant's RBCs,** to which the Rh antibody has been attached in utero, and noting any agglutination. An **indirect test** involves measuring these same weak antibodies in the **maternal circulation** by adding the mother's serum to Rh^+ RBCs in vitro. The addition of antihuman immunoglobulin results in agglutination of the sensitized RBCs.

C. **Transplantation immunology** is governed mainly by allogeneic differences in histocompatibility antigens (ie, HLAs) between donor and recipient. The genes for the HLAs are located in the MHC on chromosome 6.
  1. HLAs have two major functions:
     a. To bind and present processed, foreign antigenic peptides to T cells, thus initiating the immune response.
     b. To identify and distinguish the MHC membrane antigens on a transplanted donor organ from those of the recipient.
  2. Class I and class II HLA genes, which encode the histocompatibility antigens, exhibit enormous polymorphism since multiple alleles exist at each locus.
     a. **Class I antigens are found on all nucleated cells.** They have three gene loci—HLA-A, HLA-B, and HLA-C—identified serologically with anti-HLA antibodies. Their function is to present foreign antigenic peptides to $CD8^+$ **cells.**
     b. **Class II antigens are found on immunologic effector cells** (eg, macrophages, dendritic cells, B cells, activated epithelial cells). They have three gene loci within the D region— HLA-DP, HLA-DQ, and HLA-DR—defined by cellular reactions. Their function is to present foreign antigenic peptides to $CD4^+$ **cells.**
  3. **Matching the donor and recipient at the HLA locus** improves graft acceptance.
     a. Both donor and recipient are typed for HLA profiles with anti-HLA antisera and for ABO and Rh antigens with their respective antisera.
     b. The donor must be tested for preexisting anti-HLA antibodies and CMI since sensitization to HLAs can occur as a result of prior blood transfusions, pregnancy, or other organ grafts.
  4. The degree of genetic disparity between donor and recipient governs the vigor and speed of rejection of the graft. $CD8^+$ T_c cells and macrophages (activated by $CD4^+$ T cells) mediate most rejections.
     a. **Acute rejection** is characterized by swelling and tenderness over the allograft. It is initiated by HLAs on allografts stimulating recipient $CD4^+$ T cells, which respond by secreting cytokines and inducing adhesion molecules and inflammation. Injury to the renal vasculature by the T_c cells and their products follows, with resulting ischemia of the renal parenchyma.

b. A **second allograft** from the same donor as the initial allograft (second set rejection) is rejected more quickly than the initial allograft (the memory response).

c. **Chronic rejection** is characterized by episodic bouts of rejection occurring months to years after transplantation. Both cellular and humoral mechanisms are active, eventually resulting in interstitial fibrosis, vascular occlusion, and loss of function.

d. **Hyperacute rejection** occurs when a graft is never taken because of preexisting sensitivity (**white graft**). Rejection occurs within minutes.

5. **Graft-versus-host reactions** can occur when **immunocompetent** tissues (eg, bone marrow, thymus, spleen, organs harboring passenger leukocytes) are allografted. If they recognize the recipient as foreign, CMI damage results. If the recipient is *immunocompetent*, a host-versus-graft reaction can take place. Immunosuppressive therapy can reduce this occurrence.

6. **Immunosuppression** is used to prolong graft acceptance; however, it predisposes the individual to infection. Consequently, appropriate killed (but not live) vaccines should be administered before transplantation. **Major organisms** that cause infections are:

a. Cytomegalovirus, present in more than 50% of donors.

b. *Candida*, present in more than 90% of donors.

c. Epstein-Barr virus, present in more than 90% of donors.

d. *Aspergillus*.

e. Respiratory syncytial virus.

7. **Immunosuppressive agents** include cyclosporine A, tacrolimus (FK 606), mycophenolate mofetil, azathioprine, corticosteroids, and antilymphocyte globulin (ALG).

● ● ● **Clinical Pearl**

Primary immunodeficiencies are often genetic, while secondary immunodeficiencies can result from infections, medications, or underlying medical conditions.

D. Immunologic aspects of cancer

1. **Oncogenes:** Cancers arise from cells in which growth-regulating and repair genes (**proto-oncogenes**) have become ineffective as a result of random mutation or following viral infection or chemical damage. When proto-oncogenes become altered or damaged, they are termed **oncogenes,** and their actions are capable of causing neoplastic growth. Examples of oncogenes and their actions include the following:

a. **p53 gene:** As a proto-oncogene, p53 encodes a nuclear phosphoprotein that inhibits cell division, thus suppressing tumor growth. Mutations in p53 result in uncontrolled growth.

b. *ras*: As a proto-oncogene, *ras* controls a guanosine triphosphate (GTP)-binding protein involved in signal transduction. Mutation results in failure of guanosine triphosphatase (GTPase) inactivation of *ras* and continuous *ras* activity.

c. *c-myc*: When this proto-oncogene is translocated onto a different chromosome (eg, as in Burkitt lymphoma), it becomes oncogenic, resulting in the loss of regulation of B-cell growth and B-cell lymphoma.

d. **Bcl-2** gene: The cellular protein produced by this gene inhibits apoptosis at normal concentrations. At high concentrations in B cells, Bcl-2 promotes cell expansion and follicular lymphoma.

e. **bcr/abl** gene fusion results in a protein with increased tyrosine kinase activity, which is involved in chronic myeloid leukemia.

2. **Cancer cells arise from normal cells.** For the immune system to attack cancer cells, they need to be distinguished from normal cells (ie, they need to possess antigens).

a. **Tumor-associated antigens** exist, but are not found exclusively on cancer cells; however, they are generally present in higher amounts in patients with cancer and aid in diagnosis. Examples are:

(1) **Carcinoembryonic antigen (CEA)**, which is present on fetal GI and liver cells, but normally disappears at birth. It reappears in the serum of most patients with colorectal cancer.

(2) β-**Fetoprotein** attains high levels in patients with hepatomas and testicular teratocarcinomas. Values are lower in adults without cancer.

    b. Tumor-specific antigens (TSAs) are unique to cancer cells. They can be induced by viruses (eg, papovaviruses, herpesviruses, adenoviruses) or chemical or physical carcinogens.

        (1) Virus-induced TSA is cross-reactive (ie, the genome of a particular virus synthesizes the same viral antigens in whatever cell that virus infects). Consequently, immunotherapy should be applicable to all individuals infected by the same virus.

        (2) Carcinogen-induced TSA induces random mutations in the genome of affected cells. Consequently, each mutated gene product (antigen) differs depending on which gene has been affected by the carcinogen, and immunologic cross-protection is not feasible.

3. Immune response to cancer antigens

    a. Immunocompromised hosts with diminished CD4 and CD8 **T-cell functions** have a higher incidence of lymphoproliferative cancers, implicating a T-cell protective function.

    b. Macrophages are found frequently in the bed of regressing tumors. They must be activated by macrophage-activating factor (MAF) (eg, IFN-γ) to eradicate tumor cells via the respiratory burst, nitric oxide, and TNF-α.

    c. NK cells kill cancer cells through ADCC and lysis following contact. Their cytolytic activity is increased by IL-2, IL-12, and IFN-γ.

    d. Monoclonal antibodies directed to tumor-associated antigens and TSAs can be infused into a patient either directly or conjugated with a toxin, drug, or radioisotope to kill the tumor (eg, humanized anti-CD20 for B-cell lymphomas).

    e. Immunotherapies for cancer treatment

        (1) Immune checkpoint inhibitors such as anti–PD-1 and anti–CTLA-4 antibodies block negative feedback loops by preventing these checkpoint proteins from interactions with their partner proteins to maintain signaling pathways alerting the immune system to a problem.

        (2) Chimeric antigen receptor T-cell (CAR-T) therapy involves genetically modifying a patient's T cells via methods such as CRISPR-Cas9 to facilitate precise changes that result in the T-cell's ability to express receptors that target cancer cells.

> **• • • Clinical Pearl**
>
> The tumor microenvironment consists of various immune cells, stromal cells, soluble factors, extracellular matrix components, blood vessels, and signaling molecules within the tumor, in addition to cancer cells that exhibit heterogeneity in different subpopulations. The overall composition of this environment can influence tumor progression and response to therapy.

XII. HOST DEFENSES TO VIRUSES

> **• • • Clinical Pearl**
>
> Along with IFNs, a number of host antiviral proteins serve to recognize viruses that result in phosphorylation, ubiquitination, deamination, and degradation activities on viral proteins to prevent replication.

A. Host defense mechanisms are responsible for the self-limiting nature of most viral infections.

    1. Defense mechanisms have both immune and nonimmune aspects.

    2. They operate during all stages of a viral infection and may contribute to the clinical pattern of disease (immunopathology).

B. Nonimmune defenses

    1. Innate immunity includes anatomic barriers (dead cells of the epidermis) and chemical barriers (mucous layers) that limit contact of the virus with susceptible cells. They are dependent on the complex parameters associated with the age and physiologic status of the host.

    2. Cellular resistance involves nonpermissive cells, which lack factors (eg, viral receptor sites) necessary for virus replication.

    3. Inflammation limits the spread of virus from an infection site and results in unfavorable environmental conditions for viral replication (eg, antiviral substances, low pH, elevated temperature).

4. IFN is a host-specific, viral-induced glycoprotein that inhibits viral replication by inducing the synthesis of several antiviral proteins including $2',5'$-oligoadenylate synthetase and specific protein kinases.

   a. Although it is not viral specific, IFN is fairly species specific.

   b. IFN is the first viral-induced defense mechanism at the primary site of infection in individuals without immunity.

5. Interfering RNA (iRNA)

   a. Formation: Double-stranded viral RNA interacts with ribonuclease DICER to form short interfering RNAs (siRNA), which interact with argonaute proteins to form RISC (RNA-inducing silencing complexes).

   b. RISC binds to viral mRNA and inhibits viral gene expression by repressing translation or degrading the viral mRNA.

C. Humoral immunity: This defense mechanism involves the production by B lymphocytes of neutralizing and nonneutralizing antibodies against viral-specific antigens. It is the defense mechanism most important against cytolytic viral infections accompanied by viremia and viral infections of epithelial surfaces.

   1. Neutralizing antibodies inhibit a virus's ability to replicate by inhibiting viral attachment, penetration, or uncoating, or all three processes.

   a. Lesions may also be induced in the viral envelope with the aid of a complement.

   b. These antibodies are most protective if they are present at the time of infection or during viremia.

   2. Nonneutralizing antibodies enhance phagocytosis of virion degradation by acting as opsonins.

D. Cell-mediated immunity involves cytotoxic T lymphocytes (CTLs), antibody-dependent cell-mediated cytotoxicity, NK cells, and activated macrophages.

   1. Soluble factors from T lymphocytes (lymphokines) and macrophages (monokines) regulate cellular immune responses.

   2. This form of immunity is the most important defense mechanism against noncytolytic infection in which the membrane of the virus-infected cell is antigenically altered by the virus.

E. Viral-induced immunopathology can result from various immunologic interactions, including immediate hypersensitivity, antibody-antigen complexes (as in HBV), and tissue damage due to cytotoxic cells or antibody and complement. These reactions can contribute to the disease process and are a common feature of persistent viral infections.

F. Viral-induced immunosuppression can occur during cytolytic or noncytolytic infection when infecting viruses alter the immune responsiveness or decrease the number of lymphocytes. It is frequently observed as a transient consequence of disseminated viral infections that involve lymphocyte infection by the virus.

Review Test

Directions: Select the one lettered answer that is best in each case. Commit to and write down your answers before checking the answers and explanations. Each of the numbered items in this section is followed by answers with explanations, in the following section.

1. Which of the following cell types express $CD3^+$, $CD25^+$, and $FoxP3^+$?

(A) NK T cell
(B) T_c cell
(C) T_h cell
(D) Treg cell
(E) $(\gamma\delta)$ T cell

2. Which of the following T-cell types is located at the epithelial barrier of the gut?

(A) NK T cell
(B) T_c cell
(C) T_h cell
(D) Treg cell
(E) $(\gamma\delta)$ T cell

3. Which of the following $CD3^+$ cell types is CD1 restricted to glycolipids?

(A) NK T cell
(B) T_c cell
(C) T_h cell
(D) Treg cell
(E) $(\gamma\delta)$ T cell

4. Which of the following $CD3^+$ cell types secretes perforin and granzyme?

(A) NK T cell
(B) T_c cell
(C) T_h cell
(D) Treg cell
(E) $(\gamma\delta)$ T cell

5. Which of the following $CD3^+$ cell types secretes IL-2 when activated?

(A) NK T cell
(B) T_c cell
(C) T_h cell
(D) Treg cell
(E) $(\gamma\delta)$ T cell

6. Which of the following cell types is produced as a result of vaccination?

(A) B-1 cells
(B) Centrocytes
(C) Memory B cells
(D) Naive mature B cells
(E) Plasma cells

7. Which of the following cell types secretes antibodies that recognize polysaccharides?

(A) B-1 cells
(B) Centrocytes
(C) Memory B cells
(D) Naive mature B cells
(E) Plasma cells

8. Which of the following cell types performs somatic hypermutation?

(A) B-1 cells
(B) Centrocytes
(C) Memory B cells
(D) Naive mature B cells
(E) Plasma cells

9. Which of the following cell types secretes large quantities of antibody but does not express surface immunoglobulin?

(A) B-1 cells
(B) Centrocytes
(C) Memory B cells
(D) Naive mature B cells
(E) Plasma cells

10. Which of the following cell types expresses both IgM and IgD on the cell surface?

(A) B-1 cells
(B) Centrocytes
(C) Memory B cells
(D) Naive mature B cells
(E) Plasma cells

11. Which of the following cell types resides in the liver and is a part of the reticuloendothelial system?

(A) Foam cell
(B) Giant cell
(C) Kupffer cell
(D) M1 macrophage
(E) M2 macrophage

12. Which of the following cell types is directed by IL-4 to promote tissue repair, angiogenesis, and tumor growth?

(A) Foam cell
(B) Giant cell
(C) Kupffer cell
(D) M1 macrophage
(E) M2 macrophage

13. Which of the following cell types is derived from monocytes that attach to the arterial intima and accumulate lipids?

(A) Foam cell
(B) Giant cell
(C) Kupffer cell
(D) M1 macrophage
(E) M2 macrophage

14. Which of the following cell types is directed by IFN-γ to promote reactive oxygen species (ROS) production and cytolysis?

(A) Foam cell
(B) Giant cell
(C) Kupffer cell
(D) M1 macrophage
(E) M2 macrophage

15. Which of the following is a syncytial cell found within granuloma?

(A) Foam cell
(B) Giant cell
(C) Kupffer cell
(D) M1 macrophage
(E) M2 macrophage

16. Which of the following cell types secretes IL-4, temporarily resides in draining lymph nodes, and promotes the T_h2 response?

(A) Basophil
(B) Eosinophil
(C) Mast cell
(D) Neutrophil
(E) Plasmacytoid cell

17. Which of the following cell types is a short-lived phagocytic cell recruited to inflammatory sites by macrophage secretion of CCL8?

(A) Basophil
(B) Eosinophil
(C) Mast cell
(D) Neutrophil
(E) Plasmacytoid cell

18. Which of the following cell types is a tissue-resident cell that responds to PAMPs and releases histamine and eicosanoids?

(A) Basophil
(B) Eosinophil
(C) Mast cell
(D) Neutrophil
(E) Plasmacytoid cell

19. Which of the following cell types found in the circulation secretes IFN-α and IFN-β?

(A) Basophil
(B) Eosinophil
(C) Mast cell
(D) Neutrophil
(E) Plasmacytoid cell

20. Which of the following cell types expresses Fcε receptors and is recruited to sites of helminth infections?

(A) Basophil
(B) Eosinophil
(C) Mast cell
(D) Neutrophil
(E) Plasmacytoid cell

21. Which of the following proinflammatory cytokines has a major role in asthma?

(A) IFN-γ
(B) IL-4
(C) IL-6
(D) IL-10
(E) IL-17

22. Which of the following cytokines promotes humoral immunity and is produced by T_h2 cells?

(A) IFN-γ
(B) IL-4
(C) IL-6
(D) IL-10
(E) IL-17

23. Which of the following cytokines promotes CMI and is produced by T_h1 cells?

(A) IFN-γ
(B) IL-4
(C) IL-6
(D) IL-10
(E) IL-17

24. Which of the following cytokines is anti-inflammatory?

(A) IFN-γ
(B) IL-4
(C) IL-6
(D) IL-10
(E) IL-17

25. Which of the following cytokines is produced by macrophages to induce liver production of acute phase proteins?

(A) IFN-γ
(B) IL-4
(C) IL-6
(D) IL-10
(E) IL-17

26. Which of the following cell types produces cytotoxic compounds following T_h1 cell activation?

(A) B cell
(B) FDC
(C) Immature mDC
(D) Macrophage
(E) Mature mDC

27. Which of the following cell types expresses cell surface MHC class II and CD80/88 and secretes IL-12?

(A) B cell
(B) FDC
(C) Immature mDC
(D) Macrophage
(E) Mature mDC

28. Which of the following cell types is captured by endocytosis using transmembrane immunoglobulin?

(A) B cell
(B) FDC
(C) Immature mDC
(D) Macrophage
(E) Mature mDC

29. Which of the following cell types has a majority of MHC class II located within intracellular compartments?

(A) B cell
(B) FDC
(C) Immature mDC
(D) Macrophage
(E) Mature mDC

30. Which of the following epithelial-derived cell types expresses cell surface C3 antigen?

(A) B cell
(B) FDC
(C) Immature mDC
(D) Macrophage
(E) Mature mDC

31. Which of the following is the first viral-induced defense mechanism in an individual without immunity ?

(A) Generation of CTLs
(B) Production of IFN
(C) Synthesis of lymphokines
(D) Synthesis of neutralizing antibodies

Answers and Explanations

1. **The answer is D.** [IX A 2 c] All T cells express CD3, and activated T cells and Treg cells express CD25$^+$. FoxP3 is unique to Treg cells.

2. **The answer is E.** [IX C 5 d] A characteristic of $\gamma\delta$ T cells is to surface on the mucosal barrier of the gut.

3. **The answer is A.** [IX C 5 f (2)] The invariant TCR of NK cells recognizes glycolipids expressed on CD1 molecules.

4. **The answer is B.** [Table 10.10] Several leukocytes use perforin and granzyme to perform cell-mediated cytotoxicity, but only T_c cells express this activity from the given choices.

5. **The answer is C.** [Table 10.10] The committing step for T_h cell activation is the simultaneous expression of the high-affinity IL-2 receptor subunit CD25 and the release of IL-2 to provide autocrine stimulation of proliferation.

6. **The answer is C.** [X A 2, X E and F] Vaccinations are used to establish immunologic memory to a particular pathogen.

7. **The answer is A.** [IX C 3 a] B-1 lymphocytes search and produce antibodies to recognize polysaccharides found on bacteria.

8. **The answer is B.** [IX B 5 j] Centrocytes are located in the germinal center at a site populated with T_h cells that promote antibody editing by somatic hypermutation and class switching.

9. **The answer is E.** [IX C 3 b] Plasma cells are terminal and dedicated to producing immunoglobulin; no surface receptor is needed to direct further development.

10. **The answer is B.** [IX A 1 b] Both IgD and IgM are expressed on mature B cells when exiting the bone marrow. The IgD expression is lost when the B cell begins development in the germinal center.

11. **The answer is C.** [V D 5 g] The liver plays a vital role in clearance of immune complexes from the circulation using a resident macrophage called a Kupffer cell.

12. **The answer is E.** [X C 2] IL-4 produced by T_h2 cells or basophils during inflammation promotes macrophage development into the M2 phenotype.

13. **The answer is A.** [Table 10.2] Monocytes attaching to the arterial intima are influenced by chronic inflammation to accumulate lipids, in particular the low-density lipoprotein (LDL) particle containing cholesterol.

14. **The answer is D.** [V D 5] T_h1 lymphocytes recognize nonself-antigen expressed in MHC class II molecules on the surface of the macrophage. The T cell then triggers macrophage activation of cytolytic mechanisms.

15. **The answer is B.** [V D 5] Syncytial cells are commonly found in granulomas as a result of macrophage fusion to form giant cells.

16. **The answer is A.** [V D 2 b] Basophils are short-lived cells in the circulation but will take longer term residence in draining lymph nodes and will direct inflammatory responses.

17. **The answer is D.** [III C 1 j, V D 1 e] The initial recruitment of neutrophils to an inflammatory site requires CCL8 release by resident macrophage or mast cells to initiate cellular extravasation.

18. **The answer is C.** [V A 1, Figure 10.4] Mast cells express toll-like receptors to recognize the initial stages of infection. Recognition of a PAMP results in a degranulation to release histamines and lipolysis to release eicosanoids.

19. **The answer is E.** [IX C 5 g (7)] Both IFN-α and IFN-β are produced by viral infected cells infected as a localized event, but the plasmacytoid cell is responsible to produce large quantities during a viral infection to enhance MHC class I expression on a broader scale.

20. **The answer is B.** [V D 3 i, VII D 2 d] Eosinophils are the principal agent for responding to reaginic antibody.

21. **The answer is E.** [Table 10.5] IL-17 promotes inflammatory action, such as the development of M2 macrophage and recruitment of eosinophils.

22. **The answer is B.** [VII D 1 d] IL-4 regulates humoral defenses.

23. **The answer is A.** [X C 1 b] IFN-γ regulates cell-mediated defenses.

24. **The answer is D.** [Tables 10.5, 10.10] IL-10 is produced by Treg cells to suppress immunity.

25. **The answer is C.** [III E 3] IL-6 stimulates hepatocytes to secrete acute phase proteins.

26. **The answer is D.** [X C 1] CMI is regulated by T_h1 cells secreting IFN-γ when engaging macrophages that display intracellular nonself-antigen on MHC class II molecules.

27. **The answer is E.** [V D 6 b (3)] Immature dendritic cells at the infection site are triggered to mature and migrate to the lymph node. Immature dendritic cells have low expression of MHC class II, but mature cells have high expression levels of both MHC class II and CD80/88.

28. **The answer is A.** [X D] Only B cells express transmembrane immunoglobulins.

29. **The answer is C.** [V D 6 a (2), (3)] Immature mDCs are positioned in tissues to continuously sample extracellular debris for PAMPs and loading of intracellular MHC class II.

30. **The answer is B.** [IX B 5 e] FDCs are the only choice to not be bone marrow derived.

31. **The answer is B.** [XII B 4 b] The production of IFNs that induce the synthesis of antiviral replication proteins in neighboring cells occurs before the appearance of any other viral-induced immune defense mechanisms.

11

System-Based and Situational Immunologic Disorders

I. OVERVIEW

Although the immune system functions efficiently in protecting the vast majority of the population, a small percentage of individuals react in an aberrant manner or lack some of the basic elements necessary for an adequate response. These individuals exhibit (1) hypersensitivity to certain antigens, (2) inadequate or unresponsiveness to microbial or other antigenic exposure, or (3) loss of mechanisms regulating the immune system's reaction against self. The role of the immune system in transplantation, cancer, and vaccination is included in this chapter.

II. HYPERSENSITIVITY DISEASES

There are four types of hypersensitivity diseases (Table 11.1).

A. **Anaphylaxis (type I)** reactions occur in genetically susceptible individuals who respond rapidly and excessively to the release of mediators following the complexing of an allergen with mast cell–bound immunoglobulin (Ig)-E. During the initial sensitization phase, IgE is formed in excess and binds avidly via its Fc domain to its receptor (FcFRε, CD23) on the surface of mast cells and basophils. The F(ab')2 domains containing the antigen-binding sites remain free to bind the allergen. When an allergen is reintroduced, it aggregates several cell-bound IgE molecules, causing membrane perturbations and triggering degranulation of mast cells and basophils, which subsequently release pharmacologically active agents systemically or locally (**atopy**).

1. **Anaphylactic shock** is a rapid, severe, generalized reaction that occurs when the allergen-IgE complex–induced mediators are released systemically (eg, histamine, leukotrienes, tumor necrosis factor [TNF]-α, interleukin [IL]-1, IL-6, serotonin, bradykinin, and platelet-activating factor [PAF]).

   a. These agents rapidly contract smooth muscle, increase vascular permeability and secretions, alter coagulability, and induce hypotension, leading to multiple organ failure and death.

   b. Common inducers of IgE and subsequent triggers include *Hymenoptera* venom, foods, drugs, and antibiotics (eg, penicillin).

2. **Urticaria** (hives) is an IgE-mediated, cutaneous form of immediate hypersensitivity characterized by vasodilation and increased vascular permeability of the skin. Histamine release following the allergen-IgE union is mainly responsible for the wheal and flare lesion and pruritus (Figure 11.1).

3. **Asthma** is characterized by airway obstruction and acute respiratory distress caused by mucus secretion and mediator-induced constriction of the smooth muscle surrounding the bronchioles following allergen-IgE complex formation. Symptoms include wheezing, dyspnea, chest tightness, and cough.

   a. An influx of mast cells, CD4$^+$ cells, T$_h$2 cells, basophils, and eosinophils results in cytokine release and inflammation.

Table 11.1	Hypersensitivity Classifications	
Type	**Conditions**	**Distinguishing Characteristics**
I: Anaphylaxis	Atopy (local reactions)	IgE Fc adherence to mast cells and basophils
	Urticaria	
	Asthma	Degranulation and histamine release
	Allergic rhinitis	Smooth muscle contraction
	Anaphylactic shock (systemic reactions)	
II: Cell surface Ag-Ab Cytotoxicity	Hemolytic disease of the newborn	Exogenous cell antigens
	Transfusion reactions	Complement-induced target cell lysis
	Goodpasture syndrome	Phagocytosis
	Glomerulonephritis	ABO, Rh blood loss
		Endogenous cell antigens
		Autoimmunity
		Neutrophil influx and damage
III: Ag-Ab complex Disease	Arthus reaction	Precipitating antibody
	Serum sickness	Vasculitis
	Polyarteritis nodosa	Complement-mediated neutrophil influx and damage
	Glomerulonephritis	
	Systemic lupus erythematosus	dsDNA-anti-dsDNA complexes
	Rheumatoid arthritis	Rheumatoid factor
IV: Delayed-type hypersensitivity	Tuberculosis	Cell-mediated immunity
	Granulomatous reactions	Activated macrophages
	Contact dermatitis	Epithelioid cells
		TDTH, T_h1, $CD8^+$ cells
		Haptens

Ag-Ab, antigen-antibody; CD, cluster of differentiation; dsDNA, double-stranded DNA; Ig, immunoglobulin; TDTH, T-cell–mediated delayed-type hypersensitivity effector cells; T_h1, T-helper cell type 1.
From Johnson A, Clarke B. *High-Yield Immunology*. 2nd ed. Lippincott Williams &Wilkins; 2006:60.

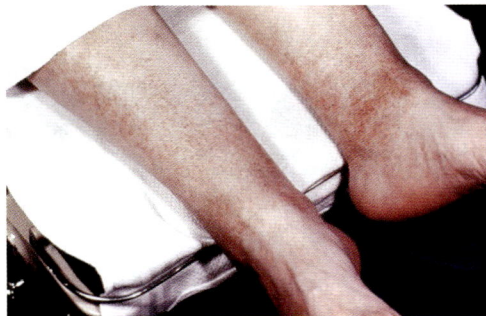

FIGURE 11.1. Urticaria pigmentosa. Red punctate lesions on a patient's legs and feet. (Courtesy of Centers for Disease Control Public Health Image Library [PHIL], image 18952.)

b. Important mediators are leukotrienes, PAF, eosinophil chemotactic factor (ECF), and histamine; important triggers include respiratory infections, environmental pollutants, aspirin, and nonsteroidal anti-inflammatory drugs.

c. Chronic exposure to occupational, environmental, and food allergens results in extrinsic asthma, whereas intrinsic asthma can be induced by nonimmunologic means (cold, exercise).

4. **Allergic rhinitis** is the most common clinical expression of atopy. Inflammation of the mucous membranes of the nose occurs, leading to profuse rhinorrhea, paroxysmal sneezing, nasal obstruction, itching, and conjunctivitis (eg, hay fever).

a. Common allergens involved are pollens, fungal spores, house dust, and animal dander.

b. Binding of the allergen to cell-bound IgE releases cytokine mediators, including histamine, leukotrienes, prostaglandin D2, and ECF.

c. With certain allergens, a **hyposensitive state** can be achieved by repeated parental injection of the agent in subliminal doses. Desensitization is associated with an increase in **IgG** antibody, which combines avidly with the allergen in the circulation, thus blocking union with cell-associated IgE and mediator release.

B. **Cellular antigen-antibody cytotoxicity (type II)** occurs when the antibody is directed against epitopes present on the cellular surface membranes of organs and tissues. Subsequent damage results from (a) the osmotic, lytic action of activated complement; (b) opsonization by phagocytic cells or killing by antibody-dependent cellular cytotoxicity (ADCC); and (c) killing of the target cell by T_c lymphocytes, natural killer (NK) cells, or both. Destruction of the target cell mainly results from the release of perforins and serine proteases (granzymes), which cause pore formation and osmotic lysis. Examples include:

1. **Transfusion reactions** mainly occur following the transfusion of blood containing red blood cell (RBC) antigens foreign to the recipient (Table 11.2). ABO incompatibility reactions are the most common; Rh reactions are the most severe.

a. Preformed antibodies in the recipient clump (agglutinate) the donor's blood cells, resulting in complement-mediated RBC lysis or rapid phagocytosis.

b. Fever is the most common reaction; in severe reactions, chest pain, hypotension, and disseminated intravascular coagulation (DIC) may occur.

2. **Hemolytic disease of the newborn** (**erythroblastosis fetalis**) can occur following the placental transfer of a nonsaline agglutinating maternal anti-Rh IgG antibody (usually anti-RhD), which binds to RhD+ fetal erythrocytes. The presence of this antibody in either the mother's circulation or on the infant's cells can be detected by the Coombs test.

a. Complement-mediated lysis or rapid phagocytosis follows, resulting in hemolysis and hemoglobinuria, which then convert to toxic indirect bilirubin.

b. Accumulation of the latter causes **kernicterus** (jaundice) with respiratory and brain damage.

c. Injection of the Rh– mother with anti-Rh antibody (RhoGAM) within 1 to 2 days following delivery prevents this disease. Anti-RhD antibody neutralizes the fetal Rh+ antigens entering the mother's circulation following spillage during removal of the placenta and prevents stimulation of the maternal immune system and injury to future Rh+ newborns.

Table 11.2	Blood Grouping					
ABO System			**Rh**		**Genotype**	
RBC Genotype	**Phenotype**	**Serum Antibody**	**Terminal Epitope**		**Rh+**	**Rh−**
OO	O	Anti-A and anti-B	Fucose, galactose		DCe	Dce
AA or AO	A	Anti-B	N-Acetylgalactosamine		DcE	dCe
BB or BO	B	Anti-A	Galactose		DCE	dcE
AB	AB	Neither	—		Dce	dCE

RBC, red blood cell.
From Johnson A, Clarke B. *High-Yield Immunology*. 2nd ed. Lippincott Williams & Wilkins; 2006:62.

3. **Autoimmune reactions** occur in genetically susceptible individuals who produce antibodies against their own cellular membrane antigens by unknown mechanisms. An example is **Goodpasture syndrome**, characterized by glomerulonephritis (GLN) and pulmonary hemorrhage (also termed Masugi type GLN in the animal model). Goodpasture syndrome is included in the spectrum of GLN diseases referred to as anti-glomerular basement membrane disease.
   a. The inciting antigen is a glycoprotein dispersed uniformly on the glomerular basement membrane (GBM).
   b. Susceptible hosts produce an IgG antibody, which binds to the membrane antigen and activates complement, releasing the potent chemotactic factor C5a.
   c. Neutrophils are attracted to the antibody-GBM complex where they release lysosomal enzymes, causing severe necrosis of the glomeruli and a loss of filtration capacity.
   d. Increased risk of disease is associated with human leukocyte antigen (HLA) type DR2 (Table 11.3).

C. **Antigen (ag)-antibody (ab) complex reactions (type III)** occur when circulating ag-ab complexes of small size, with antigen in slight excess, escape phagocytosis and deposit in tissues or on the surface of blood vessels. These complexes cause damage by activating complement and releasing the chemotactic factor C5a, anaphylatoxins, and clotting factors. Neutrophils are attracted to the area of deposition, releasing lysosomal enzymes that destroy tissue. Examples include:
   1. **Arthus reaction** is a rare inflammatory response to gross, intravascular ag-ab precipitates of intermediate size, occurring when highly sensitized humans or animals are injected with antigen. Complement-activated chemotactic factors, polymorphonuclear (PMN) infiltration, and platelets result in thrombi and hemorrhagic, necrotic lesions.
   2. **Serum sickness** occurs following injection of foreign serum or its products. It is characterized by a complement-dependent, systemic reaction with fever, pruritic rash, lymphadenopathy, and joint pains.
      a. The incidence of this condition is rare since the use of such products is restricted to several toxic diseases and immunosuppression.
      b. A similar but milder allergic vasculitis can be elicited by drugs (eg, sulfonamides, penicillin, cephalosporins, Dilantin, and thiourea).
   3. **Polyarteritis nodosa (PAN)** is characterized by continuous trauma to arteriolar walls due to the deposition of circulating ag-ab complexes, causing thrombosis and interruption of blood flow. Hepatitis B antibody complexes are frequently involved.

Table 11.3 Association of Human Leukocyte Antigens With Disease

Disorder	HLA Type	Risk[a]
Ankylosing spondylitis	B 27	87
Dermatitis herpetiformis	DR 3	56
Reactive arthritis	B 27	40
Insulin-dependent diabetes	DR 3/DR 4	33
Psoriasis vulgaris	C 6	13
Goodpasture syndrome	DR 2	13
Rheumatoid arthritis	Dw 4/DR 4	10
Systemic lupus erythematosus	DR 3	5
Pernicious anemia	DR 5	5

HLA, human leukocyte antigen.
[a]Times more likely to acquire the disorder than a person who does not have the specific HLA type.
From Johnson A, Clarke B. *High-Yield Immunology.* 2nd ed. Lippincott Williams & Wilkins; 2006:23.

4. **GLN** is characterized by soluble ag-ab complexes depositing on and behind the basement membrane of the kidney, causing an inflammatory response.
   a. Complexes can be detected with fluorescent antibody against either the antigen, antibody, or complement, as a lumpy-bumpy pattern of fluorescence due to the random deposition of the complexes.
   b. Antigens implicated most often are DNA, insulin, thyroglobulin, and group A nephritogenic streptococci.
   c. Damage is due to the release of lysosomal enzymes by PMNs attracted by chemotactic agents, which destroy the glomeruli, resulting in loss of filtration.

5. **Systemic lupus erythematosus** (**SLE**) is a chronic, exacerbating inflammatory disease usually presenting in women ages 20 to 45. Its cause is unknown, but it may be initiated by an antibody response against bacterial or viral DNA followed by the loss of regulatory control of self-tolerance. The clinical pattern is mainly associated with polyarthralgia or arthritis. An ultraviolet light–induced skin rash, facial "butterfly rash," can be seen (Figure 11.2). Pleurisy, pericarditis, vasculitis, and rheumatoid factor may also be present.
   a. SLE is characterized by the formation of autoantibodies to many **endogenous** antigens, including RBCs, white blood cells (WBCs), platelets, double-stranded (ds) RNA, and various nuclear antigens (antinuclear antibodies), with anti-dsDNA predominating.
   b. anti-dsDNA, anti-dsRNA, and other circulating complexes in slight antigen excess lodge randomly in the kidney, giving rise to the **cardinal lesion of GLN**.
   c. A lumpy-bumpy pattern of fluorescence distinguishes lupus GLN from the smooth pattern seen in the **Masugi** type of GLN, in which the kidney antigen is dispersed uniformly.

6. **Rheumatoid arthritis** is a chronic, recurrent inflammatory disease thought to be initiated by an unknown antigen that stimulates local antibody formation in the synovium. Approximately 70% of patients possess the HLA-DR4 haplotype. Inflammation of the pannus and loss of cartilage characterize the joint lesions.
   a. Union of the antigen with the local antibody alters the tertiary structure of the latter, revealing "buried" amino acid sequences now recognized as foreign by the immune system.
   b. These newly available epitopes stimulate the production of an antibody, usually IgM, termed **rheumatoid factor**, which reacts with the Fc domain of IgG molecules (ie, an antibody against a now "foreign" antibody). As a consequence, IgM-IgG complexes form in synovial fluid, activate complement, and release chemokines. PMNs are attracted, which, while attempting to phagocytize the complexes, release lysosomal enzymes that destroy articular cartilage.
   c. T-cell–mediated delayed-type hypersensitivity (TDTH) cells predominate and contribute to the damage, as do macrophages, which release IL-1, IL-6, and TNF. Osteoclasts emerge, which injure bone.
   d. Rheumatoid factor, as one diagnostic sign, can be detected by latex agglutination tests employing IgG-coated latex particles added to the patient's serum.
   e. Rheumatoid arthritis is also classified as an autoimmune disease.

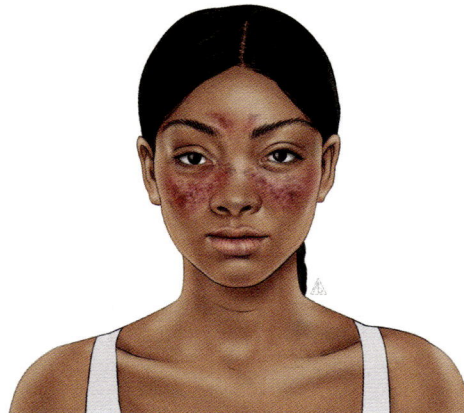

FIGURE 11.2. Systemic lupus erythematosus (SLE). Pattern of the "butterfly" rash often observed with SLE. (Image credit to Audrey Bell.)

D. Delayed-type hypersensitivity (type IV) reactions are effected by sensitized T cells, macrophages, and NK cells on direct contact with the target cell. Antibody is not involved. The basic lesion is an inflammatory response induced by activated macrophages, cytotoxic T lymphocytes, and NK cells to intracellular-dwelling microorganisms as well as reactivity to small molecular chemical irritants.

1. The **tuberculin skin test** exemplifies delayed-type hypersensitivity reactions in internal organs (eg, lungs). It identifies humans exposed to, or actively infected with, *Mycobacterium tuberculosis* and epitomizes delayed-type hypersensitivity activity to other intracellular-dwelling organisms.

   a. The patient suspected of having been exposed to the organism is injected intradermally with an antigenic extract of *M. tuberculosis* (called purified protein derivative [PPD]).

   b. A contained lesion of induration and erythema, peaking in 1 to 2 days, results from the inflammatory response induced by sensitized T-cell action at the site of PPD deposition.

   c. The skin lesion is initiated by Langerhans cell presentation of antigen to **previously sensitized TDTH** cells that have been recruited to the site of antigen deposition by chemokines.

   d. Subsequent antigen-presenting cells (APCs) and T-cell–secreted cytokines and chemokines attract PMNs followed by CD4$^+$ T cells. A nonspecific perivascular accumulation of monocytic or macrophage cells results in the destruction of the organisms, tissue, or both.

2. **Granulomatous reactions** occur if the microbial antigens persist in the tissues and continue to stimulate host reactivity.

   a. IL-1 and IL-8 are released in response and attract an influx of inflammatory cells.

   b. IL-4 and interferon (IFN)-γ promote the retention of macrophages and cause the fusion of monocytes at the site, leading to the formation of an **epithelioid cell granuloma** derived from macrophages, histiocytes, and epithelioid cells.

3. **Contact dermatitis** can occur following the deposition of small molecular weight chemicals (haptens) or other irritants into the skin of a previously sensitized individual, causing a cell-mediated immunity (CMI) reaction (**Figure 11.3**).

   a. The haptenic agent becomes antigenic by combining with intradermal host proteins as carriers via NH_3 or sulfhydryl (S) groupings. Langerhans cells and endothelial cells serve as APCs.

   b. Subsequent re-exposure to the agent results in the release of chemokines and cytokines, monocytic or macrophage infiltration, and the formation of a **vesiculating lesion** with erythema and induration.

   c. Common eliciting agents include nickel, dinitrochlorobenzene, rubber, poison ivy, and poison sumac.

• • • Clinical Pearl

An interdisciplinary approach involving specialists, such as rheumatologists, dermatologists, and endocrinologists, is necessary to manage complex diseases and ensures comprehensive care for patients with immunologic disorders.

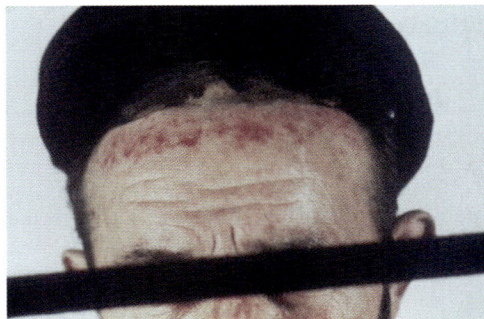

FIGURE 11.3. Contact dermatitis. Forehead rash caused by an irritant in the patient's cap. (Courtesy of Centers for Disease Control Public Health Image Library [PHIL], image 4486.)

III. IMMUNODEFICIENCY DISEASES

A. These conditions occur mainly during the prenatal period or early childhood. A depressed immune response is also associated with the aging process.

1. The child presents with a history of **recurrent infections** verified by below-normal levels of IgG, IgM, or IgA, or abnormal T cell:B cell or CD4:CD8 ratios, as well as a diminished response to standard vaccines in vivo.

2. Since both T and B cells possess specific membrane markers (CD3 on T cells and membrane-bound IgM or CD19 or CD20 on B cells), they can be counted with a fluorescent microscope following the addition of the respective fluorescent-labeled, monoclonal antibody to a blood smear.

3. Monoclonal antibodies against CD4 and CD8 differentiate T-helper and suppressor subtypes, respectively.

B. Transient physiologic hypogammaglobulinemia occurs **normally** in infants aged approximately 3 to 6 months. Although infants are born with adult levels of placentally transferred IgG, this level diminishes due to:

1. The slow disappearance of maternal antibody, which has a half-life of 22 to 28 days.

2. The infant's early low rate of synthesis of secretable immunoglobulins.

C. X-linked agammaglobulinemia (Bruton disease) is a sex-linked (male) disorder that affects infants around the ages of 5 to 6 months. These patients present with recurrent pyogenic infections (eg, *Streptococcus* and *Hemophilus*) and digestive tract disorders. Although the thymus, CMI, and reactivity to viral infections appear normal, very few mature B cells are found.

1. The defect has been found to occur in the transition from pre-B to B cells in the bone marrow and involves the loss of a tyrosine kinase gene.

2. The absence of tonsils and germinal centers, as well as B cells and antibodies, is diagnostic.

3. Treatment involves prophylactic transfer of adult serum immunoglobulin to diminish infections.

D. Dysgammaglobulinemia describes an immunoglobulin deficiency in which the patient has decreased levels of a selective immunoglobulin class (usually IgA, with 1 in 600-800 individuals affected). Mucosal surface protection is diminished or lost.

1. Although the number of IgA-bearing cells is normal, they fail to differentiate into secreting plasma cells.

2. An increased susceptibility to autoimmune diseases is seen.

E. Patients with **congenital thymic aplasia (DiGeorge syndrome)** exhibit poorly developed or absent thymus and parathyroid glands, resulting in depressed CMI. Infections caused by opportunistic organisms (eg, *Candida, Pneumocystis,* viruses) occur in the absence of T cells. The disorder is not hereditary but is caused by an unknown intrauterine injury to the third and fourth pharyngeal pouches that occurs around week 12 of development.

1. The germinal centers, plasma cells, and serum immunoglobulins appear normal.

2. The absence of parathyroid glands results in hypocalcemia and tetany.

3. Vaccination with live vaccines (eg, measles) is contraindicated.

F. Chronic mucocutaneous candidiasis is a highly specific T-cell disorder characterized by an absence of immunity to *Candida*. Patients have apparently normal T-cell and B-cell absolute numbers and functions. Approximately 50% of patients also have endocrine dysfunctions (eg, hypothyroidism) (Figure 11.4).

G. Wiskott-Aldrich syndrome is a sex-linked (male) disorder occurring mainly in children. It features thrombocytopenia (bleeding), eczema, and recurrent infections. A poor response to bacterial capsular polysaccharide antigens is seen. An increased incidence of lymphoreticular malignancies or lymphomas may occur.

1. Depressed CMI and a low serum IgM level are seen, but IgG and IgA levels appear normal.

2. The primary defect is on the short arm of the X chromosome and may result in an absence of specific glycoprotein receptors on cells and platelets.

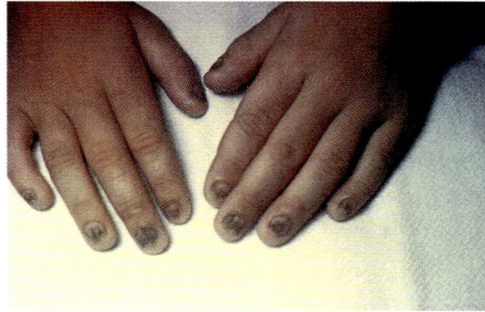

FIGURE 11.4. Cutaneous candidiasis. Persistent *Candida* infection of the nailbeds, apparent by the malformation and darkened coloration and the nail. (Courtesy of Centers for Disease Control Public Health Image Library [PHIL], image 15633.)

H. Severe combined immunodeficiency disease (SCID) is a rare disorder characterized by a genetic defect in stem cells that results in the absence of the thymus gland and T and B cells. Affected children are extremely susceptible to infections and have a very short lifespan.
   1. A deficiency in the enzyme adenosine deaminase (ADA) occurs in 50% of patients. This deficiency results in the accumulation of toxic deoxyadenosine triphosphate (DATP), which inhibits ribonucleotide reductase and prevents DNA synthesis.
   2. A mutation in the γ chain of the IL-2 receptor gene is found in other patients with SCID.

I. Chronic granulomatous disease (CGD) results from a genetic defect in the nicotinamide adenine dinucleotide phosphate (NADPH) oxidase system in neutrophils. Patients are inordinately susceptible to infections by age 2 years, especially to organisms of low virulence.
   1. Neutrophil bactericidal activity (ie, respiratory burst) is defective due to depressed NADPH oxidase, superoxide dismutase activity, and decreased hydrogen peroxide levels.
   2. Diagnosis is based on the failure of neutrophils and macrophages to reduce a nitroblue tetrazolium dye.
   3. Treatment with IFN-γ has been successful.

J. Acquired immune deficiency syndrome (AIDS) is caused by the human immunodeficiency virus (HIV) (see Chapters 4 and 5), whose major target cell is the $CD4^+$ T_h cell and its lysis. Macrophages, astrocytes, and dendritic cells with much lower membrane levels of CD4 can also be infected. Depletion of the T_h cell population results in a loss of cytokines and the capacity to activate other immunocompetent cells. Consequently, infections by endogenous and nosocomial agents predominate.
   1. Common infecting organisms include *Pneumocystis*, cytomegalovirus (CMV), *Toxoplasma*, *Candida*, *Mycobacterium*, herpesvirus, and *Cryptococcus*.
   2. HIV binds to the CD4 receptor and an obligate chemokine coreceptor (CXCR4 or CCR5) via gp120. Membrane fusion and entry of the virus through the cell membrane are mediated by gp41 (**Figure 11.5**).
   3. A viral reverse transcriptase transcribes the viral RNA into DNA, and its integration into the target cell genome is facilitated by an integrase.
   4. Following activation of the infected T cell by other viruses or antigens, the now provirus is transcribed, translated into viral proteins, assembled, and replicated, leading to lysis of the host cell by extensive viral budding.
   5. The indirect enzyme-linked immunosorbent assay (ELISA) test detects the antibody to HIV in a patient's serum, which is confirmed by Western blot testing, differentiation immunoassay or nucleic acid testing.

K. Functional deficiencies in any of the many cytokines and chemokines or their receptors could contribute to an immunodeficient state.

L. HLAs determine individual susceptibility to immunologic disorders and infectious agents (Table 11.3).

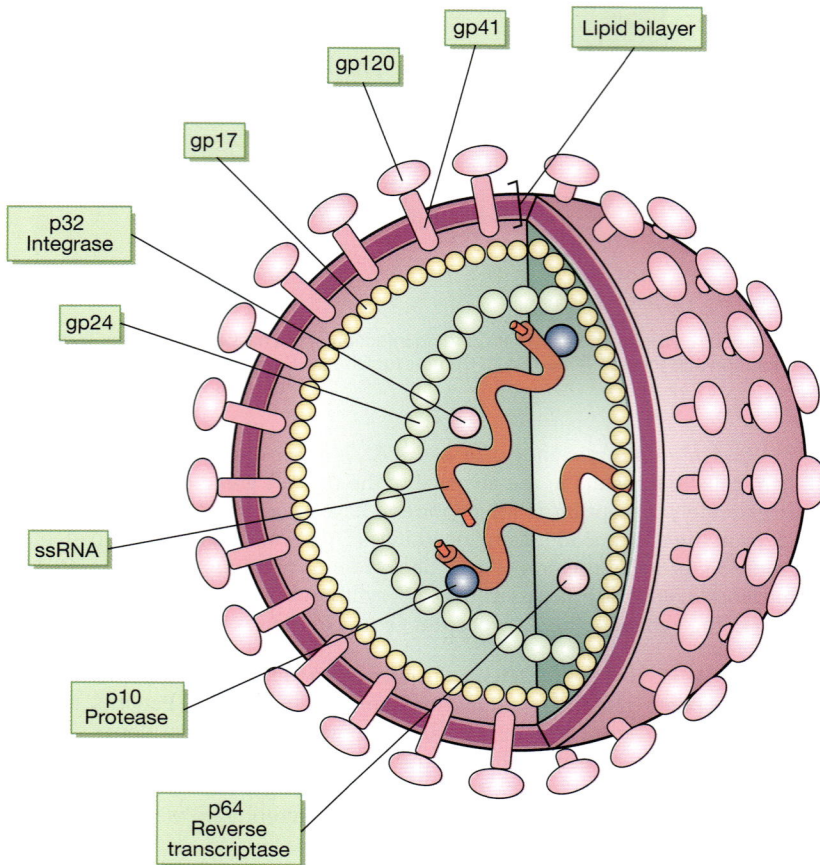

FIGURE 11.5. Components of the human immunodeficiency virus (HIV). The virus consists of an envelope formed from glycoproteins (eg, gp120 and gp41) that houses several core proteins. The virus has several genes that code for enzymes (eg, integrase, reverse transcriptase, protease) that play a role in integrating viral DNA into the host genome and degrading polyprotein precursors into smaller proteins and peptides. (Redrawn from Johnson A, Clarke B. *High-Yield Immunology.* 2nd ed. Lippincott Williams & Wilkins; 2006.)

● ● ● **Clinical Pearl**

Exercise caution when vaccinating patients with immunodeficiency disorders. Live attenuated vaccines can pose a risk of secondary infections due to vaccination strains. Another consideration may be the possibility of a suboptimal response to vaccine antigens.

IV. AUTOIMMUNE DISORDERS

A. These occur as a result of a breakdown in the regulation of the self-tolerant state characteristic of healthy humans.
   1. Humoral immunity (HI) or CMI against their own tissues results. Tolerance to self-antigens is specific for the inducing epitope and is more readily induced and lasts longer in T cells than in B cells.
   2. Suppression of autoreactive T lymphocytes has recently been ascribed to the convergence of $CD4^+$ T lymphocytes into regulatory T cells (Tregs) by FoxP3, a suppressive protein. Their impact on preventing certain autoimmune disorders is being assessed.

B. Self-tolerance is hypothesized to be caused by clonal deletion, clonal anergy, or peripheral suppression.

1. **Clonal deletion** is thought to occur when immature CD4$^+$ T cells, which bear receptors for endogenous molecules, are deleted after contact with self-antigens in the neonatal thymus gland. Similarly, immature B cells with self-reactive receptors are eliminated after contact with potential self-antigens in the bone marrow.

2. **Clonal anergy** describes the loss of T-cell and B-cell functions after exposure to antigens in the absence of mandatory costimulatory signals or following exposure to cells lacking major histocompatibility complex (MHC) class II molecules.

3. **Peripheral suppression** can occur if CD8$^+$ T cells or macrophages secrete cytokines (eg, transforming growth factor [TGF]-β), which downregulate the immune response, or if high-dose or low-dose antigen produces an anergic state.

C. The occurrence of an autoimmune disorder in a previously healthy individual can be reasoned to occur in several different ways, varying with the disorder.

1. **Microbial antigens** that cross-react with human tissue antigens have been demonstrated in *Streptococci*, which cross-react with sarcolemmal heart muscle and the kidney. Antimicrobial DNA antibodies react with cells from patients with SLE. Although an "autoimmune" reaction against the patient's tissues is induced, the antigenic stimulus is of exogenous origin.

2. **"Hidden" antigenic determinants** that were unavailable during fetal clonal deletion can become available following damage by surgery. Illustratively, patients with rheumatoid arthritis who form rheumatoid factors, mainly IgM antibodies, against the Fc fragment of IgG.

3. **Adsorption of a foreign hapten** (eg, quinidine, sulfathiazole) onto an endogenous molecule or cell (eg, platelets) leads to the formation of an antigenic hapten-carrier complex. Antibodies to the drug are formed and react with the drug on the platelet membrane. Complement activation occurs, resulting in platelet lysis.

4. If the normally occurring **suppression by T regulatory cells** of B-cell clones that arise with idiotype specificity for self-antigens is lost or diminished, autoantibodies may result. An inordinate switch from T_h1 to T_h2 cell activation during antigenic stimulus may favor autoantibody synthesis.

D. Systemic autoimmune disorders

1. **SLE** is an episodic multisystemic disease with major lesions including an erythematous rash, vasculitis, arthritis, and nephritis. Multiple autoreactive antibodies against diverse cellular constituents are formed.

2. **Rheumatoid arthritis** is a chronic, systemic inflammatory disease characterized by granulation tissue (pannus) formation and subcutaneous nodules in joints. IgG-IgM complexes activate complement, resulting in lesions.

3. **Sjögren syndrome** is characterized by autoantibodies formed against salivary duct antigens, lymphocytic infiltration, and immune complex formation in the salivary glands. Clinical features primarily occur in postmenopausal women and include dryness of the mouth, trachea, bronchi, eyes, nose, vagina, and skin. It may occur secondary to rheumatoid arthritis and SLE.

4. **Polyarteritis nodosa** is one of several human vasculitides of varying causes. The condition often involves hepatitis B ag-ab complexes, which are found in the vessel walls of 30% to 40% of patients. Similar lesions can be reproduced in animals using other ag-ab complexes.

● ● ● **Clinical Pearl**

Be aware of atypical presentations of infections in patients who are immunocompromised. Consider broader differential diagnoses when evaluating patient cases, including opportunistic infections.

E. Organ-specific autoimmune disorders

1. **Blood disorders**

   a. **Anemia, leucopenia, and thrombocytopenia** are disorders characterized by antibodies that react with RBCs, WBCs, and platelets, respectively.

b. Multiple myeloma is characterized by the malignant transformation of a single clone of plasma cells, resulting in an excess of IgG or other immunoglobulin class (termed paraproteins). Patients secrete Bence-Jones proteins (monoclonal light chains) in their urine.

2. Central nervous system (CNS) disorders
 a. Allergic encephalomyelitis is a demyelinating disease that can occur after infection or immunization. A nonapeptide isolated from an extract of brain has been implicated as the antigen, since the disorder can be mimicked in animals by injection of the peptide in adjuvant.
 b. Multiple sclerosis is a chronic, relapsing disease of unknown etiology that is characterized immunologically by mononuclear cell infiltrates and demyelinating lesions (plaques) in the white matter of the CNS. A decrease in suppressor cell function and elevated titers to measles and other viruses appear in the cerebrospinal fluid, suggesting a viral etiology.
 c. Patients with **myasthenia gravis** often exhibit thymic hyperplasia or a thymoma, along with muscle weakness and fatigue. A defect in neuromuscular transmission is indicated by the presence of **anti-acetylcholine receptor antibodies**, which bind to the receptor at the postsynaptic membrane of the neuromuscular junction. This results in an inability to transmit the acetylcholine-induced signal to muscle fibers, leading to clinical signs.

3. Endocrine disorders
 a. Chronic thyroiditis (Hashimoto disease, hypothyroidism) is a self-limiting disease with a probable genetic basis that mainly affects women. It is characterized by autoantibodies and CMI to thyroglobulin or thyroid peroxidase, leading to progressive destruction of the thyroid gland. ADCC may be responsible for tissue damage.
 b. Graves disease (hyperthyroidism) is characterized by a diffuse goiter and thyrotoxicosis. T and B cells infiltrate the thyroid gland, leading to the formation of autoantibodies against the thyroid-stimulating hormone (TSH) receptor. These autoantibodies compete with TSH, binding to the TSH receptor site and inducing uncontrolled TSH-like activity.
 c. Type 1 diabetes mellitus (insulin-dependent diabetes, juvenile-onset diabetes) is characterized by the destruction of insulin-producing cells in the pancreas. Both HI and CMI against islet cells may play a role. There is no evidence for an autoimmune pathogenesis for non–insulin-dependent (maturity onset, type 2) diabetes.

4. Gastrointestinal (GI) tract disorders
 a. Pernicious anemia is caused by impaired GI absorption of vitamin B_{12}, resulting in weakness and chronic fatigue. It occurs secondary to T-cell damage in the gastric parietal cell. The latter normally synthesizes intrinsic factor, the agent responsible for the transport of vitamin B_{12} into the blood. Antiparietal cell and anti-intrinsic factor antibodies, which block the transport function of intrinsic factor, are found in most patients. Vitamin B_{12} injections bypass the need for gastric absorption and correct the deficiency.
 b. Ulcerative colitis is characterized by chronic inflammatory lesions that are confined to the rectum and colon, accompanied by infiltration of monocytes, lymphocytes, and plasma cells. Patients' lymphocytes exert cytotoxicity against colonic epithelial cells in culture, and some may have antibodies that cross-react with *Escherichia coli*, but the disease is of unknown etiology.
 c. Crohn disease is a chronic inflammatory granulomatous disease that involves T and B cells, macrophages, and neutrophils. The disease usually occurs in the submucosal area of the terminal ileum. While microbial involvement has been suspected, no definitive microbial etiology has been established.

● ● ● Clinical Pearl

Be aware of the differences in pediatric and adult presentations of immunologic disorders. Differentiate children who may present with recurrent infections or failure to thrive from adults who may present with autoimmune manifestations or malignancies.

Review Test

Directions: Select the one lettered answer that is best in each case. Commit to and write down your answers before checking the answers and explanations. Each of the numbered items in this section is followed by answers with explanations, in the following section.

1. A 22-year-old female student presents with excessive fatigue for the past 2 months. Polyarthralgia and vasculitis are noted on examination. Laboratory tests reveal multiple autoantibodies, including anti-dsDNA. Which of the following is the most logical diagnosis?

(A) Hashimoto thyroiditis
(B) Multiple myeloma
(C) Sjögren syndrome
(D) SLE

2. A 42-year old female presents with chronic fatigue, difficulty sleeping, a rapid heartbeat, and bulging eyes. Laboratory tests reveal autoantibodies to TSH. Which of the following is the most likely diagnosis?

(A) Cancer of the thyroid
(B) Graves disease
(C) Hashimoto disease
(D) Pernicious anemia

3. A 19-year-old pregnant student presents at her health service allergy clinic with rhinorrhea, sneezing, itching, and conjunctivitis. A radioallergosorbent test finds IgE antibodies to ragweed antigens. Which of the following characteristics is typical of this condition?

(A) Desensitization can occur with repeated injection of small doses of IgE.
(B) Drugs that elevate cGMP can reduce symptoms.
(C) IL-4-mediated IgE synthesis has increased.
(D) Placental transfer of ragweed antibody can sensitize her unborn child.

4. Goodpasture syndrome is characterized by GLN in genetically susceptible individuals. Which of the following is the responsible antigen?

(A) Circulating antigen-antibody complex
(B) Complement (C5a)-induced influx of neutrophils
(C) Glycoprotein dispersed uniformly on the GBM
(D) Rheumatoid factor

5. If myasthenia gravis is suspected in a 48-year-old female presenting with muscle weakness and a thymoma, which autoantibody should laboratory tests reveal?

(A) Acetylcholine receptor
(B) Intrinsic factor
(C) Rheumatoid factor
(D) TSH

6. Which of the following is a characteristic of patients with SLE?

(A) Absence of antibodies to dsDNA
(B) Antibody against the thyroid receptor
(C) Linear deposition of immunoglobulin on the GBM
(D) Vasculitis
(E) All of the above

7. What is the underlying defect in a 5-year-old with CGD?

(A) Dysgammaglobulinemia
(B) Inability of PMNs to ingest bacteria
(C) Inability of PMNs to kill already-ingested bacteria
(D) Reduced levels of C′5a

8. Which autoimmune disease is characterized by demyelinating lesions, increased IgG in the spinal fluid, and chronic relapsing occurrences?

(A) Congenital thymic aplasia
(B) Multiple sclerosis
(C) Myasthenia gravis
(D) SLE
(E) Ulcerative colitis

9. A neonate is diagnosed with SCID, especially considering a previous sibling's death from the same condition. Which of the following would confirm the diagnosis?

(A) Absence of neutrophils
(B) Deficiency in adenosine deaminase and loss of this enzyme activity
(C) Deficiency in the NADPH oxidase system
(D) Presence of the thymus but absence of the bursal equivalent

10. Which of the following characterizes chronic inflammatory disease confined to the rectum?

(A) Graves disease
(B) Myasthenia gravis
(C) SLE
(D) Ulcerative colitis
(E) Wiskott-Aldrich syndrome

11. What autoimmune disease is characterized by antibodies against intrinsic factor?

(A) Congenital agammaglobulinemia
(B) Dysgammaglobulinemia
(C) Graves disease
(D) Pernicious anemia
(E) Wiskott-Aldrich syndrome

12. Which of the following is an autoimmune disease characterized by absence of T cells, hypocalcemia, and tetany with lowered CMI?

(A) CGD
(B) Congenital thymic aplasia
(C) Multiple sclerosis
(D) SLE
(E) Ulcerative colitis

13. Which of the following is an autoimmune state characterized by a triad of thrombocytopenia, eczema, and recurrent infections?

(A) Congenital agammaglobulinemia
(B) Myasthenia gravis
(C) Pernicious anemia
(D) SCID
(E) Wiskott-Aldrich syndrome

14. Which of the following would be found in the urine of a patient with multiple myeloma?

(A) Bence-Jones proteins
(B) Complement components
(C) Heavy chains
(D) Fc chains

15. A 25-year-old man presents to his primary care physician with episodic shortness of breath, wheezing, chest tightness, and coughing, especially at night and early morning. He reports a similar history occurred during his childhood. The symptoms have worsened recently, being triggered by exposure to cold air, strong odors, and pet dander. He has no significant history and is a nonsmoker. Pulmonary function tests show reversible airflow limitation after administration of albuterol. Which of the following conditions would be responsible for this person's symptoms?

(A) Anaphylaxis
(B) Asthma
(C) Bruton disease
(D) Rhinitis
(E) SLE

Answers and Explanations

1. **The answer is D.** [II C 5] These signs and symptoms are characteristic of SLE (systemic lupus erythematosus), with antibodies to dsDNA being selective for SLE. Although autoantibodies are present in Hashimoto thyroiditis, anti-dsDNA is absent.

2. **The answer is B.** [IV E 3 b] The autoantibodies to TSH in Graves disease compete with TSH for its receptor site and mimic TSH activity. Pernicious anemia is characterized by antibodies to the gastric parietal cell and intrinsic factor, resulting in an inability to absorb vitamin B_{12}.

3. **The answer is C.** [Table 11.1] The cytokine IL-4 is necessary for the switch to IgE synthesis. Desensitization can occur with repeated injections of allergen, not IgE. IgE antibody does not cross the placenta. Drugs that elevate cGMP enhance symptoms.

4. **The answer is C.** [Table 11.1, II B 3] In contrast to GLN in SLE (where circulating antigen-antibody complexes deposit randomly in the kidney in a lumpy-bumpy pattern), the antigen in Goodpasture syndrome is part of the GBM, and its reaction with antibody produces a linear fluorescent pattern.

5. **The answer is A.** [IV E 2 c] Autoantibodies against acetylcholine receptors are characteristic of myasthenia gravis and are not present in the other conditions.

6. **The answer is D.** [II C 5] Vasculitis is a prominent feature of SLE.

7. **The answer is C.** [III I 2] Patients with CGD lack the enzyme superoxide dismutase and have depressed hydrogen peroxide levels, functional entities in eliminating already-ingested bacteria.

8. **The answer is B.** [IV E 2 b] These symptoms are characteristics of multiple sclerosis. Myasthenia gravis is associated with an anti-acetylcholine receptor antibody, resulting in muscle weakness. Congenital thymic aplasia, SLE, and ulcerative colitis do not have a brain component.

9. **The answer is B.** [III H 1] Absence of adenosine deaminase results in the accumulation of adenosine interfering with DNA synthesis. Although lymphocytes are severely depressed, myeloid cells are present in normal numbers. The thymus does not develop.

10. **The answer is D.** [IV E 4 b] Ulcerative colitis is the only syndrome listed whose chronic inflammation is confined to the rectum.

11. **The answer is D.** [IV E 4 a] Patients with pernicious anemia give rise to antibodies against intrinsic factor that inhibit the transfer of vitamin B_{12} from the stomach to the bloodstream.

12. **The answer is B.** [III E] Congenital thymic aplasia is caused by an unknown intrauterine injury to the third and fourth pharyngeal pouches around week 12 of development. Failure of the parathyroid glands to develop results in tetany and hypocalcemia. Injury to the thymus accounts for the absence of T cells.

13. **The answer is E.** [III G] A primary defect in the short arm of the X chromosome results in thrombocytopenia, eczema, and recurrent infections. Depressed CMI and serum Ig levels along with a poor response to capsular polysaccharide antigens complete the syndrome.

14. **The answer is A.** [IV E 1 b] Bence-Jones proteins are light chains found in the urine of patients with myeloma whose plasma cells are secreting light chains in excess.

15. **The answer is B.** [II A 3] The clinical presentation, reported triggers, and response to albuterol are consistent with asthma. This patient's reversible airflow restriction is a key feature of asthma.

12

Vaccination, Immunization, and Viral Therapeutics

I. IMMUNIZATION

A. Immunization is the most cost-effective weapon available against infectious diseases, as shown in the current (2024) recommended Department of Health and Human Services, Centers for Disease Control and Prevention schedules for children and adolescents (Figures 12.1 and 12.2).

B. Six types of vaccines are currently in use or undergoing testing:
1. **Live attenuated vaccines** permit replication of the organism in the host, increasing antigenic stimulation. Attenuation occurs mainly by passages in cell culture, growth in embryonic tissue or at low temperatures, or by selective deletion of genes involved in pathogenesis.
2. **Killed vaccines** contain organisms that have been inactivated by chemical or physical means. Multiple doses must be given, and adjuvants might be required for a protective response.
3. **Recombinant vaccines** (eg, hepatitis B vaccine): Formulation requires identification of an epitope involved in the organism's pathogenicity. Synthesis of the vaccine antigen follows isolation and expression of the gene coding for the epitope in an appropriate host cell.
4. **Plasmid DNA vaccines** are under development based on the isolation of microbial DNA containing the genes coding for an antigen involved in pathogenicity. Potential advantages of DNA vaccines include stability, low cost, ease of production, and long-lasting protection.
5. **Toxoid vaccines** are made from deactivated toxins. They raise immune responses to toxins released by pathogens instead of the pathogen itself. Toxins can be small molecules or peptides. Boosters are required of unconjugated toxoid vaccines. They are also used in vaccines where they are conjugated to bacterial polysaccharides to make the polysaccharide more immunogenic.
6. **mRNA vaccines**, having long been under development, made a debut with the advent of the COVID vaccines. The vaccine design is based on the **ability of cells to act on modified mRNA transcripts to produce target proteins that elicit an immune response.**

C. Safety concerns
1. Live attenuated vaccines include insufficient attenuation, reversion to wild type, contamination by live organisms or toxins, and patients with unsuspected immunodeficiency.
2. Killed vaccines include contamination by live organisms or toxins, autoimmune or allergic reactions, or incomplete killing.
3. Recombinant vaccines to date are associated with few safety concerns.
4. Plasmid DNA vaccines' continuous stimulus may lead to tolerance or autoimmunity.
5. Toxoid vaccines have very rarely caused seizures, Guillain-Barré syndrome (GBS), or acute disseminated encephalomyelitis (ADEM). A poor immune response may occur in those that are immunocompromised.
6. mRNA vaccines appear to be associated with rarely occurring safety concerns that at present are specific to the COVID vaccines, including thrombosis, stroke, and myocarditis. These may be due to the vaccine viral target.

These recommendations must be read with the notes that follow. For those who fall behind or start late, provide catch-up vaccination at the earliest opportunity as indicated by the green bars. To determine minimum intervals between doses, see the catch-up schedule (Table 2).

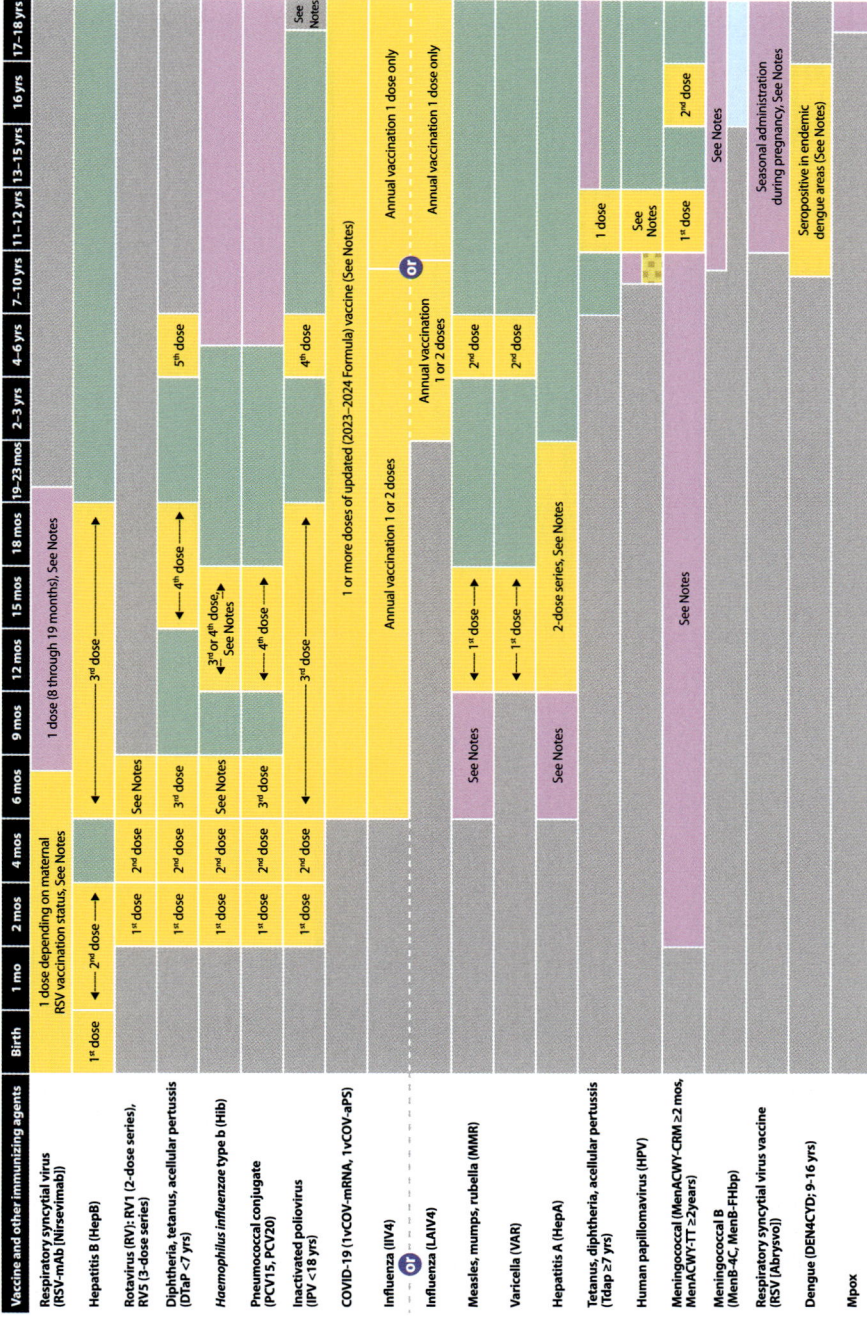

FIGURE 12.1. Recommended immunization schedule for persons aged 18 years or younger, Table 1, United States, 2024. (Access notes referenced in the table at https://www.cdc.gov/vaccines/schedules/hcp/imz/child-adolescent.html)

Source: Centers for Disease Control and Prevention.

The table below provides catch-up schedules and minimum intervals between doses for children whose vaccinations have been delayed. A vaccine series does not need to be restarted, regardless of the time that has elapsed between doses. Use the section appropriate for the child's age. **Always use this table in conjunction with Table 1 and the Notes that follow.**

Vaccine	Minimum Age for Dose 1	Minimum Interval Between Doses			
		Dose 1 to Dose 2	Dose 2 to Dose 3	Dose 3 to Dose 4	Dose 4 to Dose 5
Children age 4 months through 6 years					
Hepatitis B	Birth	4 weeks	**8 weeks and at least 16 weeks after first dose** minimum age for the final dose is 24 weeks		
Rotavirus	6 weeks Maximum age for first dose is 14 weeks, 6 days.	4 weeks	**4 weeks** maximum age for final dose is 8 months, 0 days		
Diphtheria, tetanus, and acellular pertussis	6 weeks	4 weeks	4 weeks	6 months	**6 months** A fifth dose is not necessary if the fourth dose was administered at age 4 years or older *and* at least 6 months after dose 3
Haemophilus influenzae type b	6 weeks	**No further doses needed** if first dose was administered at age 15 months or older. **4 weeks** if first dose was administered before the 1st birthday. **8 weeks (as final dose)** if first dose was administered at age 12 through 14 months.	**No further doses needed** if previous dose was administered at age 15 months or older **4 weeks** if current age is younger than 12 months *and* first dose was administered at younger than age 7 months *and* at least 1 previous dose was PRP-T (ActHIB*, Pentacel*, Hiberix*), Vaxelis*) or unknown **8 weeks *and* age 12 through 59 months (as final dose)** if current age is younger than 12 months *and* first dose was administered at age 7 through 11 months; **OR** if current age is 12 through 59 months *and* first dose was administered before the 1st birthday *and* second dose was administered at younger than 15 months; **OR** if both doses were PedvaxHIB* and were administered before the 1st birthday	**8 weeks (as final dose)** This dose only necessary for children age 12 through 59 months who received 3 doses before the 1st birthday.	
Pneumococcal conjugate	6 weeks	**No further doses needed** for healthy children if first dose was administered at age 24 months or older **4 weeks** if first dose was administered before the 1st birthday **8 weeks (as final dose for healthy children)** if first dose was administered at the 1st birthday or after	**No further doses needed** for healthy children if previous dose was administered at age 24 months or older **4 weeks** if current age is younger than 12 months *and* previous dose was administered at <7 months old **8 weeks (as final dose for healthy children)** if previous dose was administered between 7–11 months (wait until at least 12 months old); **OR** if current age is 12 months or older *and* at least 1 dose was administered before age 12 months	**8 weeks (as final dose)** This dose is only necessary for children age 12 through 59 months regardless of risk, or age 60 through 71 months with any risk, who received 3 doses before age 12 months.	
Inactivated poliovirus	6 weeks	4 weeks	**4 weeks** if current age is <4 years **6 months (as final dose)** if current age is 4 years or older	**6 months (minimum age 4 years for final dose)**	
Measles, mumps, rubella	12 months	4 weeks			
Varicella	12 months	3 months			
Hepatitis A	12 months	6 months			
Meningococcal ACWY	2 months MenACWY-CRM 2 years MenACWY-TT	8 weeks	See Notes	See Notes	
Children and adolescents age 7 through 18 years					
Meningococcal ACWY	Not applicable (N/A)	8 weeks			
Tetanus, diphtheria; tetanus, diphtheria, and acellular pertussis	7 years	4 weeks	**4 weeks** if first dose of DTaP/DT was administered before the 1st birthday **6 months (as final dose)** if first dose of DTaP/DT or Tdap/Td was administered at or after the 1st birthday	**6 months** if first dose of DTaP/DT was administered before the 1st birthday	
Human papillomavirus	9 years	**Routine dosing intervals are recommended.**			
Hepatitis A	N/A	6 months			
Hepatitis B	N/A	4 weeks	**8 weeks and at least 16 weeks after first dose**		
Inactivated poliovirus	N/A	4 weeks	**6 months** A fourth dose is not necessary if the third dose was administered at age 4 years or older *and* at least 6 months after the previous dose.	A fourth dose of IPV is indicated if all previous doses were administered at <4 years **OR** if the third dose was administered <6 months after the second dose.	
Measles, mumps, rubella	N/A	4 weeks			
Varicella	N/A	3 months if younger than age 13 years. 4 weeks if age 13 years or older			
Dengue	9 years	6 months	6 months		

FIGURE 12.2. Recommended immunization schedule for children and adolescents who have been delayed in their vaccine administration, Table 2, United States, 2024. (Access notes referenced in the table at https://www.cdc.gov/vaccines/schedules/hcp/imz/child-adolescent.html)
Source: Centers for Disease Control and Prevention.

D. Protection tests

   1. Used to determine the potency of vaccines.

   2. Active: Following immunization with the vaccine that is being tested, groups of animals are challenged with increasing numbers of microorganisms. The lowest number of microorganisms lethal for 50% of the animals (ie, LD50) is determined and compared to the LD50 in non-vaccinated animals in order to measure the protective power of the vaccine.

   3. Passive: Graded amounts of serum from immunized individuals are transferred to normal animals, which are then challenged with the infectious agent. The highest dilution of serum effective at protecting 50% of the animals (ie, ED50) is determined as a measure of the efficacy of the vaccine.

II. BACTERIAL VACCINES

Prevention has been a major means to reduce many infections. Bacterial vaccines with their immunogens are presented in Table 12.1. Vaccines are listed by the preferred age of administration or special use, certain occupations, or for US travelers to other countries.

Table 12.1 Bacterial Vaccines	
Vaccine and Type[a]	**Contents**
Pediatric vaccines	
Diphtheria, tetanus, acellular pertussis (DTaP) (all inactivated toxins or components)	Diphtheria toxoid
	Tetanus toxoid
	Pertussis toxoid and filamentous hemagglutinin plus one other purified *Bordetella pertussis* component, inactivated pertactin or fimbriae
Haemophilus influenzae type b (conjugate PS-protein vaccine)	Type b polysaccharide (polyribitol) capsule chemically complexed to protein
Pneumococcal conjugate vaccine	13 Capsular polysaccharides from the most common pediatric strains of *Streptococcus pneumoniae* complexed to protein
Special risk groups: children and adults	
Meningococcal polysaccharide: conjugate vaccine (polysaccharide and protein)	Polysaccharides of four capsule (Y, W-135, C, A) types of *Neisseria meningitidis* for those who have late complement component deficiencies or who are asplenic or at risk of becoming asplenic
Vaccines for 11- to 12-year-olds	
Tetanus and diphtheria toxoids and acellular pertussis vaccine ([Tdap]; also give once to adults)	
Meningococcal polysaccharide conjugate vaccine (MCV4) (polysaccharide and protein)	Same as above but to all not previously vaccinated; recommended for college freshmen not vaccinated
Adult vaccines[b]	
Tetanus-diphtheria absorbed (inactivated proteins) (Td)	Toxoids of tetanus and diphtheria (every 10 y)
Pneumococcal polysaccharide	23 Serotypes of capsular polysaccharides for those age >65 y plus many other groups

(continued)

Table 12.1 Bacterial Vaccines (*continued*)	
Vaccine and Type[a]	**Contents**
Anthrax vaccine (only special groups)	Cell-free filtrate of an attenuated strain of *Bacillus anthracis* that makes the protective antigen but not the lethal factor or edema factor ($PA^+LF^-EF^-$)
Cholera vaccine (only special groups)	Live attenuated oral vaccine. Travelers to areas of cholera transmission ages 2-64 y
Salmonella typhi vaccine (only special groups)	In travelers; inactivated vaccine for age 2 y and older with booster every 2 y; live vaccine for age 6 y and older with booster every 5 y
Mycobacterium tuberculosis BCG vaccine (only special groups)	Infants and small children or health care workers in TB endemic areas

BCG, bacillus Calmette-Guérin; TB, tuberculosis.
[a]Live attenuated vaccines are generally contraindicated in women who are immunocompromised or pregnant.
[b]There are many special situations of underlying medical conditions that are not presented here.

III. VIRAL VACCINES AND ANTIVIRALS

A. Immunotherapy

1. **Viral vaccines** lead to **active immunization** and are effective in preventing infections caused by viruses with few antigenic types. Vaccines may use **live virus, killed virus, virion subunits, viral polypeptides, viral DNA, or mRNA** (Table 12.2).
   a. **Live virus vaccines** use **attenuated virus strains** that are relatively avirulent.
      (1) **Advantages:** may be administered in a single dose by the natural route of infection; induces a wide spectrum of antibodies and cytotoxic cells.
      (2) **Disadvantages:** limited shelf life, possible reversion to virulence, and possible production of persistent infection.
      (3) Examples include vaccines for **measles, mumps, rubella, chickenpox, rotavirus, yellow fever**, and some **adenovirus strains**.
   b. **Killed virus vaccines** are prepared from whole virions by **heat** or **chemical inactivation** of infectivity.
      (1) They stimulate antibodies only to surface antigens of the virus.
      (2) **Advantage:** easily combined into **polyvalent vaccines** (vaccines containing virions from several virus strains).
      (3) **Disadvantages:** lack of development of secretory immunoglobulin (Ig)-A, need for boosters, poor cell-mediated response, and possible hypersensitivity reactions.
      (4) Examples include vaccines for **poliovirus (Salk vaccine), rabies, influenza,** and **hepatitis A virus (HAV)**.
   c. **Virion subunit vaccines** are purified proteins (viral receptors) obtained from virions.
      (1) Advantages and disadvantages are the same as those for killed vaccines.
      (2) Example is the **adenovirus vaccine**.
   d. **Viral polypeptides** are **polypeptide sequences of virion receptors** that have been synthesized or result from the purification of proteins made from cloned genes.
      (1) Advantages and disadvantages are the same as those for killed vaccines.
      (2) Examples include hepatitis B virus (**HBV**), hepatitis E virus (**HEV**), and human papillomavirus (**HPV**) vaccines.
   e. **DNA vaccines** are plasmid DNA expression vectors containing **specific viral genes** (usually envelope genes).
      (1) These vaccines elicit both humoral and cell-mediated immune responses.
      (2) DNA vaccines are being evaluated for human use to protect against **human immunodeficiency virus (HIV)** and **influenza viruses**.

Table 12.2   Viral Immunotherapy: Active Immunization (Vaccines)

Virus	Passive Immunization[a]	Live Strain	Killed	Recombinant Viral Protein
Adenovirus	No	Yes (previous military use; no longer available)	No	No
Ebola	No	ERVEBO	No	No
Dengue	No	Dengvaxia	No	No
Hepatitis A virus	Yes	No	Vaqta or Havrix Twinrix	No
Hepatitis B virus	Yes	No	No	Engerix-B or Recombivax-HB Twinrix
Hepatitis E virus	No	No	No	Recombinant capsid protein
Human papilloma virus (types 6, 11, 16, and 18)	No	No	No	Quadrivalent Gardasil or Bivalent Cervarix (types 16 and 18)
Influenza virus	No	Yes	Yes	Flublok Quadrivalent
Japanese encephalitis virus	No	No	IXIARO	No
Measles virus	Yes	Enders	No	No
Mumps virus	No	Jeryl Lynn	No	No
Poliovirus	No	Sabin[b]	Salk	No
Rabies virus	Yes	No	Yes (human diploid cell)	No
Respiratory syncytial virus	Yes	No	No	ABRYSO RSVpreF A/B AREXVY RSVpreF3
Rotavirus	No	Rotarix RotaTeq	No	No
Rubella	No	Ra 27/3	No	No
SARS-CoV-2	No	No	No	Comenity (mRNA) Spikevax (mRNA) Novavax Spike protein
Smallpox (variola) virus Mpox	No	Vaccinia	No	No
Tick-borne encephalitis virus	No	No	Ticovac Neudörf strain	No
Varicella-zoster virus	Yes	Oka	No	Shingrix glycoprotein E
Yellow fever virus	No	17D	No	No

[a]Commercial preparations available.
[b]No longer recommended.

f. mRNA vaccines are transcripts that have been engineered to produce viral proteins of interest, such as SARS-CoV-2 spike protein. The mRNA is contained in lipid nanoparticles that are taken up by dendritic cells that produce the protein from the mRNA and present it on the cell surface to elicit an immune response.

   (1) Advantages are the induction of high neutralizing antibody titers and activation of T-cell responses. They can be quickly designed and produced and made in response to adaptations by the pathogen. Safety profiles are better than those of DNA vaccines in that they cannot integrate into the host cell.

   (2) Disadvantages are not fully known at present but appear to include a short duration of protection, reduced efficacy to variants, and the potential for allergy or cytokine storms. Also, there are storage and stability issues.

2. Passive immunization is acquired by injection of pooled human plasma or γ-globulin fractions from immune individuals into high-risk individuals.

   a. This form of immunization is valuable in the **prevention of some viral diseases but has little value after disease onset.**

   b. Passive immunity is used to prevent **rubella, measles, mumps, HAV, HBV, rabies, and varicella-zoster virus (VZV) infections.** Note that passive immunity can also be used for some bacterial infections such as *Clostridium botulinum, Clostridium tetani,* and *Corynebacterium diphtheriae.*

B. Antiviral agents

1. General characteristics

   a. Antiviral agents must selectively inhibit viral replication without affecting the viability or normal functions of the host cell (**selective toxicity**) (Figure 12.3 and Tables 12.3-12.6).

••• Clinical Pearl

Antiviral therapy is most effective when initiated early in the course of the viral infection, preferably within the first 48 hours of symptom onset.

   b. They work by inhibiting the viral nucleic acid replication process, the penetration and uncoating process, or specific viral enzyme function.

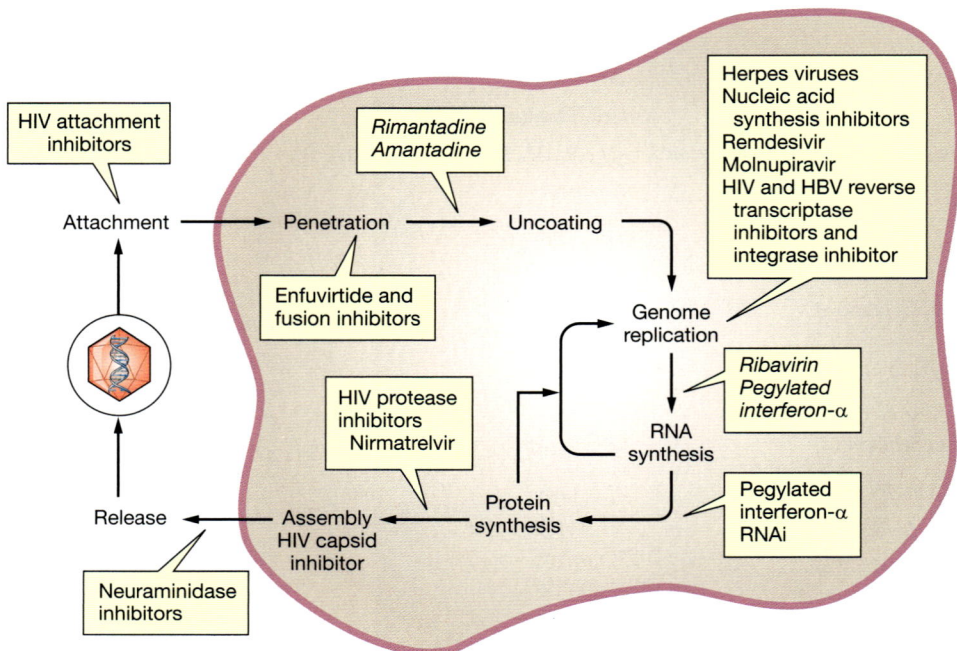

FIGURE 12.3. Sites of antiviral action. HBV, hepatitis B virus; HIV, human immunodeficiency virus.

Table 12.3 Inhibitors of Herpesviruses

Drug	Administration Route	Mechanism of Action	Indications
Acyclovir	Topical or oral	Inhibits HSV and VZV DNA synthesis	Primary genital herpes (HSV), encephalitis and keratitis
			Primary varicella infections
			Localized or ophthalmic zoster
			HSV and VZV in patients who are immunocompromised or have undergone transplant procedures
Cidofovir	Parenteral	Inhibits CMV DNA synthesis	CMV retinitis in patients with AIDS
Famciclovir	Oral	Inhibits HSV and VZV DNA synthesis	Zoster
Foscarnet	Parenteral	Inhibits herpesvirus DNA polymerase	Acyclovir-resistant HSV and VZV infections
			Ganciclovir-resistant CMV retinitis
Ganciclovir	Oral and parenteral	Inhibits herpesvirus DNA synthesis	CMV retinitis
			Disseminated CMV infection of immunocompromised or patients with AIDS
			Prophylaxis for disseminated CMV infections in transplant patients
Penciclovir	Topical	Inhibits herpesvirus DNA synthesis	Herpes cold sores
Trifluridine	Topical	Inhibits herpesvirus DNA polymerase	HSV / Keratoconjunctivitis
Valacyclovir	Oral	Inhibits HSV and VZV DNA synthesis	Herpes labialis, genital herpes, and zoster
Vidarabine	Topical or parenteral	Inhibits herpesvirus DNA polymerase	HSV keratitis and encephalitis (acyclovir is the drug of choice)

AIDS, acquired immunodeficiency syndrome; CMV, cytomegalovirus; HSV, herpes simplex virus; VZV, varicella-zoster virus.

Table 12.4 Inhibitors of Human Immunodeficiency Virus

Drug[a]	Administration Route	Mechanism of Action
A. Nucleoside inhibitors of reverse transcriptase		
Abacavir		
Emtricitabine[b]	Oral	Block incorporation of natural nucleosides to inhibit HIV DNA synthesis
Lamivudine[b]		
Zalcitabine		
B. Nonnucleoside inhibitors of reverse transcriptase		
Delavirdine		
Doravirine	Oral	Noncompetitive blocking of RT catalytic site to inhibit HIV DNA synthesis

(continued)

Table 12.4   Inhibitors of Human Immunodeficiency Virus (*continued*)

Drug[a]	Administration Route	Mechanism of Action
Efavirenz	Oral	Noncompetitive blocking of RT catalytic site to inhibit HIV DNA synthesis
Etravirine		
Nevirapine		
Rilpivirine		
C. Nucleotide inhibitor of reverse transcriptase		
Tenofovir[b]	Oral	Nucleotide that inhibits HIV DNA synthesis
D. Integrase inhibitor		
Bictegravir	Oral	
Cabotegravir	Intramuscular injection	
Dolutegravir	Oral	Inhibits HIV-1 integrase by preventing strand transfer activity
Elvitegravir	Oral	
Raltegravir	Oral	
E. Protease inhibitor		
Atazanavir		
Darunavir		
Fosamprenavir		
Lopinavir	Oral	Inhibits HIV protease to prevent virus maturation
Nelfinavir		
Ritonavir		
F. Attachment inhibitor		
Fostemsavir	Oral	Binds to gp120 blocking attachment to CD4
Maraviroc	Oral	Binds to CCR5 coreceptor for some HIV strains
G. Cell fusion inhibitor		
Enfuvirtide	Subcutaneous injection	Inhibits HIV fusion protein gp41
H. Capsid inhibitor		
Lenacapavir	Oral and subcutaneous injection	Inhibits capsid p24 to prevent protein activities
I. Biologics		
Ibalizumab	Intravenous	Monoclonal antibody causing steric hindrance of HIV interactions with CD4 receptor

AIDS, acquired immunodeficiency syndrome; CCR5, C-C chemokine receptor type 5; CD, cluster of differentiation; HIV, human immunodeficiency virus; RT, reverse transcriptase.
[a]Many of these drugs are formulated into multidrug, multiclass, single-pill combinations to form a simpler antiretroviral therapy (ART) regimen.
[b]Also used for chronic HBV infections.

Table 12.5   Inhibitors of Other Viruses

Drug	Administration Route	Mechanism of Action	Indications
Adefovir	Oral	Inhibits HBV reverse transcriptase	Chronic HBV infection
Baloxavir marboxil	Oral	Inhibits influenza polymerase acidic protein in RNA polymerase complex	Influenza A and B virus infections
Entecavir	Oral	Inhibits HBV reverse transcriptase	Chronic hepatitis B infections
Interferon-α	Parental	Induces antiviral proteins like 2,5-synthase that activates endoribonuclease to degrade viral and cellular RNAs	Chronic HBV and HCV infections
Molnupiravir	Oral	Nucleoside analogue that inhibits nucleic acid synthesis	SARS-CoV-2/COVID
Nirmatrelvir	Oral	Inhibits SARS-CoV-2 main protease	SARS-CoV-2/COVID
Oseltamivir	Oral	Inhibits influenza A and B virus neuraminidase	Influenza A and B virus infections
Peramivir	Intravenous	Inhibits neuraminidase activity	Influenza A and B virus infections
Remdesivir	Oral	Inhibits viral RNA polymerase	Developed for Ebola but has been used for treatment of COVID
Ribavirin	Oral or inhalation	Inhibits nucleic acid polymerases	Severe RSV infection Chronic HCV and IFNs Lassa fever
Rimantadine	Oral	Inhibits influenza virus penetration or uncoating	Prophylaxis for influenza A virus
Telbivudine	Oral	Inhibits HBV reverse transcriptase	Chronic HBV infection
Zanamivir	Inhalation	Inhibits influenza A and B virus neuraminidase	Influenza A and B virus infections

HBV, hepatitis B virus; HCV, hepatitis C virus; IFNs, interferons; RSV, respiratory syncytial virus.

Table 12.6   Direct-Acting Antiviral Oral Agents for Curable Hepatitis C Virus

Drug	Mechanism of Action
Elbasvir	Prevents transcription by targeting NS5A protein
Glecaprevir	Inhibits NS3/4A protease activity
Grazoprevir	
Ledipasvir	Prevents transcription by targeting NS5A protein
Pibrentasvir	
Sofosbuvir	Inhibits NS5B activity
Velpatasvir	Prevents transcription by targeting NS5A protein
Voxilaprevir	Inhibits NS3/4A protease activity

c. Only a few viral infections have antiviral agents (herpesviruses, influenza viruses, hepatitis B and C viruses, respiratory syncytial virus [RSV], and HIV).

d. There are no broad-spectrum antivirals.

● ● ● **Clinical Pearl**

As with antibiotics, adherence to the prescribed regimen and completion of the antiviral course will reduce the occurrence of viral resistance.

2. Inhibitors of attachment, fusion, and uncoating

    a. Maraviroc binds to CCR5 coreceptor of some HIV strains.

    b. Fostemsavir binds to HIV gp120 to block attachment to the CD4$^+$ cell.

    c. Rimantadine and amantadine (no longer recommended) bind to the M2 protein of influenza A virus, which inhibits this ion pore in the virion envelope, thus preventing H$^+$ ion influx and uncoating.

    d. Enfuvirtide inhibits HIV viral fusion protein gp41.

3. Inhibitors of nucleic acid synthesis

    a. Ribavirin is an **analogue of the nucleoside guanosine;** its action varies for different viruses.

      (1) This drug alters cellular nucleotide pools, inhibits viral RNA synthesis, and may cause lethal RNA mutations.

      (2) It is used for severe RSV infections and in combination with IFNα (interferon-α) for chronic hepatitis C virus (HCV) infections.

    b. Acyclovir, valacyclovir, penciclovir, famciclovir, ganciclovir, entecavir, cidofovir, adefovir, abacavir, zalcitabine, tenofovir, emtricitabine, lamivudine, remdesivir, molnupiravir, and telbivudine are **analogues** of **nucleosides/-tides** that prevent DNA chain elongation after recognition and base pairing.

      (1) These drugs are activated by phosphorylation by cellular or viral kinases.

      (2) They are selective inhibitors because (1) there is a higher binding affinity for viral DNA polymerase or (2) DNA synthesis is more rapid in infected cells.

      (3) Examples include many herpes simplex viruses (HSV), VZV, cytomegalovirus (CMV), SARS-CoV-2, and HIV antivirals.

    c. Idoxuridine, trifluorothymidine, and fluorouracil are **analogues of thymidine**, which either (1) inhibit thymidine biosynthesis or (2) replace thymidine in DNA, which leads to misreading of the DNA and mutations.

    d. Foscarnet is a nonnucleoside nucleic acid polymerase inhibitor that binds to and inhibits the DNA polymerase of all herpesviruses and the reverse transcriptase of HIV.

    e. Nevirapine, delavirdine, doravirine, efavirenz, etravirine, and rilpivirine are **nonnucleoside HIV reverse transcriptase inhibitors** that are used in combination therapy with various nucleoside analogue inhibitors of that enzyme.

    f. Bictegravir, cabotegravir, dolutegravir, elvitegravir, and raltegravir inhibit HIV integrase, preventing HIV provirus formation by blocking the copy (c)DNA viral strand from integrating into the host DNA strand.

    g. Sofosbuvir is an inhibitor of HCV NS5B polymerase activity by binding Mg$^+$ ions in the enzyme's active site.

    h. Elbasvir, ledipasvir, pibrentasvir, and velpatasvir are inhibitors of HCV NS5A protein that is involved in the formation and activity of the replication complex.

4. Protease inhibitors

    a. These drugs include **ritonavir, nelfinavir, atazanavir, darunavir, fosamprenavir, and lopinavir for HIV.**

    b. They inhibit the action of HIV protease; used in combination with nucleoside reverse transcriptase inhibitor (NRTI) or non-nucleoside reverse transcriptase (NNRT) or integrase (IN) inhibitors as "cocktail" therapy for HIV.

    c. Glecaprevir, grazoprevir, and voxilaprevir are inhibitors of HCV NS3/4A serine protease activity by blocking the catalytic site of NS3.

    d. Nirmatrelvir is a peptidomimetic that inhibits the main protease activity of SARS-CoV-2 by interfering with the processing of polyprotein precursors.

5. The **HIV capsid inhibitor** lenacapavir prevents p24 protein interactions and thereby blocks its activities.
6. **HIV biologics** are being developed that interfere with HIV virion interactions with its target cell receptor. An example is the monoclonal antibody ibalizumab that blocks HIV from efficiently binding to the CD4 receptor.
7. **Neuraminidase inhibitors**
   a. These drugs include **oseltamivir**, **peramivir**, and **zanamivir.**
   b. They inhibit the neuraminidase of **influenza A and B** viruses; they may be used for prophylaxis as well as treatment.
8. **mRNA inhibitors**
   a. **Fomivirsen** is a synthetic oligonucleotide complementary to a sequence in CMV RNA (an antisense compound). It prevents transcription of early CMV genes.
   b. Was approved for intravitreal therapy of CMV retinitis after other therapies have failed. It is no longer available in the United States.

••• Clinical Pearl

A combination of antiviral drugs can often increase the efficiency of an antiviral therapy such as in the case of HIV.

Directions: Select the *one* lettered answer that is *best* in each case. Commit to and write down your answers before checking the answers and explanations. Each of the numbered items in this section is followed by answers with explanations, in the following section.

1. A 35-year-old man with an AIDS diagnosis is hospitalized with a serious pneumonia. His x-ray shows an interstitial pattern of infection, and laboratory analysis of his sputum indicates the presence of giant cells. Which drug is best to treat this infection?

(A) Foscarnet
(B) Ganciclovir
(C) Ribavirin
(D) Trifluridine
(E) Voxilaprevir

2. An outbreak of respiratory disease that leads to pneumonia occurs in a nursing home. It is characterized by an interstitial x-ray pattern, and zanamivir is an effective treatment. What is the causative agent?

(A) HIV
(B) Influenza A virus
(C) *Legionella pneumonia*
(D) Metapneumovirus
(E) *Mycoplasma pneumonia*

3. For which of the following reasons is a live attenuated vaccine not available for protection from HPV-associated cancer?

(A) E6 and E7 viral proteins are associated with oncogenesis.
(B) The virus does not survive in the mouth and oropharynx.
(C) The virus only grows in human cells.
(D) Viral membrane receptor glycoprotein is very unstable.

4. An emerging pathogen has been associated with serious lower respiratory tract disease. Both atazanavir and darunavir have been demonstrated to be effective in treating the infection. What step in the pathogenesis of the infectious agent is affected by these drugs?

(A) Cross-linking of the agent's cell wall
(B) Inhibition of the agent's DNA replication
(C) Inhibition of the agent's reverse transcriptase
(D) Premature release of the agent's mRNA from the translation complex
(E) Processing of polyproteins

5. A new reverse transcriptase has been discovered. In addition to its effect on HIV disease, which of the following conditions should also be checked for its potential to treat?

(A) Infectious hepatitis
(B) Infectious mononucleosis
(C) Measles
(D) Serum hepatitis
(E) Shingles

6. A recent immigrant from Asia was found to be positive for the tuberculin skin test. To which of the following can the positive result most likely be attributed?

(A) Activation of previously sensitized natural killer (NK) cells
(B) Antibody against mycobacteria plus complement
(C) Niacin production by PPD
(D) Previous Bacillus Calmette-Guérin (BCG) vaccination

7. A strain of influenza A virus is resistant to treatment with oseltamivir. Which of the following is the most likely mechanism for this resistance?

(A) Decreased affinity for the M2 protein
(B) Inability to phosphorylate the antiviral
(C) Mutation in the neuraminidase gene
(D) Synthesis of a β-lactamase

8. A 10-month-old child presents with a temperature of 39.8 °C (103.6 °F) and lethargy. Both Brudzinski and Kernig signs are present. A gram stain of sediment from cerebrospinal fluid (CSF) showed gram-negative rods. Which of the following vaccines could have prevented this disease?

(A) 13-Valent polysaccharide-protein conjugate vaccine
(B) Covalently linked protein-polysaccharide vaccine
(C) Polysaccharide vaccine with 23 different antigens
(D) Quadrivalent capsular-conjugate vaccine
(E) Trivalent killed viral vaccine

9. Which of the following is a nonnucleo-side analogue that inhibits herpesvirus DNA replication?

(A) Acyclovir
(B) Amantadine
(C) Foscarnet
(D) Interferon
(E) Tenofovir

10. The antiviral 2-5A synthetase is induced by which of the following agents?

(A) Acyclovir
(B) Amantadine
(C) Bictegravir
(D) Foscarnet
(E) Interferon
(F) Ribavirin

11. A 1-year-old girl who has received no vaccines because of parental concern of autism develops *Streptococcus pneumoniae* meningitis. Which of the following vaccines might have prevented this infection?

(A) 13-Valent capsular vaccine
(B) 23-Valent polysaccharide vaccine
(C) Conjugate (protein-polysaccharide) vaccine
(D) Toxoid vaccine

12. Which of the following advantages is attributed to live, attenuated vaccines?

(A) The viral strain does not revert to virulent forms.
(B) They do not produce persistent low-grade infections.
(C) They have an unlimited shelf life.
(D) They induce a wide spectrum of antibodies.

13. Which of the following childhood vaccines is most likely to prevent otitis media in young children?

(A) *Haemophilus influenzae*
(B) Measles, mumps, and rubella
(C) Meningococcal
(D) VZV

14. A patient with a chronic cough is given a tuberculin skin test, which shows a zone of induration greater than 15 mm. What is the significance of these results?

(A) Active infection with *Mycobacterium tuberculosis*
(B) Active infection with any of the nontuberculous mycobacteria
(C) Anergy
(D) Antibody titer to *M. tuberculosis*
(E) Previous infection with *M. tuberculosis*
(F) Vaccination with BCG vaccine

15. A 12-day-old neonate is brought in because of parental concern about eye redness and "watering" associated with the conjunctiva of both eyes. Visual examination confirms and also detects several vesicles. Which of the following would be the most appropriate topical treatment?

(A) Acyclovir
(B) Foscarnet
(C) Ribavirin
(D) Zanamivir

16. Which of the following microbes has both a live attenuated vaccine and an inactivated vaccine recommended for those who are immunocompromised, younger than age 2 years, or older than age 60 years?

(A) Diphtheria, tetanus, pertussis
(B) Hepatitis B
(C) Influenza virus
(D) Poliovirus
(E) *S. pneumoniae*

Answers and Explanations

1. **The answer is B.** [III B 3 b (3), Table 12.3] The pneumonia is caused by CMV and is best treated with the CMV antiviral ganciclovir.

2. **The answer is B.** [Figure 12.3; III B 7, Table 12.5] Zanamivir inhibits the viral neuraminidase of both influenza A and B viruses.

3. **The answer is A.** [Chapter 4, VIII B 2] HPV viral proteins E6 and E7 are involved in the normal replication of the virus, but are also associated with the oncogenic properties of the virus. This association makes a live attenuated virus an inappropriate vaccine candidate.

4. **The answer is E.** [Figure 12.3; III B 4 a, b; Table 12.4 E] Both atazanavir and darunavir are antivirals that inhibit the HIV protease, which is involved in the cleavage of HIV polyproteins.

5. **The answer is D.** [Figure 12.3; III B 3 b, Table 12.5] Serum hepatitis is the only disease listed in which the causative agent has a reverse transcriptase involved in replication.

6. **The answer is D.** [Table 12.1] Many individuals from Asia have been immunized against TB with BCG vaccines. Neither sensitized NK cells, niacin, or antibodies are participants in the tuberculin test.

7. **The answer is C.** [Figure 12.3; III B 7 a; Table 12.5] The most common mechanism of resistance to antivirals is a genetic mutation in the viral gene coding for the viral protein that interacts with the antiviral so that the antiviral no longer interacts and is effective.

8. **The answer is B.** [Table 12.5] Based on the description of the disease, the child has bacterial meningitis. The gram stain suggests *H. influenzae* is the causative agent, which is confirmed by latex particle agglutination. The vaccine is a conjugate polysaccharide-protein vaccine as described in choice C. The other vaccines described belong to poliovirus (A), the adult *S. pneumoniae* vaccine (B), the infant *S. pneumoniae* vaccine (D), and the *Neisseria meningitidis* vaccine.

9. **The answer is C.** [Figure 12.3; III B 3 d; Table 12.3] Foscarnet inhibits herpesvirus DNA polymerase directly.

10. **The answer is E.** [Table 12.5] Interferon, a host-encoded glycoprotein that is produced in response to virus infection, induces the synthesis of several antiviral proteins, including 2, 5A synthetase.

11. **The answer is C.** [Table 12.1] The pediatric vaccine is 13-valent; however, it is a 13-valent conjugate vaccine, so the best answer is the protein-polysaccharide conjugate vaccine. The 23-valent polysaccharide (choice B) is the vaccine used for the older and high-risk people.

12. **The answer is D.** [III A 1 a (1)(2)] A live attenuated vaccine has the advantage of producing persistent infection, thus continuously stimulating the immune system with different antigens. A few viral strains in vaccines may revert to virulent form. A disadvantage is their limited shelf life.

13. **The answer is A.** [Table 12.1; Chapter 3, II E 2 a] Of the organisms listed, *H. influenzae* is the one most likely to cause otitis media.

14. **The answer is E.** [Table 12.1; Chapter 11, II D 1] The tuberculin test indicates previous infection with *M. tuberculosis* or *Mycobacterium bovis* from between several weeks to 5 years. It does not provide proof of current active infection with *M. tuberculosis*. The tuberculin test detects cell-mediated immunity and not antibody. If a person is infected with a nontuberculous strain of mycobacteria, usually the skin reaction is smaller. Specific skin tests for some of these nontuberculous strains of mycobacteria are available. Vaccination with BCG vaccine should not result in this large a zone of induration. The newer whole-blood interferon-γ release assays (IGRAs), which also do not distinguish latent tuberculosis infection from tuberculosis disease, are superior to distinguish infected from BCG vaccinated.

15. **The answer is A.** [Table 12.3] This is conjunctivitis caused by HSV-1 or -2, which should be treated by an ophthalmologist with the anti-herpes drug acyclovir. But the child should also be receiving IV acyclovir for potential systemic infection.

16. **The answer is C.** [Table 12.1] Besides the clues of both alive and killed vaccines in routine use, the question noted the vaccine was given across the spectrum of ages. Of the vaccines listed, only pneumococcal, DTP, and influenza fit that criterion. Two influenza vaccines are in current use. The live (attenuated) one is given intranasally and the killed (inactivated) one is injected. *S. pneumoniae* does have two vaccines, but neither is live attenuated; the pediatric pneumococcal vaccine is 13 (used to be 7)-capsular polysaccharides chemically complexed to protein. The 23-valent polysaccharide pneumococcal vaccine is used for anyone 65 years and older. Choice C is poliovirus; in the United States, the attenuated strains were routinely used to vaccinate (Sabin vaccine given orally), but the incidence of vaccine-associated polio became too high. The United States then switched to an injectable, inactivated tetravalent polio vaccine. Hepatitis B vaccine is a recombinant, single-component vaccine with only the hepatitis B surface antigen (HbsAg) present.

13

Clues for Distinguishing Causative Infectious Agents

The infectious agents discussed in this chapter are not intended to be comprehensive lists of pathogens for the diseases, but rather the most common (or at least, with a few exceptions, the most likely to be encountered in the United States). They are most likely to appear in the case-based questions on the United States Medical Licensing Examination (USMLE) step 1 examination. The clues listed relate to clinical symptoms, common laboratory data, and epidemiology. In the flowcharts, the **most common causes are in bold font.**

I. CONJUNCTIVITIS

Various types of infectious agents including viruses, bacteria, chlamydia, and protozoa can infect the eye and cause inflammation of the cornea. Viruses are the most common causative agents. Some of these infections occur in neonates (infants <2 weeks old) following passage through an infected birth canal. Red, irritated eyes are present in all cases. Diagnosis involves the presence or absence of pus, an examination of the conjunctiva for follicles or papillae, and Gram staining of discharge on conjunctival scrapings.

A. Neonate (ophthalmia neonatorum): Neonates can become infected during birth from infected mothers or by normal flora bacteria. Causative organism identification is important because of its potential for further systemic involvement (Figure 13.1).

B. Postnatal: Postnatal infections are usually **self-limiting,** except for those caused by *Staphylococcus aureus, Neisseria gonorrhoeae, Chlamydia*, and herpes simplex virus (HSV), which penetrate into the deeper layers of the eye. Viral infections usually begin unilaterally. **Preauricular adenopathy is present on the involved side in adult viral and adult chlamydia infections and in amoeba infections. Bacterial infections usually produce sticky eyelids.** *S. aureus* and *Moraxella* may produce chronic conjunctivitis (Figure 13.2).

II. PNEUMONIAS

Pneumonias may be classified in several different ways. One common classification is based on the time interval between infection and clinical symptoms (eg, acute and chronic pneumonias). Acute pneumonias include community-acquired and nosocomial pneumonia, determined by where the infectious agents are acquired. Acute pneumonias may also be classified as typical or atypical, depending on their clinical symptoms. The following information combines important aspects of these classifications as well as other (eg, geographic) considerations.

A. Community-acquired pneumonia (CAP): Considerable overlap and patient-dependent variability occur, although some generalizations can be made. Viruses are more common causes of acute disease in children younger than age 2 years.
   1. Acute, typical: Symptoms (abrupt onset, fever higher than 39 °C/102 °F, chills, productive cough, and chest pain) develop 1 to 2 days following infection (Figure 13.3).

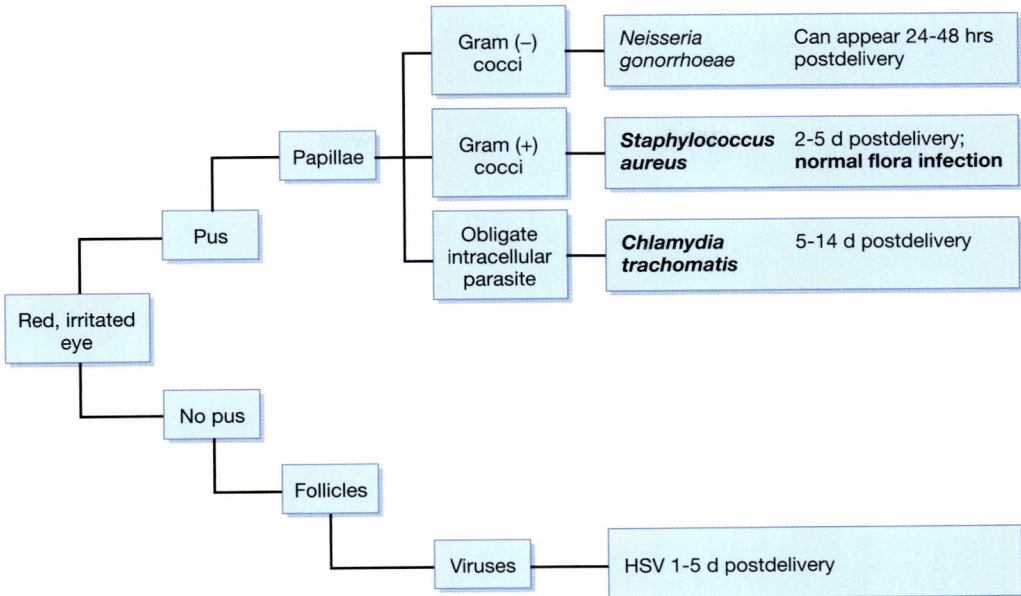

FIGURE 13.1. Neonatal conjunctivitis. HSV, herpes simplex virus.

2. **Acute, atypical:** Symptoms (slower onset, fever <39 °C (102 °F), nonproductive cough, headache, sore throat, and gastrointestinal [GI] symptoms) develop 2 to 10 days following infection; **Gram staining is not helpful in diagnosis** (Figure 13.4).
3. **Chronic pneumonia:** Symptoms are variable; primary infection may be asymptomatic; progresses or reactivates in some individuals to severe pneumonia; some fungal infections are associated with specific geological regions.
   a. **Cavitary lesions on x-ray**
      (1) *Mycobacterium tuberculosis*
         (a) **Primary infection** is **mild** but may cause **Ghon lesions** (areas of fibrosis on x-ray).
         (b) Reactivation or secondary tuberculosis occurs in 10% to 15% of those infected, particularly in middle-aged individuals. Findings include apical cavitary lesions and acid-fast bacilli (AFB) in sputum.
      (2) *Histoplasma capsulatum* causes a progressive nodular to cavitary disease restricted to the Ohio and Mississippi River valleys and related to soil containing bird and bat droppings.
   b. **Variable x-ray patterns** are characteristic of *Nocardia asteroides* and several fungal infections where findings frequently depend on the stage of the **fungal disease**.
      (1) *Blastomyces dermatitidis* (central and eastern North America): Large yeast cells are present in potassium hydroxide (KOH) preparations of sputum.
      (2) *Coccidioides immitis* (**"valley fever"**) (Arizona, Nevada, New Mexico, western Texas, and parts of central and southern California): Upper lobe nodules are frequently visible on x-ray; restricted to thick-walled "spherules" in KOH preparation of sputum; joint pain involved in disease process.
      (3) *Cryptococcus neoformans*: sometimes a single nodule on x-ray; organism is found in pigeon and bird droppings.
      (4) *N. asteroides*: Weakly gram-positive rods are present in branching filaments in sputum.

B. **Nosocomial pneumonia:** These pneumonias are the leading cause of death from nosocomial infections. Risk factors include endotracheal intubation, malnutrition and underlying disease, metabolic acidosis, medications (particularly antibiotics and immunosuppressants), and advanced age (age >70 years). Clinical aids to the identification of specific pathogens are found in the CAP information.
   1. *S. aureus.*
   2. Gram-negative bacilli (*Escherichia coli*, *Klebsiella pneumoniae*, and *Pseudomonas aeruginosa*).

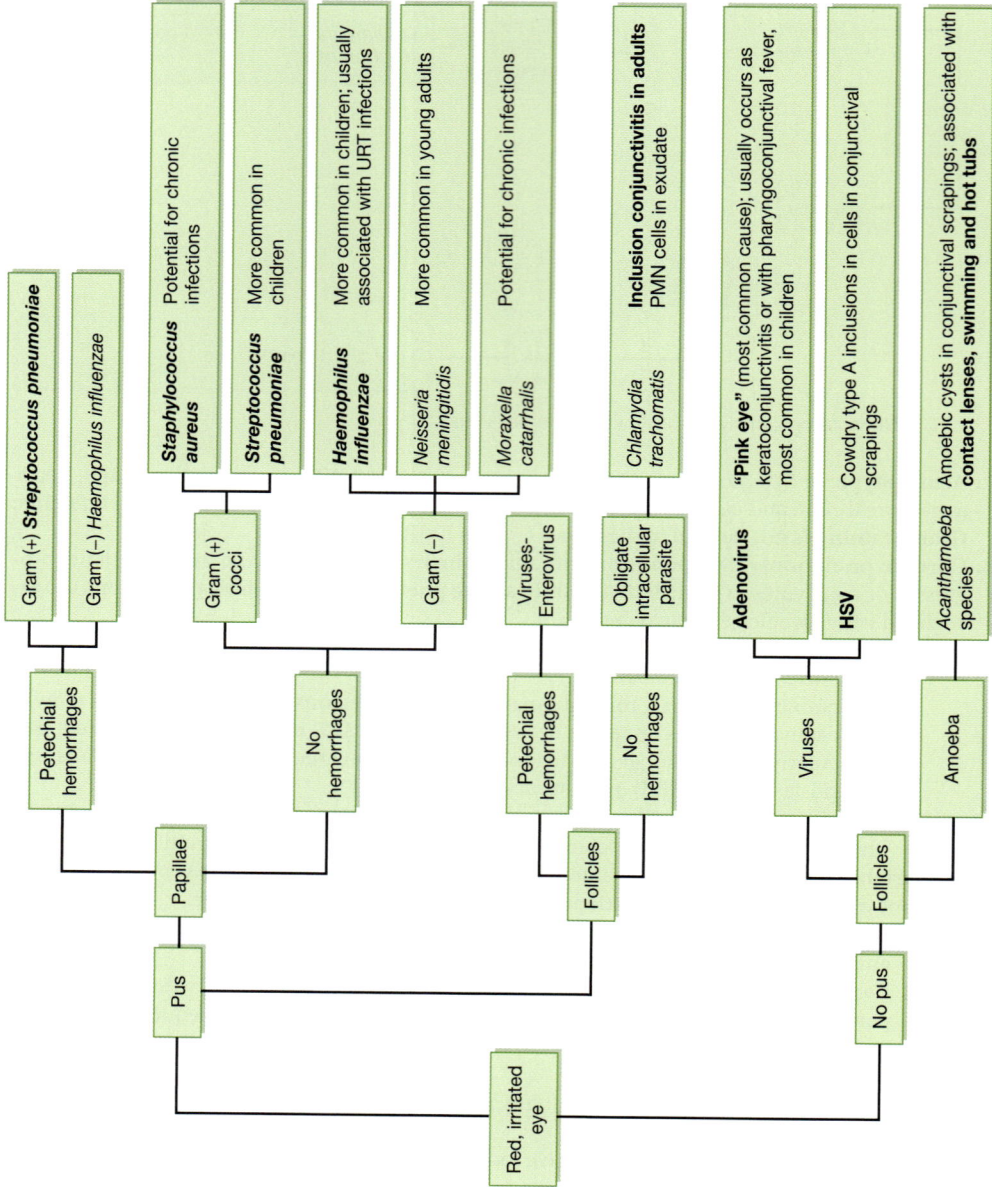

FIGURE 13.2. Postnatal conjunctivitis. HSV, herpes simplex virus; PMN, polymorphonuclear neutrophil; URT, upper respiratory tract.

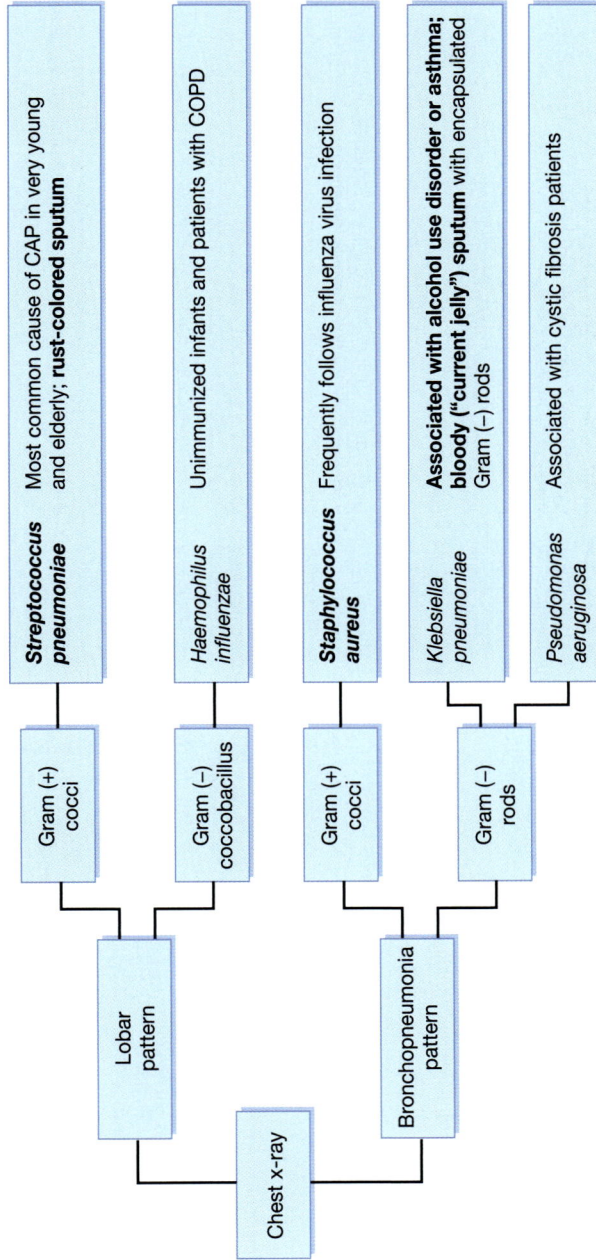

FIGURE 13.3. Acute community-acquired typical pneumonia (CAP). COPD, chronic obstructive pulmonary disease.

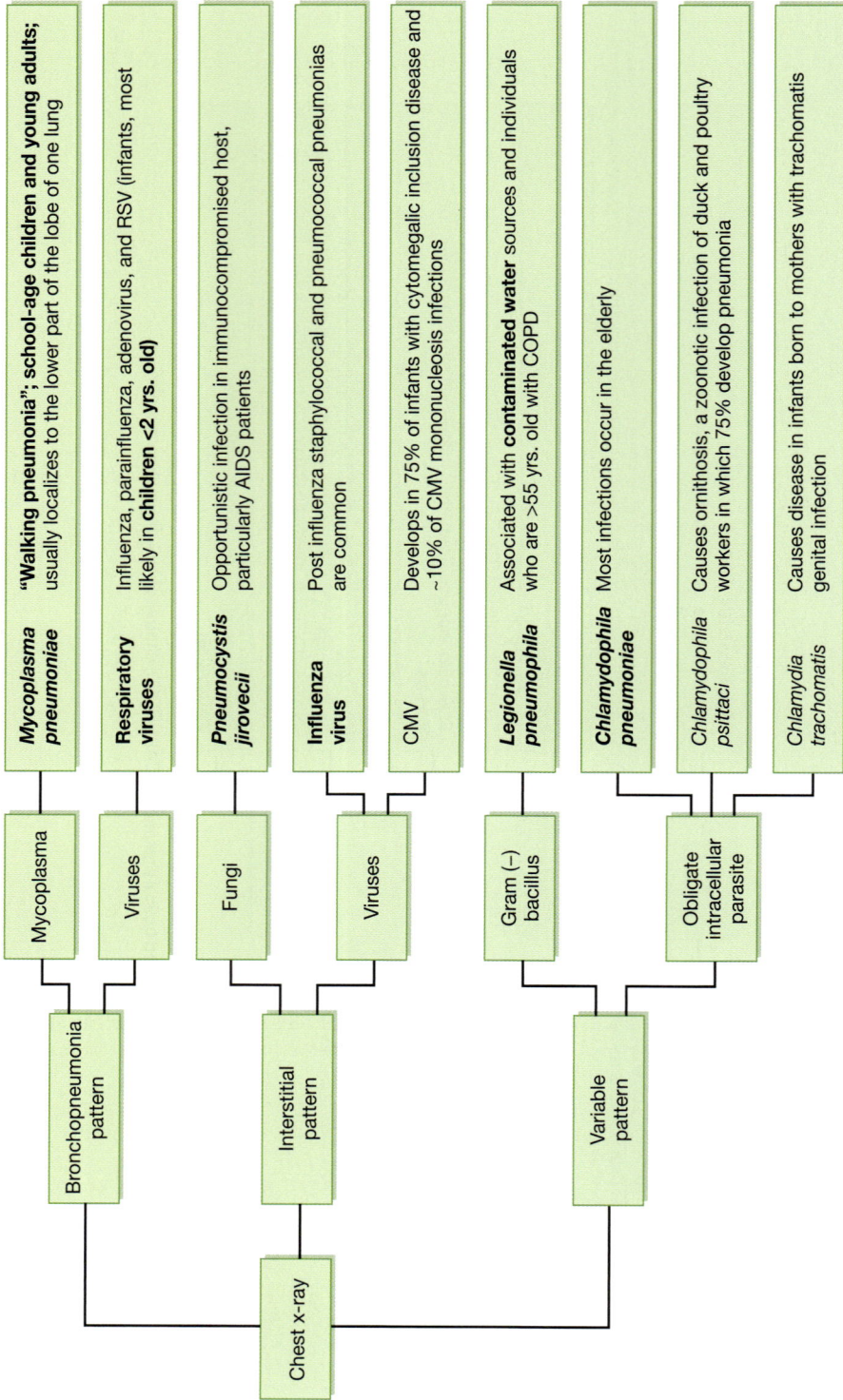

FIGURE 13.4. Acute community-acquired atypical pneumonia. CMV, cytomegalovirus; COPD, chronic obstructive pulmonary disease; RSV, respiratory syncytial virus.

C. Aspiration pneumonia: Aspiration pneumonia results in excessive aspiration of contaminated fluids or the loss of the reflexes utilized to protect the lungs from accumulating fluids or secretions. These situations occur in individuals who have a poor gag reflex or difficulty swallowing for various reasons or who have lost consciousness. They may result from aspiration of gastric contents or mouth flora during various conditions, such as endotracheal intubation, GI endoscopy, general anesthesia, and seizures. Older patients with stroke are particularly vulnerable.

1. **Anaerobic streptococci** infections are characterized by foul-smelling sputum containing no other leading CAP bacteria; frequently associated with periodontal disease.
2. *S. aureus* **and gram-negative bacilli** are the most frequent causes of nosocomial aspiration pneumonia.

D. Pneumonia in an immunocompromised host: In addition to being susceptible to the usual pneumonia-causing pathogens mentioned above, individuals with compromised immunity are also at risk for infection from several opportunistic pathogens.

1. *Aspergillus fumigatus:* X-rays show fungus balls, nodules, and cavitation; aspirates or biopsy materials contain large, branching septate hyphae.
2. *Pneumocystis jirovecii:* X-rays indicate a bilateral diffuse alveolar disease; silver staining of bronchoalveolar lavage material shows sporocytes (cysts).
3. **Cytomegalovirus (CMV):** This pathogen is an important consideration as the causative agent of pneumonias in organ transplant patients receiving immunosuppressive therapy.

III. DIARRHEAS AND DYSENTERY

Diarrheas are characterized by frequent and fluid stools that result from small intestine disease involving fluid and electrolyte loss. **Dysentery** is an inflammatory disease of the large intestine with blood or pus in the stool. Diarrhea can be classified on the basis of the nature of the diarrhea, which reflects the pathology and the site of infection.

The sources of infectious agents are food, water, zoonotic, or person-to-person transfer by the fecal-oral route. Toxins play a major role in the development of the symptoms observed with some bacteria and rotavirus infections, and the incubation times depend on whether a preformed toxin, colonization and toxin synthesis, or tissue invasion is involved. Many infections are self-limiting, but some, particularly in children without proper rehydration, can be fatal. Since it is impossible to clinically diagnose causative agents, recent food and travel history as well as examination of the stool is important. Specific diagnosis is dependent on laboratory analysis of the stool involving Gram staining for bacteria, staining for polymorphonuclear neutrophils (PMNs), and bacterial culture and immunologic-based or molecular tests for specific pathogens. Another important consideration related to diagnosis is whether the pathogen is associated with an epidemic; infection is frequently location dependent. An identification scheme initially based on the nature of the diarrhea and the presence or absence of vomiting is described.

A. **Watery diarrheas and/or vomiting:** Causative pathogens are viruses and several bacteria, the majority of which synthesize **enterotoxins** involved in the pathogenesis of the disease. Some produce fever, but all have relatively **short incubation times, ranging from several hours to a few days**, due to the associated toxins or virus multiplication in the small intestine (Figure 13.5).

B. **Watery diarrhea with no vomiting:** One bacterium and two protozoa are in this group. A variety of toxins contribute to the bacterial disease, which has a short (<24 hours) incubation period. The protozoa have longer (1-4 weeks) incubation periods with disease that is usually moderate, but it can become chronic and serious in individuals who are immunocompromised. **No fever** is associated with these infections (Figure 13.6).

C. **Bloody diarrhea with vomiting:** Two types of *E. coli* cause this form of diarrhea. Enterohemorrhagic *E. coli* (EHEC) strains release a verotoxin that is cytotoxic to intestinal villi and colon epithelial cells. Enteroinvasive *E. coli* (EIEC) strains invade and destroy colon epithelial cells. Both have incubation periods of 2 to 5 days (Figure 13.7).

D. **Bloody diarrhea with no vomiting:** Both bacillary and amoebic dysentery cause this form of diarrhea. Gram-positive and gram-negative rods and a protozoan are involved. PMNs in the stool and fever occur with most infections. Tissue invasion is common (Figure 13.8).

IV. ACUTE MENINGITIS

Meningitis is both an acute and chronic disease. Bacteria and viruses cause acute disease, while **M. tuberculosis and fungi (*Cryptococcus* and *Coccidioides*) cause a chronic form.** Both types are preceded by infections that lead to meningeal invasion. Acute infections are usually preceded by a throat, ear, or lung infection. Clinical presentation and history, cerebrospinal fluid (CSF) characteristics, age of the patient, and time of the year are helpful in diagnosis.

A. **Bacterial meningitis:** Bacterial meningitis can be acquired either in the community or in the hospital. The symptoms (fever, severe headache, stiff neck, and **some cerebral dysfunction** such as confusion or delirium) may develop in a few hours or a few days. Nausea, vomiting, and photophobia frequently occur. Specific pathogens need to be identified as quickly as possible so that appropriate intravenous administration of bacterial antibodies may be started (Figure 13.9).

B. **Viral (aseptic) meningitis:** Acute viral meningitis is a milder disease than bacterial meningitis. There is usually **less neck stiffness and no cerebral dysfunction.** It is the **most common form of acute meningitis** and is frequently a component of common viral diseases, such as chickenpox. In temperate climates, the disease is usually observed in summer or early fall. Identification of the causative virus is rarely done (Figure 13.10).

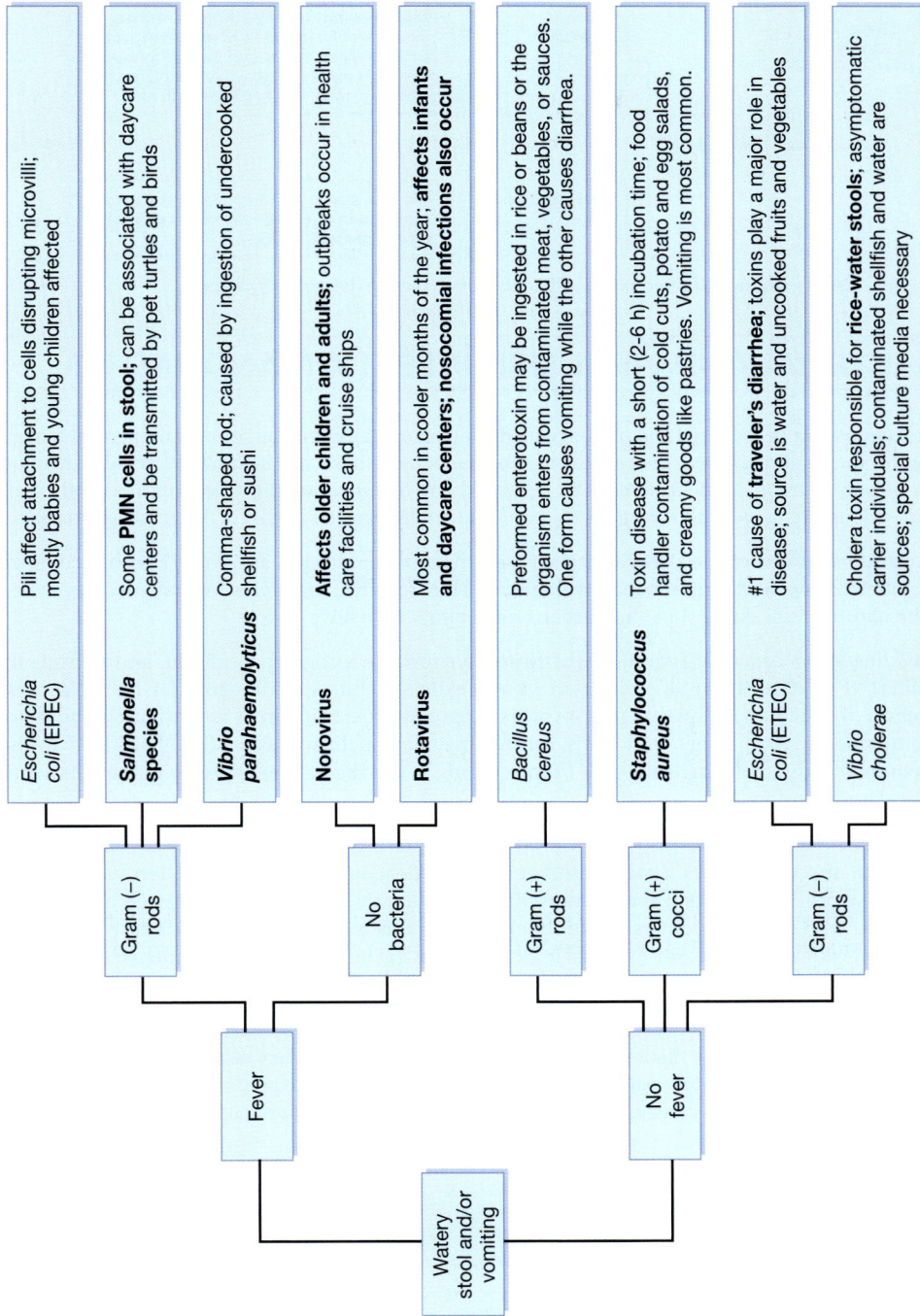

FIGURE 13.5. Watery stools and/or vomiting. EPEC, enteropathogenic *Escherichia coli*; ETEC, enterotoxigenic *E. coli*; PMN, polymorphonuclear neutrophil.

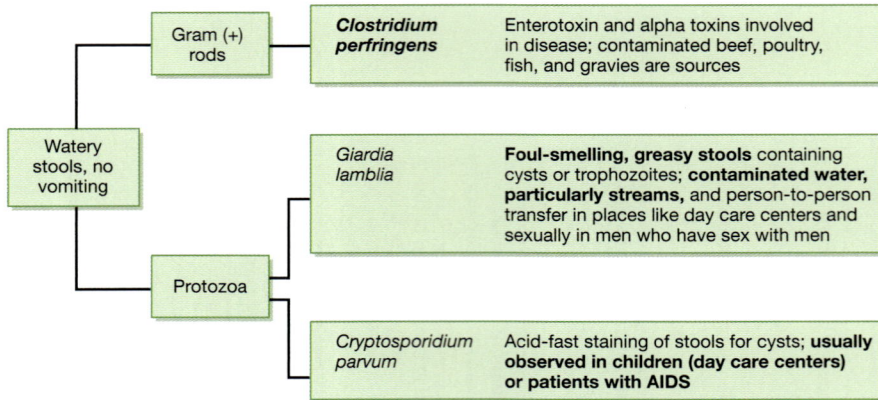

FIGURE 13.6. Watery stools with no vomiting. AIDS, acquired immune deficiency syndrome.

V. BACTERIAL AND VIRAL SKIN INFECTION AND RASHES

These infections may be localized and present with distinctive symptoms at the site of pathogen entry or attachment, or they may result from their spread to subcutaneous tissues or the action of bacterial toxin upon the skin. Group A streptococci (*Streptococcus pyogenes*) and *S. aureus* are the most common pathogens in skin infections. Many systemic infectious diseases also produce rashes as part of their disease process.

A. Localized infections of the skin: Several viruses infect the epidermis, and some bacteria colonize the epidermis, sweat glands, sebaceous glands, and hair follicles. Diagnosis is usually accomplished by the nature of the skin lesion and perhaps recent patient history (**Figure 13.11**).

B. Spreading skin infections: Two classes of these infections are recognized: cellulitis and necrotizing fasciitis (NF). **Cellulitis** is a skin infection with an extension into subcutaneous fat. **NF** is a serious infection of subcutaneous tissue that involves progressive destruction of fat and fascia. Both are accompanied by pain, fever, and chills, but NF may have delirium as well. A "hard feel" to the subcutaneous tissue distinguishes NF from cellulitis. It is a medical emergency that may involve surgical intervention (**Figure 13.12**).

C. Toxin-associated skin shedding: Toxin-producing strains of **S. aureus** can cause a **"scalded skin"** **syndrome** and **toxic shock syndrome** that includes desquamation of the epidermis as part of the disease process. "Scalded skin" syndrome occurs mainly in infants and children and may be associated with small epidemics. Toxic shock syndrome is a serious systemic disease frequently associated with a skin abscess or vaginal infection involving tampon use during menstruation. The rash observed with the disease resembles the scarlet fever rash.

D. Rashes: Many systemic bacterial, rickettsial, and viral infections, and some localized viral infections (cited previously), produce rashes as part of their disease process. They can be classified into four types: (1) maculopapular, (2) vesicular, (3) petechial purpuric, and (4) diffuse erythroderma. They are helpful in identifying causative agents. Common pathogens found in the United States are listed in **Tables 13.1** to **13.4**.

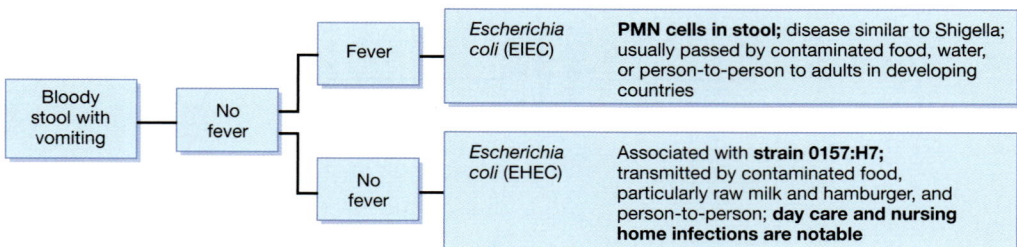

FIGURE 13.7. Bloody stools with vomiting. PMN, polymorphonuclear neutrophil.

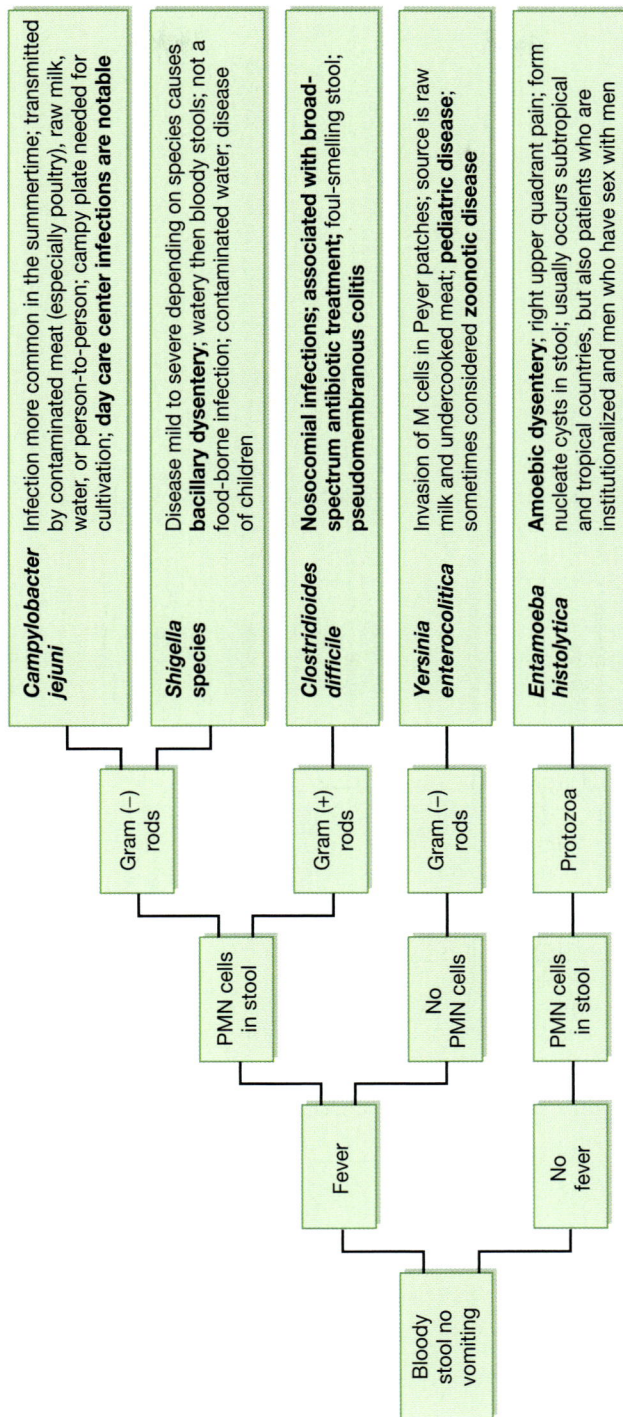

FIGURE 13.8. Bloody stools with no vomiting. PMN, polymorphonuclear neutrophil.

The flowchart starts at "Bloody stool no vomiting" which branches into "Fever" and "No fever."

Fever branches into:
- **PMN cells in stool**
  - **Gram (−) rods** → *Campylobacter jejuni*: Infection more common in the summertime; transmitted by contaminated meat (especially poultry), raw milk, water, or person-to-person; campy plate needed for cultivation; **day care center infections are notable**
  - **Gram (−) rods** → *Shigella species*: Disease mild to severe depending on species causes **bacillary dysentery**; watery then bloody stools; not a food-borne infection; contaminated water; disease of children
  - **Gram (+) rods** → *Clostridioides difficile*: **Nosocomial infections; associated with broad-spectrum antibiotic treatment;** foul-smelling stool; **pseudomembranous colitis**
- **No PMN cells**
  - **Gram (−) rods** → *Yersinia enterocolitica*: Invasion of M cells in Peyer patches; source is raw milk and undercooked meat; **pediatric disease;** sometimes considered **zoonotic disease**

No fever branches into:
- **PMN cells in stool**
  - **Protozoa** → *Entamoeba histolytica*: **Amoebic dysentery;** right upper quadrant pain; form nucleate cysts in stool; usually occurs subtropical and tropical countries, but also patients who are institutionalized and men who have sex with men

295

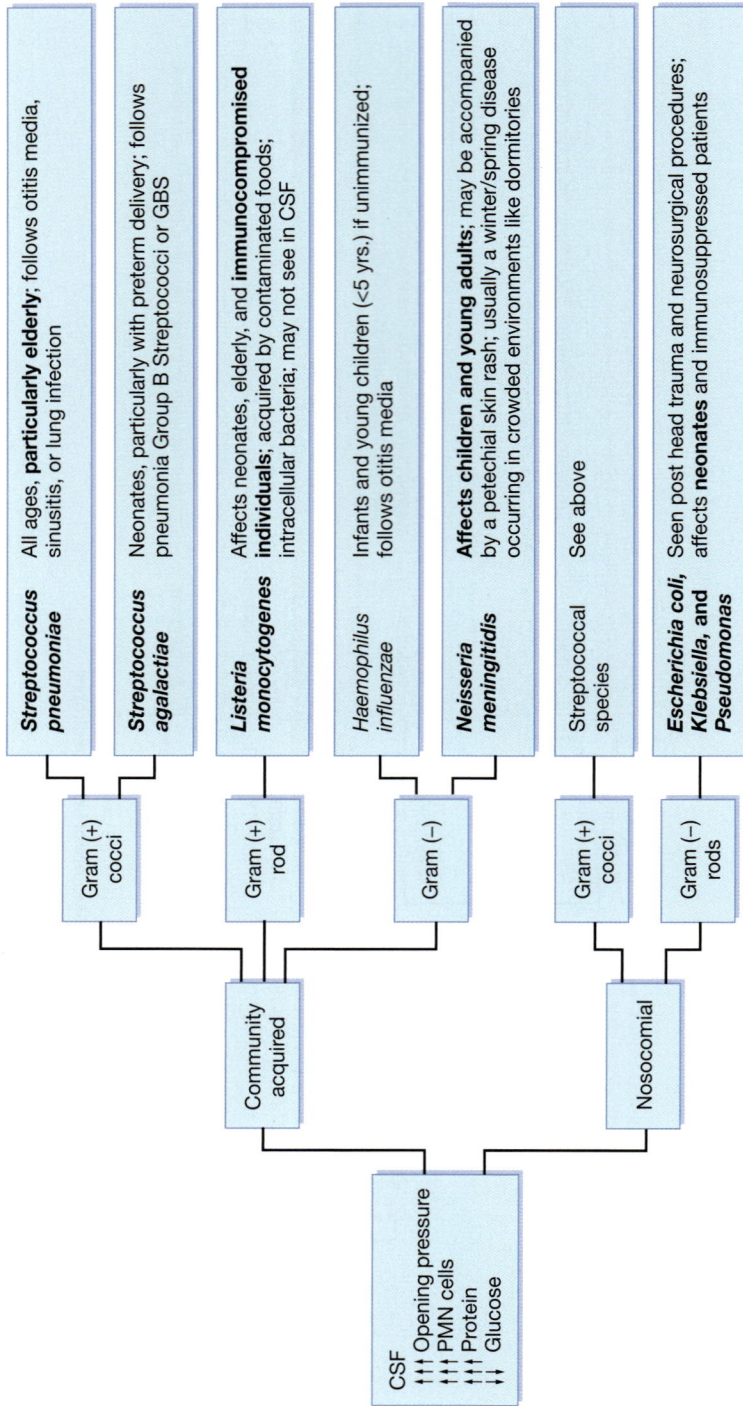

FIGURE 13.9. Acute bacterial meningitis. CSF, cerebrospinal fluid; PMN, polymorphonuclear neutrophil.

Enteroviruses (Echo and Coxsackie)	**Most common cause** is fecal-oral spread; **summer and early fall infections;** may be mini-epidemics. Usually part of systemic disease; enanthem and exanthems (rashes) observed
HSV-2	Seen after preceding genital infection
Lymphocytic choriomeningitis virus	Transmitted to humans by urine of mice or hamsters; more frequent in the winter
Mumps virus	Unimmunized 5- to 9-year-olds show symptoms as part of the mumps disease process
VZV EBV CMV	Part of the systemic disease associated with these virus infections

CSF
Normal opening pressure
↑ Cells (lymphocytes)
↑ Protein
Normal glucose

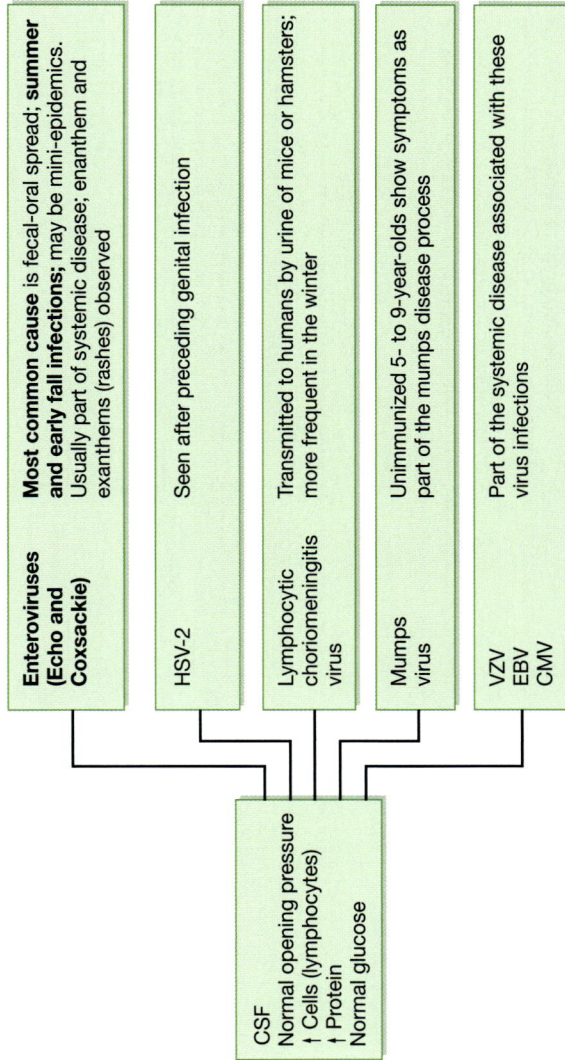

FIGURE 13.10. Acute viral (aseptic) meningitis. CMV, cytomegalovirus; CSF, cerebrospinal fluid; EBV, Epstein-Barr virus; HSV, herpes simplex virus; VZV, varicella-zoster virus.

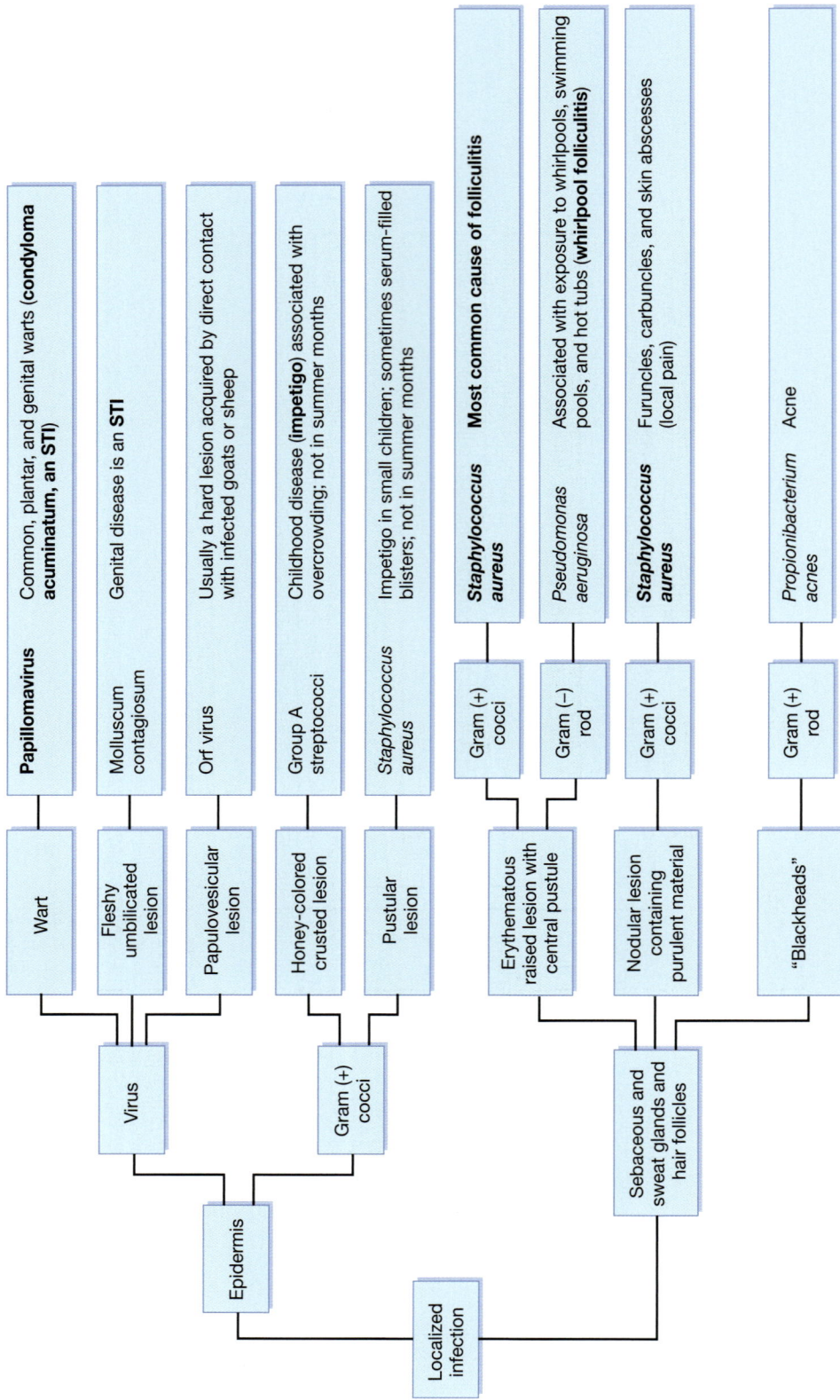

FIGURE 13.11. Localized skin infections. STI, sexually transmitted infection.

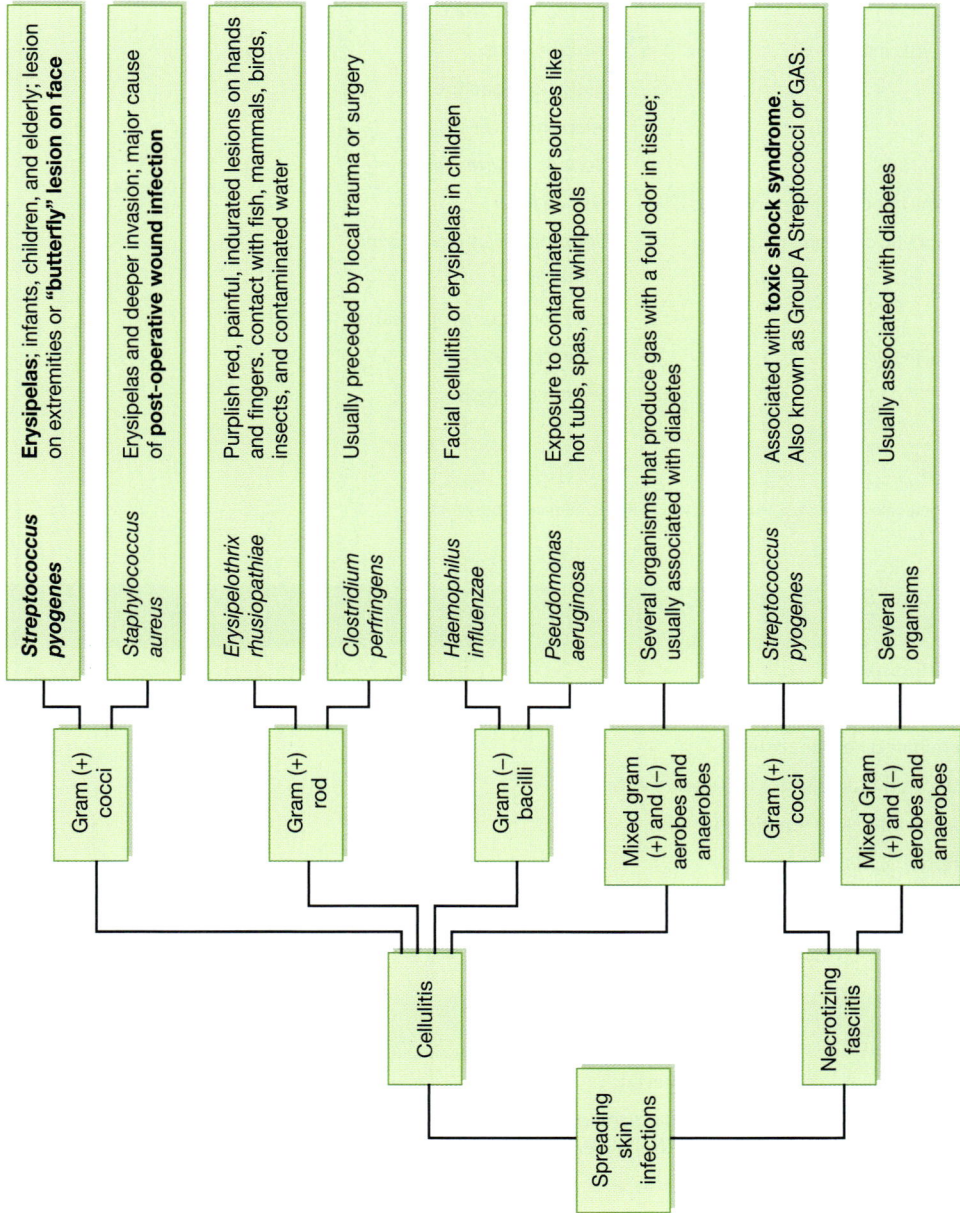

FIGURE 13.12. Spreading skin infections.

299

Table 13.1   Maculopapular Rashes

Viral	Bacterial	Rickettsial
Colorado tick fever	*Leptospirosis*	Ehrlichia infections
CMV mononucleosis	Lyme disease (*Borrelia burgdorferi*)	Rickettsial infections
Dengue	*Meningococcemia*	
Enterovirus infections	*Pseudomonas aeruginosa* bacteremia	
EBV	Relapsing fever (*Borrelia recurrentis*)	
Erythema infectiosum (parvovirus B19)	Rat bite fever	
Lymphocytic choriomeningitis	(*Streptobacillus moniliformis*)	
	Scarlet fever (*Streptococcus pyogenes*)	
Roseola (HHV-6)	Typhoid fever (*Salmonella typhi*)	
Rubella		
Rubeola		

CMV, cytomegalovirus; EBV, Epstein-Barr virus; HHV-6, human herpesvirus 6.

Table 13.2   Vesicular Rashes (All are Viral)

Chickenpox (VZV)

Disseminated herpes simplex virus (HSV)

Disseminated herpes zoster

Hand-foot-mouth disease (Coxsackie A16)

Echovirus infections (enterovirus 11)

Smallpox

VZV, varicella-zoster virus.

Table 13.3   Petechial Purpuric Rashes

Viral	Bacterial	Rickettsial
Congenital cytomegalic inclusion disease	Acute meningococcemia (*Neisseria meningitidis*)	Epidemic typhus (*Rickettsia prowazekii*)
Congenital rubella	Rat bite fever (*Streptobacillus moniliformis*)	Rocky Mountain spotted fever (*Rickettsia rickettsii*)
Echovirus 9 infections	Relapsing fever (*Borrelia recurrentis*)	
Infectious mononucleosis (Epstein-Barr virus)	*Staphylococcus aureus* bacteremia	
Yellow fever (Yellow Fever Virus)		

| Table 13.4 | Diffuse Erythroderma Rashes (All are Bacterial) |

Scarlet fever (*Streptococcus pyogenes*)

Scalded skin syndrome (*Staphylococcus aureus*)

Toxic shock syndromes (*S. aureus* and *S. pyogenes*)

> **• • • Clinical Pearl**
>
> Pay attention to the morphology, configuration, and distribution of the rash, as these can aid in identifying triggers or conditions relevant to diagnosis.

VI. GENITOURINARY TRACT INFECTIONS

These infections are frequently classified according to the site of infection (ie, urethritis, cervicitis, vaginitis, etc). They produce some type of **exudate**, which usually contains the infectious agent; several form **genital lesions, which can be diagnostic** and some cause sexually transmitted infections (STIs).

A. Urethritis: Urethritis is characterized by dysuria and urethral exudate. Coinfections with *Neisseria* and *Chlamydia* are common (Figure 13.13).

B. Epididymitis: Infection is painful with acute unilateral swelling of the testicle. Causative organism is found in urethral specimens or epididymal aspirates (Figure 13.14).

C. Cervicitis: Infection produces a mucopurulent discharge containing PMNs. The cervix is inflamed and friable. Causative agents are found in the exudate (Figure 13.15).

D. Vaginitis: Certain invading organisms can cause infection, but overgrowth of the normal vaginal flora, including anaerobic bacteria and *Gardnerella vaginalis*, cause disease. Organisms in vaginal discharge are diagnostic (Figure 13.16).

E. Genital lesions: Some infectious agents cause visible lesions (warts and ulcers) on the genitalia. The nature of these lesions is diagnostic (Figure 13.17).

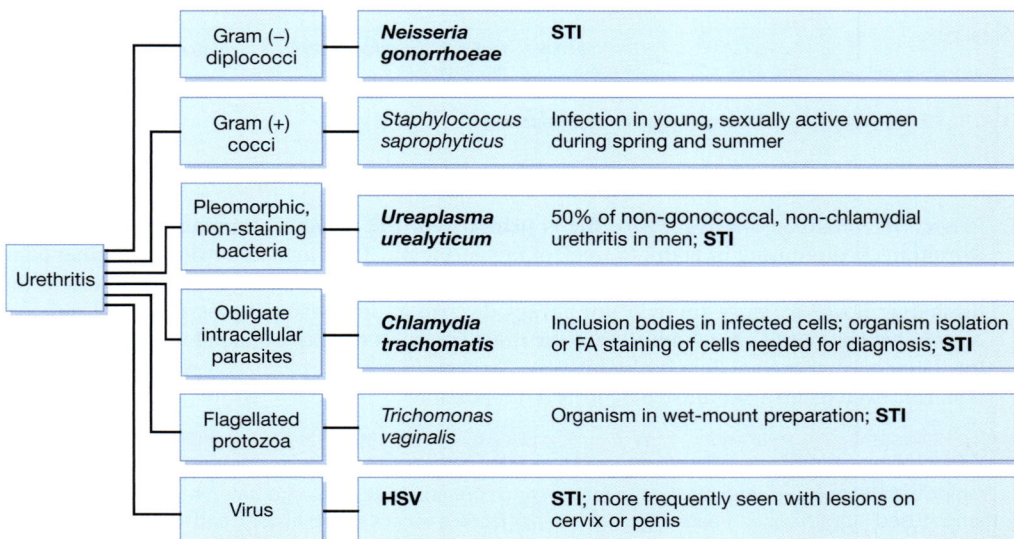

FIGURE 13.13. Urethritis. FA, fluorescent antibody; HSV, herpes simplex virus; STI, sexually transmitted infection.

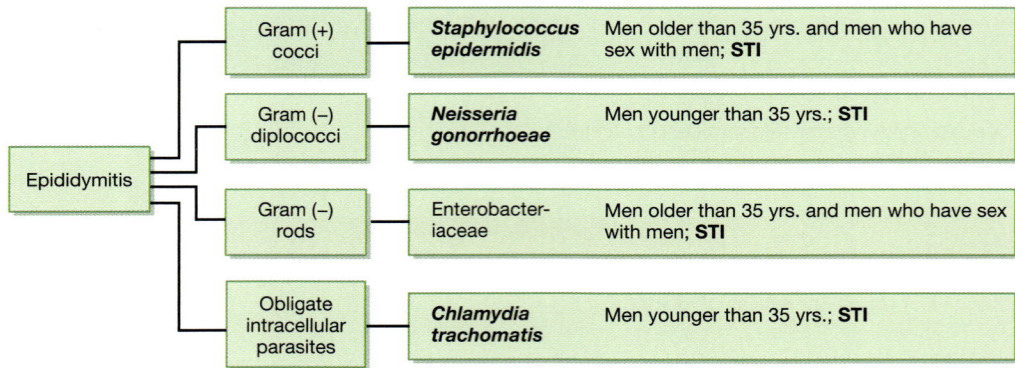

FIGURE 13.14. Epididymitis. STI, sexually transmitted infection.

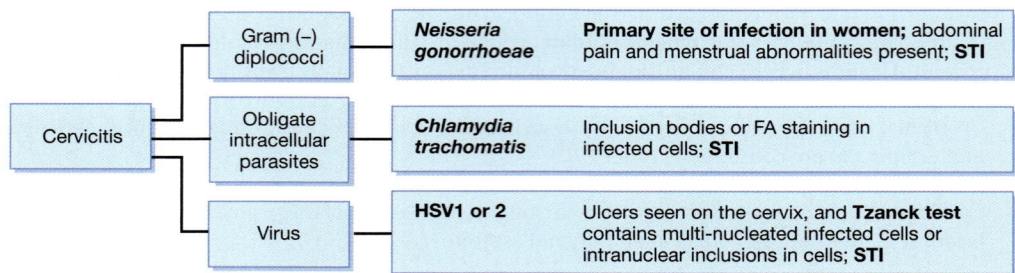

FIGURE 13.15. Cervicitis. FA, fluorescent antibody; HSV, herpes simplex virus; STI, sexually transmitted infection.

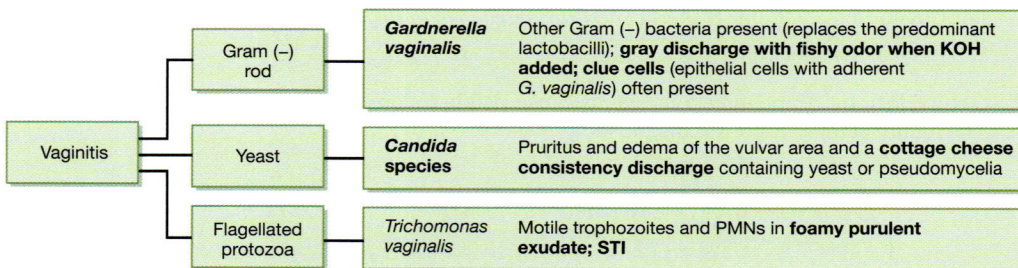

FIGURE 13.16. Vaginitis. STI, sexually transmitted infection.

F. Pelvic inflammatory disease (PID): PID is **primarily a STI of young sexually active women.** Symptoms begin during or within a week of menstruation. They include lower abdominal pain, fever, and vaginal discharge in 50% of those infected. Causative organisms may be found in the discharge; however, since there is not always discharge, definitive diagnosis may be difficult. *N. gonorrhoeae* and *C. trachomatis* **are the most common causes**, but a polymicrobial etiology involving normal vaginal flora is also possible. To prevent complications and sequelae, treatment is started even when a definitive diagnosis is not possible.

● ● ● **Clinical Pearl**

Empiric broad-spectrum antibiotic treatment covering common bacterial pathogens is recommended and then focused individualized treatment based on risk factors, recent sexual history, and local antibiotic resistance patterns is warranted.

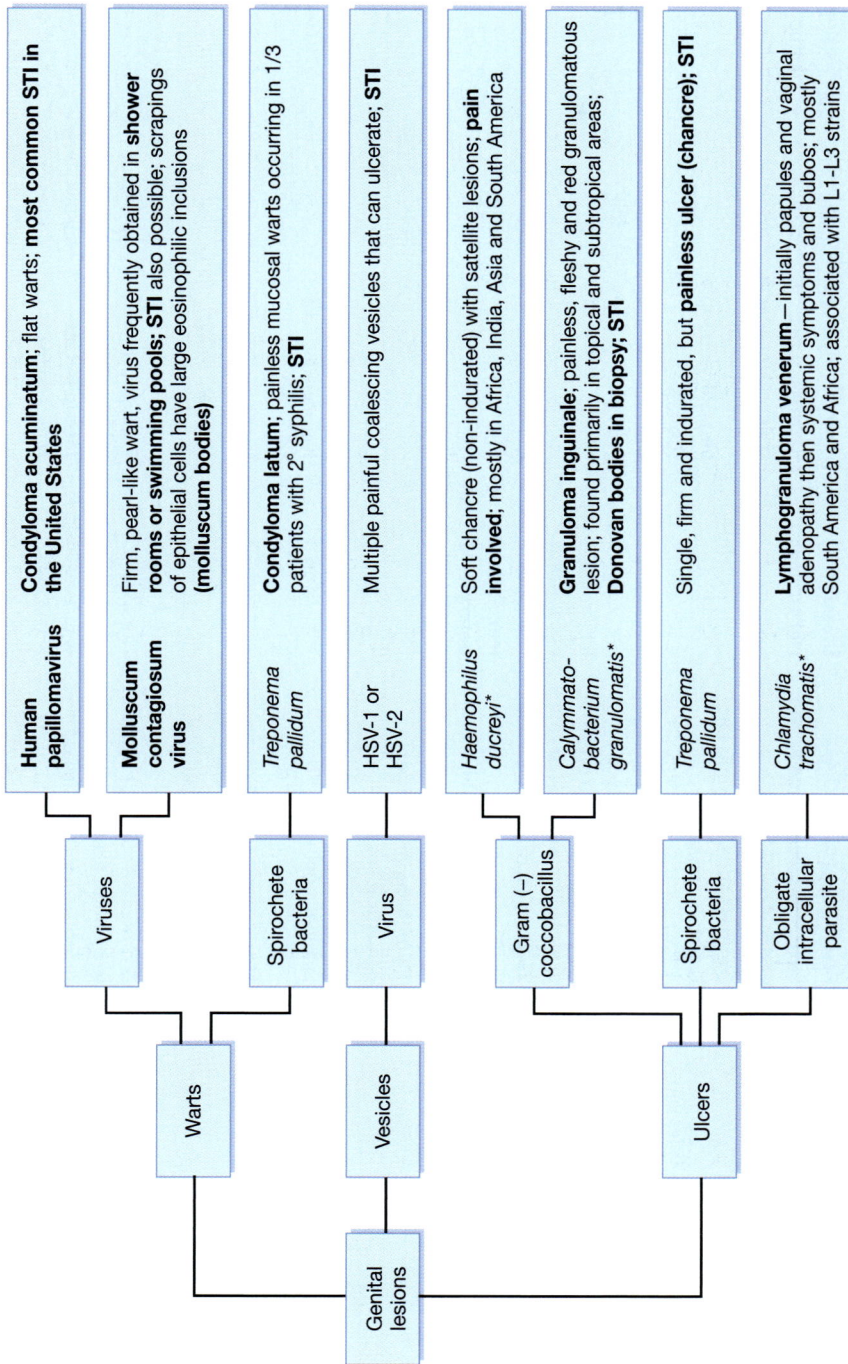

Genital lesions

- **Warts**
  - **Viruses**
    - **Human papillomavirus** — **Condyloma acuminatum**; flat warts; **most common STI in the United States**
    - **Molluscum contagiosum virus** — Firm, pearl-like wart, virus frequently obtained in **shower rooms or swimming pools; STI** also possible; scrapings of epithelial cells have large eosinophilic inclusions **(molluscum bodies)**
  - **Spirochete bacteria**
    - *Treponema pallidum* — **Condyloma latum**; painless mucosal warts occurring in 1/3 patients with 2° syphilis; **STI**
- **Vesicles**
  - **Virus**
    - HSV-1 or HSV-2 — Multiple painful coalescing vesicles that can ulcerate; **STI**
- **Ulcers**
  - **Gram (–) coccobacillus**
    - *Haemophilus ducreyi** — Soft chancre (non-indurated) with satellite lesions; **pain involved**; mostly in Africa, India, Asia and South America
    - *Calymmato-bacterium granulomatis** — **Granuloma inguinale**; painless, fleshy and red granulomatous lesion; found primarily in topical and subtropical areas; **Donovan bodies in biopsy; STI**
  - **Spirochete bacteria**
    - *Treponema pallidum* — Single, firm and indurated, but **painless ulcer (chancre); STI**
  - **Obligate intracellular parasite**
    - *Chlamydia trachomatis** — **Lymphogranuloma venerum** — initially papules and vaginal adenopathy then systemic symptoms and bubos; mostly South America and Africa; associated with L1-L3 strains

FIGURE 13.17. Genital lesions. HSV, herpes simplex virus; STI, sexually transmitted infection. *Mostly observed outside the United States.

303

VII. SYSTEM SUMMARIES OF INFECTIOUS AGENTS

A. Characteristics of Important Causes of Encephalitis

Infection	Type of Microorganism	Microorganism	Virulence or Epidemiologic Factors	Associated Disease	Prominent Groups	Diagnosis	Prevention/ Treatment
ENCEPHALITIS	Viruses	Mosquito-borne arboviruses (EEE and WEE viruses, La Crosse virus, and St. Louis virus)	**Birds 1° reservoir for EEE, WEE, and St. Louis virus** **Squirrels and chipmunks for La Crosse virus**	Flulike illness	**La Crosse virus: children (mean age 7.5 y). St. Louis virus: older people (>60 y)**	ELISA test for IgM in CSF for each virus	Supportive
		West Nile virus	**Birds, particularly jays, are 1° reservoir**, but breastfeeding, blood transfusion, and organ transplant transmission can occur.	80% asymptomatic, 20% acute febrile illness, <1% **encephalitis**	**Older persons (>60 y)**	ELISA for IgM in CSF	Supportive
		Tick-borne arbovirus (Colorado tick fever)	**Small forest or field mammals are 1° reservoir.**	GI symptoms and **maculopapular or petechial rash can be present.**	**Children**	ELISA for IgM in serum	Supportive
		Poliovirus	**1% of those infected get paralytic disease.**			RT-PCR of CSF for virus RNA	Salk trivalent inactivated vaccine/ supportive
		Other enteroviruses	Summer months		Neonates (<7 d old)	PCR of CSF for virus RNA	Supportive
		HSV-1 and HSV-2	**Most common cause of sporadic encephalitis in the United States,** 90% of cases are HSV-1; 1° infections are latent.		½ cases <20 y ½ cases >50 y	PCR of CSF for virus DNA	Acyclovir
		Rabies virus	**G protein of envelope attaches to nicotinic acetylcholine receptor;** infection initiated by animal bite	Nonspecific prodromal period with fever, malaise, and fatigue	**Persons bitten by skunks, dogs, raccoons, cats, bats, and foxes**	Applied to possible rabid animals; Negri bodies or FA tests of biopsy material	Active immunization with inactive rabies vaccine and passive immunization with human rabies immune globulin

Infection	Type of Microorganism	Microorganism	Virulence or Epidemiologic Factors	Associated Disease	Prominent Groups	Diagnosis	Prevention/Treatment
ENCEPHALITIS	Protozoa	*Naegleria fowleri*	Secrete cysteine proteases, form cysts; **found in warm recreational freshwater like swimming holes**; nasal inoculation	Preceding changes in taste or smell	**Children and young adults**	PCR of CSF for amoeba DNA	Amphotericin B (intrathecal and IV miconazole and rifampin)
		Acanthamoeba	Mannose surface glycoproteins, IgA protease	Cutaneous lesions **and sinus infections**	Individuals experiencing debilitation due to immunosuppression	Culture of brain biopsy, wet-mount examination of CSF	Sulfamethazine or trimethoprim/sulfamethoxazole
		Toxoplasma gondii	Forms cysts; **cyst transmission from cat feces and under-cooked meat, particularly pork and lamb**	Toxoplasmosis; **most common focal CNS infection in patients with AIDS**	**Congenitally infected fetuses and newborns;** persons who are immunosuppressed	PCR of CSF for organism DNA, ELISA of serum for IgA or IgG	Sulfadiazine plus pyrimethamine and leucovorin

CNS, central nervous system; CSF, cerebrospinal fluid; EEE, Eastern equine encephalitis; EIA, enzyme immunoassay; ELISA, enzyme-linked immunosorbent assay; FA, fluorescent antibody; GI, gastrointestinal; HSV, herpes simplex virus; Ig, immunoglobulin; IV, intravenous; RT-PCR, reverse transcription polymerase chain reaction; TB, tuberculosis; WEE, Western equine encephalitis.

Infection	Type of Microorganism	Microorganism	Epidemiologic or Virulence Factors	Associated Disease	Prominent Groups	Diagnosis	Prevention/ Treatment
ACUTE MENINGITIS	**Bacteria**	*Streptococcus pneumoniae*	**Polysaccharide capsule**, IgA protease	**Otitis media, respiratory infections**, neurologic sequence	**<2 y and older**	Gram stain and antigen latex agglutination test of CSF to be confirmed by culture	**13-valent vaccine (very young), 23-valent (Pneumovax 23) >5 y**/penicillin G (drug susceptible) and ceftriaxone plus vancomycin (drug resistant)
		Neisseria meningitidis	**Polysaccharide capsule**, IgA protease, pili, outer membrane proteins, endotoxin	**Hemorrhagic skin rash**, neurologic sequelae	**Children and adolescents**	Same as strep pneumonia	**Tetravalent meningococcal polysaccharide vaccine/**penicillin G, if susceptible, ceftriaxone if not
		Haemophilus influenzae type b	**Polysaccharide capsule**, IgA protease, pili, outer membrane proteins, endotoxin	**Otitis**, neurologic sequelae	**Infants and young children (<5 y)**	Gram stain and culture	**Polysaccharide-protein conjugate vaccine/**ceftriaxone
		Streptococcus agalactiae	**A surface protein, pili, polysaccharide capsule**	Asymptomatic in pregnant females, generalized disease in neonates	**Neonates (<7 d)**	Latex agglutination for antigen in serum or urine; culture or Gram stain of CSF	Ampicillin
		Borrelia burgdorferi	Spirochetal surface protein facilitates binding to host cells.	**Preceding rash**, arthritis succeeds rash after a variable period of time.	All bitten by infected tick	Clinical, but aided by serology and PCR of CSF or serum for bacterial DNA	Ceftriaxone

Infection	Type of Microorganism	Microorganism	Epidemiologic or Virulence Factors	Associated Disease	Prominent Groups	Diagnosis	Prevention/Treatment
ACUTE MENINGITIS		*Listeria monocytogenes*	**Grows during refrigeration, food-borne;** mother-child transmission, iron, cell surface internalin, listeriolysin	Febrile gastroenteritis, neonatal bacteremia	**Neonates (<7 d),** persons who are immunocompromised including patients with AIDS	CSF Gram stain and culture	Ampicillin
	Viruses	Enteroviruses, echoviruses, and Coxsackie viruses	**Causes 80% of meningitis cases**	Pharyngitis	Infants, young children; also adults	RT-PCR of CSF for viral RNA	Supportive
		HSV-2 (rarely other herpesviruses)	Viral glycoproteins C, B, and D	**1° genital infection with HSV-2**	All with 1° HSV-2 infection	PCR of CSF for virus DNA	Acyclovir
		Mumps virus	Envelope glycoproteins	Mumps	Males 2-5 times greater than females; peak incidence in children 5-9 y	Clinical, also IgM serology possible	**Jeryl Lynn strain of attenuated virus vaccine/** supportive
		Lymphocytic choriomeningitis virus		Nonspecific febrile illness	**Contact with rodents or their excreta, especially young adults**	IgM serology of serum aid CSF	Elimination of infected rodents/ supportive
CHRONIC MENINGITIS	Bacteria	*Mycobacterium tuberculosis*	**Waxy coat**	**Miliary TB**	Individuals with HIV infection	PCR of CSF for bacterial DNA, lung lesions culture	**Four-drug therapy: isoniazid, rifampin, pyrazinamide, and ethambutol;** adjunctive corticosteroids
		Treponema pallidum		2° syphilis, neurosyphilis	**2° individuals with syphilis**	EIA tests for abs, microhemagglutination test	Penicillin G

(continued)

Infection	Type of Microorganism	Microorganism	Epidemiologic or Virulence Factors	Associated Disease	Prominent Groups	Diagnosis	Prevention/Treatment
CHRONIC MENINGITIS	*Bacteria*	*Borrelia burgdorferi* (see Acute Meningitis)					
	Fungi	*Cryptococcus neoformans*	Polysaccharide capsule	Cryptococcosis	**Individuals who are immunosuppressed, particularly patients with AIDS**	Cryptococcal latex agglutination on CSF	Amphotericin B plus flucytosine
		Coccidioides immitis	Formation of endospores	Coccidioidomycosis	**Persons living or traveling in the southwest United States;** individuals who are immunosuppressed	Fungal immunodiffusion test on serum; complement fixation test on CSF; culture	Fluconazole
		Histoplasma capsulatum	**Bird or bat guano**	Histoplasmosis	Individuals who are immunosuppressed; **persons living/traveling in Ohio or Mississippi River Valleys**	EIA for ag in CSF and culture of CSF	Liposomal amphotericin B (4-6 wk), followed by itraconazole for a year
	Protozoa	*Acanthamoeba*	Mannose surface glycoproteins, IgA protease	**Cutaneous lesions and sinus infections**	Individuals experiencing debilitation or immunosuppression	Culture of brain biopsy, wet-mount examination of CSF	Sulfamethazine or trimethoprim/sulfamethoxazole

AIDS, acquired immune deficiency syndrome; CSF, cerebrospinal fluid; EIA, enzyme immunoassay; HSV, herpes simplex virus; Ig, immunoglobulin; RT-PCR, reverse transcription polymerase chain reaction; TB, tuberculosis.

C. Characteristics of Important Causes of Pneumonia

Infection	Sub-Type	Type of Microorganism	Microorganism	Epidemiologic or Virulence Factor	Associated Disease	Prominent Groups	Diagnosis	X-Ray Pattern	Prevention/Treatment
ACUTE COMMUNITY-ACQUIRED PNEUMONIA	Typical (80%–90%)	Bacteria	*Streptococcus pneumoniae* (both drug-sensitive and drug-resistant strains)	**Estimates of 65% of CAP isolates resistant to penicillin due to alterations in PBPs;** polysaccharide capsule, pneumococcal surface protein A, pneumolysin, and neuraminidase	**Otitis media and meningitis**	**Newborns and infants (<2 y old) and older adults (>65 y old)**	Gram stain of sputum, urinary ag test, and PCR	**Single lobe lobar**	Three pneumococcal vaccines: (1) protein conjugate to 13 capsular polysaccharides (2-59 mo children and 60-71 mo children with underlying medical conditions); (2) protein conjugate to seven capsular polysaccharides (children <5 y); (3) 23-valent pneumococcal polysaccharide vaccine (>65 y old)/ empiric treatment (outpatients); amoxicillin and azithromycin; hospitalized adults; IV ceftriaxone and azithromycin
			Haemophilus influenzae (both drug-sensitive and drug-resistant strains)	Minor percent of CAP, except in older adults; **most common bacterial cause of COPD**	Otitis media and sinusitis	**Older adults**	Gram stain and culture of sputum	Patchy or lobar	**Hib polysaccharide-protein conjugate vaccine.** Drug sensitive; amoxicillin, drug-resistant ceftriaxone

(continued)

309

Infection	Sub-Type	Type of Microorganism	Microorganism	Epidemiologic or Virulence Factor	Associated Disease	Prominent Groups	Diagnosis	X-Ray Pattern	Prevention/Treatment
ACUTE COMMUNITY-ACQUIRED PNEUMONIA	Typical (80%-90%)	Bacteria	*Staphylococcus aureus*	**Minor cause of CAP;** polysaccharide capsule; lipoteichoic acids, protein A, hemolysins Panton-Valentine toxin, **pathogenicity islands, resistance to a variety of antibacterials (eg, penicillinase and active efflux) mechanism**	Soft tissue infections, endocarditis, and **20%-30% of nosocomial pneumonia**	**Hospitalized patients**	Gram stain of sputum and PCR	Patchy	MSSA: IV nafcillin MRSA: linezolid
			Moraxella catarrhalis	Minor cause of CAP, outer membrane protein, pili, lipooligosaccharide, and penicillinase; second most common bacterial cause of COPD	Otitis media sinusitis	**Older and hospitalized persons, persons with COPD**	Gram stain of sputum	Diffuse	Azithromycin
			Pseudomonas aeruginosa	**#1 cause of nosocomial pneumonia (associated with mechanical ventilation);** pili; mucoid exopolysaccharide (MEP) endotoxin extracellular cytotoxins β-lactamases and efflux pumps	"Swimmer's ear"	Patients who are immunocompromised and those with HIV and **cystic fibrosis**	Gram stain and culture of sputum	Diffuse with some nodules	IV piperacillin; tazobactam plus tobramycin (2-3 wk treatment)

(continued)

Infection	Sub-Type	Type of Microorganism	Microorganism	Epidemiologic or Virulence Factor	Associated Disease	Prominent Groups	Diagnosis	X-Ray Pattern	Prevention/Treatment
ACUTE COMMUNITY-ACQUIRED PNEUMONIA	*Atypical*	*Bacteria*	*Mycoplasma pneumoniae*	Largest number of atypicals (10%-15% of CAP); surface cytohesin protein (p1)	Bronchitis	**School-age children and young adults (5-20 y old)**	Serology for **"cold agglutinins,"** PCR of lower respiratory tract specimens	Alveolar and interstitial	Doxycycline
			Chlamydophila pneumoniae	**5%-10% of CAP; can cause persistent infections**; elementary and reticulate bodies	Pharyngitis and asthma	**School-aged children and teenagers;** more severe in older adults	PCR on nasopharyngeal swabs or sputum	Patchy subsegmental	Azithromycin
			Legionella pneumophila	**1%-5% of CAP; no** person-to-person transmission, **transmission by aerosolized bacteria from aquatic habitats (eg, cooling towers, spas, potable water)** Also multiply in free-living amoebas; Mip protein, Hsp60 (heat shock protein), endotoxin, secreted degradative enzymes, and possible toxins.	**"Pontiac Fever"**	Hospitalized individuals	RIA urine ag test	**Patchy, unilateral lower lobe**	Prevent aerosol formation; azithromycin

(continued)

Infection	Sub-Type	Type of Microorganism	Microorganism	Epidemiologic or Virulence Factor	Associated Disease	Prominent Groups	Diagnosis	X-Ray Pattern	Prevention/Treatment
ACUTE COMMUNITY-ACQUIRED PNEUMONIA	Atypical	Bacteria	Coxiella burnetii	Zoonotic disease, inhalation of small particle aerosols; reservoirs are cattle, sheep, and goats.	Fever; chronic disease featuring endocarditis	Occupational disease of farmers, veterinarians, and abattoir workers	IFA serology on paired sera	Lobar or segmented rounded alveolar	Doxycycline
		Virus	Lower respiratory tract viruses (mostly influenza, parainfluenza viruses, and RSV)	80% of infants and children but only 10%-20% of adults; likely to occur during seasonal epidemics	Predispose to 2° bacterial infection	Infants (RSV) and children		Diffuse interstitial	See individual viruses in upper and lower respiratory tract infections.
			Hantavirus (Sin Nombre virus)	Related to excreta of deer mice; most infections in the southwest United States	Hantavirus pulmonary syndrome and cardio-pulmonary syndrome		Serology test for Sin Nombre virus IgM ab or RT-PCR of plasma	Diffuse interstitial	Fluid replacement and restoration of electrolytes and supportive measures
		Fungi	Pneumocystis jirovecii	Transmission from other individuals with infection, minor source of CAP except in populations of individuals with specific immunocompromising conditions; major surface glycoprotein, protease, antigenic variation	PCP pneumonia	Malnourished and premature infants and patients with AIDS	RT-PCR and PCR on oropharyngeal washes	Diffuse alveolar	Trimethoprim-sulfamethoxazole

(continued)

Infection	Sub-Type	Type of Microorganism	Microorganism	Epidemiologic or Virulence Factor	Associated Disease	Prominent Groups	Diagnosis	X-Ray Pattern	Prevention/Treatment
NOSOCOMIAL PNEUMONIAS		Bacteria	*P. aeruginosa*	**Accounts for 50%–70% of these infections**; transmissible airborne pathogen; **found in moist microenvironments in hospitals (eg, sinks, inhalation equipment)**, pili, and extracellular polysaccharides Pel, Psl, and mucoid exopolysaccharide (MEP) endotoxin and wide variety of antimicrobial resistance factors	Bacteremia; also causes both acute (small %) and chronic pneumonia.	Hospitalized patients with neutropenia and those with CF	Culture from sputum or bronchio-alveolar lavage	Diffuse with some nodules	Piperacillin and tazobactam
			S. aureus (MRSA and MSSA)	**Accounts for 20%–30% of these infections;** capsular polysaccharide, variety of surface proteins including protein A, several cytotoxins and secreted enzymes, **pathogenicity islands, and multiple antibiotic resistance mechanisms including penicillinase**	Bacteremia; endocarditis	**Lung abscess or thoracic surgery patients**	Sputum Gram stain and culture, also PCR of sputum	Patchy	MRSA: vancomycin or linezolid MSSA: nafcillin

(continued)

313

Infection	Sub-Type	Type of Microorganism	Microorganism	Epidemiologic or Virulence Factor	Associated Disease	Prominent Groups	Diagnosis	X-Ray Pattern	Prevention/Treatment
NOSOCOMIAL PNEUMONIAS		Bacteria	Klebsiella pneumoniae	Minor percent of infections but usually associated with other nosocomial infections; polysaccharide capsule, pili, penicillinase, and other β-lactamases with extended spectrums (eg, cephalosporin)	Insertion of intravascular and other invasive devices; infections, meningitis, bacteremia	Debilitated patients	"Currant jelly" sputum, culture and Gram stain of sputum	Lobar	Susceptible organisms; IV ceftriaxone, resistant organisms; IV colistin
		Viruses	Influenza viruses, parainfluenza viruses, and RSV	2%-10% of these infections		See Listings in Upper and Lower Respiratory Tract Infections			
ASPIRATION PNEUMONIA		Bacteria	Anaerobic gram-negative bacilli (Bacteroides, Prevotella, and Fusobacterium species; some S. pneumoniae and S. aureus	Cause 60%-80% of these infections (usually polymicrobial). Capsular polysaccharides, extracellular enzymes, and a penicillinase	Periodontal disease	Patients with altered consciousness or dysphagia and older individuals (>65 y old)	Anaerobic culture of sputum and Gram stain	Patchy, unilateral or bilateral, right lung	IV metronidazole
CHRONIC PNEUMONIA		Bacteria	Mycobacterium tuberculosis	Most chronic infections due to reactivation from sites of dormancy (macrophages and lung); mycolic acid in the cell wall and lipoarabinomannan on the cell surface; also drug resistance	Previous TB infection which is usually asymptomatic; empyema	Patients with AIDS; older adults	Acid-fast stain, PCR, and culture of sputum. Tuberculin skin test	Patchy or nodular in apical regions or subapical posterior; some cavitation	Prolonged combination therapy with isoniazid, rifampin, pyrazinamide, and ethambutol

(continued)

	Organism	Characteristics	Clinical Features	Host	Diagnosis	Radiographic Findings	Treatment
Bacteria	*Mycobacterium avium-intracellulare* (MAC)	40% of patients with AIDS get it within 2 y; **naturally occurring in indoor water systems, pools, and hot tubs;** virulence factors same as TB organism	Disseminated disease in patients with AIDS	**Older men who are heavy smokers or alcoholics; patients with AIDS**	Acid-fast stain and culture of sputum but difficult to distinguish from TB organism	**Fibronodular and cavitary in upper lobes**	Same as for TB
	Nocardia asteroides	Found in soil and areas of plant decay; adhesins and mycolic acid polymers	**CNS disease** with granulomas or abscesses in the brain	**Individuals with defective T-cell immunity or immunosuppressed**	Modified acid-fast stain of sputum and culture; PCR of sputum	Diffuse with irregular nodules	IV trimethoprim and sulfamethoxazole plus imipenem
Fungi	*Aspergillus fumigatus*	Surface-binding proteins and extracellular enzymes (proteases, elastase, and phospholipases)	Aspergillus colonization and allergic bronchopulmonary aspergillosis	Patients with granulopenia	Demonstrated tissue invasion in histopathologic specimens	Multiple diffuse nodules; cavitation late	Oral voriconazole
	Blastomyces dermatitidis	**Endemic soil fungus in south central, central, and Southeastern United States;** glycoprotein adhesion (BAD1)	Skin lesions, acute pneumonia, **high incidence of subclinical infections**		**Yeast cells in KOH smears of sputum,** chemiluminescent DNA probes	Lobar or segmental alveolar, + or −	Lipid forms of amphotericin B or itraconazole

(continued)

Infection	Sub-Type	Type of Microorganism	Microorganism	Epidemiologic or Virulence Factor	Associated Disease	Prominent Groups	Diagnosis	X-Ray Pattern	Prevention/Treatment
CHRONIC PNEUMONIA		Fungi	*Coccidioides immitis*	Exposure to soil dust in **alkaline soil of semi-arid zones (AZ, NV, NM, and arid CA)**; secreted protease, and spherule outer cell wall	1° valley fever; chronic in alcoholics/poor health with or without meningitis; disseminates in patients who are immunocompromised or in late pregnancy	**Farm and construction workers**; high mortality for women in the third trimester of pregnancy	**Spherules in KOH preps of sputum or in biopsy specimens. EIA** tests for IgM or IgG antibodies	Diffuse unilateral; sometimes cavitation	Amphotericin B
			Histoplasma capsulatum	Inhalation of mold microconidia **found in soil containing bird or bat droppings (found in Ohio and Mississippi River Basins)**	Preceding interstitial pneumonitis; disseminated disease with the RES organs and adrenal glands	**Farmers, construction workers, and spelunkers, patients with AIDS**	EIA histoplasma ag test on urine bronchoalveolar lavage	Patchy upper lobes progress to cavitation	Itraconazole

AIDS, acquired immune deficiency syndrome; CAP, community-acquired pneumonia; CF, cystic fibrosis; COPD, chronic obstructive pulmonary disease; CNS, central nervous system; EIA, enzyme immunoassay; HiB, *Haemophilus influenzae* type b; HIV, human immunodeficiency virus; IFA, indirect fluorescent antibody; Ig, immunoglobulin; IV, intravenous; MRSA, methicillin-resistant *S. aureus*; MSSA, methicillin-sensitive *S. aureus*; PBP, penicillin-binding protein; RES, reticuloendothelial system; RIA, radioimmunoassay; RSV, respiratory syncytial virus; RT-PCR, reverse transcription polymerase chain reaction; TB, tuberculosis.

D. Characteristics of Important Causes of Lower Respiratory Tract Infections

Infection	Type of Microorganism	Microorganism	Epidemiologic or Virulence Factors	Associated Disease	Prominent Groups	Diagnosis	Prevention/Treatment
BRONCHITIS	Virus	Any of the cold and URT viruses can be involved.	Viruses cause 90% of infections.				
	Bacteria	*Bordetella pertussis*	Adults can get disease in spite of immunization as a child. Filamentous hemagglutinin facilitates attachment and **pertussis toxin and other cytotoxins,** including an adenylate cyclase, contribute to the disease.	**Whooping cough**	Infants and young children	PCR on nasopharyngeal swabs	**Acellular pertussis vaccine is part of DPT vaccine and Tdap vaccine given as a booster to teens and initial adult vaccine**/erythromycin.
		Chlamydophila pneumoniae	**Can cause persistent infections; elementary and reticulate bodies**	Pharyngitis and asthma	School-aged children and teenagers	PCR on nasopharyngeal swabs	Azithromycin
		Mycoplasma pneumoniae	**Account for 75% of agent's infections;** surface cytohesin protein (P1)	"Walking pneumonia" (25% of infections)	5- to 20-y-olds	Definitive diagnosis not done unless a serious infection, then PCR of lower respiratory tract specimens	Erythromycin
BRONCHIOLITIS	Virus	Respiratory syncytial virus	**Causes 50%-80% of cases (usually occurs in winter) and is the leading cause of all infant hospitalizations;** F and G surface glycoproteins important for attachment and penetration and nonstructural proteins NS1 and NS2 inhibit type 1 interferon synthesis.	**Croup (2%-10% of cases);** otitis media (children 1-3 y old). Colds or bronchiolitis in adults	Infants <1 y old	**Dipstick immunoassay for RSV antigens** in nasal washings or nasopharyngeal swabs	**Passive immunization with palivizumab monoclonal antibody for high-risk infants;** supportive, but aerosolized ribavirin for hospitalized infants
		Human metapneumovirus (hMPV)	Causes 3%-19% of cases; membrane G glycoprotein needed for attachment	Exacerbations of childhood asthma	Infants 3-24 mo old	PCR of respiratory specimens; immunofluorescence of indicator shell cultures inoculated with nasopharyngeal swab	Supportive
		Other upper respiratory viruses (see individual viruses)	Less common than RSV and hMPV				

DPT, diphtheria, pertussis, and tetanus; hMPV, human metapneumovirus; PCR, polymerase chain reaction; RSV, respiratory syncytial virus; Tdap, tetanus, diphtheria, and pertussis; URT, upper respiratory tract.

E. Characteristics of Important Causes of Upper Respiratory Tract Infections

Infection	Type of Microorganism	Microorganism	Epidemiologic or Virulence Factors	Associated Disease	Prominent Groups	Diagnosis	Prevention/Treatment
COMMON COLD	Virus	Rhinoviruses	Optimum >160 serotypes growth temperature is 33 °C and **>100 serotypes**; cellular receptor is ICAM-1.	Often exacerbate asthma attack in school-aged children and LRT infections	Adults	Clinical; but specific virus identification usually not done	Supportive
		Coronaviruses	**Infection mostly in winter and spring;** cellular receptor is aminopeptidase N.	SARS with SARS-CoV	Children	RT-PCR, but not usually done	Supportive
		Parainfluenza viruses	HN protein binds to cellular sialic acid surface molecules, but **cellular proteolytic activation of F protein is needed for entry.**	**Otitis media and croup**	Children	RT-PCR, but not usually done	Live vaccine attenuated strains of type 3 virus developed but not licensed
PHARYNGOTONSILLITIS	Bacteria	Streptococcus pyogenes	**M protein,** capsule, hyaluronic acid, lipoteichoic acids, exotoxins, **streptolysin O, streptokinase**	Epiglottis, **pneumatic fever,** and acute glomerulonephritis	Children (5-15 y)	Rapid antigen detection tests (RADTs) for wall carbohydrate ag	Oral penicillin V or amoxicillin
		Corynebacterium diphtheriae	**Diphtheria toxin**	Diphtheritic myocarditis	Unimmunized children and adults	Clinical	Diphtheria toxoid vaccine is part of DPT vaccine; penicillin G procaine or erythromycin antibacterials and diphtheria antitoxin (DAT) available for treatment
	Viruses	Cold and mouth viruses (Coxsackie A viruses, parainfluenza viruses, and HSV)	**See Mouth and Cold listings for details**				

(continued)

Infection	Type of Microorganism	Microorganism	Epidemiologic or Virulence Factors	Associated Disease	Prominent Groups	Diagnosis	Prevention/Treatment
PHARYNGOTONSILLITIS	Viruses	Infectious mononucleosis viruses (CMV and EBV)	**Throat manifestations are part of systemic infectious mononucleosis.**	Infectious mononucleosis	CMV childhood EBV: 15- to 25-y-olds	CMV hybrid capture assay on WBC; EBV PCR on sputum	Valganciclovir for CMV; supportive for EBV
		Adenoviruses	**Most infections in late winter and early spring, many serotypes, latent in lymphoid tissue;** pentons have toxic activity.	Multiple respiratory syndromes and pharyngoconjunctival fever	Children (<2 y) and military recruits	PCR of throat swabs or sputum	Supportive
EPIGLOTTITIS	Bacteria	*Haemophilus influenzae*	Polysaccharide capsule, IgA protease, pili, outer membrane proteins, endotoxin	**Otitis media**, neurologic sequelae	Unvaccinated children	Gram stain and culture	**Hib polysaccharide-protein conjugate vaccine**/ceftriaxone plus airway
LARYNGI-TIS	Viruses	*Streptococcus pyogenes*	See earlier		Adults	See earlier	
CROUP	Virus	Cold, mouth, and upper respiratory tract viruses		See those listed earlier			
	Virus	Parainfluenza virus	**Types 1 and 2 are most involved not Type 3**		See listing under Common Cold		
INFLUENZA	Virus	Influenza virus	**Hemagglutinin glycoprotein (H) is a virus receptor, neuraminidase protein (N) is important for virus release; genetic reassortment, and genetic shift and drift are important epidemiologic processes.**	1° viral pneumonia and **2° pneumonia caused by bacterial superinfection**	Children and adults	Dipstick test of respiratory secretions for viral ags	**Trivalent killed virus vaccines/influenza A only: amantadine and rimantadine; influenza A and B: zanamivir and oseltamivir,** but not all for young children (<1 y old). Some use of oseltamivir for prophylaxis.

CMV, cytomegalovirus; EBV, Epstein-Barr virus; HSV, herpes simplex virus; ICAM, intercellular adhesion molecule; Ig, immunoglobulin; LRT, lower respiratory tract; RT-PCR, reverse transcription polymerase chain reaction; WBC, white blood cell.

Review Test

Directions: Select the *one* lettered answer that is *best* in each case. Commit to and write down your answers before checking the answers and explanations. Each of the numbered items in this section is followed by answers with explanations, in the following section.

1. One week postdelivery, an infant boy becomes extremely irritable and continuously rubs his right eye, which contains a mucopurulent exudate. Examination of the eye shows papillae on the conjunctiva. No bacteria are seen in the exudate. Which of the following organisms is the most likely causative infectious agent?

(A) *Candida albicans*
(B) *C. trachomatis*
(C) CMV
(D) HSV

2. A 58-year-old male presents to the clinic with extreme pain in his right testicle. Physical examination shows considerable swelling. A small amount of urethral exudate can be aspirated. Microscopic examination and Gram staining showed the presence of bacteria. Which of the following classifications of bacteria is most likely to be visualized on microscopy?

(A) Gram-negative cocci
(B) Gram-negative diplococci
(C) Gram-positive cocci
(D) Gram-positive rods

3. A 22-year-old female presents with symptoms of vaginitis, including a yellowish discharge. They report to have not been sexually active for 18 months. When KOH is added to a sample of the discharge, a "fishy" odor appears. Which of the following organisms is the most likely cause of their symptoms?

(A) *C. albicans*
(B) *C. trachomatis*
(C) *G. vaginalis*
(D) HSV-2

4. A person with alcohol use disorder appears at the emergency department with chest pain, a 40 °C/104 °F temperature, chills, and a productive cough. They have no history of chronic pulmonary disease. There are red blood cells and encapsulated gram-negative rods in the sputum. Which of the following organisms is the most likely cause of these symptoms?

(A) *Haemophilus influenzae*
(B) *K. pneumoniae*
(C) *N. asteroides*
(D) *P. aeruginosa*

5. There is an outbreak of GI disease involving six children at a daycare center. The children all have symptoms of fever, watery stool, and vomiting. Recent activities at the center involved playing with animals, including kittens, turtles, birds, and hamsters. Which of the following types of bacteria are most likely to be observed in the stool?

(A) Gram-positive cocci
(B) Gram-negative cocci
(C) Gram-positive rods
(D) Gram-negative rods

6. A 75-year-old man is brought by his daughter to the community health center. He appears confused and has a stiff neck and severe headache. She indicates that the previous week, he had a runny nose and other symptoms consistent with sinusitis. Which of the following organisms would be expected to be found in his CSF?

(A) Coxsackie virus
(B) *H. influenzae*
(C) *Neisseria meningitidis*
(D) *Streptococcus pneumoniae*

7. While on winter semester break, a 21-year-old college student appears at his family physician's office with several skin lesions on his right arm. They consist of a central pustule within a raised erythematous area. He reports that the only recent unusual activities that have involved skin exposure have been hot tub parties at his friend's cabin during the previous two weekends. Which of the following organisms is the most likely causative infectious agent?

(A) Human papillomavirus
(B) *P. aeruginosa*
(C) *S. aureus*
(D) *S. pyogenes*

8. In July, a rural nursing home reports that several of the residents have developed a GI disease consisting of fever, vomiting, and bloody stool. Lab analysis of some of the stool samples shows the presence of PMNs and gram-negative rods. Epidemiologic discussions with the residents indicate they all shared the same raw milk brought to one resident by his child who was a farmer. Which of the following organisms is the most likely cause of this infection?

(A) *Campylobacter jejuni*
(B) *Clostridium perfringens*
(C) *S. aureus*
(D) *Vibrio parahaemolyticus*

9. An 18-month-old female infant is brought to the emergency department by her parent. The parent reports an abrupt onset of symptoms consisting of continual crying, high fever (40 °C/104 °F), and a cough producing rusty-colored sputum. Which of the following would be expected to be observed in a chest x-ray and lab finding?

(A) Bronchopneumonia pattern and gram-positive cocci
(B) Bronchopneumonia pattern and gram-negative rods
(C) Lobar pattern and gram-positive cocci
(D) Lobar pattern and gram-negative cocci

10. A 14-year-old boy is brought to the clinic with a skin infection. The causative agent is identified as gram-positive bacteria. Which of the following bacterial components would be expected to be found in the most likely causative agent, but not in gram-negative bacteria?

(A) Capsule
(B) Lipopolysaccharide
(C) Outer membrane
(D) Peptidoglycan
(E) Teichoic acid

11. A 29-year-old woman with acquired immunodeficiency syndrome has severe, nonresolving watery diarrhea. It is not gray or greasy. Acid-fast oocysts are seen in the stools. Which of the following organisms is the most likely causative agent?

(A) *Cryptosporidium*
(B) EHEC
(C) Enterotoxic *E. coli*
(D) *Giardia*
(E) *Salmonella*

12. A 22-year-old female presents with vaginal itching and erythema as well as a thick, white discharge. External erythema is also present with discrete pinpoint lesions off the edge. The discharge pH is 4.7 (normal). Amine test is negative as is the genetic probe test for *Neisseria*. Which of the following is the most likely cause of the symptoms?

(A) Bacterial vaginosis
(B) *C. albicans*
(C) *C. trachomatis*
(D) Overgrowth of *G. vaginalis*
(E) *Trichomonas vaginalis*

13. A 70-year-old man presents with a pulmonary infection caused by an organism that requires 4 weeks to grow on Löwenstein-Jensen medium. Past medical history indicates that the patient is HIV positive with a CD4$^+$ cell count of 40/mm^3, and he is nonadherent to HIV treatment. Which of the following is the best descriptor of the most likely causative agent of this patient's pulmonary infection?

(A) Acid-fast organism
(B) Dimorphic fungus
(C) Filamentous fungus
(D) Gram-positive coccus
(E) Gram-negative coccus
(F) Gram-negative rod

14. A 63-year-old woman presents to the clinic with chest pain, fever, shaking chills, cough, and myalgia. She has a previous medical history of a diagnosis of alcohol use disorder. She was very cold 2 nights ago and says she has felt "poorly" ever since. Her cough produces rust-colored, odorless, mucoid sputum. Her temperature on admission is 40 °C. Her white blood cell count is 16,000 cells/mm^3 and is predominantly neutrophils with an overall left shift. An α-hemolytic, lancet-shaped, gram-positive diplococcus is isolated on blood agar. What is the most likely causative agent?

(A) *K. pneumoniae*
(B) *Legionella pneumophila*
(C) *Mycoplasma pneumoniae*
(D) *N. meningitidis*
(E) *S. pneumoniae*

15. A neonate develops meningitis at age 7 days. The young mother reports multiple sexual partners without barrier protection and lives in the United States. The infant was born 23 hours after the mother's amniotic sac ruptured. What is the most likely causative agent?

(A) *E. coli*
(B) *H. influenzae*
(C) *Listeria monocytogenes*
(D) *N. meningitidis*
(E) *Streptococcus agalactiae*

16. In January, a 74-year-old woman was brought to the hospital emergency department by her wife, who states that she had a fever and headache during the past week. During the past 2 days, she has been confused and cannot perform her daily chores. Her physical examination indicates some weaknesses in her left side, and her head magnetic resonance imaging (MRI) shows necrosis in the right temporal lobe. What is the most likely causative agent?

(A) Coxsackie A16 virus
(B) HSV-1
(C) Rabies virus
(D) West Nile virus
(E) Western equine encephalitis virus

17. In which of the following fungal scalp infections is hair loss most likely to be permanent?

(A) Anthropophilic tinea capitis
(B) Black dot tinea capitis of adults
(C) Favus (tinea favosa)
(D) Zoophilic tinea capitis

18. Which of the following organisms cause a respiratory infection known to increase susceptibility to *S. pneumoniae* pneumonia?

(A) Epstein-Barr virus infection
(B) *H. influenzae* type b or type d infection
(C) Influenza virus infection
(D) *M. tuberculosis* infection
(E) *M. pneumoniae* infection

19. An 18-year-old who lives in Iowa presents in September with cough, malaise, low-grade fever, myalgias, and chest pain. They say that they visited the desert in the southwest 3 weeks ago for a camping and hiking trip. Rales are heard, and respiratory infiltrates are noted on radiograph. Sputum stained with calcofluor white and viewed on an ultraviolet microscope shows large blue-white fluorescing spherical structures (with a wall) and with numerous small round cells inside. Which of the following organisms is the most likely causative agent?

(A) *C. albicans*
(B) *C. immitis*
(C) *H. capsulatum*
(D) Influenza virus type A
(E) *M. pneumoniae*
(F) *S. pneumoniae*

20. Several workers in a small office develop a pseudomembranous conjunctivitis without corneal involvement. No bacteria can be identified. Which of the following organisms is the most probable cause?

(A) Acanthamoeba
(B) Adenovirus
(C) *C. trachomatis*
(D) HSV

21. A 15-year-old boy receiving antibiotics to clear up a community-acquired methicillin-resistant *S. aureus* infection has clindamycin added to his treatment regimen to slow the production of various toxins, including Panton-Valentine leukocidin. He recovers but develops *Clostridioides difficile* diarrhea. Which of the following reasons explains how *C. difficile* causes diarrhea?

(A) *C. difficile* exotoxins damage the cells, causing a disruption in transport and attracting polymorphonuclear cells to cause the appearance of a pseudomembrane.
(B) *C. difficile* multiplies and causes disease in a mechanism similar to that of *Listeria*.
(C) *C. difficile* multiplies, secreting Shiga toxin during cell lysis.
(D) *C. difficile* stacks itself on the colonic surface to cause malabsorption and the appearance of a pseudomembrane.

22. In June, an 18-year-old man developed a sore throat with a fever and a nonproductive cough that developed into pneumonia with a severe, prolonged hacking cough but little sputum production. Cryoagglutinins are present. He is treated appropriately and successfully with azithromycin. Which of the following features is related to the most likely causative agent?

(A) Acid-fast organism
(B) DNA virus
(C) Gram-negative rod
(D) Gram-positive coccus
(E) Pleomorphic no cell wall

23. A 10-year-old boy presents with an itchy scalp, with the underlying hair becoming lighter. The patch has expanded to 2 inches. A KOH-digested mount is prepared from skin scrapings taken at the infected margin of a lesion from this patient's tinea capitis. Which of the following forms would be expected to be seen in the microscope?

(A) Irregular but broad, aseptate hyphae
(B) Regular septate hyphae with little branching
(C) Septate hyphae regularly branching dichotomously at an acute angle
(D) Yeast cells, pseudohyphae, and true hyphae
(E) Yeasts only

24. A patient presents with explosive, watery, noninflammatory diarrhea along with headache, abdominal cramps, nausea, vomiting, and fever. Symptoms began the day after eating raw oysters in August. Which of the following organisms is the most likely causative agent?

(A) *Giardia lamblia*
(B) Norwalk agent
(C) Rotavirus
(D) *Salmonella enteritidis*
(E) *S. aureus*
(F) *V. parahaemolyticus*

25. A 5-year-old girl is brought to her pediatrician by her father who reports the child had a flulike illness for the past week and now has developed a rash. Examination of the rash on the face and trunk shows general redness consistent with a slapped cheek. Which of the following viruses is most likely responsible?

(A) Coxsackie A virus
(B) Echovirus
(C) JC virus
(D) Parvovirus

26. A 7-year-old boy develops watery diarrhea, which becomes bloody. He is afebrile but becoming very ill. Macroscopic examination of the feces shows no areas of pus; microscopically, there was no excess of PMNs over that expected from peripheral blood. Recent history is a trip to a Wisconsin dairy farm where he was petting cattle. Which of the following activities is most likely causing the bleeding?

(A) Invasion of intestinal cells with transit to the bloodstream and reinvasion
(B) Invasion of M cells with shallow ulceration, resulting from actin C
(C) Polymerization, "jetting" the bacterium laterally
(D) Toxin binding to G_s, shutting off protein syntheses
(E) Toxin cleaving the eukaryotic ribosome, shutting down protein synthesis and damaging the mucosa

27. Six 18-year-old women return from a recent camping trip to the Rocky mountains with abdominal cramping, gas, pain, and diarrhea that is pale, greasy, and malodorous. They drank untreated stream water on the past 2 days of the trip after losing their water filter. Which of the following organisms is the most likely causative agent?

(A) *Baylisascaris procyonis*
(B) *Entamoeba histolytica*
(C) *G. lamblia*
(D) *Norovirus*
(E) *S. enteritidis*
(F) *V. parahaemolyticus*

28. A patient presents with an inflamed itchy groin area. Which of the following antifungals would be effective as long as the causative agent is a dermatophyte but might make it worse if it is a yeast infection?

(A) Amphotericin B
(B) Griseofulvin
(C) Miconazole
(D) Nystatin
(E) Trimethoprim-sulfamethoxazole

29. A 15-month-old undervaccinated child develops meningitis. A gram-negative rod is seen in the CSF. Which of the following organisms is the most likely causative agent?

(A) Enterovirus
(B) *E. coli*
(C) *H. influenzae*
(D) *N. meningitidis*
(E) *S. agalactiae*

30. A patient with a cough of several weeks of duration but no fever has radiologic signs of a coin lesion. The needle biopsy shows large, broad-based budding yeasts with a very thick cell wall. Most of the yeasts are extracellular. Which of the following conditions is the most likely diagnosis?

(A) Aspergillosis
(B) Blastomycosis
(C) Cancer
(D) Coccidioidomycosis
(E) Histoplasmosis

31. A 17-year-old develops *N. meningitidis* meningitis. Which of the following events are most likely to have occurred first?

(A) Central nervous system (CNS) invasion directly through the cribriform plate
(B) Crossing the blood-brain barrier
(C) Meningococcemia
(D) Skin lesions
(E) Upper respiratory colonization
(F) Waterhouse-Friderichsen syndrome

Answers and Explanations

1. **The answer is B.** [I A; Chapter 3 II A] This case of neonatal conjunctivitis is most likely caused by *C. trachomatis* since no bacteria are present and papillae rather than follicles are observed. The mother was probably the source of the infection.

2. **The answer is C.** [VI B; Chapter 3 VIII E] Both *Staphylococcus epidermidis* and various Enterobacteriaceae can cause epididymitis in men older than 35 years, but gram-negative rod is not a choice; therefore, gram-positive cocci are correct.

3. **The answer is C.** [VI D; Chapter 3 XII] *G. vaginalis* and *C. albicans* are the non-STI choices. *G. vaginalis* is correct because it produces a fishy odor when KOH is added to the discharge.

4. **The answer is B.** [II B 2; Chapter 3 VI D] *K. pneumoniae* is associated with pneumonia in individuals with alcohol use disorder. The other gram-negative rod (*P. aeruginosa*) is associated with chronic pulmonary disease in the immunocompromised.

5. **The answer is D.** [III A; Chapter 3 IX L] The most likely bacteria to cause GI disease with the symptoms and circumstances provided is a species of *Salmonella*, which is gram-negative rod. Turtles are the most likely source.

6. **The answer is D.** [II C 1; Chapter 3 II D] The symptoms of confusion and severe headache point to a case of bacterial meningitis. With preceding sinusitis in an older man, *S. pneumoniae* is the most likely cause. The other two bacteria are more often observed in infants or young adults.

7. **The answer is B.** [V D; Chapter 3 I B] *P. aeruginosa* is associated with an infection known as *whirlpool* or *hot tub* folliculitis. Inappropriate care of whirlpools, hot tubs, and swimming pools can allow this organism to grow and enter the skin through small breaks.

8. **The answer is A.** [III C; Chapter 3 IX J] The symptoms and lab analysis of the stool are consistent with *C. jejuni* infection. The raw milk was most likely the source of the infection.

9. **The answer is C.** [II A; Chapter 3 II D] The most common cause of CAP in infants and older adults is *S. pneumoniae*. The symptoms in this case are consistent, and the rusty-colored sputum is suggestive of this bacteria. It is a gram-positive coccus with a lobar pneumonia on a chest x-ray.

10. **The answer is E.** [V; Chapter 2 I B 8 b] Teichoic and teichuronic acids, which are polymers containing ribitol or glycerol, are found in the cell walls or cell wall membranes of gram-positive bacteria. Capsules may be found in both gram-negative and gram-positive bacteria.

11. **The answer is A.** [III B; Table 9.3] Oocysts are only formed by protozoans, eliminating A, C, and E. Acid-fast oocysts are only found in *Cryptosporidium, Cyclospora,* or *Isospora* infections.

12. **The answer is B.** [VI D; Chapter 7 VII B] The discharge is characteristic of *Candida* overgrowth. Note that no foul odor is mentioned, and the negative amine test "rules down" bacterial vaginosis and *Trichomonas*. Both yeast vaginitis and yeast diaper rash have the described satellite lesions outside the area of major erythema. *Gardnerella* is the prominent agent in bacterial vaginosis. The normal pH range is 4.5 to 5, and yeast vaginitis is usually in that range.

13. **The answer is A.** [II A 3 a (1); Chapter 3 VI L] *Mycobacterium avium-intracellulare* or *M. tuberculosis*, both acid-fast organisms, are the most likely causes of this pulmonary infection in a patient with acquired immunodeficiency syndrome. Both can be cultured on Lowenstein-Jensen but, in general, both systems providing a similar high-lipid content for making the mycobacterial cell wall have replaced Lowenstein-Jensen. *P. jirovecii*, now considered a fungus, cannot be cultured on any medium.

14. **The answer is E.** [II B; Chapter 3 II D] *S. pneumoniae* is the most common causative agent of pneumonia in those with alcohol use disorder. *K. pneumoniae* is less common but even more deadly because of the high incidence of abscesses. (Almost all of the patients who have pneumonia caused by *K. pneumoniae* suffer from chronic lung disease or alcohol use disorder.) If foul-smelling sputum had been present, then anaerobes would most likely be involved.

Legionella and *Klebsiella* are both gram-negative rods. *N. meningitidis* is a gram-negative diplococcus. Neither *Legionella* nor *Mycoplasma* would have grown on blood agar.

15. **The answer is E.** [IV A; Chapter 3 VII A] *S. agalactiae* (group B streptococci) is the most common cause of neonatal meningitis. It is most prevalent in young females who have had multiple partners and is most likely to infect the infant during a protracted delivery. *E. coli* is the second most common cause of neonatal meningitis. *Listeria* is a less frequent cause of neonatal meningitis and other severe diseases in newborns. *H. influenzae* and *N. meningitidis* rarely cause neonatal meningitis.

16. **The answer is B.** [IV B; Chapter 5 IX A] Viral encephalitis in January, which localizes to the temporal lobe, is most likely HSV-1.

17. **The answer is C.** [V A; Chapter 7 III G] Scarring and permanent hair loss are most likely to occur with favus (tinea favosa).

18. **The answer is C.** [II D; Chapter 3 VI B] Pneumococcal pneumonia is most frequent in patients with some damage to mucociliary elevators in the upper respiratory tracts. Antecedent measles, influenza virus infections, and alcoholism predispose patients to pneumococcal pneumonia.

19. **The answer is B.** [II A 3; Chapter 7 VI D] The causative agent can only be *C. immitis* from the description of the spherules and endospores in the sputum. Note that no definitive geographic clue is given in this question. Without the results of the microscopic examination, it possibly could have been *H. capsulatum* or *Blastomyces* pneumonia. The patient is also in the right age group for *Mycoplasma* pneumonia, but again the microscopic data point instead to *Coccidioides*.

20. **The answer is B.** [I B; Chapter 5 I C 1 a] Adenovirus is easily spread, and it causes a mild conjunctivitis without corneal involvement. It can also cause pseudomembranous conjunctivitis.

21. **The answer is A.** [III A; Chapter 3 IX O] *C. difficile* causes the production of exotoxins, which cause diarrhea and the production of the pseudomembrane.

22. **The answer is E.** [II A 2; Chapter 3 VI G] *Mycoplasma* is a common cause of pneumonia in teenagers and young adults. During the course of the infection, some autoagglutinating antibodies (cold agglutinins) may be formed against red blood cells. The antibodies are inactive at normal body temperature, but agglutinate red blood cells at 4 °C.

23. **The answer is B.** [V A; Chapter 7 III B] The tineas are caused by dermatophytes that generally appear in the tissue as septate hyphae with little branching. Sometimes, arthroconidia are formed where large sections or the entire filament break up into spores.

24. **The answer is F.** [III A; Chapter 3 IX I] *V. parahaemolyticus* is the most likely causative agent. It is found in raw oysters from contaminated oyster beds from spring to fall.

25. **The answer is D.** [V D; Chapter 5 XI E 2 a] Only one virus family has single-stranded DNA as its genetic material, and that is the parvovirus family. Parvovirus B19 can cause a disease called *erythema infectiosum*, which produces signs and symptoms consistent with those described.

26. **The answer is E.** [III C; Chapter 3 IX K] The symptoms are only characteristic of EHEC. The toxin kills intestinal cells by shutting off protein synthesis, causing erosion of the intestinal wall. Hemolytic uremic syndrome (HUS) may also occur.

27. **The answer is C.** [III B; Table 9.3] Pale, greasy, malodorous stools with malabsorption after drinking untreated stream or lake water strongly suggest a *G. lamblia* infection. The organisms can be detected most reliably by a fecal antigen test because they attach to the intestinal mucosa.

28. **The answer is B.** [Chapter 6 IV E] Griseofulvin is given orally and is effective on dermatophytes but may exacerbate yeast infections. Choice A, miconazole, works on both dermatophytes and yeasts. Choice B, nystatin, works on yeasts. Of the fungi, choice D is used orally only for pneumocystis. Choice E (AMB) is incorrect as it is not used topically on the skin.

29. **The answer is C.** [IV A; Chapter 3 II E] The only gram-negative rods in the choices are *E. coli* and *H. influenzae*. The causative agent is more likely to be *H. influenzae* in a child at this age.

30. The answer is B. [II A 3; Chapter 7 VI C] The picture given is classic for the pulmonary lesions of blastomycosis, which cannot be differentiated from carcinoma without biopsy.

31. The answer is E. [IV A; Chapter 3 VII E] *N. meningitidis* is transmitted by direct oral mucosal contact or direct receipt of infected respiratory droplets on another's oropharyngeal mucosa. *N. meningitides* adheres via pili and other adhesins; in addition, IgA protease production and the capsule allow survival in an individual without immunity, allowing upper respiratory colonization that is followed by invasion of the bloodstream. This precedes the development of pneumonia or meningitis. Skin lesions develop from overproduction of the outer membrane, which is excreted without being incorporated, causing endotoxic shock and petechiae that progress to frank purpura. Waterhouse-Friderichsen syndrome is late.

14

Clinical Laboratory Diagnosis

Laboratory diagnosis is just one portion of the diagnostic algorithm for identifying causes of infectious disease. In general, the following steps are taken before laboratory tests are considered. Placing the results of these assays in the proper context increases their utility.

1. Take a detailed patient history to identify the symptoms, travel history, exposure risk to infectious agents, and relevant medical information.
2. Perform a physical examination to identify physical signs that may indicate an infectious cause of the symptoms and body system involved.
3. Develop a differential that would explain the data thus far and then order diagnostic tests based on that differential. These may include tests such as blood tests, urine tests, imaging studies, and other specialized tests to identify the underlying cause of the infection.
4. Analyze the test results to determine the most likely cause from the differential.
5. Make a diagnosis based on the patient's history, physical findings, and test results.
6. Lastly, develop a treatment plan that at best removes the infectious cause or at least relieves the symptoms of the infection.

Clinical identification of pathogens is determined by a variety of methods. New methods are continuously introduced but do not always replace older methods. In this review book, critical identification methods and standard culture media are presented along with the newer methods because many of the older methods will continue to be used by some laboratories and will appear on national examinations. This chapter identifies useful tests that are used generally as well as those tests that can be used specifically for particular microorganisms.

> **• • • Clinical Pearl**
>
> All assays work to achieve 100% specificity and 100% sensitivity. While most assays come close to this goal, there is often a tradeoff between the two. Specificity is the accuracy with which the analyte is detected to discern false positives from true positives. Sensitivity is the ability to detect all true positives.

I. IMMUNOLOGIC ASSAYS

A. **Detection of patient antibody** demonstrates current or previous exposure to a pathogen.
   1. Positive titers (levels) are expressed as the highest dilution of the serum still giving a positive test so that a titer written as 1/64 is much higher than a titer of 1/4. Titers may also be written as 1:4. A 4-fold increase or greater over a 2-week period is indicative of active infection.
   2. High immunoglobulin M (IgM) titers also suggest recent infection.
   3. High IgG titers with no IgM usually indicate previous infection.

B. **Precipitation reactions** are used to detect soluble proteins, polysaccharides, and antigen-antibody (ag-ab) complexes.
   1. Either antigen or antibody in serum can be measured **quantitatively** with analytical precision.

   a. Increasing amounts of antigen are added in separate tubes containing a constant amount of the patient's serum.
   b. The resulting precipitate in each tube is washed and analyzed by micromethods, and the precipitated antibody is plotted as a function of antigen added. Three zones result: antibody excess, equivalence, and antigen excess (Figure 14.1).
  2. Immunoelectrophoresis may be used to identify a specific antigen in a mixture and in immunologic disorders. Components of an antigen mixture are separated in agar, first by migration in an electric field, followed by their diffusion and subsequent precipitation with specific antibody diffusing from an overhead trough.
  3. Radioimmunoassay (RIA) is based on the displacement of a known, radiolabeled antigen from an ag-ab complex by an unknown, unlabeled antigen (eg, hormone) in a patient's body fluids. The extent of loss of the labeled antigen from the ag-ab complex can be measured and is a function of the concentration of the unknown antigen in the patient's fluid. Sensitivity is less than 1 ng.
  4. Immunochromatography, also identified as the lateral flow technique, is utilized in rapid diagnostic testing at the bedside or clinic.
   a. A test strip that contains antibodies specific to the target is conjugated to colored particles.
   b. The target analyte moves through the conjugated antibody and forms a complex that then reacts with a captured antibody that is immobilized on the detection zone of the test strip.
  5. Enzyme-linked immunosorbent assay (ELISA) is a highly sensitive, practical assay useful in detecting either antigens or antibodies in low concentrations in a patient's body fluids (Figure 14.2).
   a. To measure low (nanogram) concentrations of **antigen** (eg, hormones, drugs, serum proteins), dilutions of the fluid containing antigen are added to its antibody, which is adsorbed onto plastic wells. The resulting complex is washed, and an enzyme-conjugated antibody specific for a different epitope on the test antigen is added.
   b. After washing, the enzyme substrate is added, and the color reaction is measured using a spectrophotometer. The titer is recorded as the highest dilution of antigen giving a color above the background.
   c. **Specific antibodies** in low concentrations in a patient's serum (eg, HIV) can also be measured by adding dilutions of the test antibody to its antigen adsorbed onto plastic wells; the complex is washed and an enzyme-conjugated anti-isotype antibody is added. After washing, the enzyme substrate is added, the color is measured, and the titer is determined, as mentioned earlier.
   d. The use of an enzyme label eliminates problems associated with radioisotope disposal in RIAs.

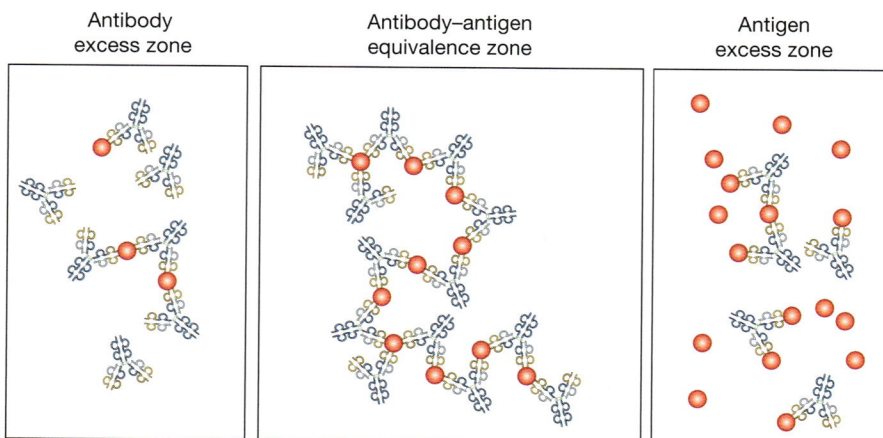

| Antibody excess zone | Antibody–antigen equivalence zone | Antigen excess zone |

FIGURE 14.1. The size of antigen-antibody (ag-ab) complexes is determined by the ratio of antigen to antibody. In vivo, larger complexes (in antibody excess and at equivalence) are phagocytosed; smaller complexes (in antigen excess) escape and lodge in blood vessels and behind the renal basement membrane, causing vasculitis and glomerulonephritis. Antigen is depicted in red circles.

ELISA

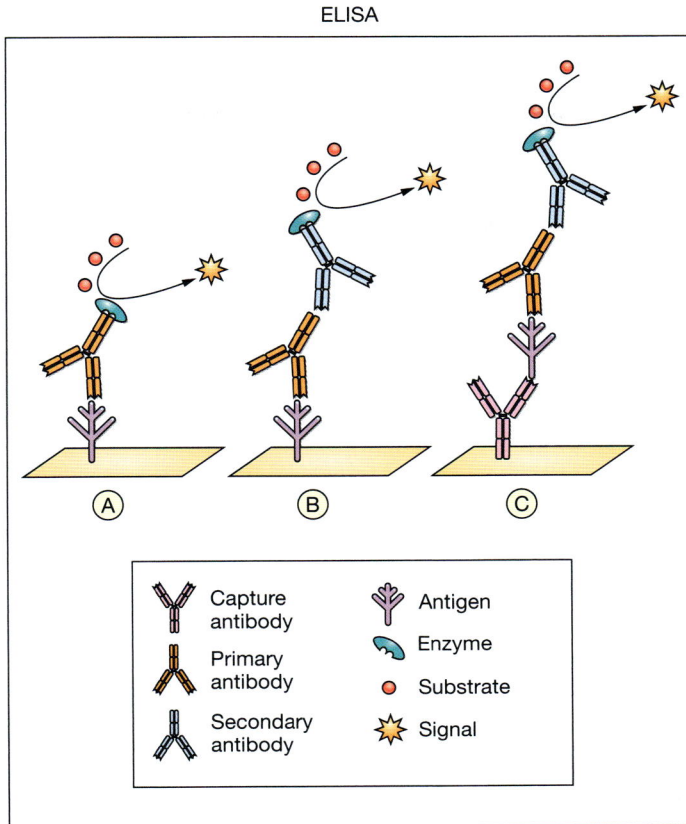

FIGURE 14.2. Enzyme-linked immunosorbent assay (ELISA). The components listed describe the mechanism for (A) direct ELISA, (B) indirect ELISA, and (C) sandwich ELISA. For (A), an unknown antigen is bound to the plate and detection antibody binds to the target. For (B), a known capture antigen is immobilized to the plate and binds to sample antibody. For (C), a known capture antibody is immobilized to the plate which binds to a sample antigen. (Image credit to Audrey Bell.)

C. Fluorescent antibody permits the visualization of either antigen or antibody in cells or tissues (Figure 14.3).

   1. In the **direct technique**, fluoresceinated (or another appropriate label) antibody to the antigen is added directly to the specimen (eg, tissue) containing antigen and visualized under ultraviolet light.

   2. The more sensitive **sandwich technique** (indirect fluorescence) is used to:

   a. Detect antigen: Its antibody is added first to the specimen, followed by fluoresceinated anti-Ig, and the specimen is visualized under ultraviolet light.

   b. Detect antibody: The antigen is added to the specimen followed by fluoresceinated antibody against the antigen, and the specimen is visualized under ultraviolet light.

D. The Western Blot technique is valuable in identifying an antigen or an antibody within a mixture (Figure 14.4).

   1. The components of the mixture are separated by electrophoresis on a sodium dodecyl sulfate-polyacrylamide gel and "blotted" (ie, transferred) onto a nitrocellulose matrix. It is then reacted with a known antibody and labeled with a secondary antibody that recognizes the ag-ab complex of interest.

   2. As a confirmatory test such as previously used for acquired immunodeficiency syndrome (AIDS), the patient's serum suspected of containing anti-AIDS antibody is added to known HIV antigens bound to a nitrocellulose matrix. Binding of a labeled, antihuman immunoglobulin antibody to the HIV-anti-HIV complex confirms exposure.

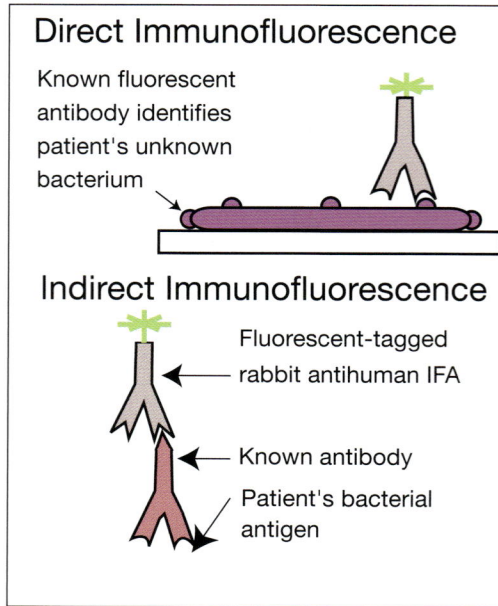

FIGURE 14.3. Immunofluorescent staining (also known as *fluorescent antibody staining*). (Top) With **direct fluorescent antibody staining**, highly specific (depending on antibody choice) fluorescent staining can be achieved by conjugating fluorescent dye (tagging) to a specific antibody. For example, because *Bordetella pertussis* is often difficult to culture after the characteristic cough has been present for a few days, a nasopharyngeal smear can be made and stained with tagged *B. pertussis* antibody. Thus, the gram-negative *Bordetella*, which on a Gram stain would be confused with nonpathogenic normal flora, can be positively identified because of the specificity of the ag-ab combination. (Bottom) With **indirect fluorescent antibody**, this test first reacts with commercially prepared antibody specific for the agent you are looking for with the fixed patient's specimen. After washing, a fluorescent dye-tagged anti-Ig is used to detect bound antibody. (Theoretically, if all of the commercially made unlabeled antibodies for this immunofluorescent "sandwich technique" were rabbit antibody, then all tests could use one fluorescent-tagged anti-rabbit antibody to "light" the bound antibody.)

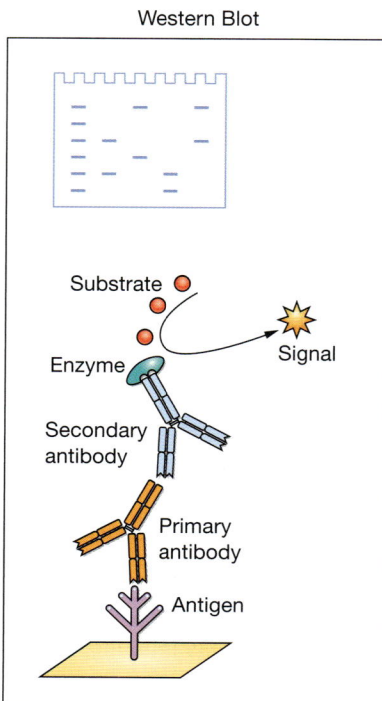

FIGURE 14.4. Western immunoblotting. Proteins of interest are subjected to electrophoresis through a polyacrylamide gel. The proteins are transferred to a membrane identified in the image as the antigen. The membrane is then exposed to a primary antibody that recognizes the target antigen. A labeled secondary antibody recognizes the ag-primary ab complex and is used for detection. Signals used can be chemiluminescent, fluorescent, or radioactive. (Image credit to Audrey Bell.)

II. NUCLEIC ACID-BASED ASSAYS

Nucleic acid detection is done with gene probes with or without amplification of target sequences or signal amplification. Newer techniques may be done directly on clinical specimens as well as cultured growth. These assays have the greatest specificity for the target.

A. Nucleic acid amplification tests (NAATs) include polymerase chain reaction (PCR), reverse transcription PCR (RT-PCR), and quantitative (aka real-time) PCR (qPCR; utilizing fluorescent dyes on probes to detect and help quantitate amplicons) (Figure 14.5).

   1. The process of NAAT requires first the denaturation of double-stranded DNA, second the annealing of short oligo sequences to prime the synthesis of new DNA strands from the template, and lastly the elongation of the new strand from the primer to create the complementary strand of the template.

   2. The elongation step requires the activity of a polymerase enzyme.

   3. This amplification process happens at three temperatures in a cycle and multiple cycles to synthesize enough DNA for detection. The amount of DNA doubles at each cycle.

   4. **RT-PCR** has an initial step at the start to convert the RNA target to DNA using a reverse transcriptase enzyme before cycling for DNA amplification.

B. Microarrays, which are microchips with hundreds of probes from different microorganisms on one slide, expand the ability of NAATs (Figure 14.6).

C. Fluorescent in situ hybridization (FISH) tests are available for clinical diagnostic use for some organisms or toxins and can be used on tissue sections, specimens such as sputum, or on gels.

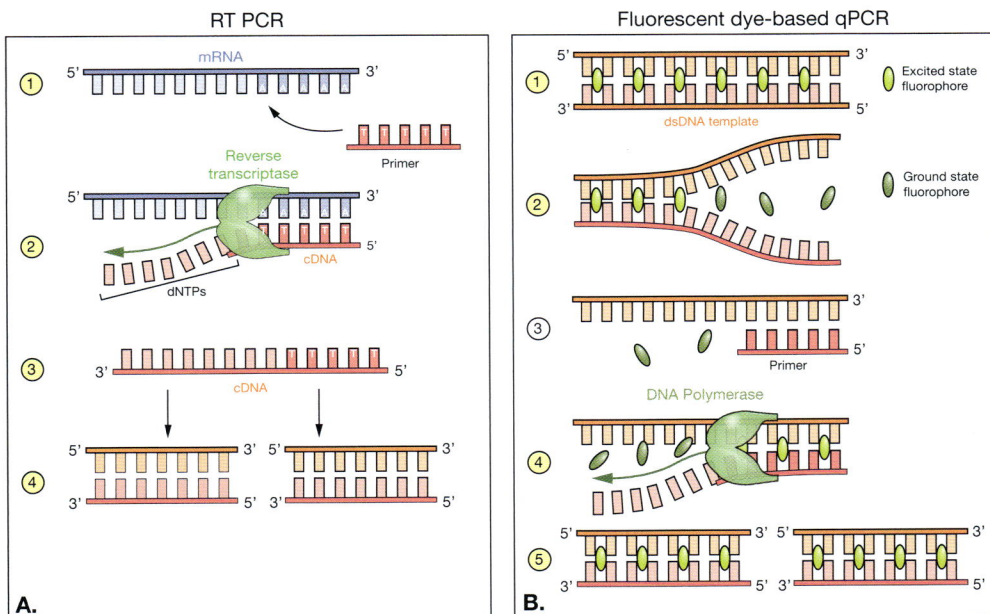

FIGURE 14.5. Polymerase chain reaction (PCR) synthesizes new strands of DNA from target templates by a process of primer annealing, dinucleotide base hybridization, and base pair extension. These steps are repeated for a number of cycles. Detection of the final amplification product occurs at the end of all PCR cycling. A. RT-PCR. In this amplification process, RNA is transcribed into copy DNA (cDNA). Step 1 shows primer annealing of a DNA primer to the mRNA. In step 2, dinucleotide base hybridization, and base pair extension occur via the enzyme Reverse Transcriptase to produce a copied DNA single strand (cDNA shown in step 3). This newly synthesized cDNA strand is then used as a template for the amplification of the DNA by PCR (step 4). B. Quantitative or real-time PCR (qPCR). A fluorescent dye marker is used to quantify the amount of DNA synthesized during each PCR cycle instead of at the end. This fluorophore is in an excited (detectable) state when bound to double-stranded DNA (step 1) and is in a ground state (undetectable) when not bound to double-stranded DNA (step 2) and 3. During PCR (step 4), a signal will not be detected, but the produces of each round of PCR (step 5) will be detected. Variations of the method exist to stimulate the ground state fluorophore to the excited state for detection, aiming to increase specificity and sensitivity. (Image credit to Audrey Bell.)

DNA Microarray

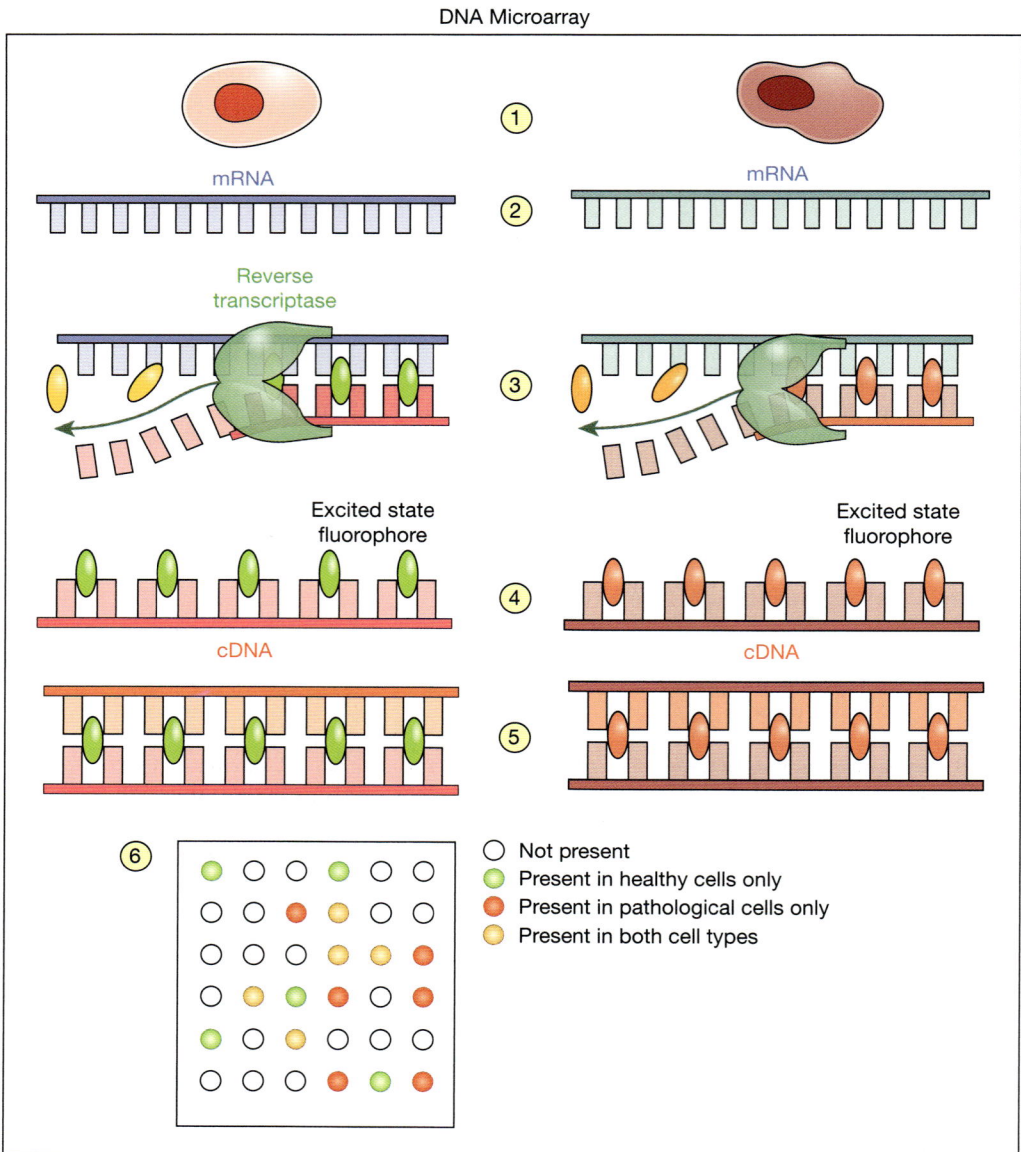

FIGURE 14.6. Microarray constructs. This image depicts the real-time detection of orders of magnitude, multiple genes or gene products for the purpose of comparing a normal healthy (left column path) state to a diseased state (right column path) (step 1). In this case, RNA from healthy cells is isolated (step 2) and reverse transcribed to copy DNA (cDNA) incorporating a unique fluorescent tag (step 3). This results in a single stranded cDNA copy (step 4). The same is done with RNA isolated from disease cells using a separate unique fluorescent tag. The cDNA amplification products are then hybridized (step 5) to a platform array with bound-specific nucleic acid capture fragments used for detection (step 6). (Image credit to Audrey Bell.)

D. **Sequencing pathogen genomes** allows for identification and fingerprinting of microorganisms. Traditional Sanger sequencing evaluates a single nucleic acid fragment at a time. Next-generation sequencing platforms can increase throughput by sequencing multitudes of fragments in parallel at the same time.

1. **Multilocus sequence typing** (**MLST**) for bacteria determines the sequence of multiple housekeeping genes for identification and species typing.
2. Mutational analysis sequencing can be utilized to determine genotypic resistance to pharmaceutical therapy such as in HIV drug monitoring.
3. Fungal sequencing is done to determine strain identity.

> **● ● ● Clinical Pearl**
>
> Assay positive and negative controls are required for every assay run to determine test performance. They must be treated the same as the patient sample to identify false results.

III. DIAGNOSTIC BACTERIOLOGY

Taxonomic relationships of the various genera of medically important bacteria are currently determined using molecular techniques and numerical taxonomy.

A. The identification of the specific causative agent of a bacterial infection is most commonly made by detecting the presence of one or more of the following:

  1. Bacteria through microscopy or culture.

  2. Bacterial components or products such as specific nucleic acid sequences, toxins, enzymes or enzymatic activities, capsules, or antigens.

  3. Patient antibodies to a specific organism or its products.

B. Diagnostic tests: Tests can be performed on the following:

  1. Clinical specimens: Some tests (eg, NAATS or microscopy) may be performed directly on clinical specimens.

  2. Isolated pathogen: Other tests require that the pathogen is isolated by culture, and the diagnostic tests then are performed on the isolated pathogen. This is especially true when identification requires running biochemical tests and most often to also be able to do antibiotic susceptibility testing.

C. Microscopy

  1. Gram stain, a differential stain, is a key starting point for etiologic diagnosis of infection.

    a. On some clinical specimens, it is used to guide initial therapy For example, lancet-shaped gram-positive diplococci in a sputum sample suggesting *Streptococcus pneumoniae.*

    b. On clinical specimens with normal flora, it may not be useful For example, gram-negative diplococci are found in normal pharyngeal flora, so a Gram stain cannot be used to diagnose gonococcal pharyngitis. However, the finding of gram-negative diplococci inside polymorphonuclear neutrophils (PMNs) from a urethral discharge is sufficient to start treatment in males.

    c. On the isolated bacterial culture, the source of the isolate, gram reaction, and oxidase or catalase test results guide the selection of additional identification tests and antibiotic susceptibilities.

    d. Gram-positive bacteria are purple.

    e. Gram-negative bacteria are red/pink because their cell envelopes lose the large purple dye complex, and so the stain pink/red counterstain is shown.

    f. Not reliably visualized on Gram stain are *Mycoplasma, Ureaplasma, Chlamydia, Rickettsia, Anaplasma, Ehrlichia, Coxiella, Legionella,* and spirochetes (especially ***Treponema***).

    g. Review the Gram stain procedure and see the provided examples (**Figure 14.7**). On direct clinical specimens (eg, pus), the background of human cells will stain pale red with red nuclei.

  2. Acid-fast stain (eg, Ziehl-Neelsen or Kinyoun stain) (**Figure 14.8**): This stain distinguishes **mycobacteria,** all of which are **acid fast (red),** from all other bacteria, all of which are **not acid fast (blue).** In addition, *Nocardia* is partially acid fast, sometimes showing some blue rods along with the red ones on the same slide; however, there will always be some red.

  3. Wet mounts are used for specific specimens such as unspun urine or for motility.

  4. Additional stains.

    a. India ink used to visualize capsules.

    b. Wright-Giemsa stain to differentially stain bacteria and human cells.

    c. Periodic acid-Schiff (PAS) reaction used to detect polysaccharides, glycoproteins, and glycolipids.

  5. Dark-field microscopy is useful for spirochetes that are too thin to be seen in a Gram stain and to show their motility.

Gram-Positive = Purple
Highly cross-linked and thick cell
walls; no outer membrane

Gram-Negative = Red
Thin peptidoglycan with little cross
linkage + phospholipid outer membrane

Step 1:
Crystal violet

| Small dye particle | | Small dye particle |

Step 2:
Iodine

| Large dye complex | | Large dye complex |

Step 3:
Alcohol decolorization

| Large dye complex trapped | | Large dye complex gets out |

Step 4:
Safranin counterstain

| Stays purple to dark blue/black | | Counterstain pale red to red |

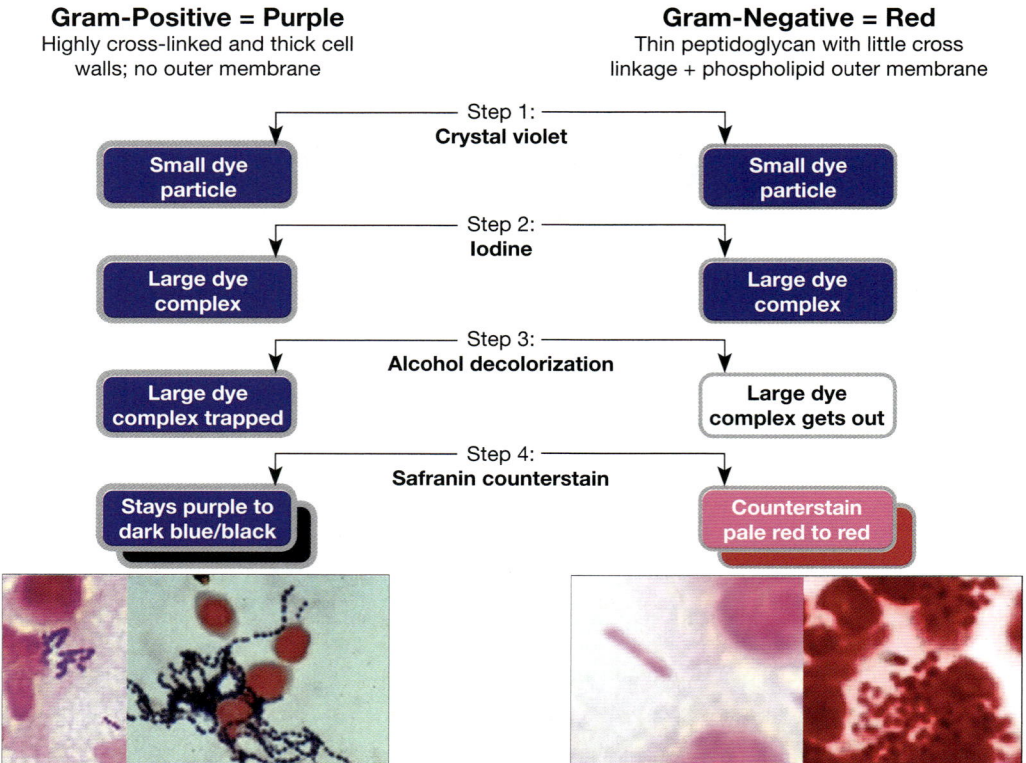

FIGURE 14.7. Gram stain. The photomicrographs at the bottom of the figure show the color variation of gram-positive cells (left) and gram-negative cells (right). (In each pair of images, the left image is from a former author (LH) and the right graciously provided by Dr Dilip K. Banerjee from *Microbiology of Infectious Diseases.* Gower Medical Publishing; 1986.)

6. **Fluorescent microscopy** may be used to examine both cultured isolates and directly on clinical specimens.
    a. **Fluorochrome dye methods** include auramine-rhodamine dyes that bind nonspecifically to waxy cell wall components of both *Mycobacterium* and relatives (**Figure 14.9**).
        (1) This stain is more sensitive because it is easier to read than an acid-fast stain. The fluorescent dyes light up the bacteria on the black background without interference from the specimen.
        (2) The fluorochrome dyes are sensitive but not specific like immunofluorescent staining because antibodies are not involved.

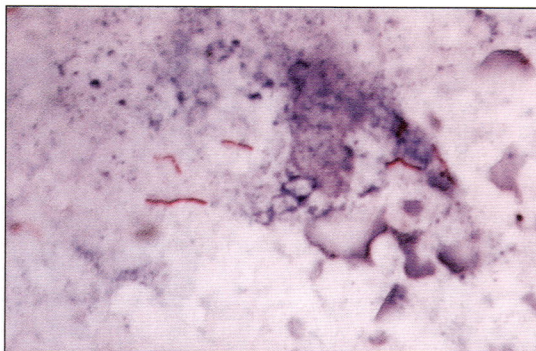

FIGURE 14.8. Acid-fast stain. Mycobacteria (acid fast = red) are shown in this sputum sample. This image has been enlarged greater than what is possible with the light or fluorescent microscope, making the images generally easier to read than on the actual microscope. Note how hard it is to see the red acid-fast bacteria. On acid-fast stains, human cells and debris are stained blue. (Image was graciously provided by Dr David Carter of St. Mary's/ Duluth Clinic, Duluth Minnesota.)

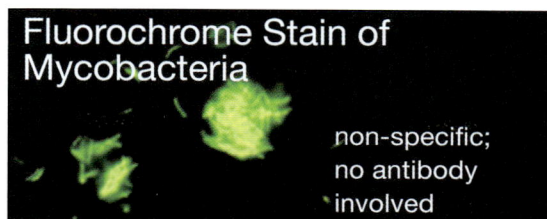

FIGURE 14.9. Fluorochrome stain. The auramine binds nonspecifically to the waxy mycobacterial cell well. Because there is no antibody involved in this binding, this is not a specific stain, but it is a sensitive screening test for sputum samples and is easy to read because of the contrast of the bound dye with everything else dark. A positive fluorochrome stain is always confirmed by an acid-fast stain or a mycobacterial fluorescent antibody stain.

D. Culture is a complex process that requires that specimens be properly obtained and transported and then grown on appropriate media under the correct conditions. Partial immunity, presence of active white cells (in blood cultures), or partial antibiotic treatment may interfere with growth.

1. The area from which the specimen is obtained influences the interpretation of results.
    a. If a specimen is obtained from a normally sterile area (eg, cerebrospinal fluid [CSF]) using aseptic technique, the finding of any microbes in the specimen is significant.
    b. If a specimen is obtained from a normally sterile area but passes through tissue with normal flora, specific specimen guidelines are used to evaluate the quality of the specimen and to interpret the results. Examples of these specimens are sputa or urine taken by the clean-catch midstream urine method.
       (1) With "sputum," the finding of many epithelial cells and lack of PMNs suggests that the specimen is saliva rather than material from the lungs.
       (2) With urine, quantitation guidelines suggest whether the patient has an infection or has normal levels of normal flora contaminating the specimen.
       (3) The finding of a specific pathogen that is not part of the normal flora is diagnostic of infection with that agent.
    c. If a specimen is obtained from an area with normal flora such as skin or mucous membranes, interpretation involves isolating pathogens or finding overgrowth of normal flora.
2. The **method** and **transport medium** of the specimen are often critical, especially if it is transported to a reference lab.
    a. Potentially anaerobic specimens such as abscess material must be obtained and transported anaerobically.
    b. Some organisms are sensitive to cold or drying.
3. **Proper culture medium** and **growth conditions** influence growth. A rich medium, often with blood, is commonly used as one isolation medium for most specimens.
    a. **Hemolysis** on blood agar may be used when identifying bacterial species (**Figure 14.10**).
       (1) α-**Hemolysins** produce **incomplete lysis,** with green pigment surrounding the colony.
       (2) Bacteria producing **no hemolysis** are said to be γ-**hemolytic** or **nonhemolytic.**
       (3) β-**Hemolysins** produce **total hemolysis** and break down the hemoglobin creating a clear area around the colony.
    b. **Differential media:** Some specific media (including blood agar) help **differentiate groups of organisms directly on the plate.** Examples are Hektoen and MacConkey agars that distinguish lactose fermenters from nonfermenters (**Figure 14.11**).
    c. **Fastidious bacteria** are those with complex nutritional requirements. These bacteria will not grow on standard laboratory agars and require special specific media. The following are **media commonly used to grow fastidious bacteria** (**Table 14.1**; also see Table 2.1):
       (1) **Chocolate agar (agar made with lysed red blood cells [RBCs])**
          (a) This medium is used for both *Haemophilus* **spp.** and *Neisseria* **spp.,** both of which are nonhemolytic but require nutrients from the lysed RBCs (**Figure 14.12**).
          (b) **Thayer-Martin** and **New York City agars** are used to grow *Neisseria* that have been obtained from body areas with competing normal flora (any mucosa). Both are chocolate agars that contain antibiotics to prevent growth of the bacteria and yeasts that are part of the normal mucosal flora. NAATs or gene probes may be used instead of cultures for diagnosis of gonorrhea.

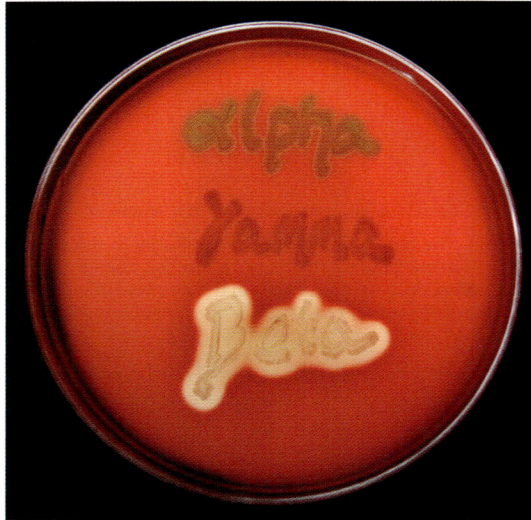

FIGURE 14.10. Hemolysis. Examples of the different types of hemolysis. Plates were inoculated in cursive writing. Note that the growth on these plates does not show up well because transmitted light was used to show the hemolysis. (Top) α-**Hemolysis** is partial hemolysis of the red blood cells (RBCs) with a change in the color of hemoglobin resulting in a translucent area with a greenish coloration. (Middle) γ-**Hemolysis** is no hemolysis. (Bottom) β-**Hemolysis** is complete lysis of the RBCs, which results in a transparent area around the colony. (From Engleberg NC, et al. *Schaechter's mechanism of microbial disease.* 5th ed. Wolters Kluwer Health; 2013.)

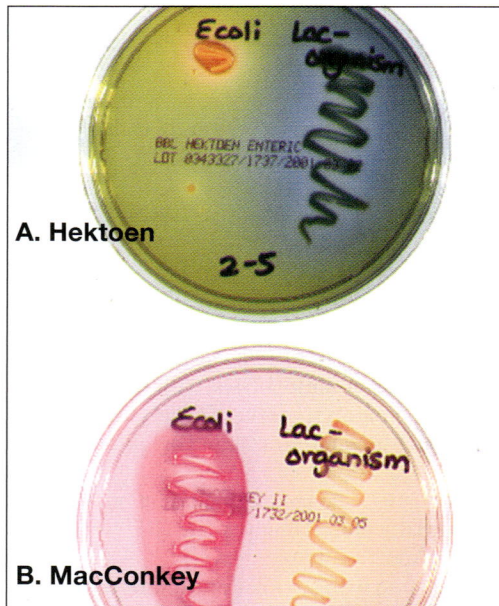

FIGURE 14.11. Differential media. These media allow the distinction of certain groups from the growth and substrate changes directly on the plate. Thus, on several of the enteric media, gram-positive bacterial growth is inhibited and gram-negative bacteria which grow and ferment lactose can be distinguished from those that do not ferment lactose. A. **Hektoen agar.** Lactose fermentation (eg, *Escherichia coli*) produces acid that turns the colonies and medium into colors in the yellow range. B. **MacConkey medium.** The pale straw color of the medium turns to red when the pH becomes acidic from the lactose fermentation products.

Table 14.1 Common Bacteriologic Media	
Common Bacteriologic Media	**Bacteria**
Charcoal-yeast extract agar	*Legionella*
Chocolate agar	*Haemophilus*
	Neisseria
New York City or Thayer-Martin	*Neisseria* from nonsterile specimens
Lowenstein-Jensen agar or Middlebrook medium	*Mycobacterium*
Regan-Lowe	*Bordetella*
Thiosulfate-citrate-bile salts-sucrose (TCBS)	*Vibrio*

(2) Regan-Lowe and **Bordet-Gengou agars**
   (a) These media are used for culture of ***Bordetella pertussis.***
   (b) Rapid, nonculture methods are replacing culture because it is difficult to culture *B. pertussis* either from a vaccinated person or after the early paroxysmal stage of whooping cough.
(3) Thiosulfate-citrate-bile salts-sucrose: Thiosulfate-citrate-bile salts-sucrose (TCBS) is an alkaline medium used to grow *Vibrio cholerae.*
(4) (Buffered) charcoal-yeast extract (BCYE) agar is used to grow ***Legionella.*** It contains needed iron and cysteine plus charcoal.
(5) Lowenstein-Jensen agar
   (a) Lowenstein-Jensen agar contains egg yolk that provides the necessary lipids for **mycobacteria.**
   (b) It is being replaced with high lipid broth cultures specifically designed for mycobacteria, allowing faster growth and machine detection of growth by quantitative PCR.

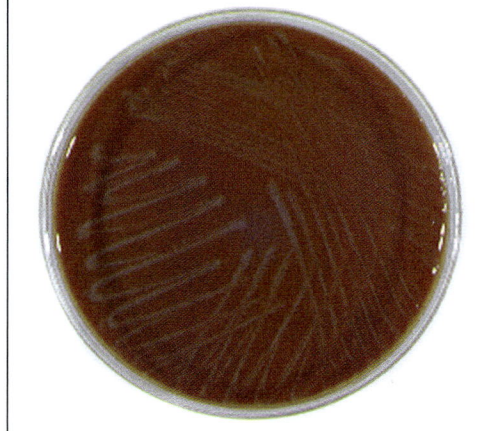

Haemophilus influenzae on chocolate agar

FIGURE 14.12. Chocolate agar. Some organisms, such as *Haemophilus influenzae* and pathogenic *Neisseria*, are nonhemolytic but require complex factors inside blood cells; therefore, they will not grow on blood agar but will grow on chocolate agar, which is made with lysed blood. *H. influenzae* will also grow on nutrient agar with added hemin and NAD (nicotinamide adenine dinucleotide, X and V factors, respectively).

E. Detection of microbial products (many require isolating the pathogen in culture)

1. **Antigen detection** requires specific antibodies and may be done by direct or indirect fluorescent microscopy or by ELISA.
2. **PCR for 16s ribosomal RNA gene sequencing.**
3. Tests demonstrating **specific enzymes** or **toxin activities**.
    a. **Nagler test for *Clostridium perfringens* α-toxin (a lecithinase):** This test uses a lecithin-containing agar to detect lecithinase activity. One side of the plate has an antibody to the *C. perfringens* α-toxin that neutralizes its activity. The test result is positive if there is a visual change around the growth on the side without antitoxin and no change in the media on the side containing the antitoxin since the antitoxin will inactivate the enzyme.
    b. Hemolysin detected on **blood agar** (see III D 3 a).
    c. Growth on media with **one major carbohydrate source.**
        (1) Growth in broths in microtiter plates where there is only one carbohydrate per well.
        (2) **MacConkey agar:** This agar has peptone and lactose; it supports the growth of all Enterobacteriaceae but only those fermenting the lactose will cause the color change from buff to hot pink red (Figure 14.11B). (It also contains bile salts and crystal violet to inhibit the growth of nonenteric organisms and gram-positive organisms.)
    d. Growth in **broths with specific substrates** for detection of specific activities: These tests are the mainstay of commonly used automated identification systems.
    e. **Rapid enzyme tests** detect the presence of the following enzymes:
        (1) **Catalase** breaks down hydrogen peroxide. This test is used to differentiate the gram-positive cocci of the genus *Staphylococcus* (catalase positive) from *Streptococcus* (catalase negative). In general, many anaerobes (and some microaerophiles) do not make catalase (Figure 14.13A).
        (2) **Oxidase (cytochrome-C oxidase)** is produced by most gram-negative bacteria but not by members of the Enterobacteriaceae. Oxidase positive rules the latter out.

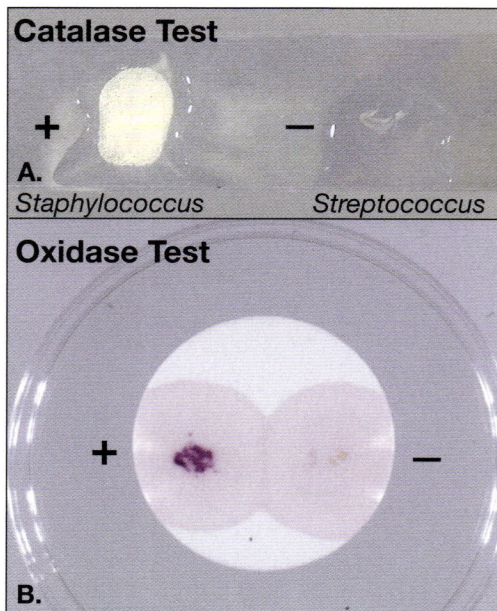

FIGURE 14.13. Important rapid tests used in early identification of some bacteria. A. **Catalase test**. Hydrogen peroxide is reacted with a small amount of the bacterial growth. The production of bubbles (oxygen) suggests that the organism contains catalase. The organism on the left side of the slide is positive; the organism (hard to see because there are no bubbles) on the right side is negative. B. **Oxidase test**. This test detects the presence of cytochrome oxidase and is used largely for gram-negative bacteria. All Enterobacteriaceae are oxidase negative. Most others are oxidase positive.

(3) Nitrate reductase reduces nitrate to nitrite. It is used to detect the presence of Entero-bacteriaceae in urine.

   (a) *Escherichia coli* and other enterobacteria produce nitrate reductase; this test requires that the bacteria remain in contact with the urine for a sufficient time.

   (b) *Staphylococcus saprophyticus* does not produce nitrate reductase.

f. Growth under specific conditions can be used to identify certain metabolic features of microbes, such as whether it is an aerobe or anaerobe.

   (1) Suspected *Campylobacter* cultures are grown in incubators at 42 °C under microaerophilic conditions.

   (2) Thioglycollate broth is a medium with reducing power that develops an oxygen gradient. The tubes of media are carefully stab inoculated the full length.

   (a) If an organism grows only at the top of the medium, the isolate is an obligate aerobe.

   (b) If an organism grows throughout the medium but grows more heavily at the top, it is a facultative anaerobe.

g. Commercial test systems are generally designed to identify a clinical isolate and determine antibiotic susceptibility simultaneously. The general steps used in these systems are as follows:

   (1) Bacterial isolates are grown from the patient specimen.

   (2) Gram stain results (often along with catalase or oxidase tests) are used to select the appropriate identification tests (a series of tests identifying specific enzyme activities such as carbohydrate utilization and urease). The plates also contain wells with antimicrobials for susceptibility determination.

   (3) Plates are read by machine; results are given as the probability that the isolate is the identified organism and gives minimal inhibitory concentrations (MICs) for the tested antibiotics.

F. Detection of immune response to a specific pathogen: Agglutination tests are used to detect antibody union with large, particulate antigens.

1. Rapid, slide identification of bacteria can occur by mixing a loopful of bacteria from the patient's culture with a battery of specific antibacterial antisera and noting which antiserum causes agglutination.

2. Semiquantitative diagnostic test for bacterial diseases involves addition of the suspect bacterium (killed) to dilutions of the patient's serum. The highest dilution that results in visible agglutination is called *the titer.* A 4-fold increase in titer is necessary for diagnosis due to low levels of "natural" antibodies occurring in the serum of most normal humans.

3. IgM complement-fixing antibodies, which agglutinate RBCs at temperatures below 37 °C, can be detected by incubation at lower temperatures. These cold agglutinins are frequently autoimmune in nature and occur commonly in patients with primary atypical pneumonia caused by *Mycoplasma pneumonia.*

4. Detection of patient antibody for *Mycobacterium tuberculosis.*

   a. A positive **skin test** (eg, tuberculin skin test) in a person who is immunocompetent may demonstrate past or current infection and, unlike serology, cannot differentiate between the two. (Remember that patients who are immunocompromised may not be able to produce antibodies or mount a positive skin test.)

   b. Detection of immune response from whole blood (QuantiFERON or ELISpot test) has replaced the tuberculin skin test in many situations.

G. Determination of antimicrobial susceptibility: Susceptibility testing is done by many methods depending on the organism.

1. Gene probes (generally with amplification methods) may be used to determine if an organism carries a specific known gene for drug resistance.

2. Rapid tests are performed on an isolate mixed with a special substrate such as a chromogenic (colored) β-lactam. If the β-lactam ring is broken by lactamase, it leads to a color change.

3. Rapid growth detection systems (such as for *M. tuberculosis*) use quantitative PCR to detect growth. These tests are performed in a series of "tubes," some of which contain antimicrobials. Growth can be assessed in the presence or absence of specific antimicrobials (at appropriate levels).

4. Minimal inhibitory concentration broth tests are used to determine the minimal concentration in the presence of a particular drug that inhibits the growth of a bacterium.

    a. Commercially prepared microtiter plates with a series of tests to identify an organism (eg, a gram negative isolated from urine) also have a series of wells in which multiple appropriate antibiotics can be tested at a range of concentrations achievable in the body (Figure 14.14A). The lowest concentration of each drug that inhibits growth is MIC for that drug. (In other words, the MIC is the level that must be achieved at the site of the infection for the antibiotic to inhibit further growth.)

    b. The killing level or **minimal bactericidal concentrations (MBCs)** are usually determined after determination of the MICs. It is the lowest concentration of antimicrobial drug that will kill the specific organism.

5. Agar gel diffusion plates (Kirby-Bauer) use paper disks containing standard concentrations of dehydrated antibiotics (see Figure 14.14B).

    a. A solid agar medium in a petri dish is spread evenly with a broth of the patient's isolate.

    b. A dispenser drops the appropriate disks containing specific amounts of dried antibiotics on each surface. The disks are tapped to lay flat. The antibiotics hydrate and begin to diffuse out, setting up a concentration gradient in the agar surrounding the disk.

    c. The plates are incubated, generally overnight, and zones of growth inhibition are then measured and interpreted using charts as to whether the organism is sensitive, has intermediate susceptibility, or is resistant to the drug.

    d. These tests are qualitative, not quantitative.

6. E-tests (named for the elliptical zone of inhibition) are also agar diffusion antibiotic susceptibility tests but are made semiquantitative through the incorporation of a small plastic "ruler" with a scale that, through testing hundreds of isolates, correlates the zone of inhibition with quantitative MIC data (see Figure 14.14C).

Drug Susceptibility Testing

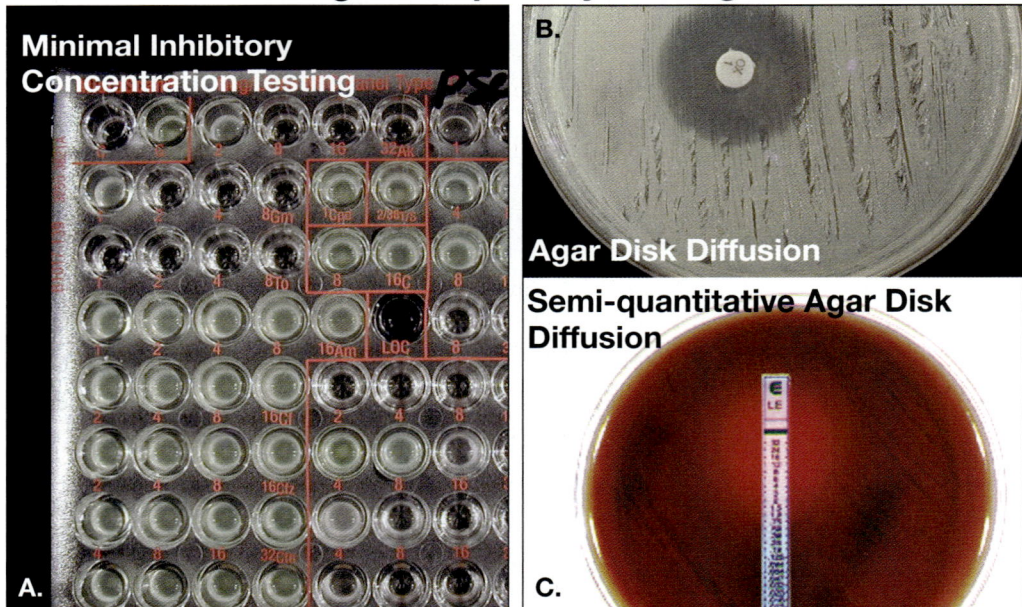

FIGURE 14.14. Drug susceptibility testing. A. **Minimal inhibitory concentration (MIC)**. Each well has a specific concentration of a single drug and the same approximate number of the patient's bacterial isolate. Drugs are tested in achievable concentration ranges in this test. Growth is measured by a variety of methods. B. **Agar disk diffusion.** A disk with a known concentration of dried antibiotic is placed on the surface of an agar plate spread inoculated with the patient's bacterial isolate. After incubation, the diameter of the zone of inhibition determines if the isolate is susceptible intermediate or resistant to that antibiotic. This is a qualitative technique. C. **E test, a semiquantitative agar disk diffusion**. A sterile plastic "ruler" with a drop of dried antibiotic on the back is placed on a plate inoculated with the patient's bacterial isolate to create a lawn of bacteria. After incubation, the zone of growth inhibition can be correlated with the expected MIC by reading the measurements on the ruler. The ruler is different for each antibiotic.

IV. DIAGNOSTIC VIROLOGY

A. Laboratory viral diagnosis involves one of three basic approaches: virus isolation; direct demonstration of virus, viral nucleic acid, or antigens in clinical specimens; or serologic testing of viral-specific antibodies.

1. Because the clinical symptoms of a virus are often distinctive, lab diagnosis is frequently not conducted.
2. If done, it begins with identification of the most likely viruses based on clinical symptoms and the patient's history.
3. It is often not possible during the first few days after infection.

B. Virus isolation

1. This technique identifies virus replication in susceptible cells. Tissue culture cells, embryonated eggs, or animal hosts are often used.
   a. In live infected tissue culture cells, replication may be detected by observing a characteristic **cytopathogenic effect** (CPE) such as polykaryocyte formation or hemadsorption (adhesion of RBCs to infected cells) (Table 14.2).
   b. In fixed infected tissue culture cells, replication may be detected by observing characteristic inclusion bodies (Table 14.2; also see Table 4.1) or performing immunohistochemical staining of viral antigens.
   c. In an embryonated egg, replication is detected by pock formation; in animals, by the development of clinical symptoms.
2. Proper collection and preservation of specimens are necessary for virus isolation.
3. It is best accomplished during the onset and acute phase of disease.

C. Direct examination of clinical specimens

1. **General characteristics**
   a. Specimens may include sections of tissue biopsies, tissue imprints or smears, blood, CSF, urine, throat swabs, feces, or saliva.
   b. Only those specimens likely to contain the virus (eg, throat swabs for respiratory tract infection) should be examined.
   c. Examples include the following assays: viral-induced CPE (see Chapter 4 IV C 5), immunohistochemical staining, nucleic acid hybridization and amplification methods, and solid-phase immunoassay.
2. **Immunohistochemical staining:** This technique uses fixed or fresh specimens and chemically labeled (fluorescein) or enzymatically labeled (peroxidase) antibodies to detect viral antigens with either a direct or an indirect staining method. May use impression slides made from specific tissues.
3. **Nucleic acid hybridization and amplification** involves the detection of viral DNA or RNA sequences in nucleic acid extracted from specimens. It is highly sensitive and specific and is a

Table 14.2 Types of Cytopathic Effect	
Cytopathic Effect	**Manifestation**
Vacuoles	Large, frothy, bubble-like forms in cytoplasm of cell
Syncytia	Large cell masses containing many nuclei resulting from fusion of infected cells
Clumping	Swelling of cells where they form rounded grapelike clusters
Stress granulations	Cells exhibit dark, rough, finely speckled appearance, composed of protein and RNA, caused by inhibition of protein synthesis
Inclusions	Areas of dark staining composed of viral components for particle assembly either being eosinophilic or basophilic

popular technique for identifying adenovirus in nasopharyngeal washings, cytomegalovirus (CMV) in urine, and HIV in the blood of seronegative individuals.

   a. PCR may be used to amplify viral genes.
   b. Dot blot hybridization techniques that usually use single-stranded, complementary nucleic acid probes may be used.
   c. Sequencing is used for strain identification or genotyping.

4. **Solid-phase immunoassays** detect viral antigens such as rotavirus and hepatitis A virus (HAV) in feces. They use specific viral antibodies and RIA or ELISA techniques. These assays are highly sensitive and specific.

D. Serologic tests
   1. **General characteristics**
      a. Serologic tests are used to determine the **titer** of specific antiviral antibodies.
      b. Paired blood samples are taken (one sample at the onset and one sample during the recovery phase of the illness); **at least a 4-fold increase in titer between the samples must be present to indicate a current infection** (see I A).
      c. The test may be diagnostic without the use of paired samples if significant levels of IgM antiviral antibodies are obtained.
      d. Techniques include virus neutralization, complement fixation, hemagglutination inhibition tests, and solid-phase immunoassays.
   2. **Virus neutralization tests** are based on the principle that certain antiviral antibodies will neutralize the cytopathic effect of the virus.
      a. Constant amounts of virus are incubated with decreasing amounts of serum added to susceptible cells.
      b. These tests are expensive to perform and must be standardized for each virus.
   3. Agglutination tests are used to detect antibody union with large, particulate antigens.
      a. A diagnostic test for myxoviruses (eg, influenza, mumps, some pox viruses, and arboviruses) involves neutralization of their ability to spontaneously agglutinate RBCs by the infected patient's serum. The patient's serum titer is determined by the highest dilution blocking the agglutination.
      b. Hemagglutination inhibition tests are based on the principle that anti-hemagglutinin antibodies in serum will inhibit viral agglutination of erythrocytes.
         (1) These tests can be performed only on viruses with hemagglutinins on their surface (influenza, measles).
         (2) They require careful standardization of erythrocytes and viral hemagglutinin preparations.
   4. **Solid-phase immunoassays** are highly sensitive and specific assays used to detect specific viral antibodies.
      a. They use viral antigens in RIA and ELISA protocols.
      b. These tests are several hundred times more sensitive than other serologic tests.

V. DIAGNOSTIC MYCOLOGY

A. Clinical manifestations suggestive of fungal infection trigger special orders to the clinical microbiology lab of a possible mycology infection.

B. Microscopic examination: rapid methods.
   1. Potassium hydroxide in a wet mount (**KOH mount**) of skin scrapings breaks down the human cells, enhancing the visibility of the unaffected fungus (Figure 14.15).
   2. A nigrosin or **India ink** wet mount of **cerebrospinal fluid** highlights the **capsule of *Cryptococcus neoformans*** but is **insensitive** (misses 50% of cases).
   3. A **Giemsa** or Wright stain of **thick blood or bone marrow smear** may detect the **intracellular *Histoplasma capsulatum.***
   4. **Calcofluor white stain** "highlights" fungal elements in exudates, small skin scales, or frozen sections under a fluorescent microscope, giving the fungus a fluorescent blue-white appearance on a black background.

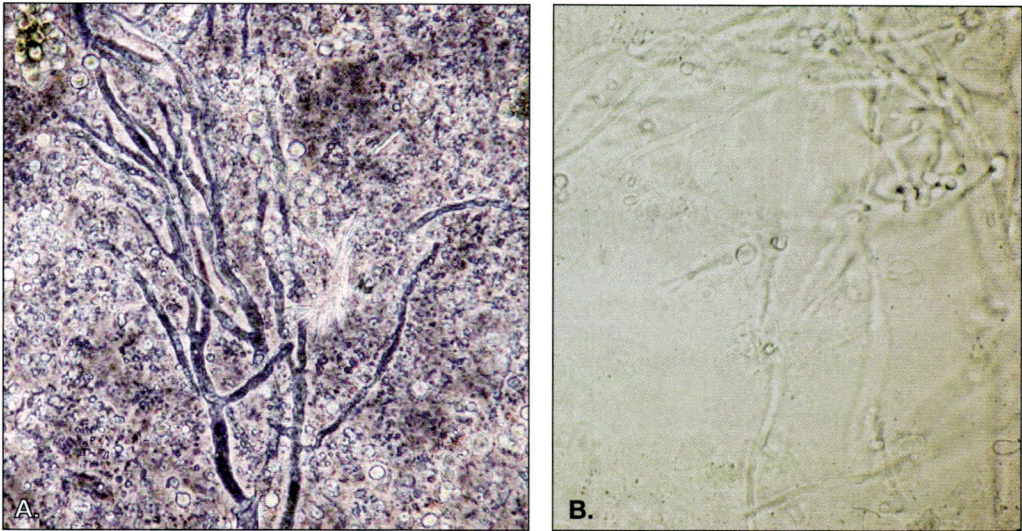

FIGURE 14.15. Wet mounts. A. Dichotomously branching hyphae released by tissue by KOH (potassium hydroxide) digestion. (Courtesy of Glenn D. Roberts, PhD, Mayo Clinic, Rochester, MN.) B. Wet mount of mucosal scrapings for vaginitis showing pseudohyphae and some yeasts.

C. Histologic staining: Special fungal stains for fixed tissues are necessary because fungi are not distinguished by color with hematoxylin and eosin (H&E) stain.
  1. Gomori methenamine-silver stain: Fungi are dark gray to black.
  2. Periodic acid-Schiff reaction: **Fungi are hot pink to red.**
  3. Gridley fungus stain: **Fungi are purplish roses** with a yellow background.
  4. Calcofluor white stain: fluorescent blue-white as mentioned earlier.
  5. Immunofluorescent stains are available for some fungal pathogens.

D. DNA probes and NAATs are available for some systemic pathogens.

E. Cultures for fungi must be specially ordered. They use special media (eg, **Sabouraud** dextrose medium), enriched media (eg, blood agar) with antibiotics to inhibit bacterial growth, and enriched media with both antibiotics and cycloheximide (which inhibits many saprobic fungi).
  1. Identification (ID) of *yeast* **cultures**
      a. Identification traditionally has been based on morphologic characteristics (presence of capsule, formation of germ tubes in serum, and morphology on cornmeal agar) and biochemical tests (urease, nitrate reduction, and carbohydrate assimilations and fermentations).
      b. Some yeast cultures may be identified with DNA probes.
      c. Speciation should be done for serious yeast infections as certain species carry drug resistance.
  2. Identification of *filamentous fungal* **cultures**
      a. Identification is based on morphologic criteria or uses an immunologic method called *exoantigen testing*, in which antigens extracted from the culture to be identified are immunodiffused against known antisera.
      b. DNA probes/nucleic acid amplification kits are available for some systemic pathogens.

F. Fungal antigen detection
  1. Known antibodies to identify circulating fungal antigens in a patient's serum, CSF, or urine. Antibodies are available for *Histoplasma* and *Cryptococcus.* These tests are important when patients are compromised, and antibodies may not be reliably detected.
  2. Galactomannan is a cell component of many fungi and identifies the presence of fungi in serum samples via agglutination assay or ELISA.

G. Serologic testing done to identify patient antibodies specific to a fungus generally requires acute and convalescent sera and is complicated by some cross-reactivity among pathogenic fungi and some patients' inability to produce antibodies.

VI. DIAGNOSTIC PARASITOLOGY

A. Laboratory parasite diagnosis depends on proper sample collection guided by the life cycle of the organism and the location of the parasite within the host. Testing involves direct detection of parasite life stages, nucleic acid or antigens, or serologic specimens containing parasite-specific antibodies.

  1. Sample sources include blood, stool, urine, CSF, sputum, and tissue biopsies.

  2. The timing of sample collection is important as many parasites have periodicity to different stages of their life cycles (eg, malaria, *Enterobius vermicularis, Giardia intestinalis*).

  3. Samples need to be collected and stored using appropriate preservatives and transport media.

  4. The quality and quantity of the specimen sample need to be appropriate to reduce false-negative results (eg, *Blastocystis* spp.).

B. Direct examination of clinical specimens

  1. Microscopic examination (see images in Chapter 9).

   a. Blood smears

    (1) Thick blood smears allow for greater sensitivity of detection, but they are not appropriate for review of morphology. A small drop of blood is placed in the center of a slide and the blood is spread until it is of proper density for evaluation.

    (2) Thin blood smears spread the blood droplet across a larger area of the slide. It allows for greater ability to observe morphology as in for speciation of malaria.

     (a) Detection of blood microfilariae utilizes fingerstick capillary blood for smears since microfilariae concentrate in the peripheral capillaries.

     (b) Fluorescence microscopy can be employed using acridine orange, benzothiocarboxypurine, or rhodamine-123 as fluorochromes.

   b. Ova and parasite

    (1) Used to detect intestinal parasites such as *Cryptosporidium* and *Giardia* in stool specimens.

    (2) Morphologies detected are:

     (a) Protozoan trophozoites, cysts, oocysts.

     (b) Helminth proglottids, scoleces, rhabditiform larvae, and eggs.

   c. Direct mount and stains

    (1) Direct wet mounting is placing the specimen directly on the slide with only water. No stain is utilized.

    (2) Methylene blue, trichrome stain, iodine, and iron-hematoxylin staining are commonly used **for intestinal protozoa (eg, *Giardia*) or helminth eggs.**

    (3) Parasitic oocysts of *Cryptosporidium, Cyclospora,* and *Isopora* are acid fast.

    (4) H&E stain may be used for visualizing worm components.

C. Molecular tests

When considering NAAT, DNA isolation methods must be amenable to extraction from parasite life stages such as eggs or cysts. They should also eliminate substances from samples that can inhibit molecular reactions such as those contained in feces.

D. Serologic tests

  1. Detection of specific antibodies to parasite infection can be done by immunologic methods such as ELISA, immunoblotting, and indirect fluorescence assay.

  2. Rapid detection tests (RDTs) utilize a lateral flow diffusion method to spread collected blood across a membrane with immobilized capture antibodies that react with parasite ag-ab complexes, producing a detection band.

   a. RDT tests can be used in the field to detect malaria parasites and speciate *Plasmodium falciparum* from other *Plasmodium* species.

   b. Other RDTs are available that utilize feces as the sample source such as for testing intestinal parasites *Giardia duodenalis* and *Cryptosporidium parvum.*

Directions: Select the *one* lettered answer that is *best* in each case. Commit to and write down your answers before checking the answers and explanations. Each of the numbered items in this section is followed by answers with explanations, in the following section.

1. A clinical microbiology laboratory is requested to identify the presence of specific pathogen antigens in a patient's clinical sample. Which of the following techniques is the most sensitive for detecting the pathogen's antigen?

(A) Culture-based methods
(B) Direct microscopic examination
(C) ELISA
(D) PCR
(E) Western immunoblotting

2. A 32-year-old woman presents to her physician with symptoms of fever, chills, malaise, and diarrhea. She reports recent travel to a tropical region. Physical examination reveals an elevated body temperature and mild hepatomegaly. Laboratory tests show leukocytosis and elevated liver enzymes. Suspecting a possible bacterial infection, the physician decides to order a molecular assay for microbial detection. Which of the following molecular assays would be most appropriate for detecting the causative agent of this patient's symptoms?

(A) Agarose gel electrophoresis
(B) Culture-based methods
(C) ELISA
(D) Ribosomal RNA (rRNA) sequencing
(E) Western immunoblotting

3. A 28-year-old man living with HIV presents to his physician for a follow-up appointment. Despite being on antiretroviral therapy (ART) for the past year, his viral load has increased. The physician suspects the development of drug resistance due to HIV mutations. Which of the following assays would be most appropriate for detecting specific mutations associated with drug resistance in this patient?

(A) ELISA
(B) Immunofluorescence microscopy
(C) Next-generation sequencing
(D) RT-PCR
(E) Western immunoblotting

4. A 42-year-old woman reports to her primary care physician for a routine health checkup. She has no significant medical history and doesn't report any recent symptoms. Laboratory tests

reveal elevated liver enzymes. Serologic assays for hepatitis B virus (HBV) markers are ordered to assess the patient's HBV natural history. Which of the following serologic profiles is most consistent with chronic hepatitis infection?

(A) HBsurface antigen(+); HBcore IgM(+); HBcore IgG(+)
(B) HBsurface antigen(+); HBcore IgG(+); HBsurface IgG(−)
(C) HBsurface antigen(−); HBcore IgG(+); HBsurface IgG(+)
(D) HBsurface antigen(−); HBcore IgG(−); HBsurface IgG(+)
(E) HBsurface antigen(−); HBcore IgG(+); HBsurface IgG(−)

5. A 55-year-old individual has symptoms consistent with a viral respiratory infection. Due to the ongoing COVID-19 pandemic, the health-care provider decides to perform testing for the presence of antibodies against SARS-CoV-2. Which of the following techniques is most appropriate for detecting these antibodies in the patient's blood?

(A) ELISA
(B) Next-generation sequencing
(C) PCR
(D) RT-PCR
(E) Western immunoblotting

6. A 35-year-old individual presents to a tropical medicine clinic with symptoms of recurrent fever, chills, and sweating. The patient reports a recent travel history to a malaria-endemic region. Which of the following assays would be most appropriate for identification of *P. falciparum*?

(A) Culture on selective media
(B) ELISA
(C) Microscopy of blood smears
(D) Next-generation sequencing
(E) RT-PCR

7. A 28-year-old man presents to his health-care provider with symptoms of persistent watery diarrhea, abdominal cramps, and weight loss. He reports recently visiting a local water park. Stool examination is performed to identify the causative agent of his gastrointestinal symptoms. Upon microscopic examination of the stool sample, the presence of oocysts is observed. Which of the following techniques should be most appropriate for confirming the diagnosis and detection of *C. parvum* in this patient's stool?

(A) Gram stain
(B) Giemsa stain
(C) India ink stain
(D) Modified acid-fast stain
(E) PAS stain

8. A 12-year-old child from a rural area presents to a community health clinic with symptoms of abdominal pain, vomiting, and intermittent diarrhea. Physical examination reveals a distended abdomen and tenderness on palpation. The child's family reports a recent history of consuming raw vegetables and uncooked fish. Stool analysis is performed to assess for possible parasitic infection. Which of the following laboratory techniques is most appropriate for detecting helminth parasites in this patient's stool?

(A) Acid-fast stain
(B) Direct wet mount
(C) Gram stain
(D) India ink stain
(E) PAS stain

9. A 45-year-old man presents to his physician with symptoms of fever, headache, and muscle aches. He mentions spending a lot of time outdoors in a region known for its bird population. The patient is concerned that he has West Nile virus. The physician orders serologic testing to assess the patient's immune response to the virus. Which of the following Igs would be most appropriate for detecting recent West Nile infection?

(A) IgA
(B) IgD
(C) IgE
(D) IgG
(E) IgM

10. A 6-month-old infant is brought to the pediatrician due to fever, irritability, and difficulty breathing. Physical examination reveals inspiratory stridor and a muffled voice. The pediatrician suspects epiglottitis, a potentially life-threatening condition caused by *Haemophilus influenzae* type b (Hib) infection. A throat swab is collected for culture to confirm the diagnosis. Which of the following selection media is most appropriate for isolating *H. influenzae* from the throat swab?

(A) Blood agar
(B) MacConkey agar
(C) Chocolate agar
(D) Sabouraud agar
(E) Mannitol salt agar

11. A 37-year-old woman presented to her physician with symptoms of abdominal pain, weight loss, and diarrhea. She reported recent travel to a tropical region. The physician suspects a parasitic infection. Which of the following assays would most likely be used to detect a parasite?

(A) Gram stain
(B) Lateral flow immunoassay
(C) Ova and parasite
(D) RT-PCR
(E) Sequencing

12. A 32-year-old man presents to a clinic with symptoms of a high fever, headache, and muscle aches. He reports recent travel to a tropical region where he was bitten by mosquitos. Given the symptoms and travel history, the clinician suspects a viral infection. To confirm diagnosis, a serum sample is collected and used to inoculate cultured cells. After a few days of incubation, the cells in the culture dish show signs of a viral infection. What technique would be utilized to detect these signs?

(A) Lateral flow immunoassay
(B) Light microscopy
(C) RT-PCR
(D) DNA microarray
(E) Western immunoblotting

13. A 42-year-old woman with a history of injection drug use presents to the emergency department with a painful, swollen abscess on her forearm. The abscess is drained, and the purulent material is sent to the microbiology lab for culture. The culture shows the growth of *Staphylococcus aureus*. Susceptibility testing is performed to determine the appropriate antibiotic therapy. The MIC of methicillin is found to be exceptionally elevated. This finding indicates that the isolated bacterial strain is which of the following?

(A) Intermediate resistant to methicillin
(B) Nonreactive to methicillin
(C) Resistant to methicillin
(D) Sensitive to methicillin
(E) Susceptible to methicillin

14. A 25-year-old woman presents to the emergency department with symptoms of fever, abdominal pain, and frequent, watery diarrhea. She reports attending a family picnic a day prior and suspects food poisoning as the cause of her symptoms. A stool sample is collected for microbiologic analysis. The sample is streaked onto an agar plate and incubated overnight. The next day, the agar plate shows colonies that are pink and mucoid. Which of the following media is most likely used for this plate?

(A) Blood agar
(B) Chocolate agar
(C) MacConkey agar
(D) Sabouraud agar
(E) Trypticase soy agar

15. A 27-year-old man presents to his primary care physician with symptoms of a painful, red swelling on his foot. Physical examination reveals an erythematous, warm, and tender lesion with a central pustule. A sample is collected from the lesion for microbiologic analysis. Upon exposure to hydrogen peroxide, the sample produces bubbles. Which of the following bacterial components is being detected by this assay?

(A) Coagulase
(B) Catalase
(C) Mycolic acid
(D) Peptidoglycan
(E) Nucleic acid

16. A 57-year-old patient presents with persistent oral thrush caused by *Candida* species. A tongue scraping is collected on a sterile swab and sent to the microbiology laboratory for analysis. Which of the following methods is best for detecting the fungal organisms in this patient?

(A) Blood agar culture
(B) Galactomannan assay
(C) India ink staining
(D) KOH prep
(E) Ova and parasite examination

17. A 30-year-old woman is suspected of having a yeast infection and a culture is planned to confirm diagnosis. Which of the following media is most suitable for cultivating fungi from a clinical specimen?

(A) Chocolate agar
(B) Lowenstein-Jensen agar
(C) MacConkey agar
(D) Thayer-Martin agar
(E) Sabouraud agar

Answers and Explanations

1. **The answer is C.** [I B 5] The most sensitive method of those listed is ELISA. The sensitivity makes it the most effective clinical method for diagnosing various microbial pathogens. However, PCR has the best specificity.

2. **The answer is D.** [II D 1, III E 2] Sequencing of the 16s ribosomal RNA gene is the best method to identify and categorize a wide range of bacterial species. It is highly specific and sensitive.

3. **The answer is C.** [IV C 3 c] HIV drug resistance genotyping by sequencing is the most appropriate assay for detecting therapy-associated mutations in the viral genome. Next-generation sequencing can detect mutations down to 1% of the amplicon population from the region of interest.

4. **The answer is B.** [IV D 4] Answer A is the profile of an acute infection. Answer C is a resolved infection. Answer D is the profile of an immunized individual. Answer E is the profile of an occult infection.

5. **The answer is A.** [IV C 4] ELISA is a highly sensitive and specific assay for detection of antibody response to a viral pathogen. It would allow for detection of IgM which would signify a recent infection versus IgG suggesting an infection that occurred in the past. B and D would detect the RNA genome of the virus.

6. **The answer is C.** [VI B 1 a] The best method listed is the evaluation of thick and thin blood smears looking for the presence of parasite trophozoites or merozoites. Point-of-care rapid diagnostic tests are also available, but they have limited utility for speciation at this time.

7. **The answer is D.** [VI B 1 c (3)] Modified acid-fast staining is the most appropriate method for detecting *C. parvum* oocysts due to a waxy outer membrane similar to mycobacteria.

8. **The answer is B.** [VI B 1 c (1)] The direct wet mount application of the sample for microscopic evaluation is the best initial method for visualizing helminth eggs, larvae, or proglottids. In some instances, stains such as iodide can be used to enhance detection.

9. **The answer is E.** [I A] IgM antibodies are the first produced in an acute infection scenario. IgG antibodies present indicate a past infection. IgA antibodies are relevant to mucosal immunity. IgE antibodies are relevant to allergy responses.

10. **The answer is C.** [III D 3 c (1)] *H. influenzae* is a fastidious organism that requires specific growth conditions. Chocolate agar provides required nutrients due to the preparation of lysed RBCs in the media, specifically making available hemin (factor X) and NAD+ (nicotinamide adenine dinucleotide, factor V).

11. **The answer is C.** [VI B 1 b] The ova and parasite evaluation is a standard test for identification of gastrointestinal parasites.

12. **The answer is B.** [IV B 1 a; Table 5.1] This vignette describes the presence of cytopathic effect (CPE) in virally infected cells. Such cytology would be visualized by light microscopy of the infected cells.

13. **The answer is C.** [III G 4 b] The MIC assay determines the concentration of drug to which a bacterial isolate is susceptible. An elevated concentration of drug needed to have an inhibitory effect on the isolate would indicate that the strain is not susceptible to the drug and thus resistant.

14. **The answer is C.** [III E 3 c (2)] Many gram-negative bacteria are often a cause of bacterial contamination of food. MacConkey agar is selective for gram-negative bacterial growth. An indication of pink colonies is that the bacteria are able to ferment lactose such as *E. coli*.

15. **The answer is B.** [III E 3 e (1)] The presence of bubbles on exposure to hydrogen peroxide indicates the presence of catalase enzyme which breaks down hydrogen peroxide into water and oxygen. This case describes a *Staphylococcus* infection, which is often associated with skin and soft tissue infections. Catalase activity is used to discern *Staphylococcus* from *Streptococcus*.

16. **The answer is D.** [V B 1] KOH preparation is helpful for microscopic examination of fungi collected from cell scrapings. Blood agar is not appropriate for selective culture of fungi as bacteria will also grow. The galactomannan assay is not specific as galactomannan is a component of the cell wall of many fungal species. India ink is used for staining *Cryptococcus* capsules. Ova and parasites are used for the detection of parasites.

17. **The answer is E.** [V E] Sabouraud agar is the most appropriate to be selective for fungal growth. It contains peptones and antibiotics which are inhibitory for bacterial growth. Chocolate agar is appropriate for fastidious bacteria but will be nonselective for fungi. Lowenstein-Jensen agar is appropriate for *Mycobacterium* species. MacConkey agar is selective for gram-negative bacteria. Thayer-Martin agar is selective for *Neisseria* species.

Directions: Perform this block under examination conditions. Please allocate 90 seconds per question: this block should take 60 minutes. Select the *one* lettered answer that is *best* in each case. Commit to and write down your answers *before* checking the answers and explanations. Each of the numbered items in this section is followed by answers with explanations, in the following section.

1. A 6-month-old infant is brought to the emergency department having woken up from a nap with a weak cry, ptosis, unreactive pupils, and the inability to lift her arms. She has had routine well-baby care. There is no sign of physical abuse or rash, and she is afebrile. The physician puts the child on a respiration monitor and calls the infectious disease consultant. Which of the following conditions is the most likely cause of her symptoms?

(A) Bacterial meningitis—*Listeria monocytogenes*
(B) Bacterial meningitis—*Streptococcus pneumoniae*
(C) Botulism from contaminated canned goods
(D) Infant botulism
(E) Viral meningitis

2. What is the mechanism of action of the toxin described in question 1?

(A) Blockage of the synapse of acetylcholine at the ganglia
(B) Blockage of the transport of choline into neurons
(C) Cleavage of terminal neuronal docking proteins preventing the release of acetylcholine
(D) Inhibition of acetylcholinesterase
(E) Inhibition of choline acetyltransferase

3. Five children in a third-grade class develop a disease that begins as a bright red rash on the face, turns violet after a few days, and then disappears; then, a maculopapular rash appears on their trunk, buttocks, and extremities. It soon fades from the trunk but persists on the thighs and forearms. Two children have also had a slight fever and a sore throat but neither was severely sick. Which of the following nucleic acids best describes the genetic material of the most likely causative agent?

(A) Double-stranded DNA
(B) Double-stranded RNA
(C) Segmented single-stranded RNA
(D) Single-stranded DNA
(E) Single-stranded RNA

4. A researcher creates a single antigen vaccine that would have prevented the outbreak from question 3 that can be used as a vaccine in females before pregnancy. Which of the following viral molecules is most likely to lead to the production of successful neutralizing antibodies?

(A) Capsid protein
(B) Matrix protein
(C) Polymerase
(D) Surface glycopeptide

5. A 34-year-old presents to the hospital with an infection. A new resident proclaims that the causative agent acts by colonizing a surface in the body. Which of the following bacterial components is most important for this patient's infection?

(A) Calcium dipicolinate
(B) Diaminopimelic acid
(C) Pilin
(D) Porins
(E) O-antigens

6. A pathogenic bacterium is being studied in a research laboratory and found to be facultative. These bacteria are also found to contain cyclic adenosine monophosphate (cAMP)-binding proteins. What is the function of these cAMP-binding proteins?

(A) Decrease levels of elongation factors
(B) Enhance RNA polymerase activity
(C) Facilitate binding of repressor proteins
(D) Increase transcription initiation
(E) Suppress the Pasteur effect

7. An 18-year-old male college student came to the Student Health Services, reporting a sore throat, fatigue, and difficulty in swallowing. Physical examination showed an enlarged spleen; a palpable, tender liver; and swollen cervical lymph nodes. His blood is positive for heterophile antibodies. Which of the following entities would be expected to be seen in a blood smear?

(A) Atypical T cells (Downey cells)
(B) Gram-negative rods
(C) Gram-positive rods
(D) Mononuclear cells with Cowdry type A inclusions
(E) Multinucleated giant cells

8. A 17-year-old female presents to the gynecology clinic with recurring pelvic pain. A probable diagnosis of pelvic inflammatory disease (PID) is made. The patient states that they do not do drugs and drink alcohol occasionally. They have been dating the same person for the past 9 months, and 6 months ago they had unprotected sex on three occasions. What is the most likely causative agent of this patient's infection?

(A) *Candida albicans*
(B) *Chlamydia trachomatis*
(C) *Haemophilus ducreyi*
(D) *Neisseria gonorrhoeae*
(E) *Treponema pallidum*

9. A 26-year-old man presents to the clinic with cellulitis for the previous 2 days. He reports that 2 days prior, he was bitten by his friend's cat. What is the most likely dominant organism involved in the infection?

(A) *Bartonella henselae*
(B) *Calymmatobacterium granulomatis*
(C) *Clostridium tetani*
(D) *Pasteurella multocida*
(E) *Toxoplasma gondii*

10. The parents of an 18-month-old girl appear at the emergency department of a hospital with their daughter, who had an abrupt onset of vomiting and incidences of watery diarrhea. The symptoms began 2 days previously at her day care center. She refuses to eat or drink and is very lethargic. A vaccine-preventable illness is diagnosed. Which of the following features allowed for the production of a vaccine for the most likely causative agent?

(A) Ability to survive as a temperature-sensitive mutant
(B) Identification of an enterotoxin
(C) Loss of colonization factors
(D) Manipulation of O-antigens
(E) Segmented genetic material

11. A 50-year-old woman from Key West Florida presents with a mosquito-borne viral disease in which her antiviral antibodies from an infection nearly a decade ago were thought to have an "enhancing" effect so that the current reinfection with the virus caused a more serious

bleeding disease. Which of the following viruses is the most likely causative agent?

(A) Coxsackie A virus
(B) Dengue virus
(C) Hantavirus
(D) Rubella virus
(E) West Nile virus

12. A bacterial infection is diagnosed, and the treatment includes an antibiotic that has a β-lactam ring in its structure. Which of the following is the most likely prescribed treatment?

(A) Bacitracin
(B) Cephalosporin
(C) Erythromycin
(D) Griseofulvin
(E) Streptomycin
(F) Tetracycline

13. A new antibiotic-resistant strain of bacteria is identified and studied in a research lab. Which bacterial gene transfer process would be inhibited by free extracellular exonucleases?

(A) Conjugation
(B) Generalized transduction
(C) Specialized transduction
(D) Transformation
(E) Transposition

14. After a trip to Peru to adopt a 6-month-old infant, a 32-year-old man and his new child both develop profuse, watery diarrhea with flecks of mucus. Both are hospitalized due to the severity and rapidity of the dehydration but neither are febrile. What is the most likely causative agent?

(A) *Campylobacter jejuni*
(B) *Escherichia coli* O157
(C) *Salmonella typhi*
(D) *Shigella dysenteriae*
(E) *Vibrio cholerae*

15. A 19-year-old woman presents to her primary care physician with recurrent respiratory infections. On further questioning, she reports frequent episodes of sinusitis, otitis media, and upper respiratory tract infections. Physical examination reveals no significant abnormalities, and the patient's overall health is otherwise good. Laboratory studies show normal serum immunoglobulin (Ig) levels, and immunoelectrophoresis demonstrates the presence of IgA in the serum. IgA is largely responsible for protection of the respiratory and intestinal mucosal tract. Effective protection depends on the action of a secretory piece that acts by which of the following mechanisms?

(A) Facilitating the passage of IgA out of the plasma cell
(B) Facilitating the formation of the IgA dimer
(C) Being released by IgA causing an inflammatory response
(D) Being a poly Ig transport receptor on mucosal epithelial cells

16. A 45-year-old man with a history of hepatitis B virus (HBV) infection presents for a follow-up evaluation. He was initially diagnosed with acute HBV infection 5 years ago. He has no evidence of active liver disease, with normal liver function tests and an absence of cirrhosis on imaging studies. Repeat testing reveals undetectable HBV DNA levels. Which of the following serologic markers should be monitored to determine if the blood contains the infectious virus?

(A) HBcAg
(B) HBeAg
(C) HBsAg
(D) IgG HBs
(E) IgM HBc

17. Which of the following individuals is most likely to progress to chronic liver disease following an acute infection?

(A) 50-year-old who becomes HBsAg positive
(B) Infant born to a chronically active infected HBV mother
(C) Patient with a liver transplant infected with hepatitis C virus (HCV)
(D) Recent immigrant who is hepatitis E virus (HEV) positive
(E) Young adult coinfected with HBV and hepatitis D virus (HDV)

18. A 10-year-old male presents to the pediatric clinic with recurrent, severe respiratory tract infections, oral thrush, and poor growth. He has experienced multiple episodes of pneumonia and sinusitis since early childhood and has failed to thrive. Physical examination reveals no significant abnormalities, except for the presence of oral thrush. Laboratory tests show a normal complete blood count, but immune studies reveal a selective deficiency of human leukocyte antigen class II (HLA II) expression. Which of the following is one of the functions of HLA II molecules?

(A) Interact with an epitope on the membranes of most nucleated cells
(B) Interact with the gene regions DP, DQ, DR
(C) Present peptidic epitopes to CD4$^+$ T helper cells
(D) Present peptidic epitopes to CD8$^+$ T helper cells

19. A 41-year-old man presents to the emergency department with headache, confusion, and memory impairment. His family reports personality changes and agitation over the past several weeks. Neurologic examination reveals a decreased level of consciousness and focal weakness in the left hand. Brain imaging shows abnormal signal intensity and enhancement in the right temporal lobe. A cerebrospinal fluid analysis demonstrates increased white blood cell count, predominantly lymphocytes, and elevated protein levels. Which of the following features is one of the hallmarks of viral infections of the temporal lobe of the brain?

(A) Holes in the parenchyma
(B) Koplik spots
(C) Maculopapular rash along dermatomes
(D) Perivascular cuffing

20. Which of the following outcomes will occur due to pepsin digestion of the IgG antibody against tetanus toxoid?

(A) Fab (fragment antigen-binding) two molecules and destruction of the Fc (fragment crystallizable) fragment
(B) Loss of the ability to form a lattice with the toxoid
(C) Loss of the Ch 1 heavy chain constant domain
(D) Production of two Fab molecules and one Fc fragment

21. A 33-year-old man presents to a clinic with subcutaneous nodular lesions along his lymphatics (see image) from the initial site of trauma 3 weeks ago, caused by a plum thorn puncture. The man makes his living harvesting fruit for local orchards. What is the best morphologic description of the most likely causative agent of this man's lesions?

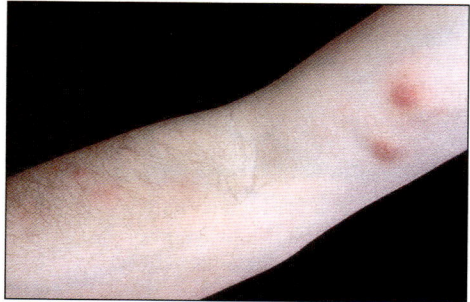

(A) Acid-fast organism
(B) Dimorphic fungus
(C) Filamentous fungus
(D) Gram-negative rod
(E) Gram-positive coccus
(F) Helminth

22. The Pap smear of a 19-year-old female college soccer player contains koilocytotic cells. The disease associated with the appearance of the cells would most likely have been prevented by previous administration of which of the following vaccines?

(A) Inactivated virus vaccine
(B) Inactivated whole-cell vaccine
(C) Live attenuated virus vaccine
(D) Recombinant vaccine containing viruslike particles
(E) Toxoid vaccine

23. A 9-year-old girl is brought to the clinic with bloody diarrhea following a neighborhood barbeque. Her guardian said that the hamburgers seemed undercooked. Ultimately, a diagnosis of infection by the O157 strain of *E. coli* is made. Where are the O-antigens (the "O" in "O157") located?

(A) Capsule
(B) Lipopolysaccharide
(C) Lipoprotein
(D) Mesosome
(E) Peptidoglycan
(F) Teichoic acid

24. Two bacterial cells undergo the process of conjugation. What is transferred when an F^+ cell is crossed with an F^- cell?

(A) Both plasmid and chromosomal genes
(B) Entire bacterial chromosome
(C) Fertility factor DNA
(D) No genes
(E) Some bacterial chromosomal genes

25. In March, a nursery school reported an outbreak among the children of a disease characterized by a high-grade fever of 100.9 to 104 °F (38.8-40 °C) that starts suddenly and rapidly falls. The children developed a short-lived (1-2 days) maculopapular rash that began on the trunk and spread to the extremities; the face was spared. The children had mild malaise but otherwise did not appear ill. Which of the following viruses is the most likely causative agent?

(A) Coxsackie A16 virus
(B) Human herpesvirus 6 (HHV-6)
(C) Parvovirus B19
(D) Rubella virus
(E) Varicella-zoster virus (VZV)

26. Which of the following clusters of differentiation antigens is a receptor for the human immunodeficiency virus (HIV)?

(A) CD2
(B) CD3
(C) CD4
(D) CD8
(E) CD25

27. A 28-year-old woman presents to her primary care physician with seasonal nasal congestion; sneezing; and itchy, watery eyes. She reports experiencing these symptoms every spring and fall for the past several years. Her symptoms tend to worsen when she spends time outdoors, particularly in grassy fields and parks. Physical examination shows no signs of sinusitis or respiratory distress. She is diagnosed with hay fever. Which of the following interleukins initiates a switch from IgG formation to IgE production in a patient with hay fever?

(A) IL-1
(B) IL-2
(C) IL-3
(D) IL-4
(E) IL-5

28. Which of the following is the principal Ig in exocrine secretions?

(A) IgA
(B) IgD
(C) IgE
(D) IgG
(E) IgM

29. A 3-year-old child develops acute glomerulonephritis following impetigo. The causative bacteria are β-hemolytic, Gram-positive cocci that have M12 surface proteins. The results of a catalase test are shown in the image. What is the most likely causative agent?

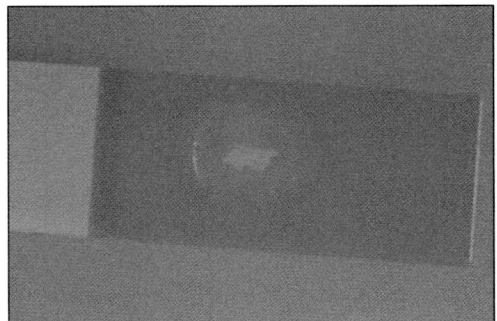

(A) *Enterococcus faecalis*
(B) *Staphylococcus aureus*
(C) *Staphylococcus epidermidis*
(D) *Streptococcus agalactiae*
(E) *Streptococcus pneumoniae*
(F) *Streptococcus pyogenes*

30. After extensive oral surgery, a 68-year-old patient subsequently developed subacute infective endocarditis. Past medical history indicates that the patient had rheumatic fever as a child and did not take the prescribed perioperative prophylactic antibiotics before the oral surgery. Which of the following is the most likely causative agent of this patient's endocarditis?

(A) *E. faecalis*
(B) *S. aureus*
(C) *S. agalactiae*
(D) *S. pneumoniae*
(E) *S. pyogenes*
(F) Viridans group *Streptococci*

31. A 37-year-old woman is admitted to the hospital in respiratory distress. Past medical history indicates that she is currently taking chemotherapy treatments. She had signs of focal central nervous system (CNS) lesions early in the day and is now in a comatose state. Both the CNS and pulmonary biopsies show dichotomously branching, septate hyphae. What is the patient's most likely underlying condition that facilitated the infection?

(A) CD4$^+$ cell count less than 200
(B) Ketoacidotic diabetes
(C) Multiple myeloma
(D) Severe neutropenia
(E) Sickle cell disease

32. Bacteria in which of the following categories can use fermentation pathways but also contain superoxide dismutase?

(A) Aerobic heterotrophs
(B) Facultative anaerobes
(C) Obligate aerobes
(D) Obligate anaerobes

33. When IgG is cleaved by papain, which of the following fragments appears?

(A) Two Fab fragments that contain only the variable section of the heavy chain
(B) Two Fab fragments that contain only the variable section of the light chain
(C) Two Fc and one Fab
(D) Two monovalent Fab

34. A 5-year-old child is brought to the physician by the parents with a severe sore throat for the past few days. Physical exam reveals a low fever, and the throat has a grayish exudate on the sides of the pharynx. The child also has a swollen neck. On questioning, the family reveals that the child is not vaccinated and that they recently returned from a trip to Africa. Clinical suspicion is of a disease with a circulating toxin inhibiting protein synthesis. What additional tissues are most frequently involved?

(A) Ears and sinuses
(B) Heart and nerves
(C) Kidneys
(D) Liver and kidneys
(E) Skin

35. In which of the following bacterial structures is *N*-acetylmuramic acid located?

(A) Lipopolysaccharide
(B) Lipoprotein
(C) Outer membrane
(D) Peptidoglycan
(E) Teichoic acid

36. A 24-year-old Peace Corps worker is sent back to the United States from East Africa with a very high fever. African sleeping sickness is diagnosed. How is the causative agent transmitted?

(A) Invasion of skin in water
(B) Mosquito bite
(C) Reduviid bug bite
(D) Respiratory droplets and direct mucosal contact
(E) Sandfly bite
(F) Tsetse fly bite

37. A 43-year-old patient presents with a boil on his neck for the past week. Past medical history indicates that he has a previous diagnosis of diabetes and has been hospitalized twice in the last year. The boil is drained, but, because of his hospitalizations, a drug-resistant strain is suspected, so a sample is sent to the lab for Gram stain, susceptibility testing, and aerobic and anaerobic culture. The preliminary report comes back with gram-negative cocci in clusters, but the lab supervisor indicates that this is likely an error as the stain was done by a new lab technician. Retesting indicates that it is *S. aureus*. What mistake in the Gram stain did the new lab technician most likely make to produce pink cocci with no hint of purple?

(A) Decolorized too quickly
(B) Forgot the decolorization step
(C) Forgot the Gram iodine
(D) Forgot the safranin
(E) Left the safranin on too long

38. An asymptomatic 35-year-old male missionary has returned to the United States following 12 years in rural Mexico. His routine physical examination shows elevated transaminases. His medical history in Mexico was unremarkable except for a vehicle accident requiring a blood transfusion of 3 pints of blood. Which definitive lab test should be performed to determine the most effective treatment?

(A) Blood culture on MacConkey agar
(B) Differential cytology of the blood
(C) Electron microscopy for Dane particles
(D) Molecular genotyping of circulating virus
(E) Serology for levels of IgG HEV

39. Which of the following virulence factors is produced by several genera of bacteria that are notable mucosal colonizers including *S. pneumoniae*?

(A) Elastase
(B) Hemagglutinin
(C) IgA protease
(D) Mucinase

40. A 25-year-old male presents to a sexual health clinic for evaluation. He reports engaging in high-risk sexual behaviors, including multiple sexual partners and inconsistent condom use. He is concerned about his risk for sexually transmitted infections and requests a comprehensive screening. Which of the following is a sexually transmitted virus with no genital signs or symptoms?

(A) Epstein-Barr virus (EBV)
(B) HBV
(C) Herpes simplex virus
(D) Parvovirus B19

Answers and Explanations

1. **The answer is D.** [Chapter 3, IX D 3] The symptoms are classic for infant botulism. Common sources of botulinum toxin include canned home goods, and, in cases of infant botulism, household dust or honey. It is most likely that this is from the ingestion of environmental spores (dust or honey) rather than from canned goods, although that is a less likely possibility. Listeria meningitis would be very uncommon this long after birth, and the child would probably be febrile and not have the descending paralysis. She should not have Streptococcal meningitis, as she is vaccinated, and it would present as a febrile disease with a stiff neck. The listed symptoms are also not typical for viral meningitis.

2. **The answer is C.** [Chapter 2, Table 2.5] Botulinum toxin (a metalloprotease) acts at the neural synapse to cleave docking proteins and block exocytosis of acetylcholine from storage vesicles, producing a flaccid paralysis. Choline acetyltransferase, choice E, is an enzyme catalyzing the synthesis of acetylcholine from an acetate and choline. Sodium-dependent transport of choline can be blocked by hemicholinium (choice B). Enzyme acetylcholinesterase is responsible for catalyzing hydrolysis of acetylcholine (choice D). Acetylcholine synapses at the ganglia of many neurons and tissues, and this step is not blocked by botulinum toxin (choice A).

3. **The answer is D.** [Chapter 4, II A 1] The disease is most probably erythema infectiosum (slapped cheek syndrome) caused by parvovirus B19, a single-stranded DNA virus.

4. **The answer is A.** [Chapter 4 V A 3] The disease is most likely erythema infectiosum (slapped cheek syndrome) caused by parvovirus B19, a single-stranded DNA virus. Parvovirus B19 is a naked virus, so protective neutralizing antibodies would be to the viral capsid (on the outer surface of each virus particle). It does not carry a polymerase but uses cellular polymerases, which is why it requires replicating cells for viral replication. It is not enveloped, so it does not produce glycoproteins or matrix proteins.

5. **The answer is C.** [Chapter 2, I B 10 b (1)] Pilin is the main protein component of the pili involved in bacterial adherence.

6. **The answer is B.** [Chapter 2, VII C 3 d] cAMP-binding proteins bind to specific DNA sequences near promoters, which facilitate RNA polymerase binding to the promoters, thus enhancing transcription of genes associated with those promoters. An example of this type of cAMP-binding protein is the CAP (catabolic activator protein) of the *lac* operon.

7. **The answer is A.** [Chapter 5 III C 2 (2)] The patient has infectious mononucleosis caused by EBV, which produces a heterophile antibody that is the basis of the monospot test, and the Downey cells, which are reactive T cells.

8. **The answer is B.** [Chapter 3, XII A 2] *C. trachomatis* and *N. gonorrhoeae* are the only two choices listed that are associated with commonly causing PID. However, *C. trachomatis* is about 4 times more common; in fact, it is the most common bacterial sexually transmitted infection in the general population.

9. **The answer is D.** [Chapter 3, Table 3.4; XI; and XI D] *P. multocida* is a dominant organism in the cat's mouth. Choice A, *Bartonella*, is the causative agent of cat scratch fever and is less common in bites. Choice B, *Calymmatobacterium*, causes a sexually transmitted infection, and *Toxoplasma* (choice E) is associated with cats but transmitted by their feces, not bites. Choice C, tetanus, is not likely unless the man has not been vaccinated.

10. **The answer is E.** [Chapter 5, V A] Rotaviruses (which are segmented, dsRNA viruses) are the most frequent cause of diarrheas in infants. RotaTeq and Rotarix vaccines are available for prevention.

11. **The answer is B.** [Chapter 5 XVI C] Dengue virus is an arbovirus that causes a disease sometimes known as *break-bone fever* because of the muscle and joint pain associated with it. Infection by a different virus serotype following a primary infection causes a more serious disease that is thought to be due to the enhancing effect that antibodies to the initial virus have on the second virus's infection properties.

12. The answer is B. [Chapter 2, IX B 2 a (1) and Figure 2.11] Cephalosporin drugs have the β-lactam ring, as do the penicillins. These antibiotics inhibit cell-wall biosynthesis and are inactivated by some β-lactamases.

13. The answer is D. [Chapter 2, VII B 4 and Figure 2.10] In transformation, the DNA is extracellular before it is picked up by the competent cells; during this period, the DNA is subject to the extracellular exonucleases. Because the DNA in generalized and specialized transduction is protected extracellularly by the virus capsid, it is not subject to extracellular exonucleases. In conjunction, the DNA is never outside of a cell. Transposition is a mechanism of inserting a transposon into another molecule of DNA and has no extracellular transport mechanism associated with it.

14. The answer is E. [Chapter 3, IX H and Table 3.4] The symptoms described raise suspicion of cholera. (Rotavirus would have to be ruled out for the infant, but it is not one of the choices.) The loss of fluids and electrolytes is rapid and most severe with *V. cholerae.* The lack of fever and lack of pus and blood in the stools suggest that the causative agent is not *Campylobacter, Salmonella,* or *Shigella.* The lack of blood also decreases the chance of *E. coli* O157. If untreated, cholera may lead to dehydration, hemoconcentration, and hypovolemic shock.

15. The answer is D. [Chapter 10, VII C1 a (1)] The secretory piece is part of a poly Ig transport receptor facilitating transfer of IgA to mucosal epithelial cells.

16. The answer is B. [Chapter 5, VI B 1 b (5)] Levels of HBeAg are monitored to determine if blood contains infectious HBV.

17. The answer is B. [Chapter 5, VI B 3 b (1)] Progression to chronic disease is inversely related to the age of infection with HBV, and 90% of neonates can become chronically ill. HCV infection progression is also high but is 70% rather than 90%.

18. The answer is C. [Chapter 10, VIII D 4 a] HLA-2 presents epitopes to $CD4^+$ Th cells. HLA-1 presents epitopes to $CD8^+$ Th cells.

19. The answer is D. [Chapter 5, IX] Lymphocytes and plasma cells surround the brain's blood vessels as they exit to combat the virus in the brain parenchyma.

20. The answer is A. [Chapter 10, VII A 1 d (2) (a)] Because a Fab 2 results, pepsin-digested antibody will still be able to form a lattice.

21. The answer is B. [Chapter 7, V A and Table 7.3] *Sporothrix schenckii*, a dimorphic fungus, is found in the environment on various plant materials. Subcutaneous infections begin with traumatic implantation of contaminated plant material, such as slivers from mine timbers, thorns, or the combination of wires and sphagnum moss (used by floral designers). The resulting sporotrichosis is characterized by a fixed nodular subcutaneous lesion or lesions along the lymphatics from the initial trauma site. When found in tissues, the fungus grows as an oval to cigar-shaped yeast. It grows as sporulating filaments in the environment and has a worldwide distribution. Cases are most common in tropical regions because people are less likely to wear protective clothing (eg, long pants, long-sleeved shirts).

22. The answer is D. [Chapter 5, XIII C] Koilocytotic cells have enlarged nuclei, and cytoplasmic vacuoles are produced from human papillomavirus (HPV)-infected epithelial cells. The Gardasil vaccine employed to prevent HPV genital disease is a recombinant quadrivalent vaccine containing viruslike particles of types 6, 11, 16, and 18 HPV.

23. The answer is B. [Chapter 2, I B 8 h] O-antigen or O-specific side chains are major surface antigens in the polysaccharide component of lipopolysaccharide.

24. The answer is C. [Chapter 2, VII B 2 and Figure 2.7A] An F^+ cell contains the fertility factor in the plasmid state. In the cross between an F^+ cell and an F^- cell, chromosomal genes are not transferred because they are not covalently linked to the plasmid. Only the plasmid genes are transferred.

25. The answer is B. [Chapter 5, XI F] The disease is most likely roseola caused by HHV-6 since it has a short duration and the face, palms, and soles are not affected.

26. The answer is C. [Chapter 6 b (2) a] CD4 is a prominent receptor for gp120.

27. The answer is D. [Chapter 10, VII D 1 d] IL-4 (interleukin-4) causes the switch from IgG to IgE.

28. The answer is A. [Chapter 10, VII C 2 a] IgA is the principal Ig in exocrine secretions in the oral and gastric cavities.

29. The answer is F. [Chapter 3, I D 3 and Table 3.1] *S. pyogenes* is a group A *Streptococcus* that has an M protein on its outer cell walls that interferes with phagocytosis in the immunologically naïve individual. M12 strains are often nephritogenic.

30. The answer is F. [Chapter 3, III A and VIII B] Viridans group *Streptococci*, which are part of the normal oral flora in humans, are noted for their ability to attach to damaged heart valves when they enter the circulation after oral surgery. *S. pyogenes* was the original trigger for rheumatic fever as an untreated *S. pyogenes* pharyngitis. Each additional exposure creates the risk of additional damage. However, the question asks about major dental work, so the correct answer is the bacteria that are a part of the normal oral flora.

31. The answer is D. [Chapter 7, VII A 3 and VII E 3 c] The disease is invasive aspergillosis, which is found primarily in patients with neutrophil counts less than $500/mm^3$.

32. The answer is B. [Chapter 2, II C 1 b and II C 4] Facultative anaerobes grow in the presence or absence of oxygen; a respiratory mode is used when oxygen is present, and fermentation occurs when it is not. Facultative anaerobes contain the enzyme superoxide dismutase, which aids aerobic growth by preventing the accumulation of the superoxide ion. Obligate aerobes do not have fermentative pathways and require oxygen for growth; obligate anaerobes lack superoxide dismutase. The heterotrophs require preformed organic compounds for growth.

33. The answer is D. [Chapter 10, VII A 1 d (1)] Papain cleaves IgG into two monovalent antigen-binding fragments containing both a heavy and light chain.

34. The answer is B. [Chapter 3, V B and Figure 3.1] The disease is diphtheria. *Corynebacterium diphtheriae* remains localized to the surface of the oropharynx throat and does not invade tissues; rather, the exotoxin enters the bloodstream and affects tissues, primarily the heart and nerves, causing myocarditis and recurrent laryngeal neuropathy.

35. The answer is D. [Chapter 2, I B 8 c (1)] Peptidoglycan (mucopeptide and murein) is a complex cell-wall polymer containing *N*-acetylglucosamine and *N*-acetylmuramic acid and associated peptides.

36. The answer is F. [Table 9.1] African trypanosomiasis (African sleeping sickness) is transmitted by tsetse flies.

37. The answer is C. [Chapter 2, IV A 1] It is most likely that she forgot to put the iodine on, so the dye does not form the large complex; in this situation, the uncomplexed crystal violet will decolorize even Gram-positive organisms. It was also a sharp physician who realized that there are no Gram-negative cocci arranged in clusters and that abscesses are either *Staphylococci* or rod-shaped anaerobes or mixed infections.

38. The answer is D. [Chapter 5, VI B 3] The man was infected with HCV during his blood transfusion. Molecular genotyping of circulating virions is necessary since effective treatment with α-interferon and ribavirin occurs in only two genotypes (2 and 3) of the six genotypes.

39. The answer is C. [Chapter 3, II D 1 c; VI B b; and VII E 3] Organisms that colonize mucosal surfaces such as the *Neisseria meningitidis* and *S. pneumoniae* generally produce immunoglobulin A proteases (also called *IgA proteases*).

40. The answer is B. [Chapter 5, XIII] HBV infection has no genital signs or symptoms but is considered one of the sexually transmitted infections.

Comprehensive Examination: Block 2

Directions: Perform this block under examination conditions. Please allocate 90 seconds per question: this block should take 60 minutes. Select the *one* lettered answer that is *best* in each case. Commit to and write down your answers before checking the answers and explanations. Each of the numbered items in this section is followed by answers with explanations, in the following section.

1. There is an outbreak of watery diarrhea in 6 members of a party of 20 who ate at a Chinese restaurant the day before. Fried rice is implicated. What is the most likely causative agent?

(A) *Bacillus cereus*
(B) *Giardia lamblia*
(C) Norovirus
(D) Rotavirus
(E) *Salmonella enteritidis*
(F) *Staphylococcus aureus*

2. In January, a 4-month-old girl is seen by her family physician. The girl's father noted that she has been coughing and has had a slight fever for 3 days and recently developed difficulty breathing characterized by wheezing. She has a runny nose composed of clear fluid with some cells present. X-rays show her lungs are clear of infection. Which of the following entities is most likely to be observed in the nasal discharge and would confirm diagnosis?

(A) Eosinophilic cytoplasmic inclusions in cells
(B) Gram-negative coccobacilli
(C) Gram-positive cocci
(D) Multinucleated giant cells
(E) Secretory immunoglobulin (Ig)A heterophile antibody

3. Which of the following best describes mobile genetic elements that code for antibiotic resistance genes in bacteria but are incapable of self-replication?

(A) Mesosomes
(B) R-factor
(C) Temperate RNA phages
(D) Transposons
(E) Virulent DNA phages

4. What is the mechanism of action of the aminoglycosides?

(A) Blocking initiation complex
(B) Damaging the membrane
(C) Inhibiting the DNA gyrase
(D) Inhibiting mycolic acid synthesis
(E) Inhibiting peptide chain elongation

5. Which of the individuals listed below is the most likely to develop a serious disease from West Nile virus?

(A) 4-month-old hospitalized with a serious respiratory syncytial virus (RSV) infection
(B) 3-year-old with croup
(C) 21-year-old college student returning from a vacation in Costa Rica
(D) 24-year-old tour guide in the four corners of the southwestern United States
(E) 55-year-old camper returning from a 2-week wilderness experience in Minnesota

6. Which of the following pairs of organisms is easiest to distinguish from each other by Gram stain?

(A) *Bacillus* and *Clostridium*
(B) *Corynebacterium* and *Lactobacillus*
(C) *Haemophilus* and *Escherichia*
(D) *Listeria* and *Proteus*
(E) *Salmonella* and *Shigella*

7. Two physicians traveling in Central America developed what they self-diagnosed as enterotoxigenic *Escherichia coli* (ETEC) infection. What virulence factor is responsible for the fluid and electrolyte disruption they experienced?

(A) Adherence causing palisade layers of the bacterium on the surface of the small intestine
(B) Entrance through intestinal M cells and migration through the tissue via actin polymerization/"jetting"
(C) Exotoxin that causes an increase in cyclic adenosine monophosphate (cAMP)
(D) Exotoxin that inhibits protein synthesis by blocking elongation factor 2
(E) Exotoxin that inhibits protein synthesis by cleaving 60S ribosomal subunits

8. In a high-frequency recombination (Hfr) cross with an F⁻ bacterial cell, each having a single DNA molecule, what is the most likely outcome?

(A) Bacterial genes will be transferred from the Hfr cell to the F⁻ cell, but there will be no change in the "sex" of either cell.
(B) Each cell may acquire genes from the other.
(C) Only plasmid genes will be transferred.
(D) Some genes will be transferred and the recipient cell will become Hfr.

9. A 60-year-old man who traveled to Haiti took prophylactic chloroquine. He stopped the medication just as he left the region and now has developed *Plasmodium vivax* malaria. Which of the following parasite stages was/were not eliminated because he stopped taking the drug early?

(A) Bradyzoites
(B) Erythrocytic schizonts/merozoites
(C) Gametocytes
(D) Liver schizonts/merozoites
(E) Sporozoites

10. A 57-year-old man presents to the hospital with paranasal swelling, hemorrhagic exudates in the eyes and nares, and mental lethargy. Nonseptate hyphae (see image) are found invading the tissues. Rhinocerebral *Mucor* infection (zygomycosis) is diagnosed. Which of the following is this patient's most likely underlying condition?

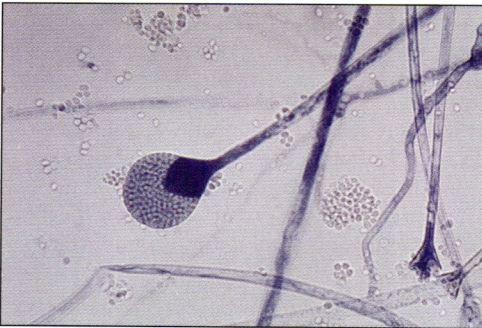

(A) C5 to C8 deficiencies
(B) Epstein-Barr virus (EBV) infection
(C) Hepatitis A infection
(D) Hepatitis B infection
(E) Ketoacidotic diabetes
(F) Severe neutropenia

11. An 18-year-old develops a severe headache, neck stiffness, and fever. He is a college freshman living in a university residence hall. When he cannot be aroused, his roommate brings him to the hospital. Centrifuged cerebrospinal fluid (CSF) is Gram stained, and the results are shown in the image. A latex particle agglutination (LPA) test confirms the etiologic cause of the bacterial

meningitis. Which causative agent is the most likely?

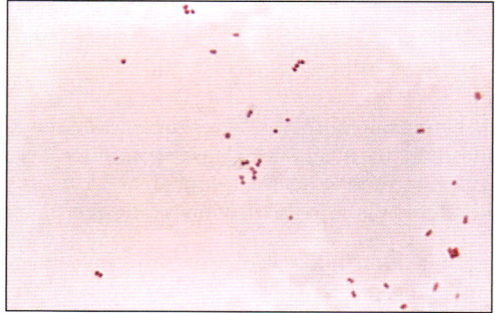

(A) *Escherichia coli*
(B) *Haemophilus influenzae*
(C) *Listeria monocytogenes*
(D) *Neisseria meningitidis*
(E) *Streptococcus pneumoniae*

12. In question 11, the substance found in the patient's CSF that gives the positive agglutination test also plays a role in the pathogenesis. What is that role?

(A) Allowing binding to the vascular endothelium, triggering uptake and passage into the central nervous system (CNS)
(B) Causing a strong inflammatory response loosening tight junctions, allowing CNS invasion
(C) Enhancing opsonization
(D) Inhibiting phagocytic uptake in the bloodstream of a nonimmune individual
(E) Promoting invasion of the bloodstream

13. Repeated *N. meningitidis* septicemias in an individual should raise suspicion of what underlying condition?

(A) C5 to C8 deficiencies
(B) Chronic hepatitis B infection
(C) Ketosis-prone diabetes
(D) Multiple myeloma
(E) Severe neutropenia

14. A 35-year-old woman presents to the emergency department with a high fever, severe headache, and muscle aches. She reports that her symptoms began abruptly and have worsened over the past 12 hours. Physical examination reveals a temperature of 102.5 °F (39.2 °C), and she appears acutely ill. Laboratory studies show an elevated white blood cell (WBC) count with left shift, and lumbar puncture reveals an increased WBC count, elevated protein levels, and normal glucose levels in the CSF. Which of the following interleukins (ILs) is an endogenous pyrogen?

(A) IL-1
(B) IL-2
(C) IL-3
(D) IL-4
(E) IL-5

15. A 28-year-old woman who is hospitalized with *Pseudomonas aeruginosa* septicemia develops shock. She is also neutropenic. Which bacterial component triggered the shock?

(A) Catalase
(B) Flagella from gram-negative bacteria
(C) Lipid A
(D) O-specific polysaccharide side chain of endotoxin
(E) Teichoic acid–peptidoglycan fragments

16. A 5-year-old girl presented to the local Family Medicine Clinic with a 2-day history of headache, earache, and swallowing difficulty. Physical examination showed bilateral swelling of the parotid glands. She is from Somali and immigrated to this country 4 months earlier and started her childhood vaccinations 2 weeks ago. Which of the following genomes belong to the pathogen that is causing her disease?

(A) Double-stranded DNA
(B) Double-stranded RNA
(C) Negative-sense RNA
(D) Positive-sense RNA
(E) Single-stranded DNA

17. A female infant is born to a 16-year-old mother. The infant shows signs and symptoms of hepatosplenomegaly, jaundice, low birth weight, chorioretinitis, and microcephaly. The mother appears healthy and reports an unremarkable pregnancy except for a period during the third month when she developed a fever, sore throat, and extreme fatigue for a period of 10 days. Which of the following organisms is the most likely causative pathogen for the infant's disease?

(A) Cytomegalovirus (CMV)
(B) *L. monocytogenes*
(C) Parvovirus B19
(D) Rubella virus
(E) *Treponema pallidum*

18. An outbreak of pneumonia occurs in a pediatric intensive care facility. A negative single-stranded RNA virus lacking hemagglutinating and neuraminidase activity is isolated. Which of the following viruses is described by these characteristics?

(A) Adenovirus
(B) Influenza A virus
(C) Parainfluenza virus
(D) RSV

19. Infection with which of the following organisms is more often noted for the production of lymphocytosis rather than mononucleosis?

(A) *Bordetella pertussis*
(B) EBV
(C) Human immunodeficiency virus
(D) *Listeria monocytogenes*

20. A 7-year-old boy develops vesicular skin lesions on his trunk, which quickly spread to his extremities and appear on the scalp. Scrapings from the vesicles show multinucleated cells and Cowdry type A inclusion bodies. Which of the following entities could have been used in a vaccine that would have prevented this disease?

(A) Capsid protein
(B) Inactivated virions
(C) Live attenuated virus strain
(D) Live reassortment virus
(E) Vaccinia virus carrying capsid protein gene

21. A 26-year-old woman presents with high fever, painful and frequent urination, and left flank pain. The isolate is a facultative anaerobe that is oxidase negative and ferments both glucose and lactose. A Gram stain is shown in the image. From these data, what genus is the most likely cause?

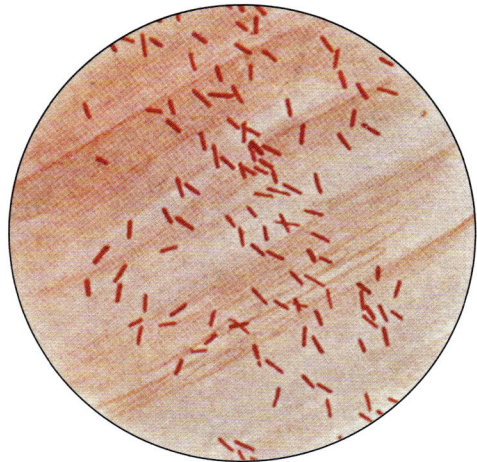

(A) *Campylobacter*
(B) *Escherichia*
(C) *Neisseria*
(D) *Proteus*
(E) *Vibrio*

22. The agent in question 21 is a pathogen causing ascending urinary tract infections and pyelonephritis. Other strains of this pathogen are normal flora. What virulence factor do urinary tract pathogen strains synthesize that normal flora strains lack, even though both are the same organism?

(A) Capsule
(B) Flagellum
(C) Lipoteichoic acid
(D) LT (heat-labile toxin)
(E) P-pili

23. A 32-year-old woman presents to her health care provider with fever, chills, headache, and joint pain. She recently returned from a tropical vacation where she spent a significant amount of time outdoors and was bitten by mosquitos. Physical examination reveals a temperature of 102.0 °F (38.9 °C) and generalized lymphadenopathy. Laboratory studies show leukopenia and thrombocytopenia. Which of the following viruses is transmitted by an arthropod vector?

(A) Arenavirus
(B) Bunyavirus
(C) Parainfluenza virus
(D) Parvovirus
(E) Reovirus

24. A 6-month-old child has had watery diarrhea for 6 days. The stools have no blood and no pus. The causative agent has double-stranded RNA as genetic material. Which of the following pathogens is the most likely causative agent?

(A) *B. cereus*
(B) *G. lamblia*
(C) Norovirus
(D) Rotavirus
(E) *S. enteritidis*
(F) *S. aureus*

25. A 26-year-old male who is heterozygous for Rh factor marries an Rh− female. Which of the following outcomes would be predicted for their offspring?

(A) No offspring would be Rh+
(B) 25% of their offspring would be Rh+
(C) 50% of their offspring would be Rh+
(D) 100% of their offspring would be Rh+

26. Which of the following Igs has the highest level in a normal 1-day-old infant?

(A) IgA
(B) IgG
(C) IgM
(D) IgD
(E) IgE

27. A 19-year-old college freshman has a sore throat, sore and enlarging cervical lymph nodes, and a fever. The student is also greatly fatigued. A diagnosis of infectious mononucleosis is made. Which of the following components of the causative agent would be present in this patient's blood?

(A) δ hemagglutinin
(B) E1A protein
(C) Large T antigen
(D) TAT protein
(E) VCA protein

28. Which of the following cluster of differentiation antigens binds to class II histocompatibility antigens?

(A) CD2
(B) CD3
(C) CD4
(D) CD8
(E) CD25

29. A child presents to the clinic and is diagnosed with impetigo with bullae. The causative agent is found to be β-hemolytic, catalase positive, and coagulase positive. A Gram stain is shown in the image. Which of the following is the most likely causative organism?

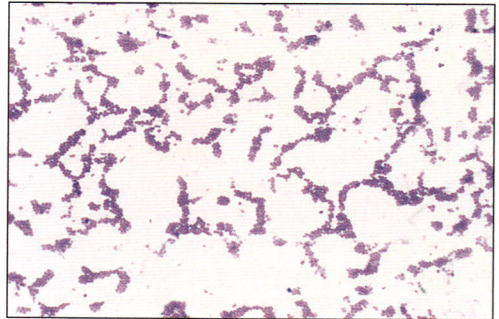

(A) Group A streptococcus
(B) Group B streptococcus
(C) *Staphylococcus aureus*
(D) *Staphylococcus epidermidis*

30. Intracellular survival and replication are the major virulence factors rather than exotoxin production for which of the following organisms?

(A) *Bordetella*
(B) *B. pertussis*
(C) ETEC
(D) *Vibrio cholerae*
(E) *Yersinia pestis*

31. An 18-year-old woman who lives in New York presents in September with cough, malaise, low-grade fever, myalgias, and chest pain. She indicates that she recently returned from a visit to the Mississippi River Valley. Physical exam reveals rales, and respiratory infiltrates are noted on x-ray. Sputum stained with calcofluor white and viewed with an ultraviolet microscope shows hundreds of small yeast cells inside WBCs. When cultured at room temperature, hyphae with small microconidia and tuberculate macroconidia grow. What is the most likely causative agent?

(A) *Aspergillus fumigatus*
(B) *Candida albicans*
(C) *Coccidioides immitis*
(D) *Histoplasma capsulatum*
(E) *Mycoplasma pneumoniae*
(F) *Streptococcus pneumoniae*

32. If a series of drug resistance genes are transferred together, what is the most likely method of transfer?

(A) Generalized transduction
(B) Plasmid-mediated conjugation
(C) Specialized transduction
(D) Transformation

33. A patient hospitalized with severe burns develops an infection with *P. aeruginosa*. The circulating exotoxin has activity that is similar to what other bacterial exotoxin?

(A) Botulinum toxin
(B) Diphtheria toxin
(C) Pertussis toxin
(D) Shiga toxin
(E) Tetanus toxin

34. A 92-year-old man presents to the clinic with a cough of several months' duration. He states that he has been coughing up brownish "stuff." The man is 5′6″ tall and he has lost 10 lb in the past 2 months without trying (starting weight was 150 lb). Past medical history indicates that a tuberculin skin test has been >10 mm the 3 times he has been tested over the past 25 years. The chest x-ray is consistent with reactivation tuberculosis. *Mycobacterium tuberculosis* testing and susceptibilities are ordered, and the patient is started on standard therapy. Luminescent real-time polymerase chain reaction confirms *M. tuberculosis* infection. What has been the standard medium used to grow the causative agent?

(A) Blood agar
(B) Buffered charcoal yeast extract agar
(C) Chocolate agar
(D) Löwenstein-Jensen medium
(E) Tellurite-containing medium such as Regan-Lowe

35. A 17-year-old visiting his grandparents in Louisiana in August develops a severe unrelenting headache that is not relieved by analgesics. He is very sleepy and reports an odd odor that he thinks is in the whole house. Primary amebic meningoencephalitis is diagnosed. Which of the following modes of transmission most likely explains how he acquired this infection?

(A) Diving or swimming in contaminated water
(B) Eating undercooked crayfish
(C) Intravenous drug abuse
(D) Handling cat litter
(E) Use of horse dung as vegetable fertilizer

36. A 4-year-old boy has a yearlong history of repeated staphylococcal and streptococcal infections. He was referred to the genetic counseling unit, where he was found to have depressed superoxide dismutase activity. Which of the following treatments would most likely be successful in alleviating his condition?

(A) CD4$^+$ T helper cells
(B) Insertion of the gene for adenosine deaminase
(C) Interferon γ
(D) Transforming growth factor β (TGF-β)

37. A 23-year-old who just returned from a 2-week missionary trip to rural Haiti presents with a 2-day history of watery diarrhea. Which of the following best describes the pathogenesis of the most likely causative bacteria?

(A) Enterotoxin that is also an endotoxin
(B) Enterotoxin that is also an exotoxin
(C) Invading tissue with no toxin production
(D) Invading tissue and producing an exotoxin

38. A 43-year-old woman develops cervical carcinoma. Which of the following viral proteins played a role in the development of the carcinoma?

(A) E1A protein
(B) E6 protein
(C) Large T antigen
(D) TAX protein

39. A 35-year-old woman develops aortitis. She has no mucosal ulcerations or exanthems. Social history indicates she injects drugs and has been employed as a sex worker for the past 20 years, where she routinely has unprotected sex. Her VDRL (Venereal Disease Research Laboratory) test is negative, and her fluorescent treponemal antibody absorption (FTA-abs) test is positive. What is the most likely diagnosis?

(A) Lyme disease
(B) Early primary syphilis
(C) Secondary syphilis
(D) Latent syphilis
(E) Tertiary syphilis

40. A 30-year-old man visits his physician experiencing difficulty in breathing, headache, and joint and lower back pain in August. He has a 101 °F (38.33 °C) fever and a prominent cough. A patient history indicates that he conducted a thorough cleaning of an old hunting shack. The cleaning involved removal of old food containers, pots, and bedding, plus some rodent nests. He also deployed new mouse traps. Based on this history, which of the following agents is most likely causing his symptoms?

(A) *Chlamydophila pneumoniae*
(B) Influenza A virus
(C) *Legionella pneumonia*
(D) *Pneumocystis jiroveci*
(E) Sin Nombre virus

Answers and Explanations

1. **The answer is A.** [Chapter 3, IX B] *B. cereus*, found in rice, is not killed by steaming. The addition of eggs and other ingredients to make fried rice encourages growth if the fried rice is not held at a high enough temperature to inhibit it. Onset of watery diarrhea may occur within 2 hours or as long as 18 hours after consumption and is in response to the presence of toxin.

2. **The answer is D.** [Chapter 4, VI B 3 e (3) and Chapter 5, IV B] The signs and symptoms of the girl's infection are consistent with bronchiolitis. The most common cause of bronchiolitis in infants is RSV. Syncytia are multinucleated cells.

3. **The answer is D.** [Chapter 2, I B 7] Transposons are incapable of independent replication but may contain antibiotic resistance genes as well as insertion sequences that provide for transfer of genetic information to bacterial chromosomes or plasmids.

4. **The answer is A.** [Chapter 2, IX B 3 a and Table 2.4] Aminoglycosides bind to multiple sites on both the 30S and 50S ribosomes, thereby preventing the transfer RNA from forming initiation complexes. They are bactericidal for many aerobic gram-negative bacteria.

5. **The answer is E.** [Chapter 5, IX B 3 a ii (b)] West Nile virus is an arbovirus transferred to humans by a mosquito vector. The most serious consequences following infection occur in those individuals older than 50 years who can develop life-threatening encephalitis.

6. **The answer is D.** [Chapter 2, III B 7 and IV B 8] *Listeria* is a gram-positive rod, whereas *Proteus* is a gram-negative rod. *Clostridium*, *Lactobacillus*, *Corynebacterium*, and *Bacillus* are all gram-positive rods, whereas *Haemophilus*, *Escherichia*, *Salmonella*, and *Shigella* are all gram-negative rods.

7. **The answer is C.** [Chapter 3, IX G b] Traveler's diarrhea is most frequently caused by enterotoxigenic strains of *E. coli* that produce the heat-labile (LT) and heat-stable (ST) toxin. LT is an exotoxin that causes an increase in cAMP. It is not invasive, making choice B incorrect. Choice E is also incorrect; it is the mechanism of Shiga toxin and the O157 Shiga-like toxin, also known as verotoxin.

8. **The answer is A.** [Chapter 2, VII B 2 a (2) and Figure 2.7B] The donor cell, which transfers part of one of the two strands of its DNA, will duplicate any areas of single-stranded DNA and so will not change genotype, including its "maleness." Only a portion of the integrated fertility factor and some bacterial genes on that strand of DNA will be transferred, so the recipient cell may pick up some new bacterial genes. But because the last thing to be transferred would be the rest of the fertility factor, the cell almost never becomes Hfr.

9. **The answer is D.** [Table 9.2] Chloroquine kills only the erythrocytic schizonts/merozoites, so you must take the chloroquine for 4 weeks after leaving the malarial area to allow all stages to continue past the liver stages into the sensitive forms.

10. **The answer is E.** [Chapter 7 VII F 1] Ketoacidotic diabetes is a major predisposing condition for zygomycosis, although lymphoma and leukemia also predispose the patient to zygomycosis.

11. **The answer is D.** [Chapter 3, VII E; Table 3.4; and Figure 3.2] In the specific patient (young adult; new stresses; crowded living conditions such as residence halls and, potentially, college bars), the first suspicion even before the Gram stain and LPA tests should be *N. meningitidis*, which was confirmed by the Gram stain. *E. coli* would be unlikely unless the patient had a CNS shunt or was a neonate. *H. influenzae* would be unlikely in anyone except a 3-month-old to a 5-year-old child who had not been vaccinated as a child.

12. **The answer is D.** [Chapter 13, III F] In addition to a Gram stain of sediment of CSF, another rapid diagnostic tool for CNS infection is a panel of LPA tests for polysaccharide of the common extracellular bacterial agents of meningitis. The capsular polysaccharide on the bacteria in the body inhibit phagocytic uptake until opsonized.

13. **The answer is A.** [Chapter 10, III D 7] The killing of *N. meningitidis* primarily depends on complement-mediated cell lysis. Patients with genetic deficiencies in C5 to C8 cannot carry out

complement-mediated lysis of bacterial cells and have repeated septicemias with
N. meningitidis.

14. **The answer is A.** [Chapter 10, IV B 4] IL-1 is an endogenous pyrogen along with IL-6 and tumor necrosis factor α (TNF-α).

15. **The answer is C.** [Chapter 2, IV B 6 and VIII C 1] *Pseudomonas* is a gram-negative organism; therefore, the patient has a gram-negative septicemia. Endotoxic activity is associated with lipid A. No toxicity is associated with the O polysaccharides, the flagella from gram-negative bacteria, or catalase. If it had been a gram-positive bacterium, teichoic acid–peptidoglycan fragments can trigger a similar process.

16. **The answer is C.** [Table 4.4] The girl is infected with the mumps virus, a single-stranded negative-sense RNA virus.

17. **The answer is A.** [Chapter 5, XII B 1] CMV is the most likely pathogen; it was probably passed to the infant during a primary CMV infection of the mother during her first trimester of pregnancy. The baby has congenital CMV infection.

18. **The answer is D.** [Chapter 4, VI B 3 a (2) (a) 1] Only influenza A virus, parainfluenza virus, and RSV are single-strand negative-sense RNA viruses. RSV lacks a hemagglutinin and neuraminidase activity.

19. **The answer is A.** [Chapter 3, VI A] *B. pertussis* is unusual among bacterial infections in that it causes a lymphocytosis (due to pertussis toxin). A mononucleosis-like presentation may occur during the first year of human immunodeficiency virus infection. EBV is a causative agent of mononucleosis.

20. **The answer is C.** [Chapter 5, V B 2 b (3) (b)] The boy has chickenpox caused by varicella zoster virus (VZV); it can be prevented by immunization with the live attenuated Oka strain of the virus.

21. **The answer is B.** [Chapter 2, IV B 8 b] *Neisseria* are diplococci, vibrios are comma shaped, and *Campylobacter* are spiral shaped. *Neisseria* and vibrios are all oxidase positive. Because *Campylobacter* is grown under unique conditions and temperature, it is identified by just growing under those conditions. It has both a poorly functioning oxidase and catalase. *Proteus* and *Escherichia* are rod shaped and both are oxidase negative. *Escherichia* is the only one of the two that is a lactose fermenter.

22. **The answer is E.** [Chapter 2, IV B 8 b (3) and Chapter 3, X A] Common pili of *E. coli* bind to the colonic mucosa but not to the uroepithelium; therefore, in order to cause ascending urinary tract infections and not just be washed out by periodic urine flow, the *E. coli* has to have either x-adhesins (not a choice) or pyelonephritis-associated pili (P-pili).

23. **The answer is B.** [Chapter 4, VI B 1 c (2)] The California and La Crosse viruses, which have mosquito vectors, are both bunyaviruses.

24. **The answer is D.** [Chapter 4, VI D 1 d] The patient's age, symptoms, and nucleic acid indicate that rotavirus is the primary suspect.

25. **The answer is C.** [Chapter 11, A 2 b; Table 11.2] Since the male is heterozygous for the Rh+ gene and Rh+ is dominant, the possibility exists for Rh+ offspring. Since the father's sperm will be half Rh+ and half Rh−, and the mother's eggs will be all Rh−, genetic theory predicts that 50% of the offspring will be Rh+.

26. **The answer is B.** [Chapter 10, VII A 2 d and Table 10.8] A 1-day-old infant has a maternal level of IgG due to cross-placental transfer of the mother's IgG. The other Igs are slowly being synthesized by the infant.

27. **The answer is E.** [Chapter 4, V B 2 d (2) (a)] The VCA protein, or viral capsid antigen, is the main component of the EBV capsid. EBV is the causative agent of infectious mononucleosis.

28. **The answer is C.** [Chapter 10, VIII C 1 b (2)] CD4 binds to class II histocompatibility antigens, resulting in humoral immunity; CD8 binds to class I histocompatibility antigens, resulting in cell-mediated immunity.

29. **The answer is C.** [Chapter 2, III B 1; Chapter 3, XI and Table 3.2] Although groups A and B streptococci and *S. aureus* are β-hemolytic, only the streptococci are catalase negative. Only *S. aureus* is both β-hemolytic and coagulase positive.

30. The answer is E. [Chapter 3, XIV C and Table 3.4] The virulence of *Y. pestis* in humans depends on a variety of factors, the most important of which is its ability to proliferate intracellularly. Associated with this ability and virulence are Ca^{2+} dependence; V and W antigens; *Yersinia* outer membrane proteins; F1 envelope antigen; coagulase and fibrinolysin production; and pigment absorption. The other choices listed produce exotoxin as a major component of pathogenesis.

31. The answer is D. [Chapter 7, VI B and Table 7.1] This condition was probably transmitted in the Midwest when the patient was visiting the Mississippi River Valley. (They may have stirred up dried bird excreta dust from starlings, chickens, or bats that contained *H. capsulatum*.) This best describes *H. capsulatum*.

32. The answer is B. [Chapter 2, VII B 2] Genes for drug resistance may reside individually on the bacterial chromosome or on plasmids. Clusters of multiple drug resistance genes are occasionally on chromosomes but are more commonly on plasmids. Also, plasmid DNA is generally entirely transferred in a conjugal cross of F^+ cells with F^- cells. R-factors are like those F^+ cells with just a few extra, closely linked drug resistance genes. So the conjugal transfer of an R-factor is the process most likely to transfer multiple drug resistance.

33. The answer is B. [Table 2.3; Chapter 3, I B 2 c and V B 1] Diphtheria toxin and *Pseudomonas* exotoxin A are both adenosine diphosphate–ribosylating toxins that irreversibly inactivate elongation factor 2 and inhibit protein synthesis. Although they have similar modes of action, they differ in their cellular targets and antigenicity.

34. The answer is D. [Table 2.2; Chapter 3, VI L 3 b] Standard cultures for *M. tuberculosis* may be set up on Löwenstein-Jensen agar. Palmitic acid–containing broths (some with anti-TB drugs) have replaced solid agars, and growth detection systems now allow more rapid diagnosis. (The mycobacteria have limited numbers of ribosomal genes slowing their growth.) Choice B (buffered charcoal yeast extract) is the media for *Legionella* spp.; chocolate agar is required to grow either *Neisseria* spp. or *H. influenzae* from sterile sites like CSF. Thayer-Martin is a chocolate agar with antibiotics used to culture *Neisseria* spp. from any mucosal surface preventing overgrowth of the normal flora. Tellurite (choice E) is a medium for culturing *C. diphtheriae*.

35. The answer is A. [Table 9.1] Swimming/diving/jumping in warm contaminated waters may cause infection with *Naegleria*, which rapidly develops into primary amebic meningoencephalitis, which is generally fatal. It is thought that the organism enters through the cribriform plate.

36. The answer is C. [Chapter 11, B 8 a] Repeated infections with depressed superoxide activity characterize chronic granulomatous disease. Interferon-γ has been successful in treatment. Loss of adenine deaminase is the lesion found in patients with severe combined immunodeficiency (SCID). TGF-β inhibits T-cell and B-cell proliferation.

37. The answer is B. [Chapter 3, IX G b] With no mention of high fever or vomiting, the disease is most likely "traveler's diarrhea," commonly caused by ETEC. ETEC produces two exotoxins (LT and ST), both acting on the intestine, so they can also be called enterotoxins. It is common that when bacteria invade the gastrointestinal tract tissue, inflammation and prostaglandins are triggered, causing higher fever, abdominal pain, and diarrhea. Choice D (incorrect) describes type I *Shigella dysenteriae*, which is both invasive and produces the Shiga toxin.

38. The answer is B. [Chapter 4, V A 2 d (3)] Cervical carcinoma is caused by oncogenic strains of the human papillomavirus (most commonly 16, 18, and 31). The early protein E6 is associated with the oncogenic potential of human papillomavirus.

39. The answer is E. [Chapter 3, XII C 7 (2) (b) and XII C 2 5] The FTA-abs test detects specific anti-treponemal antibody. The FTA-abs remains positive for life with or without antibiotic therapy. The VDRL test detects less specific reaginic antibodies, which decline with successful treatment, but also sometimes decline without treatment in tertiary syphilis. Therefore, based on the serologic data, this patient could have very early primary syphilis or untreated tertiary syphilis. The symptoms are consistent with tertiary syphilis.

40. The answer is E. [Chapter 4, VI B 1 c (3)] Although several of the organisms could result in these clinical signs and symptoms, the interactions of the patient in an old hunting shack containing rodent feces point toward the Hantavirus, Sin Nombre, as the cause.

Comprehensive Examination: Block 3

Directions: Perform this block under examination conditions. Please allocate 90 seconds per question: this block should take 60 minutes. Select the *one* lettered answer that is *best* in each case. Commit to and write down your answers *before* checking the answers and explanations. Each of the numbered items in this section is followed by answers with explanations, in the following section.

1. A neonate with very low Apgar scores dies 2 hours after birth. Autopsy reveals disseminated granulomatous lesions throughout; some are caseating, but they are not calcified. During her pregnancy, the mother most likely had septicemia caused by which of the following microorganisms?

(A) *Escherichia coli*
(B) Group B streptococci
(C) *Listeria monocytogenes*
(D) Parvovirus B19
(E) *Toxoplasma gondii*

2. A 7-year-old child presents to the pediatrician with perianal itching and discomfort. The child's parent reports that the symptoms have been present for several weeks, especially at night. On examination, there are no signs of inflammation or rash in the perianal region. The pediatrician suspects *Enterobius vermicularis* infection. Which of the following is the most appropriate diagnostic test for confirming this infection?

(A) Adhesive tape test
(B) Chest x-ray
(C) Ova and parasite test
(D) Serum antibody test
(E) Skin scraping for microscopy

3. In which of the following phases of growth is a gram-positive bacterium most susceptible to the action of penicillin?

(A) Death
(B) Decline
(C) Exponential
(D) Lag
(E) Stationary

4. What is the genetic mechanism responsible for the conversion of a nontoxigenic strain of *Corynebacterium diphtheriae* to a toxigenic strain?

(A) Conjugation
(B) In vivo transformation
(C) Lysogenic phage conversion
(D) Reciprocal genetic recombination

5. A 28-year-old male presents with recurrent episodes of painful vesicular eruptions on his lips. He reports that these outbreaks are often triggered by stress or sunlight exposure. Physical examination reveals clustered vesicles with erythematous bases on the vermillion border of the lower lip. His physician explains that these episodes are due to reactivation of latent virus from neurons that innervate the area. Which of the following viruses is capable of a latent infection of neurons and fits these symptoms?

(A) Cytomegalovirus
(B) Herpes simplex virus
(C) Measles virus
(D) Poliomyelitis virus
(E) Rabies virus

6. A patient with sickle cell anemia is most likely to have repeated septicemias and possible osteomyelitis with which agent?

(A) *Candida albicans*
(B) Nontypeable *Haemophilus influenzae*
(C) *Mycobacterium avium-intracellulare*
(D) *Salmonella enteritidis*
(E) *Staphylococcus aureus*

7. The parent of a 9-year-old who is in the same school as another child just diagnosed with meningitis called the pediatrician, requesting that her child be prophylactically treated (even though the child did not know nor had any direct contact with the infected child). The physician suggests vaccinating the child, doing surveillance cultures, and watching the child for symptoms. The medium that the lab will use for cultures has antibiotics in it. Which of the following best describes the media that will be used?

(A) Differential medium
(B) Inhibitory medium
(C) Minimal medium
(D) Selective medium

8. A 32-year-old patient presents to the emergency department with sudden-onset fever, cough, sore throat, and myalgia. The patient is visibly unwell and appears to be in respiratory distress. The medical team suspects an influenza infection, and a nasopharyngeal swab is collected for diagnostic testing. Further analysis of the influenza virus isolated from the patient's respiratory sample reveals a novel strain that contains genetic material from both human influenza A (H1N1) and avian influenza A (H5N1) viruses. Which of the following characteristics of the influenza A virus allows genetic reassortment to occur?

(A) Defective chaperone proteins
(B) Poor editing by the RNA-dependent RNA polymerase
(C) Poor editing function of the reverse transcriptase
(D) Presence of the *rec-A* gene product
(E) Segmented genome

9. A patient has been living with human immunodeficiency virus (HIV) for the past 6 years. His disease has been slowly progressing. His only partner for the past 3 years is not infected with the virus. Which of the following situations best explains the partner's lack of infection?

(A) CD4/CD8 ratio probably >2
(B) High concentration of natural killer (NK) cells that kill the virus
(C) Lacks the coreceptor CXCR4
(D) Buildup of a high titer of anti-GP160 antibody

10. A 27-year-old man who recently immigrated from Central Africa presents with occasional swelling and pain in the lower leg. He also has eye pain and sensitivity to light. On examination, a visible intraocular worm is observed to cross the conjunctiva. The worm is elongated, white, and about 2 to 3 cm in length. Which of the following is the most likely causative organism of his condition?

(A) *Ascaris lumbricoides*
(B) *E. vermicularis*
(C) Loa loa
(D) *Strongyloides stercoralis*
(E) *Wuchereria bancrofti*

11. Which of the following best describes a prophage?

(A) Intracellular temperate phage DNA
(B) Phage attached to the cell wall that has released its DNA
(C) Phage that lacks receptors
(D) Newly assembled intracellular phage particle

12. A 26-year-old man presents with an infected foot from stepping on a nail 2 days earlier. The nail penetrated the sole of his tennis shoe. He sprayed some antiseptic on it and did not seek medical help because he had his last tetanus booster about 1 year ago and thought that would take care of the wound. Now the foot is quite inflamed around the wound with blue-green pus on the bandage. The organism isolated is Gram stained, and the results are shown in the image. Further testing reveals that the organism is oxidase positive and does not ferment any carbohydrates. Which organism is the most likely causative agent?

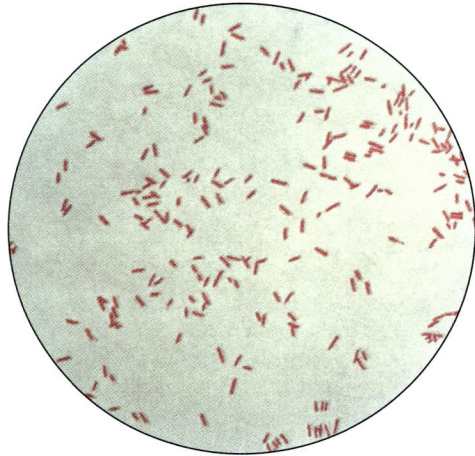

(A) *Clostridium tetani*
(B) *Escherichia coli*
(C) *Klebsiella pneumoniae*
(D) *Proteus vulgaris*
(E) *Pseudomonas aeruginosa*

13. In addition to interleukin (IL)-1, which of the following factors is an inflammation-inducing cytokine?

(A) IL-2
(B) IL-5
(C) Tumor necrosis factor α (TNF-α)
(D) Transforming growth factor β (TGF-β)

14. A Peace Corps volunteer who recently returned from rural Africa develops symptoms of liver damage and a blocked bile duct after general anesthesia for a knee replacement. Which of the following pathogens is the most likely causative agent?

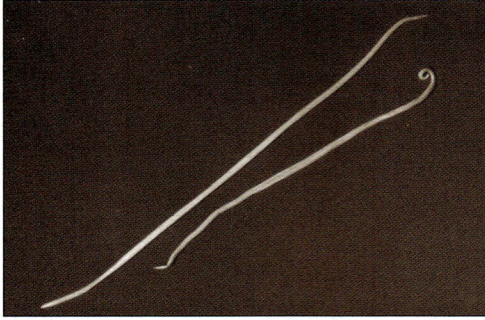

(A) Cestode
(B) Dimorphic fungus
(C) Filamentous fungus
(D) Fluke
(E) Nematode
(F) Protozoa

15. A 3-day-old newborn is brought to the pediatrician for evaluation. The parents report that the child has been experiencing recurrent infections and is failing to thrive. Physical examination reveals no apparent abnormalities in the child's appearance. Laboratory tests demonstrate severe lymphopenia, and a chest x-ray reveals an absent thymic shadow due to a thymectomy performed shortly after birth to correct a congenital heart defect. Which of the following situations would be expected following a neonatal thymectomy?

(A) Depletion of the periarteriolar region of the spleen
(B) Elimination of germinal center formation
(C) Increased ability to reject skin grafts
(D) Increased autoimmunity

16. *C. diphtheriae* is isolated from a patient with pharyngitis. What is the best predictor that the strain is pathogenic?

(A) Chromosomal *inv*+ genes
(B) Lysogenized by corynebacteriophage-β
(C) Plasmid with *tox*+ genes
(D) Producing the blackest colonies on tellurite medium

17. A 47-year-old patient presents to the neurology clinic with a 6-month history of progressive weakness in the lower extremities. The patient reports difficulty walking and frequent falls. Physical examination reveals increased muscle tone, hyperreflexia, and sustained clonus in the lower limbs. Additionally, the patient exhibits impaired vibratory sensation below the level of the umbilicus. Which of the following

organisms is an RNA tumor virus associated with the neurologic disease tropical spastic paraparesis?

(A) Human herpesvirus-8
(B) HIV
(C) Human papillomavirus
(D) Human T-lymphotropic virus type 1

18. Which of the following chemotactic factors for neutrophils is released when complement is fixed by antigen-antibody complexes?

(A) C1
(B) C2
(C) C3a
(D) C4b
(E) C789 complex

19. A 28-year-old female presents to the emergency department with sudden-onset dyspnea, wheezing, and diffuse urticaria shortly after receiving an intravenous medication. The patient has a history of allergies to various medications and foods. Physical examination reveals generalized hives, bronchospasm, and angioedema of the lips and face. Her symptoms are most likely due to the systemic release of anaphylatoxins. Which of the following complement components is most closely related to anaphylatoxin?

(A) C1qrs
(B) C2b
(C) C4b2a
(D) C5a
(E) C5b

20. A 30-year-old woman presents to her physician with an inflamed, itchy, expanding cutaneous lesion on the side of her body (see image). She suspects she might have picked it up from her dog because the lesion is located where the dog sleeps next to her, and the dog is losing fur. The woman is prescribed a topical drug from one of the major drug families commonly used to treat the infection. What is the mechanism of action of that drug class?

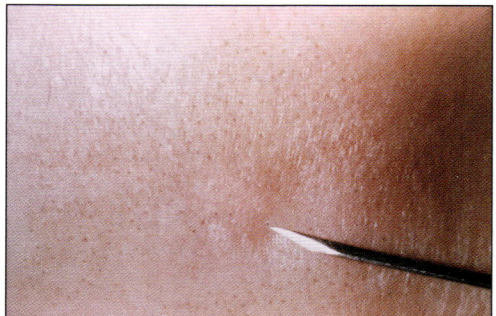

(A) Cleavage of 60S ribosomes
(B) Inhibition of chitin synthesis
(C) Inhibition of ergosterol synthesis
(D) Inhibition of formation of the peptide bond and peptide chain elongation on 70S ribosomes
(E) Inhibition of microtubule formation
(F) Inhibition of mycolic acid synthesis

21. A researcher studying emerging infectious diseases in a tropical region encounters a previously uncharacterized viral pathogen. Further analysis reveals that this virus belongs to a known viral family. The genomic characteristics of this newly discovered virus show an unusual feature, where its RNA genome consists of segments employing an ambisense coding strategy. Which of the following viruses possesses a segmented, ambisense genome?

(A) Arenavirus
(B) Parainfluenza virus
(C) Parvovirus
(D) Reovirus
(E) Respiratory syncytial virus

22. A 25-year-old presents to the emergency department with severe eye pain. She is a medical resident and had not been home for 2 days. She had the current pair of contacts in her eyes continuously for 6 weeks. Which of the following is a natural major protective mechanism of the eye that could not prevent infection due to contaminated contact lenses?

(A) B cells
(B) NK cells
(C) Lysozyme
(D) T cells
(E) Teichoic acids

23. Organisms from what genus are the most likely causative agents of the resident's eye infection in question 22?

(A) *Acanthamoeba*
(B) *Aspergillus*
(C) *Fusarium*
(D) *Pseudomonas*
(E) *Staphylococcus*

24. A 35-year-old male presents with a 3-week history of fever, malaise, and a persistent dry cough. He reports occasional unprotected sexual intercourse with multiple partners. On physical examination, he appears ill, with mild cervical lymphadenopathy. Laboratory results reveal a significantly elevated CD4/CD8 ratio. Which of the following characteristics is attributed to CD8?

(A) Recognizes class I human leukocyte antigen (HLA)
(B) Recognizes class II HLA
(C) Is a marker for T helper cells
(D) Is strongly chemotactic

25. Which of the following viruses possesses an oncogene that codes for the latent membrane-1 protein that mimics CD40 signaling?

(A) Epstein-Barr virus
(B) Hepatitis B virus
(C) Hepatitis C virus
(D) Human papillomavirus
(E) Human T-lymphotropic virus

26. Which of the following viruses is a cofactor in Burkitt lymphoma?

(A) Cytomegalovirus infection
(B) Epstein-Barr virus infection
(C) Hepatitis A virus infection
(D) Hepatitis B virus infection
(E) Influenza virus type A infection

27. Which of the following characteristics is attributed to IL-1?

(A) Inhibits T cells
(B) Initiates the acute phase reactant response
(C) Suppresses tumor necrosis factor
(D) Synthesis is restricted to phagocytic cells

28. Which of the following descriptions characterizes the γ2κ2 antibody?

(A) Contains a hypervariable region
(B) Contains a J chain
(C) Contains a secretory piece
(D) Initial antibody synthesized after antigen

29. A 45-year-old man had mental degeneration after a prolonged but inapparent infection. At autopsy, subacute spongiform encephalopathy is found. What is the nature of the most likely causative agent?

(A) Acid-fast organism
(B) Dimorphic fungus
(C) DNA virus
(D) Prion
(E) Viroid

30. Anti-A isohemagglutinins are present with which of the following blood types?

(A) Type A
(B) Type B
(C) Type AB

31. Bacterial surface polysaccharide plays a critical role in which of the following infections?

(A) Gonorrhea
(B) Meningitis with no underlying trauma
(C) *Mycoplasma* pneumonia
(D) Pyelonephritis
(E) Urinary tract infection (UTI)

32. A 36-year-old who injects drugs presents with an abscess on her jaw where she lost a tooth from being struck in the face 2 weeks earlier. She did not get medical help at that time. The physician lances the lesion to express some lumpy material with difficulty and sends a swab of the expressed material to the lab for Gram stain, routine culture, and susceptibility testing. The predominant organism in the Gram stain is a filamentous bacterium that is gram-positive, yet nothing grows in the routine cultures. What is the most likely explanation for the lack of growth on cultures?

(A) Organism is an obligate aerobe
(B) Organism is an obligate anaerobe
(C) Organism is a facultative anaerobe
(D) Organism is microaerophilic
(E) Organism was not grown on the correct media

33. Which of the following are required for the division and differentiation of B cells leading to production of plasma cells?

(A) CD4 and CD8 cells
(B) IL-1 and IL-3
(C) IL-1 only
(D) IL-4 and IL-6

34. A 65-year-old female Peace Corps worker is sent back to the States from East Africa because she had had a very high fever, and African sleeping sickness is suspected. What characteristic of the organism makes it a fatal infection unless treated properly?

(A) Ability to turn on a T2 response
(B) Damage to neutrophils
(C) Highly sialylated surface proteins
(D) Polysaccharide capsule
(E) Surface antigenic variation

35. A 2-year-old infant's mother reported her son has had three infections in the past 6 months. Which of his serum values (mg%) would indicate he had an immunodeficiency disease?

(A) Immunoglobulin (Ig)A → 350
(B) IgG → 650
(C) IgM → 150
(D) IgE → 0.05

36. What bacterial organism is noted for antigenic variation that leads to the ability to repeatedly reinfect the same individual and cause disease and has led to difficulty in vaccine development?

(A) *Chlamydia trachomatis*
(B) *Neisseria gonorrhoeae*
(C) *Neisseria meningitidis*
(D) *Streptococcus pneumoniae*
(E) *Treponema pallidum*

37. A 26-year-old woman presents with diarrhea containing both blood and pus. The lab culture shows the causative organisms on special medium incubated at 42 °C under microaerophilic conditions. A Gram stain of the isolated organism is shown in the image. What is the genus of the most likely causative agent?

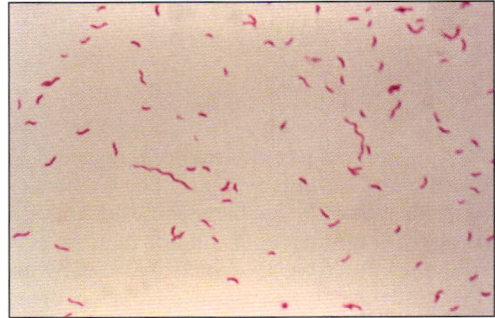

(A) *Campylobacter*
(B) *Helicobacter*
(C) *Salmonella*
(D) *Shigella*
(E) *Vibrio*

38. A 23-year-old woman presents to her physician with urinary urgency and frequency along with pain on micturition. The patient is otherwise healthy. What is the most likely causative agent?

(A) *Bacteroides* species
(B) *Clostridioides difficile*
(C) *Clostridium perfringens*
(D) *Clostridium tetani*
(E) *Escherichia coli*
(F) *Staphylococcus saprophyticus*

39. Which of the following viral proteins would be capable of disrupting calcium homeostasis within infected cells?

(A) Capsomeres
(B) Effluxions
(C) Matrix proteins
(D) Viroporins

40. A preschool day care has reported that the majority of the children have very sore throats. A closer examination of the situation indicates that they also have slight fevers and vesicular lesions (some of which have ulcerated) on their tonsillar and pharyngeal mucosa. Which of the following viruses is the most likely cause of these symptoms?

(A) Adenovirus
(B) Coronavirus
(C) Coxsackie A virus
(D) Parainfluenza virus
(E) Respiratory syncytial virus

1. **The answer is C.** [Chapter 3 XIII; VII B; Table 3.4] *Listeria* may cause in utero infections or may infect the neonate during delivery. In utero *Listeria* infections are generally severe and are characterized by caseating, granulomatous lesions. Except for *Toxoplasma* and parvovirus, the other organisms listed cause infections acquired during birth (perinatal). *Toxoplasma* usually manifests with calcified central nervous system lesions in the baby. Parvovirus B19 can cause anemia and hydrops fetalis when it crosses the placenta.

2. **The answer is A.** [Table 9.3] The adhesive tape test is the most appropriate test for determining pinworm infection. The female worm lays the eggs on the perianal folds in the very early hours of the morning. The adhesive tape is used to collect the eggs that are then identified microscopically.

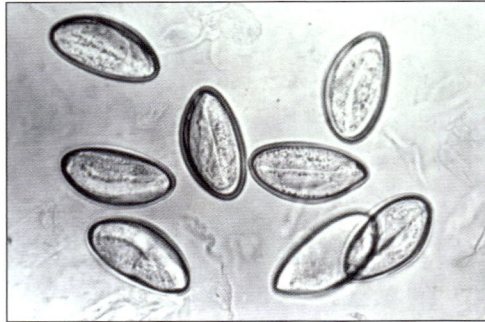

3. **The answer is C.** [Chapter 2, II A 3 c (2); Figure 2.3] Gram-positive bacteria would be most susceptible to penicillin in the exponential phase, because this is the phase in which the rate of cell wall synthesis is greatest.

4. **The answer is C.** [Chapter 2, VI C 3 d (2); Chapter 3, V B 1] A toxigenic strain of *C. diphtheriae* is produced as a result of lysogenic phage conversion after a temperate bacteriophage infects a nontoxigenic strain of the organism.

5. **The answer is B.** [Chapter 4, V B 2 a (3) (a)] Herpes simplex viruses have the ability to become latent in neurons and reactivate (replicate) under certain conditions that are not well understood.

6. **The answer is D.** [Chapter 3, IX L; XI; and Table 3.4] Patients with sickle cell anemia have problems with septicemias with encapsulated organisms, such as pneumococcus and *Klebsiella*. Of those listed, *S. enteritidis* has a prominent capsule and is noted for causing repeated infections in sickle cell carriers. *S. aureus* (often unencapsulated but sometimes with a microcapsule) is also a cause of osteomyelitis but is much less common as a causative agent of osteomyelitis in sickle cell disease (SCD) than *Salmonella*.

7. **The answer is D.** [Chapter 2, Table 2.2; II E 4; and V B 1; Chapter 13, III D] A selective medium permits growth in the presence of agents that inhibit other bacteria, in this case the normal oropharyngeal flora. A minimal medium contains the minimum quantity and number of nutrients capable of sustaining growth of the organism. A differential medium differentiates among organisms on the basis of color due to different fermentation or pH. Although you are inhibiting some bacteria, this name is not used as you are setting conditions to selectively grow the *Neisseria*.

8. **The answer is E.** [Chapter 5, VI 2 a (2) (a) 3] Influenza A virus, which causes a localized respiratory infection, has a segmented genome composed of eight pieces of negative-sense, single-stranded RNA, which can "reassort" when two different strains infect the same cell.

9. **The answer is C.** [Chapter 5, VII A 6 b (1)] The absence of the obligate coreceptor CXCR4 for HIV prevents viral entry into $CD4^+$ cells. There is no evidence that NK cells, a high CD4/CD8 ratio, or anti-GP160 antibodies are protective.

10. The answer is C. [Table 9.1] Loa loa is a filarial worm from Central Africa transmitted by the bite of a fly. The worm moves subcutaneously and can cause pain and swellings. When in the region of the eye, it can result in calabar swellings. The worm can also be seen to cross the conjunctiva.

11. The answer is A. [Chapter 2, VI C 3 b and VII B 3 b] The integrated intracellular form of the DNA of a temperate phage is called a prophage.

12. The answer is E. [Chapter 2, IV B 6 a; Chapter 3, I B and XI C] From both the genus description and the epidemiology, it is most likely *P. aeruginosa*. The rubber soles of tennis shoes generally clean off nails as they enter, so it is the flora of the inside of the tennis shoe, frequently *P. aeruginosa*, causing these infections.

13. The answer is C. [Chapter 10, X C 1 c] Both IL-1 and TNF-α are released following tissue injury and induce inflammation.

14. The answer is E. [Table 9.3] Adult *A. lumbricoides* is a roundworm that maintains its position in the gastrointestinal tract by continual movement "upstream," not by attaching. It is noted for migration into the bile duct, gallbladder, and liver, producing severe tissue damage. This process is often exacerbated by fever, antibiotics, or anesthetics.

15. The answer is A. [Chapter 10, IX B] T cells mainly home to the periarteriolar regions of the spleen and lymph nodes. B cells and macrophages make up the major cell populations in the germinal centers.

16. The answer is B. [Chapter 2, VI C 3 d (2); Chapter 3, V B 1] Only toxin-producing strains of *C. diphtheriae* cause diphtheria. The genes directing the production of the toxin are located on molecules of corynebacteriophage-β DNA, which may infect and lysogenize *C. diphtheriae*, causing production of the toxin. Neither plasmids nor the chromosome contain the genes to direct the synthesis of the toxin. Repressor molecules for the *tox*+ gene are on the chromosome, however. Both toxigenic and nontoxigenic strains of *C. diphtheriae* will be gray to black on tellurite medium.

17. The answer is D. [Chapter 5, VI A 6 c] Human T-lymphotropic virus type 1 causes adult acute T-cell leukemia, but is also associated with tropical spastic paraparesis, a slowly progressive (10 or more years) neurologic disease endemic in some areas of the Caribbean.

18. The answer is C. [Chapter 10, V E 1 a (2)] C3a and C3b are the prime components released following the action of C3 convertase. C3a along with C5a are strong chemotactic agents.

19. The answer is D. [Table 10.4] C5a binds to mast cells and basophils to induce histamine, smooth muscle contraction, and other mediators, which increase vascular permeability.

20. The answer is C. [Chapter 6, IV C; Chapter 7, III D] The infection is most likely tinea corporis (ringworm on the body), transferred by direct contact from the dog to the human. The drug most likely to be used is a topical imidazole, which inhibits the synthesis of ergosterol needed for fungal membranes. The other drugs commonly used include terbinafine, for which the answer would be the same, or griseofulvin, which inhibits cell division by disrupting microtubules.

21. The answer is A. [Chapter 4, VI B 1 c (4)] The short genome RNA molecule of arenavirus is ambisense—that is, the 3′ half has negative sense and the 5′ half has positive sense.

22. The answer is C. [Chapter 2, I B 8 c i (3)] Lysozyme found in tears is one of the major protective mechanisms of the eye. It is, in general, more effective against Gram-positive organisms.

23. The answer is D. [Chapter 3, I B and II F] Three of the causative agents listed in the question—*Aspergillus*, *Fusarium*, and *Pseudomonas*—are involved in eye trauma. *Pseudomonas*, the most common, is associated with wearing extended wear contact lenses too long and not taking them out at night. *Aspergillus* and *Fusarium* are both fungi, so they can be eliminated on the basis of the description. *Acanthamoeba* is an amoeba and does cause eye infection but is generally associated with homemade contact lens solution. *Staphylococcus* is gram-positive and mainly associated with styes.

24. The answer is A. [Chapter 10, XI C 2 a] CD8 on the T-cell membrane binds to HLA class I antigens, initiating the process leading to cell-mediated immunity (CMI).

25. The answer is A. [Chapter 5, III C 2 b] The *LMP-1* gene of Epstein-Barr virus codes for a protein that simulates activated CD40 receptor signaling.

26. The answer is B. [Chapter 4, XI B 3] Antecedent Epstein-Barr virus infection in a malarial region is associated with Burkitt lymphoma.

27. The answer is B. [Chapter 10, X C 1 c] Following tissue injury, IL-1 along with TNF-α initiates the acute phase reactant response.

28. The answer is A. [Chapter 10, VII A 1 b] γ2κ2 antibody describes an IgG antibody. It does not require a J chain, as do IgM and IgA, nor does it need a secretory piece, as does IgA. IgM is the initial antibody synthesized after antigen stimulation. All antibodies possess a hypervariable region.

29. The answer is D. [Chapter 5, IX G 3] Creutzfeldt-Jakob disease is an unconventional slow virus, or prion disease.

30. The answer is B. [Table 11.2] Type B (and type O) individuals carry anti-A antibodies.

31. The answer is B. [Chapter 3, VII] For all major causative agents of meningitis that are extracellular (and these are the major ones), the capsule (polysaccharide) is important for successful hematogenous survival to reach the blood-brain barrier (BBB) and using different mechanisms to enter the central nervous system; examples include the yeast *Cryptococcus*, meningitis-causing strains of *H. influenzae* (predominantly with type b capsule), *N. meningitidis*, and *S. pneumoniae*. All of these causative agents have polysaccharide capsules that allow survival in the bloodstream in an immunologically naive individual so they can reach the BBB. The major virulence factors in urinary tract and ascending UTIs are pili or adhesions that attach to the uroepithelium. *Mycoplasma* does not have a capsule.

32. The answer is B. [Chapter 2, III B 9; Table 3.4; and Chapter 13, III D 2 a] The causative organism is most likely an anaerobe, most probably *Actinomyces*, that did not tolerate transport aerobically. Unless there is a request for specimens to be collected anaerobically (or for culture from an abscess), specimen will not be routinely cultured anaerobically, especially if the sample is on a swab. The clinical case suggests an organism from the gingival crevices and not *S. aureus* as the cause. Large-bore needle biopsy with the specimen sent in the syringe and anaerobic culture should have been done instead. The wound will likely require debridement by an oral surgeon and antibiotics for several weeks.

33. The answer is D. [Chapter 10, X C 2 a; Table 10.5] IL-4 and IL-6 are required for division and differentiation of B cells. IL-1 and IL-3 appear to play no role. CD8 cells are functional in cytotoxic cell production.

34. The answer is E. [Table 9.1] *Trypanosoma brucei gambiense* and *T. brucei rhodesiense* both have the ability to continue to change their antigenic coats so much so that if hypergammaglobulinemia is not found in the cerebrospinal fluid (CSF) of a suspected case, it rules out African sleeping sickness.

35. The answer is B. [Chapter 10, VII A 2 a] Only IgG values are less than normal (IgG1 approximately 900 mg%).

36. The answer is B. [Chapter 3, XII B 1 b] The phenomenon described is antigenic variation. It is a particular problem in *N. gonorrhoeae*. The number of different serotypes of *N. gonorrhoeae* is over 1 million.

37. The answer is A. [Chapter 2, IV B 10 c; Chapter 3, IX J 3; and Chapter 13, III E 3 f] Both *Campylobacter* and *Helicobacter* are spiral-shaped microaerophiles requiring a special medium but only *Campylobacter* grows at 42 °C. *Salmonella* and *Shigella* are facultative anaerobes, so they would grow microaerophilically, but neither will grow at 42 °C. *Vibrio* is comma shaped and requires an alkaline medium and 35 to 37 °C for good growth.

38. The answer is E. [Chapter 3, X A] *E. coli* is a common causative agent of UTI. The strict anaerobes do not cause UTIs. *S. saprophyticus* does cause UTIs in this age group, but *E. coli* is still most common.

39. The answer is D. [Chapter 4, I F] Viroporins are small hydrophobic viral-encoded proteins that form hydrophilic pores in infected cell membranes and disrupt physiologic properties.

40. The answer is C. [Chapter 5, III A 2 a] Coxsackie A viruses cause sore throats with discrete vesiculopapular lesions on the tongue, tonsils, and the roof of the mouth (herpangina).

Comprehensive Examination: Block 4

Directions: Perform this block under examination conditions. Please allocate 90 seconds per question: this block should take 60 minutes. Select the *one* lettered answer that is *best* in each case. Commit to and write down your answers *before* checking the answers and explanations. Each of the numbered items in this section is followed by answers with explanations, in the following section.

1. An 80-year-old woman is referred to her cardiologist with no fever but worsening exertional fatigue. She has had a heart murmur since she was young. It appears to have worsened recently. At her 80th birthday party 4 weeks ago, two of her great nieces were sick, and she thinks she picked up their sore throat. She was sick with fever for about a week 3 weeks ago but did not have enough energy to go to the doctor. What would be the most likely results of standard bacterial blood cultures from this patient?

(A) Growth of enterococci
(B) Growth of *Staphylococcus aureus*
(C) Growth of *Streptococcus pyogenes*
(D) Growth of viridans group *Streptococci*
(E) No growth

2. A 29-year-old woman developed erythema at the insertion site of her intravenous line. Culture of the catheter tip indicates that a biofilm is present on the catheter. Based on this limited information, what is the most likely causative agent?

(A) *Enterococcus faecalis*
(B) *Staphyloccocus aureus*
(C) *Staphylococcus epidermidis*
(D) *Streptococcus agalactiae*
(E) *Streptococcus pneumoniae*
(F) Viridans group *Streptococci*

3. Following a 12-year-old girl's birthday party, which took place in her backyard and involved summer sport games and swimming, several parents reported that their children developed red, watery, and slightly itchy eyes; a sore throat; and a slight fever. The children's eyes were examined, and no petechial hemorrhages were observed, but preauricular adenopathy was present. Which of the following organisms is the most likely causative agent?

(A) Adenovirus
(B) Herpes simplex virus (HSV)-1
(C) Influenza virus
(D) *Moraxella catarrhalis*
(E) *Streptococcus pneumoniae*

4. Which of the following is the most important characteristic of the causative agent leading to the particular transmission in question 3?

(A) Glycosylated surface proteins are less sensitive to chlorination
(B) Gram-negative bacteria are more resistant than gram-positive bacteria
(C) Naked viruses are more resistant to chlorination
(D) The virus is more common in the summer months

5. A 70-year-old woman presents with fatigue, nausea, fever, anorexia, and abdominal pains. Her travel history shows that she is recently returned from a trip to western and central rural Mexico where she ate what everyone else was eating, including raw oysters from the coast. Physical examination shows a yellow tinge to her eyes, and her urine is dark. Lab studies show elevated liver enzymes. Blood cultures are negative for *Vibrio vulnificus*. Hepatitis serologies are:

Antibody to hepatitis A virus (HAV): positive

IgM to hepatitis B core antigen: negative

IgG to hepatitis B core antigen: positive

IgM to hepatitis B surface antigen (HBsAg): negative

IgG to HBsAg: positive

HBsAg: negative

Which of the following organisms is most likely causing her current problems?
(A) Hepatitis A
(B) Hepatitis B
(C) Hepatitis C
(D) *Vibrio vulnificus*
(E) *Vibrio cholerae*

6. In question 5, the patient's medical records indicate she was vaccinated 2 years ago for hepatitis B. In light of this, which of the following events would explain the hepatitis B virus (HBV) serologic findings?

(A) She had a subclinical hepatitis B infection before she was vaccinated
(B) She has chronic hepatitis
(C) She is in the window phase of hepatitis B infection
(D) The vaccine did not take, and she has a current active infection

7. A 25-year-old presents to the emergency department with fever and evidence of mild tricuspid valve insufficiency. He states that he has recently started injecting drugs. As far as he knows, he had no previous damage to his heart. What is the most likely causative agent of this patient's condition?

(A) *Candida albicans*
(B) Coxsackie virus
(C) *Enterococcus faecalis*
(D) *Pseudomonas aeruginosa*
(E) *Staphylococcus aureus*

8. The causative agent from the patient in question 7 is isolated and cultured. In the lab, a dense mixture of the patient's isolate with plasma on a slide shows clumping. This test correlates with which early process in the pathogenesis of acute endocarditis in a healthy heart?

(A) Binding to fibronectin
(B) Binding to fibrinogen
(C) Binding of protein A
(D) Superantigen activity
(E) Triggering fibrin production

9. While playing in the forest, a 13-year-old boy was bitten in the lower left leg by a raccoon. Which of the following findings would suggest a serious neurologic disease could result from the bite?

(A) Cowdry type A inclusion bodies in skin scrapings
(B) Molluscum bodies on epithelial cells shed from raccoon's saliva
(C) Negri bodies in skin scrapings
(D) Presence of Downey cells in the boy's blood 2 weeks following the bite

10. The hospital blood bank desires to isolate stem cells from a patient with multiple myeloma for transplantation following his radiation treatment. Which of the following cell markers is important for isolating and identifying human stem cells?

(A) CD3
(B) CD4
(C) CD28
(D) CD34

11. Which of the following is the most sensitive type of serologic test?
(A) Enzyme-linked immunosorbent assay (ELISA)
(B) Hemadsorption
(C) Nucleic acid hybridization
(D) Virus neutralization

12. A 52-year-old man presents to the emergency department with abdominal discomfort and vomiting. He reports a recent history of travel to a region with poor sanitation and consumption of undercooked pork. A fecal ova and parasite test is most likely to identify which of the following entities?

(A) Cyst
(B) Miracidium
(C) Proglottid
(D) Spore
(E) Trophozoite

13. A 32-year old presents to the clinic with recurring pain suggestive of a duodenal ulcer. When the patient is tested, they are found to be positive for antibodies against *Helicobacter pylori*. What allowed *H. pylori* to survive the transit through the gastric lumen to initiate the infection?

(A) Buffering capacity generated by the CagA protein
(B) Flagella and chemotaxis that moves the organism quickly to the mucin layer
(C) Presence of a polysaccharide capsule that protects the cells
(D) Production of urease
(E) Use of antacids by the patient

14. All *shigellae* have some invasive capability limited to mucosa of the ileum and colon, but some *Shigella dysenteriae* strains cause more severe disease. What is the reason for this difference in bacterial strains?

(A) Greater resistance to stomach acid
(B) Production of capsule (Vi antigen)
(C) Strains are motile.
(D) Toxin is produced that is similar to enterohemorrhagic *Escherichia coli*.
(E) Toxin is produced that is similar to enterotoxic *Escherichia coli*.

15. Which of the following statements characterizes idiotypic determinants?

(A) They are found in the crystallizable fragment of Igs.
(B) They are found on protein antigens.
(C) They can be antigenic.
(D) They are responsible for transplant rejection.

16. A burn patient has an infected area with odiferous, blue-green pus. What is the most likely causative agent?

(A) *A. fumigatus*
(B) *P. aeruginosa*
(C) *S. aureus*
(D) *S. epidermidis*
(E) *S. pyogenes*

17. A 14-year-old girl has symptoms that include a low-grade fever, chills, headache, muscle aches, and malaise. A physical examination indicates an enlarged spleen. A Monospot test is negative. Which of the following laboratory findings would best confirm a diagnosis?

(A) Heterophile antibodies
(B) Koilocytotic cells in pharyngeal scrapings
(C) Macrophages 10 times or more in the blood
(D) "Owl's eye" cells in urine

18. A 20-year-old female has signs and symptoms consistent with genital warts. Which of the following options would have been the best approach to prevent this disease?

(A) Immunization with a live reassortment vaccine
(B) Immunization with recombinant-produced viruslike particles
(C) Passive immunization with anti-neuraminidase antibodies
(D) Prophylactic treatment with acyclovir

19. Which of the following activities is a role of macrophages in the immune response?

(A) Present microbial antigens in the context of major histocompatibility complex (MHC) class I
(B) Production of C3 convertase
(C) Production of IL-1
(D) Production of interleukin (IL)-2

20. β-Lactam drugs bind to penicillin-binding proteins (PBPs) to halt the synthesis of peptidoglycan. Where in the bacterial cell are these proteins located?

(A) Capsule
(B) Cytoplasm
(C) Cytoplasmic membrane
(D) Peptidoglycan
(E) Periplasmic space

21. A new class of pathogen appears, causing pneumonia. It appears to be some sort of budding yeast–like organism with chitin in the cell wall, but the nucleus is not membrane bound, and the protein synthesis equipment appears to be prokaryotic. Which of the following antimicrobial agents is most likely to be effective against this novel pathogen?

(A) Doxycycline
(B) Metronidazole
(C) Penicillins
(D) Third-generation cephalosporins

22. Which of the following characteristics is attributed to a typical IgG antibody molecule?

(A) It has at least two identical heavy and no light chains.
(B) It has one antigen-binding site.
(C) It has specificity for only one antigen.
(D) It has two constant domains on each of the heavy chains.
(E) It is not a glycosylated molecule.

23. A 59-year-old man presents to the emergency department with labored breathing and a sharp stabbing pain behind the breastbone. He reports being weak and tired. He has a low-grade fever, and an electrocardiogram (ECG) shows elevated ST segments. Which of the following organisms is the most likely infectious cause of these symptoms?

(A) BK virus
(B) Coxsackie B virus
(C) *Moraxella catarrhalis*
(D) *Nocardia asteroides*
(E) Rotavirus

24. A 27-year-old worker at a daycare center has recently been feeling tired, has a slight fever, and has felt nauseated and vomited several times. Yesterday, she had abdominal pain and chills, and today she voided dark urine. Lab tests for serum enzymes indicated elevated aspartate transaminase (AST) and alanine transaminase (ALT). The genetic material of the virus most likely to cause her symptoms is which of the following?

(A) Double-stranded DNA
(B) Double-stranded RNA
(C) Single-stranded DNA
(D) Single-stranded RNA

25. The T-cell antigen receptor is associated with which of the following characteristics?

(A) It is a monomeric IgM.
(B) It is associated with CD4 or CD8.
(C) It is nonspecific.
(D) It requires free antigen for triggering.

26. Which of the following cells is capable of attacking a certain tumor cell spontaneously (ie, without prior sensitization)?

(A) CD8$^+$ cell
(B) Mature B cell
(C) Monocyte-macrophage
(D) Natural killer (NK) cell
(E) Null (K) cell

27. A 40-year-old man presents to the emergency department with a painful and swollen jaw. Two days ago he had a tooth extraction, and his gums and jaw were swollen and painful. "Nodules" are felt below the surface of the tissues, which are not lymph nodes. The causative agent is found to be a member of the gingival normal flora, and a Gram stain of the organism is shown. Which of the following is the most likely causative agent?

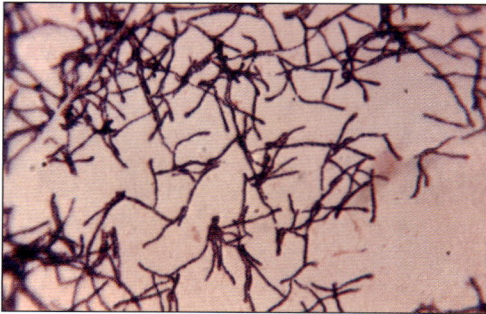

(A) *Actinomyces israelii*
(B) *Fusobacterium nucleatum*
(C) *Mycobacterium kansasii*
(D) *Nocardia asteroides*

28. Bacteria are protected from phagocytosis by which of the following bacterial structures?

(A) Capsule
(B) Lipopolysaccharide
(C) Lipoprotein
(D) Outer membrane
(E) Peptidoglycan

29. Which of the following genetic mechanisms is responsible for the conversion of nontoxigenic strains of *Corynebacterium diphtheriae* to toxigenic strains?

(A) Conjugation
(B) In vivo transformation
(C) Lysogenic phage conversion
(D) Reciprocal genetic recombination

30. Parents bring a 5-month-old to the pediatrician. The child has lost developmental ground and is no longer able to hold the head up or sit up. The parents indicate that they noticed constipation a couple of days earlier. An electroencephalogram (EEG) confirms a pattern consistent with botulism, and so appropriate treatment is initiated. Which of the following best describes the child's anticipated prognosis?

(A) Almost all cases have some permanent neurologic defects.
(B) Elevated cerebrospinal fluid (CSF) pressure occurs in over half of cases, resulting in some permanent neurologic defects.
(C) Neurologic recovery, although slow, is expected to be complete in all cases.
(D) Some permanent muscle weakness follows recovery that, like polio, may worsen late in life.

31. A 28-year-old man develops a life-threatening meningitis caused by *Histoplasma capsulatum*. Past medical history indicates that the patient is currently receiving chemotherapy. Which of the following antifungal drugs is fungicidal and appropriate for initial systemic use in this patient until the infection can be treated with maintenance therapy?

(A) Chloramphenicol
(B) Griseofulvin
(C) Itraconazole
(D) Ketoconazole
(E) Liposomal amphotericin B
(F) Nystatin

32. Which of the following complement components attaches to the crystallizable fragment of IgM?

(A) C1qrs
(B) C2a
(C) C2b
(D) C4b2a
(E) C5b

33. A 34-year-old woman presents with abdominal pain that is lessened by ingestion of bland food. A diagnosis of *H. pylori* is made. If the DNA had been analyzed, a region of unique DNA coding for the CagA protein and its type VI injection-like secretion system would be found. What is the correct term for this segment of DNA?

(A) Integron
(B) Pathogenicity island
(C) Replicon
(D) Transposon

34. A pale 6-year-old girl from a poor rural area of Appalachia presents with chronic "tiredness, upset tummy and the runs." She is found to have microcytic hypochromic anemia. Bile-stained eggs with polar plugs are found in her feces. Which of the following actions could have prevented this infection?

(A) Avoiding cat litter or taking proper care when changing litter
(B) Heating all canned foods to 60 °C for 10 minutes
(C) Not swimming in contaminated water
(D) Not using human excrement as vegetable fertilizer
(E) Wearing shoes outside in endemic regions

35. A hospitalized burn patient develops toxic shock syndrome. A strain of *Staphylococcus* spp. that secretes an enterotoxin is isolated from the burn lesion. Which of the following best describes the mechanism of action of this superantigen?

(A) Binds to the Vβ region on multiple B cells
(B) Blocks the epitope-binding region of human leukocyte antigen (HLA) molecules
(C) Decreases the numbers of polymorphonuclear cells
(D) Induces the secretion of high concentrations of cytokines

36. An 11-day-old neonate is brought to the pediatrician because the infant has developed a sharp cough. Physical examination reveals cough and mild conjunctivitis with some pus. A chest film confirms pneumonia. No organisms are seen on Gram stain of the pus. Which of the following describes the most likely causative agent?

(A) Diplococcus that has a high potential to cause blindness as well as the pneumonia
(B) Microorganism that does not have peptidoglycan or other cell wall polymer
(C) Microorganism that may be visualized by acid-fast stain and is largely intracellular
(D) Obligate intracellular organism unable to make its own adenosine triphosphate (ATP)

37. A 24-year-old man is hospitalized and in a coma for 2 weeks. He develops erythema around his catheter. The catheter is removed, the tip cultured, and a new line is started on the opposite side of his body. The culture report comes back as *S. epidermidis*, as it is noted for the production of a loose network of polysaccharide sticking to catheters. What is the layer of loosely bound polysaccharide on the bacterial cell that adheres to catheters?

(A) Biofilm
(B) Glycocalyx
(C) Peptidoglycan
(D) Pili
(E) Teichoic acids

38. A 6-month-old infant is brought to the pediatrician with watery diarrhea for the past 6 days. The parents report that he also vomited a couple of times and that the family has not traveled recently. The stools have no blood and no pus. He is dehydrated. Two other toddlers who visited for a day also are sick. What is most likely causing this?

(A) *Clostridium botulinum* toxin
(B) *Giardia lamblia*
(C) Norovirus
(D) Rotavirus
(E) *Salmonella enteritidis*
(F) *Staphylococcus aureus* enterotoxin

39. A father brings his 8-year-old son to the clinic and reports that about 10 days ago his son had a flulike disease with a minor fever. Three days ago he had a very red face that turned normal color when touched, and now he has a red rash on his arms and legs that also blanches to touch. The father states his son had all the normal childhood shots. Which of the following organisms is the most likely infectious cause of his symptoms?

(A) *C. albicans*
(B) Coxsackie A virus
(C) Parvovirus B19
(D) *S. epidermidis*

40. A 65-year-old presents to the clinic with symptoms of a sudden-onset influenza-like illness characterized by high fever, chills, backache, headache, myalgia, and retro-orbital pain. He has also had some nausea and vomiting. Which of the following is the most likely causative agent?

(A) Colorado tick fever virus
(B) Rabies virus
(C) Varicella zoster virus
(D) West Nile virus

Answers and Explanations

1. **The answer is E.** [Tables 3.3 and 3.4; Chapter 3, I D; VIII F; and V A 1 e] Without dental work or gastrointestinal or genitourinary manipulation and with the pharyngitis, the most likely explanation is rheumatic heart disease, made worse recently by an untreated strep throat. Because it is the antibodies (and, perhaps, immune cells) circulating and interacting with the heart and not an acute bacterial infection, the blood cultures would most likely be sterile. Antistreptolysin O titer would likely be positive.

2. **The answer is C.** [Table 3.2; Chapter 3, VIII E 2 and XI] *S. epidermidis* is noted for its ability to form biofilms and adhere to intravenous lines. *Streptococcus mutans* (a viridans streptococcus) is also noted for the production of a dextran biofilm; however, in this case, it adheres these organisms to dental surfaces leading to dental plaque and caries.

3. **The answer is A.** [Chapter 5, I A 2 c] The given clinical symptoms suggest viral pharyngoconjunctival fever rather than bacterial conjunctivitis, in which pus would have been present and preauricular nodes absent. Adenovirus frequently causes pharyngoconjunctival fever that can be transmitted from person to person in contaminated swimming pools.

4. **The answer is C.** [Chapter 5, I A 1 c] First you had to know that adenoviruses are naked. If chlorination is not properly maintained in pools, the virus is not sufficiently damaged to inhibit binding or viability and it leads to spread in pools. Enveloped viruses are more easily damaged by chlorination.

5. **The answer is A.** [Chapter 5, VI B 1 b v] She has hepatitis A. The lab results relating to HBV indicate that she has been previously vaccinated against HBV. Here other previous history is indicated in question 6.

6. **The answer is A.** [Chapter 5, VI B 1 b v] She probably already had a subclinical infection prior to being vaccinated; otherwise, she would not have antibody to core antigen, as the vaccine has only surface antigen in it.

7. **The answer is E.** [Table 3.4; Chapter 3, I C and VIII A] With tricuspid valve insufficiency in intravenous drug use (IVDU), the most common cause is *S. aureus*, which generally presents as an acute infection. Viridans streptococci are also common in IVDU, possibly from the practice of licking the needle to make the injection less painful.

8. **The answer is B.** [Chapter 3, VIII; VIII A; and I C] The binding of surface components to the plasma fibrinogen cross-links the staphylococci. The fibrinogen binding is probably the major reason *S. aureus* can damage the normal heart. It can also bind to fibronectin, so it is also a major causative agent of bacterial endocarditis in people with congenital defects and previously damaged hearts.

9. **The answer is C.** [Chapter 4, VI B 4 b (2)] Intracytoplasmic inclusion bodies called Negri bodies are found in nerve cells infected by the rabies virus, which can cause a serious neurologic infection unless appropriately treated. (The patient should have been immediately treated prophylactically for rabies!)

10. **The answer is D.** [Figure 10.18] CD34 is selective for human stem cells. CD3 is found on all T cells. CD28 is an accessory T-cell adhesion molecule, while CD4 is a marker for T helper cells.

11. **The answer is A.** [Chapter 13, I B 7] The ELISA test can measure nanogram amounts of hormones.

12. **The answer is C.** [Chapter 8, III B 1 a] Eating undercooked pork is a transmission risk for *Taenia solium*, the pork tapeworm. Cestodes have body segments called proglottids that can be observed in a fecal ova and parasite (O&P) test.

13. **The answer is D.** [Chapter 3, IX P] The production of urease produces ammonia, which neutralizes the stomach acid in the immediate environment of each *H. pylori* as it migrates to the mucosa. Choice B is also part of the pathogenesis, but the question asks specifically about the survival during the transit.

14. The answer is D. [Table 2.3; Chapter 3, IX M] The Shiga toxin–producing strains cleave the 60S ribosomes of the human cells, causing severe dysentery and may also cause hemolytic uremic syndrome.

15. The answer is C. [Chapter 10, VI C 3] Because idiotypic determinants on antibodies contain amino acid sequences in the (Fab') 2 variable regions that are unique to the respondent, they can be antigenic.

16. The answer is B. [Chapter 2, IV B 6 a; Chapter 3, I B and XI C] Most strains of *P. aeruginosa* produce a blue-green pigment, which is clinically notable in burn wounds infected with *Pseudomonas.* (Colonization is common but the presence of the blue-green pus is suggestive of actual presence in the tissue and infection.)

17. The answer is D. [Chapter 4, V B 2 c (1)] Symptoms are consistent with a mononucleosis disease that is usually caused by Epstein-Barr virus (EBV) or cytomegalovirus (CMV). The lack of a positive Monospot test for heterophile antibodies and presence of "owl's eye" cells would indicate CMV.

18. The answer is B. [Table 12.2] A quadrivalent recombinant vaccine (Gardasil) containing virus-like particles of Human Papilloma Virus (HPV) types 6, 11, 16, and 18 (these types cause 90% of genital warts) is available for prophylactic immunization to prevent genital warts and cervical cancer by types 16 and 18.

19. The answer is D. [Table 10.5] Macrophages produce IL-1.

20. The answer is C. [Chapter 2, I 4 a ii] The PBPs are actually in the cytoplasmic membrane, even though the substrate is the cell peptidoglycan. Thus, β-lactams must penetrate the gram-negative outer membrane through the porins and cross the peptidoglycan to bind. In the gram-positive bacteria, they just have to cross the peptidoglycan to bind in the membrane.

21. The answer is A. [Chapter 2, IX B] Metronidazole is not likely to work, as the agent is causing pneumonia, so it is probably aerobic or a facultative anaerobe. If the cell wall does not include peptidoglycan, β-lactam drugs are likely to be ineffective. However, since the ribosomes are prokaryotic, doxycycline has the best chance as long as it can penetrate the pathogen's cell wall and cytoplasmic membrane.

22. The answer is D. [Chapter 10, VII A, Table 10.7] The IgG molecule has three constant domains on the heavy chain.

23. The answer is B. [Chapter 5, VIII A] Viruses are the major infectious agents that produce symptoms similar to a heart attack. The most common of these viruses is Coxsackie B virus.

24. The answer is D. [Chapter 4, VI A 5 c] HAV is the most likely virus to cause the reported symptoms, which indicate hepatitis rather than some other disease. HAV is a positive-sense single-strand RNA virus.

25. The answer is C. [Chapter 10, X B] The T-cell antigen receptor is specific, responding only to antigen fragments bound to HLA. Choice A describes the B-cell receptor.

26. The answer is D. [Chapter 10, XI E 3 c] NK cells target cells not expressing MHC class I antigen for cytolysis. Many transformed cells and neoplastic cells lose the expression of MHC class I on their cell surface.

27. The answer is A. [Chapter 2, III B 9; Table 3.4] *A. israelii* grows contiguously in tissues, crossing anatomic barriers and causing a lumpy jaw, which is characterized by swelling and, sometimes, sinus tract formation with sulfur granules (3D colonies). It also invades bone. *M. tuberculosis* may be hematogenously spread to any tissue but is not associated with tooth extraction. *Nocardia* can also cause a similar infection, but the source is usually environmental *Nocardia* introduced by trauma; therefore, it generally involves extremities.

28. The answer is A. [Chapter 2, I B 9 b] In the immunologically naive, bacterial capsules prevent the phagocytic uptake and, therefore, the killing of the bacterium.

29. The answer is C. [Chapter 2, VI C 3 d (2)] A toxigenic strain of *C. diphtheriae* is produced as a result of lysogenic phage conversion after a temperate bacteriophage infects a nontoxigenic strain of the organism.

30. The answer is C. [Chapter 3, IX D 3] The neurotoxin involved in infant botulism, unlike bacterial meningitis, does not cause elevated CSF pressure, so recovery should be complete. The use of the recombinant human antitoxin shortens hospitalization and recovery time. However, it still requires regrowth of nerve endings.

31. The answer is E. [Chapter 6, IV A 2] Both amphotericin B (the correct answer) and nystatin are fungicidal, but nystatin is not used for systemic infections. Chloramphenicol is bactericidal. Ketoconazole and itraconazole are both fungistatic, and griseofulvin is not used systemically and localizes only in keratinized tissues.

32. The answer is A. [Chapter 10, V E 1 a (1)] C1q recognizes antibody attached to cell surfaces and binds the antibody. The antibody-C1q complex then initiates the classical complement pathway by activating two serine proteases C1s and C1r.

33. The answer is B. [Chapter 2, VII A 2 a (3); Chapter 3, IX P 1 d] Pathogenicity islands carry virulence genes and sometimes secretion systems and are often of different GC:AT ratios than most of the organism's other DNA, suggesting it was acquired from another organism.

34. The answer is E. [Table 9.3] In endemic regions, hookworm filariform larvae may grow in soil contaminated with human excrement; skin contact with soil (sitting or going barefoot) allows them to penetrate skin. Wearing shoes has been shown to greatly reduce the transmission of hookworm.

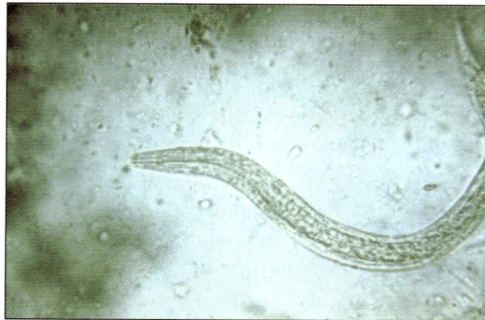

35. The answer is D. [Chapter 2, VIII C 2 a (2) and Table 2.3] The superantigen produced by *Staphylococcus* spp. simultaneously binds the T-cell receptor and the MHC class II molecule regardless of the antigen occupying the antigen-binding region. This cross-linking between an antigen-presenting cell and a T cell leads to a broad-spectrum activation of effector cells, resulting in a large-scale production of cytokines, often referred to as a "cytokine storm."

36. The answer is D. [Chapter 2, V C; Chapter 3, II A] The presentation is most likely *Chlamydia trachomatis* conjunctivitis and pneumonia. This obligate intracellular organism is unable to make its own ATP. Choice A (gonococcus) can be eliminated on Gram stain, and most would have been intracellular but not in phagosomes. Choice B describes mycoplasma, which is not intracellular and rarely causes pneumonias in neonates this young. Choice C (mycobacterium) is unlikely to cause pneumonia in someone this young and is not known to cause eye infections producing pus.

37. The answer is B. [Chapter 2, I B 9 c; Chapter 3, VIII E 2] The layer *on the cell* could be called either a glycocalyx or capsule (not a choice). The layer on the catheter is a biofilm, but the question asked for the name of the layer on the cell.

38. The answer is D. [Chapter 3, VII 3] The lack of flaccid paralysis leaves out botulinum toxin, and staphylococcal toxin is also unlikely as it is a short, self-resolving illness. The most likely is rotavirus due to his age and the length of the disease.

39. The answer is C. [Chapter 5, XI E 2 A] The clinical signs described and the fact that childhood vaccines have been administered strongly suggest that parvovirus B19 is the cause.

40. The answer is D. [Chapter 5, IX B 3 a ii (b)] Given the possible answer choices, the one that is most consistent with the patient's age and the signs and symptoms is West Nile arbovirus infections.

Index

Note: References in *italics* indicate figures; those followed by "*t*" denote tables.